DOSAGE

THIRD EDITION

CALCULATIONS
A Ratio-Proportion Approach

Gloria D. Pickar, EdD, RN

President and Chief Academic Officer
Compass Knowledge Group
Orlando, Florida

Former Academic Dean
Seminole State College of Florida
Sanford, Florida

Amy Pickar Abernethy, MD

Associate Professor of Medicine and Nursing
Duke University
Durham, North Carolina

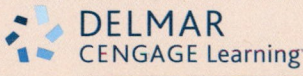
DELMAR
CENGAGE Learning™

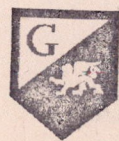

Australia • Brazil • Japan • Korea • Mexico • Singapore • Spain • United Kingdom • United States

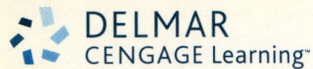
DELMAR
CENGAGE Learning™

Dosage Calculations: *A Ratio-Proportion Approach*, Third Edition
Gloria D. Pickar, EdD, RN,
and Amy Pickar Abernethy, MD

Vice President, Career and Professional Editorial: Dave Garza

Director of Learning Solutions: Matthew Kane

Senior Acquisitions Editor: Maureen Rosener

Managing Editor: Marah Bellegarde

Senior Product Manager: Elisabeth Williams

Editorial Assistant: Samantha Miller

Vice President, Career and Professional Marketing: Jennifer McAvey

Marketing Director: Wendy Mapstone

Senior Marketing Manager: Michele McTighe

Marketing Coordinator: Scott Chrysler

Production Director: Carolyn Miller

Production Manager: Andrew Crouth

Senior Content Project Manager: Kenneth McGrath

Senior Art Director: Jack Pendleton

Technology Project Manager: Erin Zeggert

For product information and technology assistance, contact us at
Professional & Career Group Customer Support, 1-800-648-7450

For permission to use material from this text or product, submit all requests online at **cengage.com/permissions**
Further permissions questions can be emailed to
permissionrequest@cengage.com

Library of Congress Control Number: 2007017012

ISBN-13: 978-1-4354-5410-1

ISBN-10: 1-4354-5410-3

Delmar
5 Maxwell Drive
Clifton Park, NY 12065-2919
USA

Cengage Learning products are represented in Canada by Nelson Education, Ltd.

For your lifelong learning solutions, visit **delmar.cengage.com**

Visit our corporate website at **cengage.com**.

Notice to the Reader

Publisher does not warrant or guarantee any of the products described herein or perform any independent analysis in connection with any of the product information contained herein. Publisher does not assume, and expressly disclaims, any obligation to obtain and include information other than that provided to it by the manufacturer. The reader is expressly warned to consider and adopt all safety precautions that might be indicated by the activities described herein and to avoid all potential hazards. By following the instructions contained herein, the reader willingly assumes all risks in connection with such instructions. The publisher makes no representations or warranties of any kind, including but not limited to, the warranties of fitness for particular purpose or merchantability, nor are any such representations implied with respect to the material set forth herein, and the publisher takes no responsibility with respect to such material. The publisher shall not be liable for any special, consequential, or exemplary damages resulting, in whole or part, from the readers' use of, or reliance upon, this material.

Printed in the United States of America
2 3 4 5 6 7 8 XXX 13 12 11 10

Contents

Preface

Introduction

Dosage Calculations: A Ratio-Proportion Approach, third edition, offers a clear and concise method of calculating drug dosages. The text is directed to students and professionals who want to increase their comfort level with mathematics and also to faculty members who prefer the ratio-proportion method for calculating dosages. Along with the companion text, *Dosage Calculations* eighth edition, the content has been classroom tested and reviewed by well over 950,000 faculty and students, who report that it has helped allay math anxiety and promote confidence in their ability to perform accurate calculations. As one reviewer noted, "I have looked at others [texts], and I don't feel they can compare."

The only math prerequisite is the ability to do basic arithmetic. For those who need a review, *Chapters 1* and *2* offer an overview of basic arithmetic calculations with extensive exercises for practice. The student is encouraged to use a three-step method for calculating dosages.

1. Convert measurements to the same system and same size units.

2. Consider what dosage is reasonable.

3. Calculate using ratio-proportion.

Dosage Calculations: *A Ratio-Proportion Approach,* third edition, is based on feedback from users of the previous editions and users of other dosage calculations texts. The new edition also responds to changes in the health care field and includes the introduction of new drugs, replacement of outdated drugs, and discussion of new or refined methods of administering medications. The importance of avoiding medication errors is highlighted by the incorporation of applied critical thinking skills based on patient care situations, and a chapter on preventing medication errors.

Organization of Content

The text is organized in a natural progression of basic to more complex information. Learners gain self-confidence as they master content in small increments with ample review and reinforcement. Many learners claim that while using this text, they did not fear math for the very first time.

The seventeen chapters are divided into four sections.

Section 1 includes a mathematics diagnostic evaluation and a mathematics review in *Chapters 1* and *2.* The *Mathematics Diagnostic Evaluation* allows learners to determine their computational strengths and weaknesses to guide them through the review of the *Section 1* chapters. *Chapters 1* and *2* provide a review of basic arithmetic procedures, with numerous examples and practice problems to ensure that students can apply the procedures.

Section 2 includes *Chapters 3* through *9.* This section provides essential information that is the foundation for accurate dosage calculations and safe medication administration, including medicine orders, labels, and equipment. *Chapters 3* and *4* introduce the three systems of measurement (metric, apothecary, and household) and outline conversion from one system of measurement to another. The metric system of measurement is emphasized because of its standardization in the health care field. The apothecary system continues to be included for recognition purposes, and the household system is included because of its implications for care at home. International, or 24-hour, time and Fahrenheit and Celsius temperature conversions are presented in *Chapter 5.*

In *Chapter 6,* users learn to recognize and select appropriate equipment for the administration of medications based on the drug, dosage, and method of administration. Emphasis is placed on interpreting syringe calibrations to ensure that the dosage to be administered is accurate. All photos and drawings have been enhanced for improved clarity with updates for state-of-the-art technology and information systems.

Chapter 7 presents the common abbreviations used in health care so that learners can become proficient in interpreting medical orders. Additionally, the content on computerized medication administration records has been updated and expanded.

It is essential that learners be able to read medication labels to calculate dosages accurately. This ability is developed by having readers interpret the medication labels provided beginning in *Chapter 8.* These labels represent current commonly prescribed medications and are presented in full color and actual size (except in a few instances where the label is enlarged to improve readability). For the first time, some labels have been substituted with generic simulated labels to demonstrate critical calculations. This ensures that the entire range of medications seen in practice is presented, and gives the learners more experience with actual generic drugs.

Chapter 9 directs the learner's attention to the risks and responsibilities inherent in receiving medication prescriptions, transcribing orders, and administering medications. It provides the rationale for the patient's rights to safe medication administration. Throughout the text, care is taken to comply with standards and recommendations for medical notation available at the time of publication by The Joint Commission and The Institute for Safe Medication Practices. The *Official "Do Not Use" List* is emphasized. Learners are directed to stay abreast of these standards as they evolve to best ensure patient safety and prevent medication administration errors.

In *Section 3,* the user learns and practices the skill of dosage calculations applied to patients across the life span. *Chapters 10* and *11* guide the learner to apply all the skills mastered to achieve accurate oral and injectable drug dosage calculations. Users learn to think through the problem logically for the right answer and then to apply ratio-proportion to double-check their thinking. When this logical but unique system is applied every time to every problem, experience has shown that decreased math anxiety and increased accuracy result.

Insulin types, species, and manufacturers have been expanded with a description of insulin action time and the addition of U-500 insulin. The 70/30 and 50/50 insulins are also thoroughly explained.

Chapter 12 introduces the concepts of solutions. Users learn the calculations associated with diluting solutions and reconstituting injectable drugs. This chapter provides a segue to intravenous calculations by fully describing the preparation of solutions. With the expanding role of the nurse and other health care workers in the home setting, clinical calculations for home care, such as nutritional feedings, are also emphasized.

The new *Chapter 13* introduces the formula and dimensional analysis methods of calculating dosages. Ample *Review Sets* and *Practice Problems* provide exposure to these methods, giving the learner an opportunity to sample other calculation methods and choose the one preferred.

Chapter 14 covers the calculation of pediatric and adult dosages and concentrates on the body weight method. Emphasis is placed on verifying safe dosages and applying concepts across the life span.

Advanced clinical calculations applicable to both adults and children are presented in **Section 4.** Intravenous administration calculations are presented in Chapters *15* through *17.* Coverage reflects the greater application of IVs in drug therapy. Shortcut calculation methods are presented and explained fully. More electronic infusion devices are included. Heparin and saline locks, types of IV solutions, IV monitoring, IV administration records, and IV push drugs are included in *Chapter 15.* Pediatric IV calculations are presented in *Chapter 16,* and obstetric, heparin, and critical care IV calculations are covered in *Chapter 17.* Ample problems help students master the necessary calculations.

Procedures in the text are introduced using **Rule** boxes and several **Examples.** Key concepts are summarized and highlighted in **Quick Review** boxes before each set of **Review Problems** to give learners an opportunity to review major concepts prior to working through the problems. **Math Tips** provide memory joggers to assist learners in accurately solving problems. Learning is reinforced by **Practice Problems** that conclude each chapter. The importance of calculation accuracy and patient safety is emphasized by patient scenarios that require careful and accurate consideration. **Critical Thinking Skills** scenarios conclude to each chapter's **Practice Problems** to further emphasize accuracy and safety.

Information to be memorized is identified in **Remember** boxes, and **Caution** boxes alert learners to critical procedures and information.

Section Self-Evaluations found at the end of each section provide learners with an opportunity to test their mastery of chapter objectives prior to proceeding to the next section. Two **Posttests** at the conclusion of the text serve to evaluate the learner's overall skill in dosage calculations. The first **Posttest** covers essential skills commonly tested by employers, and the second serves as a comprehensive examination. Both are presented in a case study format to simulate actual clinical calculations.

An **Answer Key** at the back of the text provides all answers and solutions to selected problems in the **Review Sets, Practice Problems, Section Self-Evaluations,** and **Posttests.**

Features of the Third Edition

- Content is divided into four main sections to help learners better organize their studies.

- Measurable objectives at the beginning of each chapter emphasize the content to be learned.

- More than 2,100 problems are included for learners to practice their skills and reinforce their learning, reflecting current drugs and protocols.

- More *Critical Thinking Skills* are applied to real-life patient care situations to emphasize the importance of accurate dosage calculations and the avoidance of medication errors.

- Full color is used to make the text user friendly. Chapter elements, such as *Rules, Math Tips, Cautions, Remember* boxes, *Quick Reviews,* and *Examples,* are color-coded for easy recognition and use. Color also highlights *Review Sets* and *Practice Problems.*

- Color has been added to selected syringe drawings throughout the text to *simulate a specific amount of medication,* as indicated in the example or problem. Because the color used may not correspond to the actual color of the medications named, *it must not be used as a reference for identifying medications.*

- Photos and drug labels are presented in full color; color is used to highlight and enhance the visual presentation of content to improve readability. Special attention is given to visual clarity with some labels enlarged to ensure legibility.

- The *Math Review* brings learners up to the required level of basic math competence.

- SI conventional metric system notation is used (apothecary and household systems of measurement are deemphasized though still included).

- *Rule* boxes draw the learner's attention to pertinent instructions.

- *Remember* boxes highlight information to be memorized.

- *Quick Review* boxes summarize critical information throughout the chapters before *Review Sets* are solved.

- *Caution* boxes alert learners to critical information.

- *Math Tips* serve to point out math shortcuts and reminders.

- Content is presented from simple to complex concepts in small increments, followed by *Review Sets* and chapter *Practice Problems* to assess understanding and skills and to reinforce learning.

- Many problems are included involving the interpretation of syringe scales to ensure that the proper dosage is administered. Once the dosage is calculated, the learner is directed to draw an arrow on a syringe at the proper value.

- Many more labels of current and commonly prescribed medications are presented, including a few simulated labels to help users learn how to select the proper information required to determine correct dosage. There are over 375 labels included.

- Hundreds of *Examples* are included to demonstrate the ratio-proportion, $\frac{D}{H} \times Q = X$, or dimensional analysis methods of calculating dosages.

- For the first time, dimensional analysis is included as an alternative dosage calculation method. The $\frac{D}{H} \times Q$ formula method is also included, giving learners and instructors a choice of which method they prefer to use.

- IV equipment and calculations have been expanded.

- Clear instructions are included for calculating IV medications administered in milligram per kilogram per minute.

- Clinical situations are simulated using actual medication labels, syringes, physician order forms, and medication administration records.

- Case study format of *section Exams* and *Posttests* simulates actual clinical calculations and scenarios.

- An *Essential Skills Evaluation* simulates exams commonly administered by employers for new hires. A *Comprehensive Skills Evaluation* assesses the learner's overall comprehension in preparation for a level or program assessment.

- The index facilitates learner and instructor access to content and skills.

New to the Third Edition

- A new chapter presents dimensional analysis and the formula method as alternative alternate dosage calculation methods.

- New and simulated labels are added throughout the book to reflect current drugs on the market.

- U-500 insulin is introduced.

- New questions are added throughout to reflect current drugs and protocols.

- Photographs of state-of-the-art equipment are replaced and updated.

- The number of *Critical Thinking Skills* scenarios has increased.

- An index of all drug labels is added.

- Online course formats are available in **Blackboard** and **WebCT** so that students can access their *Dosage Calculations* course content, practice activities, communications, and assessments through the Internet.

- An exciting new *Practice Software CD-ROM* is included in the book, offering a glossary review, chapter tutorials, and hundreds of practice problems.

Resources

Instructor Resources
(ISBN 1-4354-5411-1)

The *Instructor Resources (IR) to Accompany Dosage Calculations: A Ratio-Proportion Approach,* third edition, contains a variety of tools to help instructors successfully prepare lectures and teach within this subject area. The following components in the *IR* are all free to adopters of the text:

- A **Solutions Manual** includes answers and step-by-step solutions for every question in the *Review Sets, Practice Problems, Section Evaluations,* and *Posttests* from the book.

- The **Computerized Test Bank** includes approximately 500 additional questions not found in the book for further assessment. The software also allows for the creation of test items and full tests, as well as coding for difficulty level.

- Lecture slides created in **PowerPoint** ® offer a depiction of administration tools and include calculation tips helpful to classroom lecture of dosage calculations.

- An **Image Library** is an invaluable digital resource of dozens of figures, labels, and syringes from the text. With the Image Library, you can search for, copy, and save images to easily paste into slide presentations or other learning tools.

WebTutor Advantage on WebCT
(ISBN 1-4354-5413-8) and Blackboard
(ISBN 1-4354-5412-X)

WebTutor Advantage (both **WebCT** and **Blackboard** formats) accompany this new edition of *Dosage Calculations: A Ratio-Proportion Approach.* These online supplemental courses offer must-have classroom management tools such as chats and calendars, as well as additional content resources, including class notes, lecture slides, student quizzes, frequently asked questions, a glossary, and more.

Online Companion

A new online companion, accessed at http://www. delmarlearning.com/companions, is available to adopters of the text. This resource includes valuable instructor tools to facilitate lecture preparation and test administration.

Tutorial Software

Engaging **Practice Software** is available FREE to each user of *Dosage Calculations: A Ratio-Proportion Approach,* third edition. The CD-ROM packaged within the book features:

- A bank of several hundred questions that support and reinforce the content presented in the text.

- A user-friendly menu structure to immediately access the program's items.

- A tutorial for each chapter outlining instructions and approaches to safe and accurate medication calculation.

- *Quizzes, Pretest,* and *Posttest* that operate within a tutorial mode, which allows two tries before the correct answer is provided.

- Interactive exercises that ask you to fill a medicine cup or draw back a syringe to the correctly calculated dose.

- A comprehensive glossary of terms and drug names with definitions and pronunciations.

- Drop-down calculator available at a click of a button, as used on the NCLEX-RN™ examination.

Acknowledgments

Contributor

Maureen D. Tremel, MSN, ARNP
Professor of Nursing
Seminole State College of Floirda
Sanford, Florida

Reviewers

Kathleen K. Gudgel, RN, MSN
Assistant Professor
School of Health Sciences
Pennsylvania College of Technology
Williamsport, Pennsylvania

Marilyn Handley, RN, PhD
Associate Professor
Capstone College of Nursing
The University of Alabama
Tuscaloosa, Alabama

Patricia A. Roper, RN, MS
Professor Emeritus
Columbus State Community College
Columbus, Ohio

Cinda Siekbert, RN, BSN, MS
Great Oaks Institute of Technology
Georgetown, Ohio

Accuracy Reviewer

Janie Corbitt, MLS, RN
Instructor
Central Georgia Technical College
Milledgeville, Georgia

From the Authors

We wish to thank our many students and colleagues who have provided inspiration and made contributions to the production of the text. We are particularly grateful to Maureen Tremel for her careful attention to researching and updating information; to Janie Corbitt for her careful attention to accuracy; to Maureen Rosener, Elisabeth Williams, Ken McGrath, Erin Zeggert, Mary Colleen Liburdi, and Samantha Miller for their careful attention to deadlines and details; and to Roger Pickar and Steve Abernethy for their careful attention to us and our families.

Gloria D. Pickar, EdD, RN
Amy Pickar Abernethy, MD

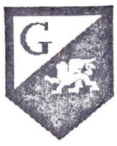

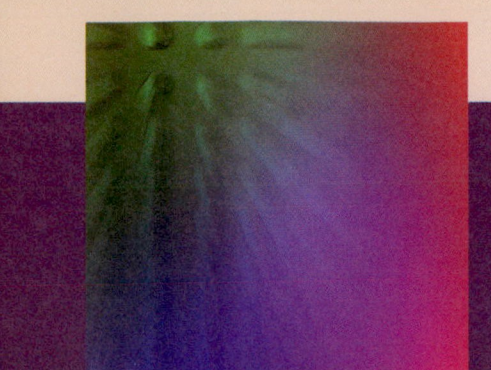

Introduction to the Learner

The accurate calculation of drug dosages is an essential skill in health care. Paracelsius (1493–1591), often referred to as the father of pharmacology, recognized that the difference between a poison, narcotic, hallucinogen, and medicine is dosage. Serious harm to the patient can result from a mathematical error during the calculation and subsequent administration of a drug dosage. It is the responsibility of those administering drugs to precisely and efficiently carry out medical orders.

Learning to calculate drug dosages need not be a difficult or burdensome process. *Dosage Calculations: A Ratio-Proportion Approach,* third edition, provides an uncomplicated, easy-to-learn, easy-to-recall three-step method of dosage calculations. Once you master this method, you will be able to consistently compute dosages with accuracy, ease, and confidence.

The text is a self-study guide that is divided into four main sections. The only mathematical prerequisite is the basic ability to add, subtract, multiply, and divide whole numbers. A review of fractions, decimals, percents, ratios, and proportions is included. You are encouraged to work at your own pace and seek assistance from a qualified instructor as needed.

Each procedure in the text is introduced by several *Examples.* Key concepts are summarized and highlighted before the *Practice Problems.* This gives you an opportunity to review the concepts before working the problems. Ample *Review* and *Practice Problems* are given to reinforce your skill and confidence.

Before calculating the dosage, you are asked to consider the reasonableness of the computation. More often than not, the correct amount can be estimated in your head. Many errors can be avoided if you approach dosage calculation in this logical fashion. The mathematical computation can then be used to double-check your thinking. Answers to all problems and step-by-step solutions to select problems are included at the back of the text.

Many photos and drawings are included to demonstrate key concepts and equipment. Drug labels and measuring devices (for example, syringes) are included to give a simulated "hands-on" experience outside of the clinical setting or laboratory. *Critical Thinking Skills* emphasize the importance of dosage calculation accuracy, and medication scenarios provide opportunities to analyze and prevent errors.

This text has helped hundreds of thousands of learners just like you to feel at ease about math and to master dosage calculations. I am interested in your feedback. Please write to me to share your reactions and success stories.

Gloria D. Pickar, EdD, RN
gpickar@cfl.rr.com

To our husbands, Roger and Steve,
whose support makes our lives possible.

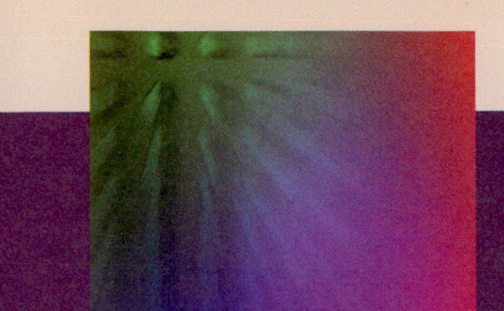

Using This Book

- Concepts are presented from simple to complex, in small increments, followed by a quick review and solved examples. *Review Sets* and *Practice Problems* provide opportunities for you to reinforce your learning.

Refer to the following label to identify the specific drug information described in questions 16 through 21.

Used with permission from Pfizer Inc.

NDC 0049-0520-83
Rx only
Buffered
Pfizerpen®
(penicillin G potassium)
For Injection
FIVE MILLION UNITS
Pfizer Roerig
Division of Pfizer Inc, NY, NY 10017

SEE ACCOMPANYING PRESCRIBING INFORMATION
RECOMMENDED STORAGE IN DRY FORM.
Store below 86°F (30°C).
Sterile solution may be kept in refrigerator for one (1) week without significant loss of potency.

05-4243-32-6

6505-00-958-3305

USUAL DOSAGE
Average single intramuscular injection: 200,000–400,000 units.
Intravenous: Additional information about the use of this product intravenously can be found in the package insert.

mL diluent added	Units per mL of solution
18.2 mL	250,000
8.2 mL	500,000
3.2 mL	1,000,000

Buffered with sodium citrate and citric acid to optimum pH.
PATIENT: _____
ROOM NO: _____
DATE DILUTED: _____

16. Generic name _____
17. Brand name _____
18. Dosage strength _____
19. Route of administration _____
20. National Drug Code _____
21. Manufacturer _____

- All syringes are drawn to full size, providing accurate scale renderings to help you master the reading of injectable dosages.

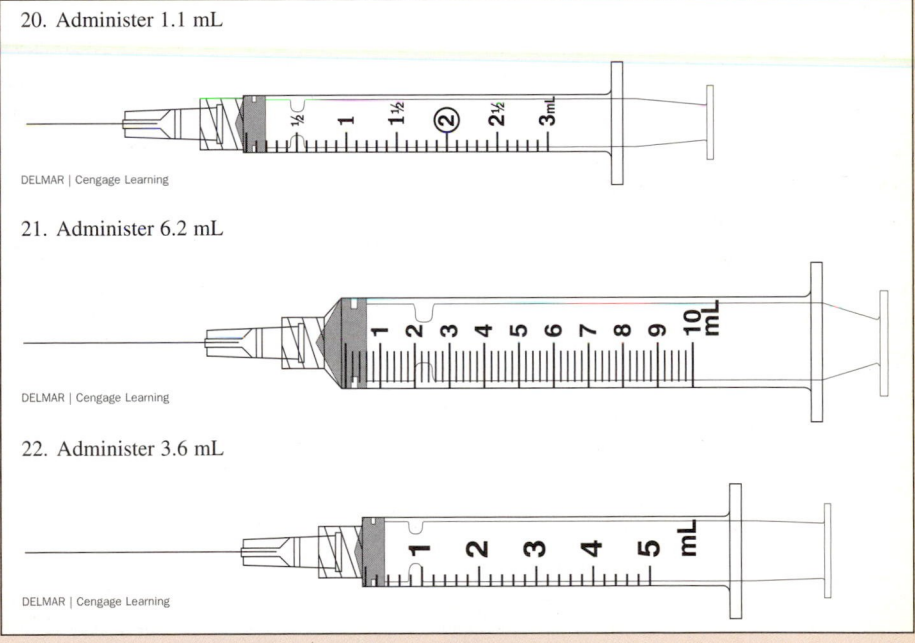

20. Administer 1.1 mL

DELMAR | Cengage Learning

21. Administer 6.2 mL

DELMAR | Cengage Learning

22. Administer 3.6 mL

DELMAR | Cengage Learning

- Photos and drug labels are presented in full color; actual size labels help prepare you to read and interpret content in its true-life format.

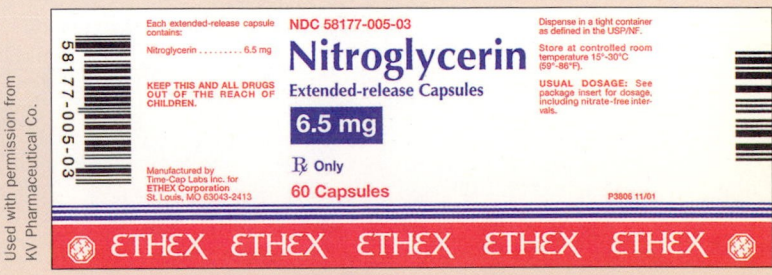

Used with permission from KV Pharmaceutical Co.

Each extended-release capsule contains:
Nitroglycerin . . . . 6.5 mg
KEEP THIS AND ALL DRUGS OUT OF THE REACH OF CHILDREN.

NDC 58177-005-03
Nitroglycerin
Extended-release Capsules
6.5 mg
℞ Only
60 Capsules

Dispense in a tight container as defined in the USP/NF.
Store at controlled room temperature 15°-30°C (59°-86°F).
USUAL DOSAGE: See package insert for dosage, including nitrate-free intervals.

Manufactured by Time-Cap Labs Inc. for **ETHEX Corporation** St. Louis, MO 63043-2413

P3806 11/01

ETHEX ETHEX ETHEX ETHEX ETHEX

Extended-release capsules

MATH TIP

Notice that to multiply 2 by 1,000, you are moving the decimal three places to the right. This is a shortcut. Sometimes to complete this operaton, you add zeros to hold the places equal to the number of zeros in the equivalent. In this case 1 g = 1,000 mg, so you add three zeros: $2 \times 1,000 = 2.000. = 2,000$

■ *Math Tip* boxes provide you with clues to essential computations.

CAUTION

If any of the seven parts is missing or unclear, the order is considered incomplete and is, therefore, not a legal drug order.

■ *Caution* boxes alert you to critical information and safety concerns.

RULE

In a proportion, the ratio for a known equivalent equals the ratio for an unknown equivalent. To use ratio-proportion to convert from one unit to another, you need to follow these three steps.

1. Recall the equivalents.

2. Set up a proportion of two equivalent ratios.

3. Cross-multiply to solve for an unknown quantity, X.

■ *Rule* boxes highlight and draw your attention to pertinent instructions.

REMEMBER

The Six Rights of safe and accurate medication administration are as follows:

The *right patient* must receive the *right drug* in the *right amount* by the *right route* at the *right time*, followed by the *right documentation*.

■ *Remember* boxes highlight information that you should memorize.

QUICK REVIEW

To use the ratio-proportion method to convert from one unit to another or between systems of measurement:

■ Recall the equivalent.

■ Set up a proportion: Ratio for known equivalent equals ratio for unknown equivalent.

■ Label the units and match the units in the numerators and denominators.

■ Cross-multiply to find the value of the unknown X equivalent.

■ Label the units in the answer to match the unknown X.

■ *Quick Review* boxes summarize critical information that you will need to know and understand to safely prepare and administer medications.

SUMMARY

At this point, you should be quite familiar with the equivalents for converting within the metric, apothecary, and household systems and from one system to another. From memory, you should be able to recall quickly and accurately the equivalents for conversions. If you are having difficulty understanding the concept of converting from one unit of measurement to another, review this chapter and seek additional help from your instructor.

Consider the two Critical Thinking Skills scenarios and work the practice problems for Chapter 4. Concentrate on accuracy. One error can be a serious mistake when calculating the dosages of medicines or performing critical measurements of health status.

■ *Summary* boxes draw out key information from the chapter as a quick study and review tool.

EXAMPLE 5 ■

Convert: 0.004 L to mL

Equivalent: 1 L = 1,000 mL

$$\frac{1\ L}{1,000\ mL} = \frac{0.004\ L}{X\ mL}$$

$$\frac{1\ L}{1,000\ mL} \quad \diagdown\!\!\!\!\diagup \quad \frac{0.004\ L}{X\ mL} \qquad \text{Cross-multiply}$$

X = 1,000 × 0.004   0.004. Move the decimal 3 places to the right to multiply by 1,000. (There are already enough places, so you do not need to add a zero to complete the operation.)

X = 4 mL   Label the units to match the unknown X

■ *Examples* walk you step-by-step through the calculation process, using different conversions, medications, and methods, to ensure that your mastery of the process is complete.

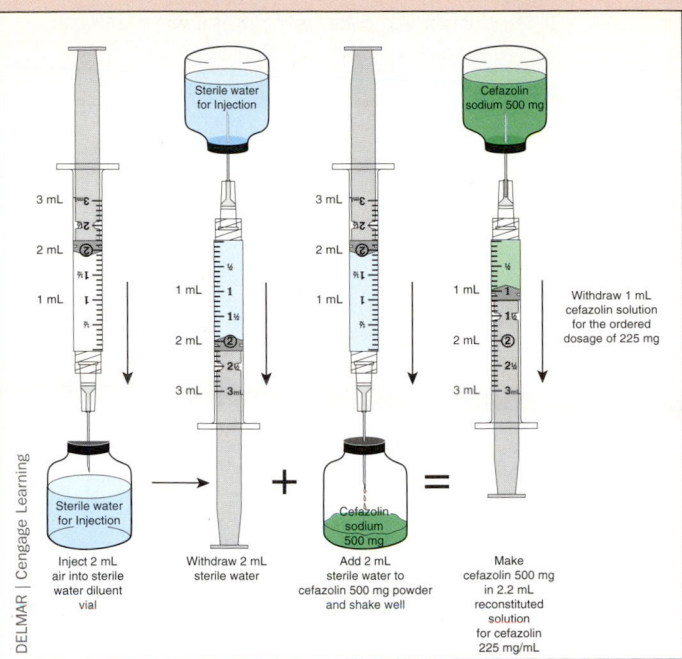

■ *Illustrations* simulate critical dosage calculation and dose preparation skills.

■ *Critical Thinking Skills* are applied to real-life patient care situations for you, emphasizing the importance of accurate dosage calculations and the avoidance of medication errors. As an added benefit, critical thinking scenarios present prevention strategies so you can learn how to avoid these errors in practice.

CRITICAL THINKING SKILLS	**ERROR**

ERROR

Incorrectly interpreting grains as grams.

Possible Scenario

A physician ordered a single dose of **15 grains of aspirin** for a patient complaining of a severe headache. Aspirin was available in *500 mg aspirin tablets*. While preparing the medication, the nurse was distracted by a visitor who fell by the nurses' station. The nurse returned to read the order as *1.5 grams* and calculated the dose this way:

If: 1 g = 1,000 mg and 0.5 g = 0.5 g × 1,000 mg/g = 500 mg
then: 1.5 g = 1,000 mg + 500 mg = 1,500 mg, so the patient was given 3 tablets.   **INCORRECT**

You know that 15 grains is equivalent to 1 g or 1,000 mg. By misreading the dose, the nurse gave 500 mg more than ordered, overdosing the patient.

Potential Outcome

The patient received $1\frac{1}{2}$ times, or 150%, of the dosage ordered. This larger dose, 1,500 mg, could cause nausea, heartburn, and gastrointestinal upset. In aspirin-sensitive patients it could result in gastrointestinal bleeding.

Prevention

This type of medication error is avoided by carefully checking the drug order at least three times: before preparing a medication, once the dose is prepared, and prior to giving the patient the medication. Also, the nurse should recognize that the ordered dose is in apothecary measurement, whereas the supply dosage is in metric measurement, and carefully convert between systems.

Review Set 14

Convert each of the following amounts to the unit indicated. Indicate the approximate equivalent(s) used in the conversion. If rounding is necessary, round decimals to two places (hundredths).

■ *Review Sets* are sprinkled throughout the chapters to encourage you to stop and check your understanding of material just presented.

	Approximate Equivalent			Approximate Equivalent
1. gr $\frac{1}{2}$ =	_____ mg _____		21. gr v =	_____ mg _____
2. gr $\frac{3}{4}$ =	_____ mg _____		22. 30 mg =	gr _____ _____
3. 3 g =	_____ kg _____		23. 1 pt =	_____ mL _____
4. gr $\frac{1}{150}$ =	_____ mg _____		24. gr x =	_____ mg _____
5. gr x =	_____ mg _____		25. 300 mg =	gr _____ _____
6. 15 mg =	gr _____ _____		26. 30 cm =	_____ in _____
7. 13 t =	_____ mL _____		27. 90 mg =	gr _____ _____

- *Practice Problems* round out each chapter. This is your opportunity to put your skills to the test, to identify your areas of strength, and also to acknowledge those areas in which you need additional study.

PRACTICE PROBLEMS—CHAPTER 11

Calculate the amount you will prepare for 1 dose. Indicate the syringe you will select to measure the medication.

1. Order: **Dilaudid 4 mg IV q.4h p.r.n., pain**

   Supply: Dilaudid 10 mg/mL

   Give: _____ mL   Select _____ syringe

2. Order: **morphine sulfate gr $\frac{1}{4}$ IV stat**

   Supply: morphine sulfate 10 mg/mL

   Give: _____ mL   Select _____ syringe

- *Section Self-Evaluations* and two *Posttests* test your mastery of concepts and critical calculation skills.

SECTION 4 SELF-EVALUATION

Chapter 15—Intravenous Solutions, Equipment, and Calculations

1. Which of the following IV solutions is normal saline? _____ 0.45% NaCl

   _____ 0.9% NaCl   _____ D_5W

2. What is the solute and concentration of 0.9% NaCl? _____

3. What is the solute and concentration of 0.45% NaCl? _____

Use the following information to answer questions 4 and 5.

Order: **D_5 0.45% NaCl 1,000 mL IV q.8h**

4. The IV solution contains _____ g dextrose.

5. The IV solution contains _____ g sodium chloride.

6. Order: **0.45% NaCl 500 mL IV q.6h.** The IV solution contains _____ g sodium chloride.

- *Drug Index* identifies each label in the text as a quick reference.

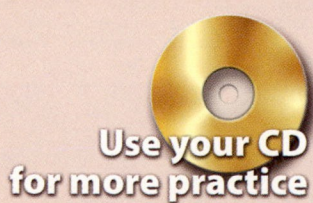

Use your CD for more practice

- *Practice Software CD-ROM* is your built-in learning tutor. As you study each chapter, be sure to also work with the in-book CD. This valuable resource will help you verify your understanding of key rules and calculations.

- *Online Resources* are available at your fingertips. Visit the **Online Companion** and **WebTutor Advantage** components for valuable course content, exercises, class notes, and case studies.

Mathematics Review

MATHEMATICS DIAGNOSTIC EVALUATION

As a prerequisite objective, *Dosage Calculations* takes into account that you can add, subtract, multiply, and divide whole numbers. You should have a working knowledge of fractions, decimals, ratios, percents, and basic problem solving as well. This text reviews these important mathematical operations, which support all dosage calculations in health care.

Set aside $1\frac{1}{2}$ hours in a quiet place to complete the 50 items in the following diagnostic evaluation. You will need scratch paper and a pencil to work the problems.

Use your results to determine your computational strengths and weaknesses to guide your review. A minimum score of 86 is recommended as an indicator of readiness for dosage calculations. If you achieve that score, you may proceed to Chapter 3. However, note any problems that you answered incorrectly, and use the related review materials in Chapters 1 and 2 to refresh your skills.

This mathematics diagnostic evaluation and the review that follows are provided to enhance your confidence and proficiency in arithmetic skills, thereby helping you to avoid careless mistakes when you perform dosage calculations.

Good luck!

Directions

1. Carry answers to three decimal places and round to two places.

   (Examples: 5.175 = 5.18; 5.174 = 5.17)

2. Express fractions in lowest terms.

   (Example: $\frac{6}{10} = \frac{3}{5}$)

Mathematics Diagnostic Evaluation

1. 1,517 + 0.63 =   _____

2. Express the value of 0.7 + 0.035 + 20.006 rounded to two decimal places.   _____

3. 9.5 + 17.06 + 32 + 41.11 + 0.99 =   _____

4. $19.69 + $304.03 =   _____

5. 93.2 − 47.09 =   _____

6. 1,005 − 250.5 =   _____

7. Express the value of 17.156 − 0.25 rounded to two decimal places.   _____

8. 509 × 38.3 =   _____

9. $4.12 × 42 =   _____

10. 17.16 × 23.5 =   _____

11. 972 ÷ 27 =   _____

12. 2.5 ÷ 0.001 =   _____

13. Express the value of $\frac{1}{4} \div \frac{3}{8}$ as a fraction reduced to lowest terms.   _____

14. Express $\frac{1,500}{240}$ as a decimal.   _____

15. Express 0.8 as a fraction.   _____

16. Express $\frac{2}{5}$ as a percent.   _____

17. Express 0.004 as a percent.   _____

18. Express 5% as a decimal.   _____

19. Express $33\frac{1}{3}\%$ as a ratio in lowest terms.   _____

20. Express 1:50 as a decimal.   _____

21. $\frac{1}{2} + \frac{3}{4} =$ _____

22. $1\frac{2}{3} + 4\frac{7}{8} =$ _____

23. $1\frac{5}{6} - \frac{2}{9} =$ _____

24. Express the value of $\frac{1}{100} \times 60$ as a fraction.   _____

25. Express the value of $4\frac{1}{4} \times 3\frac{1}{2}$ as a mixed number.   _____

26. Identify the fraction with the greatest value: $\frac{1}{150}, \frac{1}{200}, \frac{1}{100}$.   _____

27. Identify the decimal with the least value: 0.009, 0.19, 0.9.   _____

28. $\frac{6.4}{0.02} =$ _____

29. $\frac{0.02 + 0.16}{0.4 - 0.34} =$ _____

30. Express the value of $\frac{3}{12 + 3} \times 0.25$ as a decimal.   _____

31. 8% of 50 =   _____

32. $\frac{1}{2}\%$ of 18 =   _____

33. 0.9% of 24 =   _____

Find the value of X. Express your answer as a decimal.

34. $\frac{1:1,000}{1:100} \times 250 = X$ _____

35. $\frac{300}{150} \times 2 = X$ _____

36. $\frac{2.5}{5} \times 1.5 = X$ _____

37. $\frac{1,000,000}{250,000} \times X = 12$ _____

38. $\frac{0.51}{1.7} \times X = 150$ _____

39. $X = (82.4 - 52)\frac{3}{5}$ _____

40. $\frac{\frac{1}{150}}{\frac{1}{300}} \times 1.2 = X$ _____

41. Express 2:10 as a fraction in lowest terms.   _____

42. Express 2% as a ratio in lowest terms.   _____

43. If five equal medication containers contain a total of 25 tablets, how many tablets are in each container?   _____

44. A person is receiving 0.5 milligrams of a medication four times a day. What is the total amount of milligrams of medication given each day?   _____

45. If 1 kilogram equals 2.2 pounds, how many kilograms does a 66-pound child weigh?   _____

46. If 1 kilogram equals 2.2 pounds, how many pounds are in 1.5 kilograms? (Express your answer as a decimal.)   _____

47. If 1 centimeter equals $\frac{3}{8}$ inch, how many centimeters are in $2\frac{1}{2}$ inches? (Express your answer as a decimal.)   _____

48. If 2.5 centimeters equal 1 inch, how long in centimeters is a 3-inch wound?   _____

49. This diagnostic test has a total of 50 problems. If you incorrectly answer 5 problems, what percentage will you have answered correctly?   _____

50. For every 5 female student nurses in a nursing class, there is 1 male student nurse. What is the ratio of female to male student nurses?   _____

After completing these problems, see page 501 to check your answers. Give yourself 2 points for each correct answer.

Perfect score = 100   My score = _____

Minimum readiness score = 86 (43 correct)

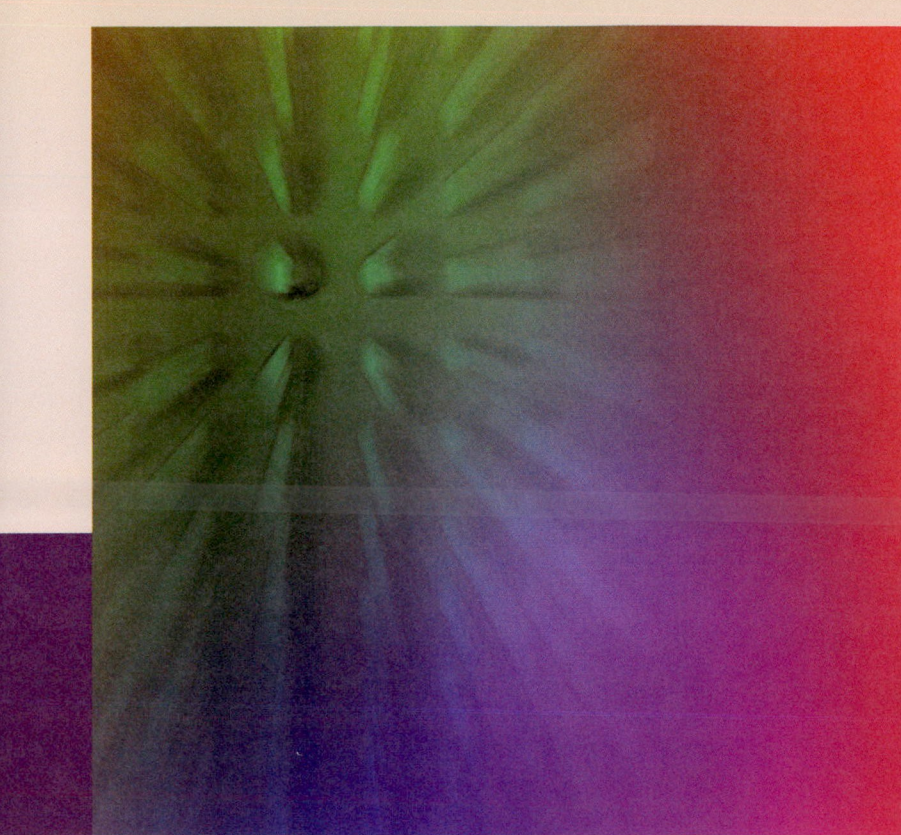
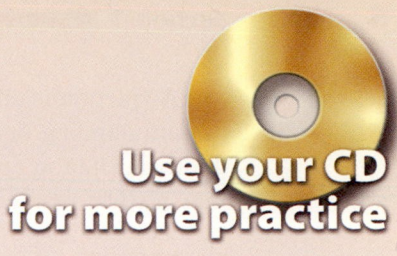

Use your CD for more practice

1

Fractions and Decimals

OBJECTIVES

Upon mastery of Chapter 1, you will be able to perform basic mathematical computations that involve fractions and decimals. Specifically, you will be able to:

- Compare the values of fractions and decimals.
- Convert between mixed numbers and improper fractions, and between reduced and equivalent forms of fractions.
- Add, subtract, multiply, and divide fractions and decimals.
- Round a decimal to a given place value.
- Read and write out the value of decimal numbers.

Health care professionals need to understand fractions and decimals to be able to interpret and act on medical orders, read prescriptions, and understand patient records and information in health care literature. The most common system of measurement used in prescription, dosage calculation, and administration of medications is the metric system. Metric measure is based on decimals. You will see fractions used in apothecary and household measures in dosage calculations. The method of solving dosage problems in this book relies on expressing relationships in fractional form. Therefore, proficiency with fractions and decimals will add to your success with a variety of medical applications.

FRACTIONS

A *fraction* indicates a portion of a whole number. There are two types of fractions: *common fractions,* such as $\frac{1}{2}$ (usually referred to simply as *fractions*) and *decimal fractions,* such as 0.5 (usually referred to simply as *decimals*).

A fraction is an expression of division, with one number placed over another number ($\frac{1}{4}$, $\frac{2}{3}$, $\frac{4}{5}$). The bottom number, or *denominator*, indicates the total number of equal-sized parts into which the whole is divided. The top number, or *numerator*, indicates how many of those parts are considered. The fraction may also be read as *the numerator divided by the denominator.*

EXAMPLE ■

$\frac{1}{4}$ $\frac{\text{numerator}}{\text{denominator}}$

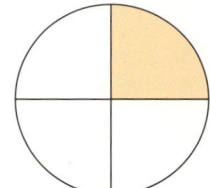

The whole is divided into four equal parts (denominator), and one part (numerator) is considered.

DELMAR | Cengage Learning

$\frac{1}{4}$ = 1 part of 4 parts, or $\frac{1}{4}$ of the whole.

The fraction $\frac{1}{4}$ may also be read as *1 divided by 4.*

MATH TIP

The *denominator* begins with *d* and is *down* below the line in a fraction.

Types of Fractions

There are four types of fractions: proper, improper, mixed numbers, and complex.

Proper Fractions

Proper fractions are fractions in which the value of the numerator is less than the value of the denominator. The value of the proper fraction is less than 1.

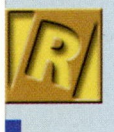

RULE

Whenever the numerator is less than the denominator, the value of the fraction must be less than 1.

EXAMPLE ■

$\frac{5}{8}$ $\frac{\text{numerator}}{\text{denominator}}$ is less than 1

Improper Fractions

Improper fractions are fractions in which the value of the numerator is greater than or equal to the value of the denominator. The value of the improper fraction is greater than or equal to 1.

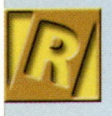

RULE

Whenever the numerator is greater than the denominator, the value of the fraction must be greater than 1.

EXAMPLE ■

$\frac{8}{5}$ is greater than 1

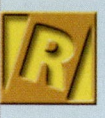

RULE

Whenever the numerator and denominator are equal, the value of the improper fraction is always equal to 1; a nonzero number divided by itself is equal to 1.

EXAMPLE ■

$\frac{5}{5} = 1$

Mixed Numbers

When a whole number and a proper fraction are combined, the result is referred to as a *mixed number*. The value of the mixed number is always greater than 1.

EXAMPLE ■

$1\frac{5}{8} = 1 + \frac{5}{8}$ $1\frac{5}{8}$ is greater than 1

Complex Fractions

Complex fractions include fractions in which the numerator, the denominator, or both contain a fraction, decimal, or mixed number. The value may be less than, greater than, or equal to 1.

EXAMPLES ■

$\dfrac{\frac{5}{8}}{\frac{1}{2}}$ is greater than 1 $\dfrac{\frac{5}{8}}{2}$ is less than 1 $\dfrac{1\frac{5}{8}}{\frac{1}{5}}$ is greater than 1 $\dfrac{\frac{1}{2}}{\frac{2}{4}} = 1$

To perform dosage calculations that involve fractions, you must be able to convert among these different types of fractions and reduce them to lowest terms. You must also be able to add, subtract, multiply, and divide fractions. Review these simple rules of working with fractions. Continue to practice until the concepts are crystal clear and automatic.

Equivalent Fractions

The value of a fraction can be expressed in several ways. This is called *finding an equivalent fraction*. In finding an equivalent fraction, both terms of the fraction (numerator and denominator) are either multiplied or divided by the same nonzero number.

MATH TIP

In an equivalent fraction, the form of the fraction is changed, but the value of the fraction remains the same.

EXAMPLES ■

$\frac{2}{4} = \frac{2 \div 2}{4 \div 2} = \frac{1}{2}$ $\frac{1}{3} = \frac{1 \times 3}{3 \times 3} = \frac{3}{9}$

Reducing Fractions to Lowest Terms

When calculating dosages, it is usually easier to work with fractions using the smallest possible numbers. Finding these equivalent fractions is called *reducing the fraction to the lowest terms* or *simplifying the fraction*.

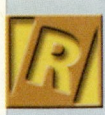

RULE

To reduce a fraction to lowest terms, divide both the numerator and denominator by the largest nonzero whole number that will go evenly into both the numerator and the denominator.

EXAMPLE ■

Reduce $\frac{6}{12}$ to lowest terms.

6 is the largest number that will divide evenly into both 6 (numerator) and 12 (denominator).

$\frac{6}{12} = \frac{6 \div 6}{12 \div 6} = \frac{1}{2}$ in lowest terms

Sometimes this reduction can be done in several steps. Always check a fraction to see if it can be reduced further.

EXAMPLE ■

$\frac{5,000}{20,000} = \frac{5,000 \div 1,000}{20,000 \div 1,000} = \frac{5}{20}$ (not in lowest terms)

$\frac{5}{20} = \frac{5 \div 5}{20 \div 5} = \frac{1}{4}$ (in lowest terms)

MATH TIP

If both the numerator and denominator cannot be divided evenly by a nonzero number other than 1, then the fraction is already in lowest terms.

Enlarging Fractions

RULE

To find an equivalent fraction in which both terms are larger, multiply both the numerator and the denominator by the same nonzero number.

EXAMPLE ■

Enlarge $\frac{3}{5}$ to the equivalent fraction in tenths.

$\frac{3}{5} = \frac{3 \times 2}{5 \times 2} = \frac{6}{10}$

Conversion

It is important to be able to convert among different types of fractions. Conversion allows you to perform various calculations with greater ease and permits you to express answers in simplest terms.

Converting Mixed Numbers to Improper Fractions

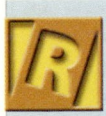

RULE

To change or convert a mixed number to an improper fraction with the same denominator, multiply the whole number by the denominator and add the numerator. Place that value in the numerator, and use the denominator of the fraction part of the mixed number.

EXAMPLE ■

$$2\frac{5}{8} = \frac{(2 \times 8) + 5}{8} = \frac{16 + 5}{8} = \frac{21}{8}$$

Converting Improper Fractions to Mixed Numbers

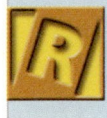

RULE
To change or convert an improper fraction to an equivalent mixed number or whole number, divide the numerator by the denominator. Any remainder becomes the numerator of a proper fraction that should be reduced to lowest terms.

EXAMPLES ■

$$\frac{8}{5} = 8 \div 5 = 1\frac{3}{5}$$

$$\frac{10}{4} = 10 \div 4 = 2\frac{2}{4} = 2\frac{1}{2}$$

Comparing Fractions

In calculating some drug dosages, it is helpful to know when the value of one fraction is greater or less than another. The relative sizes of fractions can be determined by comparing the numerators when the denominators are the same or comparing the denominators if the numerators are the same.

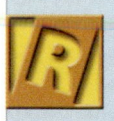

RULE
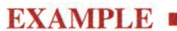
If the denominators are both the same, the fraction with the smaller numerator has the lesser value.

EXAMPLE ■

Compare $\frac{2}{5}$ and $\frac{3}{5}$

Denominators are both 5

Numerators: 2 is less than 3

$\frac{2}{5}$ has a lesser value

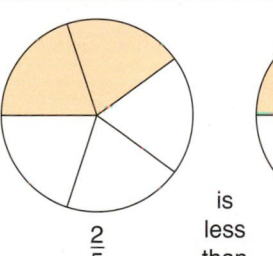

$\frac{2}{5}$ is less than $\frac{3}{5}$

DELMAR | Cengage Learning

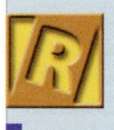

RULE
If the numerators are the same, the fraction with the smaller denominator has the greater value.

EXAMPLE ■

Compare $\frac{1}{2}$ and $\frac{1}{4}$

Numerators are both 1

Denominators: 2 is less than 4

$\frac{1}{2}$ has a greater value

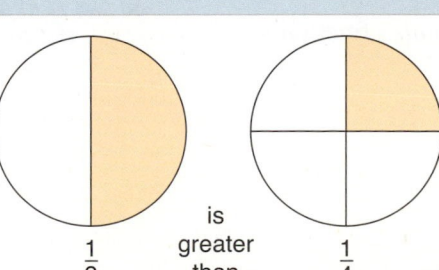

$\frac{1}{2}$ is greater than $\frac{1}{4}$

DELMAR | Cengage Learning

Note: A smaller denominator means it has been divided into fewer pieces, so each one is larger.

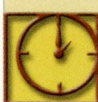

QUICK REVIEW

- Proper fraction: numerator is less than denominator; value is less than 1. Example: $\frac{1}{2}$

- Improper fraction: numerator is greater than denominator; value is greater than 1. Example: $\frac{4}{3}$

  Or numerator = denominator; value = 1. Example: $\frac{5}{5}$

- Mixed number: whole number + a fraction; value is greater than 1. Example: $1\frac{1}{2}$

- Complex fraction: numerator and/or denominator are composed of a fraction, decimal, or mixed number; value is less than, greater than, or = 1.

  Example: $\dfrac{\frac{1}{2}}{\frac{1}{50}}$

- Any nonzero number divided by itself = 1. Example: $\frac{3}{3} = 1$

- To reduce a fraction to lowest terms, divide both terms by the largest nonzero whole number that will divide both the numerator and denominator evenly. Value remains the same.

  Example: $\frac{6}{10} = \frac{6 \div 2}{10 \div 2} = \frac{3}{5}$

- To enlarge a fraction, multiply both terms by the same nonzero number. Value remains the same.

  Example: $\frac{1}{12} = \frac{1 \times 2}{12 \times 2} = \frac{2}{24}$

- To convert a mixed number to an improper fraction, multiply the whole number by the denominator and add the numerator; use original denominator in the fractional part.

  Example: $1\frac{1}{3} = \frac{(3 \times 1) + 1}{3} = \frac{3 + 1}{3} = \frac{4}{3}$

- To convert an improper fraction to a mixed number, divide the numerator by the denominator. Express any remainder as a proper fraction reduced to lowest terms.

  Example: $\frac{21}{9} = 21 \div 9 = 2\frac{3}{9} = 2\frac{1}{3}$

- When numerators are equal, the fraction with the smaller denominator is greater.

  Example: $\frac{1}{2}$ is greater than $\frac{1}{3}$

- When denominators are equal, the fraction with the larger numerator is greater.

  Example: $\frac{2}{3}$ is greater than $\frac{1}{3}$

Review Set 1

1. Circle the *improper* fraction(s).

$\frac{2}{3}$ $1\frac{3}{4}$ $\frac{6}{6}$ $\frac{7}{5}$ $\frac{16}{17}$ $\dfrac{\frac{1}{9}}{\frac{2}{3}}$

2. Circle the *complex* fraction(s).

$\frac{4}{5}$ $3\frac{7}{8}$ $\frac{2}{2}$ $\frac{9}{8}$ $\frac{8}{9}$ $\dfrac{\frac{1}{100}}{\frac{1}{150}}$

3. Circle the *proper* fraction(s).

$\frac{1}{4}$ $\frac{1}{14}$ $\frac{14}{1}$ $\frac{14}{14}$ $\frac{144}{14}$

4. Circle the *mixed* number(s) *reduced to the lowest terms.*

$3\frac{4}{8}$ $\frac{2}{3}$ $1\frac{2}{9}$ $\frac{1}{3}$ $1\frac{1}{4}$ $5\frac{7}{8}$

5. Circle the pair(s) of *equivalent* fractions.

$$\frac{3}{4} = \frac{6}{8} \qquad \frac{1}{5} = \frac{2}{10} \qquad \frac{3}{9} = \frac{1}{3} \qquad \frac{3}{4} = \frac{4}{3} \qquad 1\frac{4}{9} = 1\frac{2}{3}$$

Change the following mixed numbers to improper fractions.

6. $6\frac{1}{2} =$ _____   9. $7\frac{5}{6} =$ _____

7. $1\frac{1}{5} =$ _____   10. $102\frac{3}{4} =$ _____

8. $10\frac{2}{3} =$ _____

Change the following improper fractions to whole numbers or mixed numbers; reduce to lowest terms.

11. $\frac{24}{12} =$ _____   14. $\frac{100}{75} =$ _____

12. $\frac{8}{8} =$ _____   15. $\frac{44}{16} =$ _____

13. $\frac{30}{9} =$ _____

Enlarge the following fractions to the number of parts indicated.

16. $\frac{3}{4}$ to eighths _____   19. $\frac{2}{5}$ to tenths _____

17. $\frac{1}{4}$ to sixteenths _____   20. $\frac{2}{3}$ to ninths _____

18. $\frac{2}{3}$ to twelfths _____

Circle the correct answer.

21. Which is larger? $\frac{1}{150}$ or $\frac{1}{100}$

22. Which is smaller? $\frac{1}{1,000}$ or $\frac{1}{10,000}$

23. Which is larger? $\frac{2}{9}$ or $\frac{5}{9}$

24. Which is smaller? $\frac{3}{10}$ or $\frac{5}{10}$

25. A patient is supposed to drink a 10 fluid ounce bottle of magnesium citrate prior to his X-ray study. He has been able to drink 6 fluid ounces. What portion of the liquid remains? (Express your answer as a fraction reduced to lowest terms.) _____

26. If 1 medicine bottle contains 12 doses, how many full and fractional bottles of medicine are required for 18 doses? (Express your answer as a fraction reduced to lowest terms.) _____

27. A respiratory therapy class consists of 3 men and 57 women. What fraction of the students in the class are men? (Express your answer as a fraction reduced to lowest terms.) _____

28. A nursing student answers 18 out of 20 questions correctly on a test. Write a proper fraction (reduced to lowest terms) to represent the portion of the test questions that were answered correctly.

_____

29. A typical dose of Children's Tylenol contains 160 milligrams of medication per teaspoonful. Each 80 milligrams is what part of a typical dose? _____

30. In question 29, how many teaspoons of Children's Tylenol would you need to give an 80 milligram dose? _____

After completing these problems, see pages 501–502 to check your answers.

If you answered question 30 correctly, you can already calculate dosages!

Addition and Subtraction of Fractions

To add or subtract fractions, all the denominators must be the same. You can determine the least common denominator by finding the smallest whole number into which all denominators will divide evenly. Once the least common denominator is determined, convert the fractions to equivalent fractions with the least common denominator. This operation involves *enlarging the fractions,* which we examined in the last section. Let's look at an example of this important operation.

EXAMPLE ■

Find the equivalent fractions with the least common denominator for $\frac{3}{8}$ and $\frac{1}{3}$.

1. Find the smallest whole number into which the denominators 8 and 3 will divide evenly. The least common denominator is 24.

2. Convert the fractions to equivalent fractions with 24 as the denominator.

$$\frac{3}{8} = \frac{3 \times 3}{8 \times 3} = \frac{9}{24} \qquad \frac{1}{3} = \frac{1 \times 8}{3 \times 8} = \frac{8}{24}$$

You have enlarged $\frac{3}{8}$ to $\frac{9}{24}$ and $\frac{1}{3}$ to $\frac{8}{24}$. Now both fractions have the same denominator. Finding the least common denominator is the first step in adding or subtracting fractions.

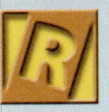

RULE

To add or subtract fractions:

1. Convert all fractions to equivalent fractions with the least common denominator.

2. Add or subtract the numerators, place that value in the numerator, and use the least common denominator as the denominator.

3. Convert to a mixed number and/or reduce the fraction to lowest terms, if possible.

MATH TIP

To add or subtract fractions, no calculations are performed on the denominators once they are all converted to equivalent fractions with the least common denominators. Perform the mathematical operation (addition or subtraction) on the *numerators* only, and use the least common denominator as the denominator of the answer. Never add or subtract denominators.

Adding Fractions

EXAMPLE 1 ■

$\frac{3}{4} + \frac{1}{4} + \frac{2}{4}$

1. Find the least common denominator. This step is not necessary in this example because the fractions already have the same denominator.

2. Add the numerators and use the common denominator: $\frac{3 + 1 + 2}{4} = \frac{6}{4}$

3. Convert to a mixed number and reduce to lowest terms: $\frac{6}{4} = 1\frac{2}{4} = 1\frac{1}{2}$

EXAMPLE 2 ▪

$$\frac{1}{3} + \frac{3}{4} + \frac{1}{6}$$

1. Find the least common denominator: 12. The number 12 is the smallest number that 3, 4, and 6 will all equally divide into.

   Convert to equivalent fractions in twelfths. This is the same as enlarging the fractions.

   $$\frac{1}{3} = \frac{1 \times 4}{3 \times 4} = \frac{4}{12}$$

   $$\frac{3}{4} = \frac{3 \times 3}{4 \times 3} = \frac{9}{12}$$

   $$\frac{1}{6} = \frac{1 \times 2}{6 \times 2} = \frac{2}{12}$$

2. Add the numerators, and use the common denominator: $\frac{4 + 9 + 2}{12} = \frac{15}{12}$

3. Convert to a mixed number, and reduce to lowest terms: $\frac{15}{12} = 1\frac{3}{12} = 1\frac{1}{4}$

Subtracting Fractions

EXAMPLE 1 ▪

$$\frac{15}{18} - \frac{8}{18}$$

1. Find the least common denominator. This is not necessary in this example because the denominators are the same.

2. Subtract the numerators, and use the common denominator: $\frac{15 - 8}{18} = \frac{7}{18}$

3. Reduce to lowest terms. This is not necessary here because no further reduction is possible.

EXAMPLE 2 ▪

$$1\frac{1}{10} - \frac{3}{5}$$

1. Find the least common denominator: 10. The number 10 is the smallest number that both 10 and 5 will equally divide into.

   Convert to equivalent fractions in tenths:

   $$1\frac{1}{10} = \frac{11}{10} \qquad \text{Note: First convert mixed numbers into improper fractions for computations.}$$

   $$\frac{3}{5} = \frac{3 \times 2}{5 \times 2} = \frac{6}{10}$$

2. Subtract the numerators, and use the common denominator: $\frac{11 - 6}{10} = \frac{5}{10}$

3. Reduce to lowest terms: $\frac{5}{10} = \frac{1}{2}$

   Let's review one more time how to add and subtract fractions.

QUICK REVIEW

To add or subtract fractions:

- Convert to equivalent fractions with the least common denominator.

- Add or subtract the numerators; place that value in the numerator. Use the least common denominator as the denominator of the answer.

- Convert the answer to a mixed number and/or reduce to lowest terms, if possible.

Review Set 2

Add, and reduce the answers to lowest terms.

1. $7\frac{4}{5} + \frac{2}{3} =$ _____

2. $\frac{3}{4} + \frac{2}{3} =$ _____

3. $4\frac{2}{3} + 5\frac{1}{24} + 7\frac{1}{2} =$ _____

4. $\frac{3}{4} + \frac{1}{8} + \frac{1}{6} =$ _____

5. $12\frac{1}{2} + 20\frac{1}{3} =$ _____

6. $\frac{1}{4} + 5\frac{1}{3} =$ _____

7. $\frac{1}{7} + \frac{2}{3} + \frac{11}{21} =$ _____

8. $\frac{4}{9} + \frac{5}{8} + 4\frac{2}{3} =$ _____

9. $34\frac{1}{2} + 8\frac{1}{2} =$ _____

10. $\frac{12}{17} + 5\frac{2}{7} =$ _____

11. $\frac{6}{5} + 1\frac{1}{3} =$ _____

12. $\frac{1}{4} + \frac{5}{33} =$ _____

Subtract, and reduce the answers to lowest terms.

13. $\frac{3}{4} - \frac{1}{4} =$ _____

14. $8\frac{1}{12} - 3\frac{1}{4} =$ _____

15. $\frac{1}{8} - \frac{1}{12} =$ _____

16. $100 - 36\frac{1}{3} =$ _____

17. $355\frac{1}{5} - 55\frac{2}{5} =$ _____

18. $\frac{1}{3} - \frac{1}{6} =$ _____

19. $2\frac{3}{5} - 1\frac{1}{5} =$ _____

20. $14\frac{3}{16} - 7\frac{1}{8} =$ _____

21. $25 - 17\frac{7}{9} =$ _____

22. $4\frac{7}{10} - 3\frac{9}{20} =$ _____

23. $48\frac{6}{11} - 24 =$ _____

24. $1\frac{2}{3} - 1\frac{1}{12} =$ _____

25. A patient weighs 50 pounds on admission and 48 pounds on day 3 of his hospital stay. Write a fraction, reduced to lowest terms, to express the fraction of his original weight that he has lost.

_____

26. A patient is on strict recording of fluid intake and output, including measurement of liquid medications. A nursing student gave the patient $\frac{1}{4}$ fluid ounce of medication at 8 AM and $\frac{1}{3}$ fluid ounce of medication at noon. What is the total amount of medication the patient consumed?

_____

27. An infant has grown $\frac{1}{2}$ inch during his first month of life, $\frac{1}{4}$ inch during his second month, and $\frac{3}{8}$ inch during his third month. How much did he grow during his first 3 months? _____

28. The required margins for your term paper are $1\frac{1}{2}$ inches at the top and bottom of a paper that has 11 inches of vertical length. How long is the vertical area available for typed information?

_____

29. A stock clerk finds that there are $34\frac{1}{2}$ pints of hydrogen peroxide on the shelf. If the fully stocked shelf held 56 pints of hydrogen peroxide, how many pints were used?

_____

30. Your 1-year-old patient weighs $20\frac{1}{2}$ pounds. At birth, she weighed $7\frac{1}{4}$ pounds. How much weight has she gained in 1 year? _____

After completing these problems, see page 502 to check your answers.

Multiplication of Fractions

To multiply fractions, multiply numerators (for the numerator of the answer) and multiply denominators (for the denominator of the answer) to arrive at the *product* or result.

When possible, *cancellation of terms* simplifies and shortens the process of multiplication of fractions. Cancellation (like reducing to lowest terms) is based on the fact that the division of both the numerator and denominator by the same nonzero whole number does not change the value of the resulting number. In fact, it makes the calculation simpler because you are working with smaller numbers.

EXAMPLE ■

$\frac{1}{3} \times \frac{250}{500}$ (numerator and denominator of $\frac{250}{500}$ are both divisible by 250)

$$= \frac{1}{3} \times \frac{\cancel{250}^{1}}{\cancel{500}_{2}} = \frac{1}{3} \times \frac{1}{2} = \frac{1}{6}$$

Also, a numerator and a denominator of any of the fractions involved in the multiplication may be cancelled when they can be divided by the same number. This is called *cross-cancellation.*

EXAMPLE ■

$$\frac{1}{8} \times \frac{8}{9} = \frac{1}{\cancel{8}_{1}} \times \frac{\cancel{8}^{1}}{9} = \frac{1}{1} \times \frac{1}{9} = \frac{1}{9}$$

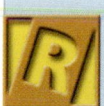

RULE

To multiply fractions:

1. Cancel terms, if possible.

2. Multiply numerators for the numerator of the answer, and multiply denominators for the denominator of the answer.

3. Reduce the result *(product)* to lowest terms, if possible.

EXAMPLE 1 ■

$\frac{3}{4} \times \frac{2}{6}$

1. Cancel terms: Divide 2 and 6 by 2

$$\frac{3}{4} \times \frac{\cancel{2}^{1}}{\cancel{6}_{3}} = \frac{3}{4} \times \frac{1}{3}$$

Divide 3 and 3 by 3

$$\frac{\cancel{3}^{1}}{4} \times \frac{1}{\cancel{3}_{1}} = \frac{1}{4} \times \frac{1}{1}$$

2. Multiply numerators and denominators:

$$\frac{1}{4} \times \frac{1}{1} = \frac{1}{4}$$

3. Reduce to lowest terms. This is not necessary here because no further reduction is possible.

EXAMPLE 2 ▪

$\dfrac{15}{30} \times \dfrac{2}{5}$

1. Cancel terms: Divide 15 and 30 by 15

$$\dfrac{\overset{1}{\cancel{15}}}{\underset{2}{\cancel{30}}} \times \dfrac{2}{5} = \dfrac{1}{2} \times \dfrac{2}{5}$$

Divide 2 and 2 by 2

$$\dfrac{1}{\underset{1}{\cancel{2}}} \times \dfrac{\overset{1}{\cancel{2}}}{5} = \dfrac{1}{1} \times \dfrac{1}{5}$$

2. Multiply numerators and denominators:

$$\dfrac{1}{1} \times \dfrac{1}{5} = \dfrac{1}{5}$$

3. Reduce to lowest terms. This is not necessary here because no further reduction is possible.

MATH TIP

When multiplying a fraction by a nonzero whole number, first convert the whole number to a fraction with a denominator of 1; the value of the number remains the same.

EXAMPLE 3 ▪

$\dfrac{2}{3} \times 4$

1. No terms to cancel. (You cannot cancel 2 and 4 because both are numerators. To do so would change the value.) Convert the whole number to a fraction.

$$\dfrac{2}{3} \times 4 = \dfrac{2}{3} \times \dfrac{4}{1}$$

2. Multiply numerators and denominators:

$$\dfrac{2}{3} \times \dfrac{4}{1} = \dfrac{8}{3}$$

3. Convert to a mixed number.

$$\dfrac{8}{3} = 8 \div 3 = 2\dfrac{2}{3}$$

MATH TIP

To multiply mixed numbers, first convert them to improper fractions, and then multiply.

EXAMPLE 4 ▪

$3\dfrac{1}{2} \times 4\dfrac{1}{3}$

1. Convert: $3\dfrac{1}{2} = \dfrac{7}{2}$

               $4\dfrac{1}{3} = \dfrac{13}{3}$

Therefore, $3\dfrac{1}{2} \times 4\dfrac{1}{3} = \dfrac{7}{2} \times \dfrac{13}{3}$

2. Cancel: not necessary. No numbers can be cancelled.

3. Multiply: $\frac{7}{2} \times \frac{13}{3} = \frac{91}{6}$

4. Convert to a mixed number: $\frac{91}{6} = 15\frac{1}{6}$

Division of Fractions

The division of fractions uses three terms: *dividend, divisor,* and *quotient.* The *dividend* is the fraction being divided or the first number. The *divisor,* the number to the right of the division sign, is the fraction the dividend is divided by. The *quotient* is the result of the division. To divide fractions, the divisor is inverted, and the operation is changed to multiplication. Once inverted, the calculation is the same as for multiplication of fractions.

EXAMPLE ■

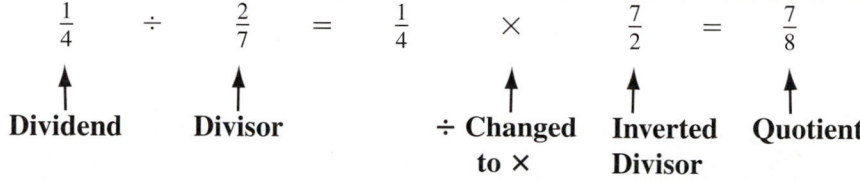

$$\frac{1}{4} \quad \div \quad \frac{2}{7} \quad = \quad \frac{1}{4} \quad \times \quad \frac{7}{2} \quad = \quad \frac{7}{8}$$

Dividend   **Divisor**   **÷ Changed**   **Inverted**   **Quotient**
                                      to ×   **Divisor**

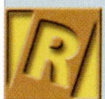

RULE

To divide fractions:

1. Invert the terms of the divisor, change ÷ to ×.

2. Cancel terms, if possible.

3. Multiply the resulting fractions.

4. Convert the result (quotient) to a mixed number, and/or reduce to lowest terms, if possible.

EXAMPLE 1 ■

$\frac{3}{4} \div \frac{1}{3}$

1. Invert divisor, and change ÷ to ×: $\frac{3}{4} \div \frac{1}{3} = \frac{3}{4} \times \frac{3}{1}$

2. Cancel: not necessary. No numbers can be cancelled.

3. Multiply: $\frac{3}{4} \times \frac{3}{1} = \frac{9}{4}$

4. Convert to mixed number: $\frac{9}{4} = 2\frac{1}{4}$

EXAMPLE 2 ■

$\frac{2}{3} \div 4$

1. Invert divisor, and change ÷ to ×: $\frac{2}{3} \div \frac{4}{1} = \frac{2}{3} \times \frac{1}{4}$

2. Cancel terms: $\frac{\overset{1}{2}}{3} \times \frac{1}{\underset{2}{4}} = \frac{1}{3} \times \frac{1}{2}$

3. Multiply: $\frac{1}{3} \times \frac{1}{2} = \frac{1}{6}$

4. Reduce: not necessary; already reduced to lowest terms.

MATH TIP

To divide mixed numbers, first convert them to improper fractions.

EXAMPLE 3 ■

$1\frac{1}{2} \div \frac{3}{4}$

1. Convert: $\frac{3}{2} \div \frac{3}{4}$

2. Invert divisor, and change $\div$ to $\times$: $\frac{3}{2} \times \frac{4}{3}$

3. Cancel: $\frac{\overset{1}{\cancel{3}}}{\underset{1}{\cancel{2}}} \times \frac{\overset{2}{\cancel{4}}}{\underset{1}{\cancel{3}}} = \frac{1}{1} \times \frac{2}{1}$

4. Multiply: $\frac{1}{1} \times \frac{2}{1} = \frac{2}{1}$

5. Simplify: $\frac{2}{1} = 2$

MATH TIP

Multiplying complex fractions also involves the division of fractions.

   In the next example the divisor is the same as the denominator, so you will invert the denominator and multiply. Multiplying complex fractions can be confusing—take your time and study this carefully.

EXAMPLE 4 ■

$\dfrac{\frac{1}{150}}{\frac{1}{100}} \times 2$

1. Convert: Express 2 as a fraction. $\dfrac{\frac{1}{150}}{\frac{1}{100}} \times \frac{2}{1}$

2. Rewrite complex fraction as division: $\frac{1}{150} \div \frac{1}{100} \times \frac{2}{1}$

3. Invert divisor and change $\div$ to $\times$: $\frac{1}{150} \times \frac{100}{1} \times \frac{2}{1}$

4. Cancel: $\frac{1}{\underset{3}{\cancel{150}}} \times \frac{\overset{2}{\cancel{100}}}{1} \times \frac{2}{1} = \frac{1}{3} \times \frac{2}{1} \times \frac{2}{1}$

5. Multiply: $\frac{1}{3} \times \frac{2}{1} \times \frac{2}{1} = \frac{4}{3}$

6. Convert to mixed number: $\frac{4}{3} = 1\frac{1}{3}$

This example appears difficult at first but when solved logically, one step at a time, it is just like the others.

QUICK REVIEW

■ To *multiply* fractions, cancel terms, multiply numerators, and multiply denominators.

■ To *divide* fractions, invert the divisor, cancel terms, and multiply.

■ Convert results to a mixed number and/or reduce to lowest terms, if possible.

Review Set 3

Multiply, and reduce the answers to lowest terms.

1. $\frac{3}{10} \times \frac{1}{12} =$ _____

2. $\frac{12}{25} \times \frac{3}{5} =$ _____

3. $\frac{5}{8} \times 1\frac{1}{6} =$ _____

4. $\frac{1}{100} \times 3 =$ _____

5. $\frac{\frac{1}{6}}{\frac{1}{4}} \times \frac{\frac{3}{2}}{\frac{2}{3}} =$ _____

6. $\frac{\frac{1}{150}}{\frac{1}{100}} \times 2\frac{1}{2} =$ _____

7. $\frac{30}{75} \times 2 =$ _____

8. $9\frac{4}{5} \times \frac{2}{3} =$ _____

9. $\frac{3}{4} \times \frac{2}{3} =$ _____

10. $4\frac{2}{3} \times 5\frac{1}{24} =$ _____

11. $\frac{3}{4} \times \frac{1}{8} =$ _____

12. $12\frac{1}{2} \times 20\frac{1}{3} =$ _____

Divide, and reduce the answers to lowest terms.

13. $\frac{3}{4} \div \frac{1}{4} =$ _____

14. $6\frac{1}{12} \div 3\frac{1}{4} =$ _____

15. $\frac{1}{8} \div \frac{7}{12} =$ _____

16. $\frac{1}{33} \div \frac{1}{3} =$ _____

17. $5\frac{1}{4} \div 10\frac{1}{2} =$ _____

18. $\frac{1}{60} \div \frac{1}{2} =$ _____

19. $2\frac{1}{2} \div \frac{3}{4} =$ _____

20. $\frac{\frac{1}{20}}{\frac{1}{3}} =$ _____

21. $\frac{1}{150} \div \frac{1}{50} =$ _____

22. $\frac{7}{8} \div 1\frac{1}{2} =$ _____

23. $\frac{\frac{3}{5}}{\frac{3}{4}} \div \frac{\frac{4}{5}}{1\frac{1}{9}} =$ _____

24. The nurse is maintaining calorie counts (or counting calories) for a patient who is not eating well. The patient ate $\frac{3}{4}$ of a large apple. If one large apple contains 80 calories, how many calories were consumed? _____

25. How many seconds are there in $9\frac{1}{3}$ minutes? _____

26. A bottle of Children's Tylenol contains 20 teaspoons of liquid. If each dose for a 2-year-old child is $\frac{1}{2}$ teaspoon, how many doses for a 2 year old are available in this bottle? _____

27. You need to take $1\frac{1}{2}$ tablets of medication 3 times per day for 7 days. Over the 7 days, how many tablets will you take? _____

28. The nurse aide observes that the patient's water pitcher is $\frac{1}{3}$ full. If the patient drank 850 milliliters of water, how many milliliters does the pitcher hold? (Hint: The 850 milliliters does not represent $\frac{1}{3}$ of the pitcher.) _____

29. A pharmacist weighs a tube of antibiotic eye ointment and documents that it weighs $\frac{7}{10}$ of an ounce. How much would 75 tubes weigh? _____

30. A patient is taking a liquid antacid from a 16 fluid ounce bottle. If the patient takes $\frac{1}{2}$ fluid ounce every 4 hours while awake beginning at 7 AM and ending with a final dose at 11 PM, how many full days would this bottle last? (Hint: First, draw a clock.) _____

After completing these problems, see pages 502–503 to check your answers.

DECIMALS

Decimal Fractions and Decimal Numbers

Decimal fractions are fractions with a denominator of 10, 100, 1,000, or any power of 10. At first glance, they appear to be whole numbers because of the way they are written. But the numeric value of a decimal fraction is always less than 1.

EXAMPLES ■

$$0.1 \ \ = \frac{1}{10}$$

$$0.01 \ \ = \frac{1}{100}$$

$$0.001 = \frac{1}{1,000}$$

Decimal numbers are numeric values that include a whole number, a decimal point, and a decimal fraction.

EXAMPLES ■

4.67 and 23.956

Generally, decimal fractions and decimal numbers are referred to simply as *decimals*.

Nurses and other health care professionals must have an understanding of decimals to be competent at dosage calculations. Medication orders and other measurements in health care primarily use metric measure, which is based on the decimal system. Decimals are a special shorthand for designating fractional values. They are simpler to read and faster to use when performing mathematical computations.

MATH TIP

When dealing with decimals, think of the decimal point as the center that separates whole and fractional amounts. The position of the numbers in relation to the decimal point indicates the place value of the numbers.

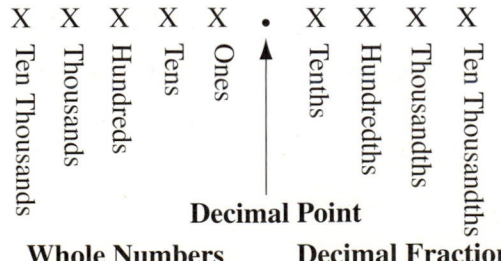

MATH TIP

The words for all decimal fractions end in *th(s)*.

EXAMPLES ▪

0.001 = one thousand*th*

0.02 = two hundred*ths*

0.7 = seven ten*ths*

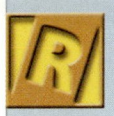

RULE

The decimal number is read by stating the whole number first, the decimal point as *and,* and then the decimal fraction by naming the value of the last decimal place.

EXAMPLE ▪

Look carefully at the decimal number 4.125. The last decimal place is thousandths. Therefore, the number is read as *four and one hundred twenty-five thousandths*.

4 .	1	2	5
Ones	Tenths	Hundredths	Thousandths

EXAMPLES ▪

The number 6.2 is read as *six and two tenths*.

The number 10.03 is read as *ten and three hundredths*.

MATH TIP

Given a decimal fraction (whose value is less than 1), the decimal number is read alone, without stating the zero. However, the zero is written to emphasize the decimal point. In fact, since 2005 this is a requirement by the accrediting body for health care organizations, The Joint Commission (2005), when writing decimal fractions in medical notation.

EXAMPLE ▪

0.125 is read as *one hundred twenty-five thousandths*.

A set of rules governs the decimal system of notation.

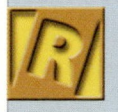

RULE

The whole number value is controlled by its position to the left of the decimal point.

EXAMPLES ▪

10.1 = ten and one tenth. The whole number is *10*.

1.01 = one and one hundredth. The whole number is *1*.

Notice that the decimal point's position completely changes the numeric value.

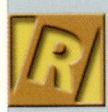

RULE

The decimal fraction value is controlled by its position to the right of the decimal point.

EXAMPLES ■

25.1 = twenty-five and one tenth. The decimal fraction is *one tenth*.

25.01 = twenty-five and one hundredth. The decimal fraction is *one hundredth*.

MATH TIP

Each decimal place is counted off as a power of 10 to tell you which denominator is expected.

EXAMPLE 1 ■

437.5 = four hundred thirty-seven and **five tenths** $(437 + \frac{5}{10})$

One decimal place indicates *tenths*.

EXAMPLE 2 ■

43.75 = forty-three and **seventy-five hundredths** $(43 + \frac{75}{100})$

Two decimal places indicate *hundredths*.

EXAMPLE 3 ■

4.375 = four and **three hundred seventy-five thousandths** $(4 + \frac{375}{1,000})$

Three decimal places indicate *thousandths*.

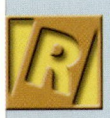

RULE

Zeros added after the last digit of a decimal fraction do not change its value and are not necessary, except when a zero is required to demonstrate the level of precision of the value being reported, such as for laboratory results.

EXAMPLE ■

0.25 = 0.25**0**

Twenty-five hundredths equals two hundred fifty thousandths.

CAUTION

When writing decimals, eliminate unnecessary zeros at the end of the number to avoid confusion. As of May 2005, The Joint Commission (2008) forbids the use of trailing zeros for medication orders or other medication-related documentation and cautions that, in such cases, the decimal point may be missed when an unnecessary zero is written. This is part of The Joint Commission's *Official "Do Not Use" List* (2005) for medical notation, which will be discussed again in Chapters 3 and 9.

Because the last zero does not change the value of the decimal, it is not necessary. For example, the required notation is 0.25 rather than 0.250 and 10 not 10.0, which can be misinterpreted as 250 and 100, respectively, if the decimal point is not clear.

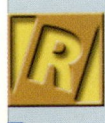

RULE

Zeros added before or after the decimal point of a decimal number *may* change its value.

EXAMPLES ■

0.125 ≠ (is not equal to) 0.**0**125

1.025 ≠ **1**0.025

However, .6 = **0.**6 and 12. = 12.**0**, but you should write 0.6 (with a leading decimal) and 12 (without a trailing zero).

Comparing Decimals

It is important to be able to compare decimal amounts, noting which has a greater or lesser value.

CAUTION
A common error in comparing decimals is to overlook the decimal place values and misinterpret higher numbers for greater amounts and lower numbers for lesser amounts.

MATH TIP
You can accurately compare decimal amounts by aligning the decimal points and adding zeros so that the numbers to be compared have the same number of decimal places. Remember that adding zeros at the end of a decimal fraction for the purposes of comparison does not change the original value.

EXAMPLE 1 ■

Compare 0.125, 0.05, and 0.2 to find which decimal fraction is largest.

Align decimal points and add zeros.

$0.125 = \frac{125}{1,000}$ or one hundred twenty-five thousandths

$0.05\mathbf{0} = \frac{50}{1,000}$ or fifty thousandths

$0.2\mathbf{00} = \frac{200}{1,000}$ or two hundred thousandths

Now it is easy to see that 0.2 is the greatest amount and 0.05 is the least. But at first glance, you might have been tricked into thinking that 0.2 was the least amount and 0.125 was the greatest amount. This kind of error can have dire consequences in dosage calculations and health care.

EXAMPLE 2 ■

Suppose 0.5 microgram of a drug has been ordered. The recommended maximum dosage of the drug is 0.25 microgram, and the minimum recommended dosage is 0.125 microgram. Comparing decimals, you can see that the ordered dosage is not within the recommended range.

0.125 microgram (recommended minimum dosage)

0.25**0** microgram (recommended maximum dosage)

0.5**00** microgram (ordered dosage)

Now you can see that 0.5 microgram is outside the allowable limits of the recommended dosage range of 0.125 to 0.25 microgram for this medication. In fact, it is twice the recommended maximum dosage.

CAUTION
It is important to eliminate possible confusion and avoid errors in dosage calculation. To avoid overlooking a decimal point in a decimal fraction and thereby reading the numeric value as a whole number, always place a zero to the left of the decimal point to emphasize that the number

continues

continued

has a value less than 1. This is another of The Joint Commission's requirements. The Joint Commission's *Official "Do Not Use" List* (2005) prohibits writing a decimal fraction that is less than 1 without a leading zero. This important concept will be emphasized again in Chapters 3 and 9.

EXAMPLES ■

0.425, **0**.01, or **0**.005

Conversion between Fractions and Decimals

For dosage calculations, you may need to convert decimals to fractions and vice versa.

RULE

To convert a fraction to a decimal, divide the numerator by the denominator.

MATH TIP

Make sure the numerator is inside the division sign and the denominator is outside. You will avoid reversing the numerator and the denominator in division if you write down the number you read first and put the division sign around that number, with the second number written outside the division sign. This will work regardless of whether is is written as a fraction or as a division problem (such as $\frac{1}{2}$ or 1 ÷ 2).

EXAMPLE 1 ■

Convert $\frac{1}{4}$ to a decimal.

$$\frac{1}{4} = 4\overline{)\begin{array}{r} .25 \\ 1.00 \\ \underline{8} \\ 20 \\ \underline{20} \end{array}} = 0.25$$

EXAMPLE 2 ■

Convert $\frac{2}{5}$ to a decimal.

$$\frac{2}{5} = 5\overline{)\begin{array}{r} .4 \\ 2.0 \\ \underline{20} \end{array}} = 0.4$$

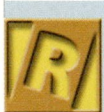

RULE

To convert a decimal to a fraction:

1. Express the decimal number as a whole number in the numerator of the fraction.

2. Express the denominator of the fraction as the number 1 followed by as many zeros as there are places to the right of the decimal point.

3. Reduce the resulting fraction to lowest terms.

EXAMPLE 1 ■

Convert 0.125 to a fraction.

1. Numerator: 125

2. Denominator: 1 followed by 3 zeros = 1,000

3. Reduce: $\frac{125}{1,000} = \frac{1}{8}$

EXAMPLE 2 ■

Convert 0.65 to a fraction.

1. Numerator: 65

2. Denominator: 1 followed by 2 zeros = 100

3. Reduce: $\frac{65}{100} = \frac{13}{20}$

MATH TIP

State the complete name of the decimal, and write the fraction that has the same name, such as $0.65 =$ "sixty-five hundredths" $= \frac{65}{100}$.

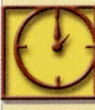

QUICK REVIEW

■ In a decimal number, whole number values are to the left of the decimal point and fractional values are to the right.

■ Zeros added to a decimal fraction before the decimal point of a decimal number less than 1 or at the end of the decimal fraction do not change the value (except when a zero is required to demonstrate the level of precision of the reported value). Example: .5 = **0.**5 = 0.5**0**. However, using the leading zero is the only acceptable notation (such as 0.5).

■ In a decimal number, zeros added before or after the decimal point *may* change the value.

Example: 1.5 ≠ 1.**0**5 and 1.5 ≠ **1**0.5.

■ To avoid overlooking the decimal point in a decimal fraction, *always* place a zero to the left of the decimal point.

Example:
.5 ← Avoid writing a decimal fraction this way; it could be mistaken for the whole number *5*.

Example:
0.5 ← This is the required method of writing a decimal fraction with a value less than 1.

■ The number of places in a decimal fraction indicates the power of 10.

Examples:
0.5 = five tenths
0.05 = five hundredths
0.005 = five thousandths

■ Compare decimals by aligning decimal points and adding zeros at the end.

Example:
Compare 0.5, 0.05, and 0.005.
0.500 = five hundred thousandths (greatest)
0.050 = fifty thousandths
0.005 = five thousandths (least)

■ To convert a fraction to a decimal, divide the numerator by the denominator.

■ To convert a decimal to a fraction, express the decimal number as a whole number in the numerator and the denominator as the correct power of 10. Reduce the fraction to lowest terms.

Example:

$$0.04 = \frac{4 \text{ (numerator is a whole number)}}{100 \text{ (denominator is 1 followed by 2 zeros)}} = \frac{\overset{1}{\cancel{4}}}{\underset{25}{\cancel{100}}} = \frac{1}{25}$$

Review Set 4

Complete the following table of equivalent fractions and decimals. Reduce fractions to lowest terms.

Fraction	Decimal	The decimal number is read as:
1. $\frac{1}{5}$	_____	_____
2. _____	_____	eighty-five hundredths
3. _____	1.05	_____
4. _____	0.006	_____
5. $10\frac{3}{200}$	_____	_____
6. _____	1.9	_____
7. _____	_____	five and one tenth
8. $\frac{4}{5}$	_____	_____
9. _____	250.5	_____
10. $33\frac{3}{100}$	_____	_____
11. _____	0.95	_____
12. $2\frac{3}{4}$	_____	_____
13. _____	_____	seven and five thousandths
14. $\frac{21}{250}$	_____	_____
15. _____	12.125	_____
16. _____	20.09	_____
17. _____	_____	twenty-two and twenty-two thousandths
18. _____	0.15	_____
19. $1,000\frac{1}{200}$	_____	_____
20. _____	_____	four thousand eighty-five and seventy-five thousandths

21. Change 0.017 to a four-place decimal. _____

22. Change 0.2500 to a two-place decimal. _____

23. Convert $\frac{75}{100}$ to a decimal. _____

24. Convert 0.045 to a fraction reduced to lowest terms. _____

Circle the correct answer.

25. Which is largest?   0.012   0.12   0.021

26. Which is smallest?   0.635   0.6   0.063

27. True or false?   0.375 = 0.0375

28. True or false?   2.2 grams = 2.02 grams

29. True or false?   6.5 ounces = 6.500 ounces

30. For a certain medication, the safe dosage should be greater than or equal to 0.5 gram but less than or equal to 2 grams. Circle each dosage that falls within this range.

    0.8 gram   0.25 gram   2.5 grams   1.25 grams

After completing these problems, see page 503 to check your answers.

Addition and Subtraction of Decimals

The addition and subtraction of decimals is similar to addition and subtraction of whole numbers. There are two simple but essential rules that are different. Health care professionals must use these two rules to perform accurate dosage calculations for some medications.

RULE
To add and subtract decimals, line up the decimal points.

CAUTION
In final answers, eliminate unnecessary zeros at the end of a decimal to avoid confusion.

EXAMPLE 1 ■
$$1.25 + 1.75 = \begin{array}{r} 1.25 \\ + 1.75 \\ \hline 3.00 = 3 \end{array}$$

EXAMPLE 2 ■
$$1.25 - 0.13 = \begin{array}{r} 1.25 \\ - 0.13 \\ \hline 1.12 \end{array}$$

EXAMPLE 3 ■
$$3.54 + 1.26 = \begin{array}{r} 3.54 \\ + 1.26 \\ \hline 4.80 = 4.8 \end{array}$$

EXAMPLE 4 ■
$$2.54 - 1.04 = \begin{array}{r} 2.54 \\ - 1.04 \\ \hline 1.50 = 1.5 \end{array}$$

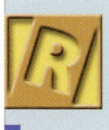

RULE
To add and subtract decimals, add zeros at the end of decimal fractions if necessary to make all decimal numbers of equal length.

EXAMPLE 1 ■
$$3.75 - 2.1 = \begin{array}{r} 3.75 \\ - 2.10 \\ \hline 1.65 \end{array}$$

EXAMPLE 2 ■
Add 0.9, 0.65, 0.27, 4.712
$$\begin{array}{r} 0.900 \\ 0.650 \\ 0.270 \\ + 4.712 \\ \hline 6.532 \end{array}$$

EXAMPLE 3 ▪

$5.25 - 3.6 = 5.25$

$$\begin{array}{r} 5.25 \\ - \ 3.60 \\ \hline 1.65 \end{array}$$

EXAMPLE 4 ▪

$66.96 + 32 = 66.96$

$$\begin{array}{r} 66.96 \\ + \ 32.00 \\ \hline 98.96 \end{array}$$

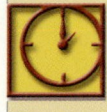

QUICK REVIEW

▪ To add or subtract decimals, align the decimal points and add zeros at the end of the decimal fraction, making all decimals of equal length. Eliminate unnecessary zeros at the end in the final answer.

EXAMPLES ▪

$1.5 + 0.05 = 1.50$

$$\begin{array}{r} 1.50 \\ + \ 0.05 \\ \hline 1.55 \end{array}$$

$7.8 + 1.12 = 7.80$

$$\begin{array}{r} 7.80 \\ + \ 1.12 \\ \hline 8.92 \end{array}$$

$0.725 - 0.5 = 0.725$

$$\begin{array}{r} 0.725 \\ - \ 0.500 \\ \hline 0.225 \end{array}$$

$12.5 - 1.5 = 12.5$

$$\begin{array}{r} 12.5 \\ - \ 1.5 \\ \hline 11.0 = 11 \end{array}$$

Review Set 5

Find the result of the following problems.

1. $0.16 + 5.375 + 1.05 + 16 =$ _____

2. $7.517 + 3.2 + 0.16 + 33.3 =$ _____

3. $13.009 - 0.7 =$ _____

4. $5.125 + 6.025 + 0.15 =$ _____

5. $175.1 + 0.099 =$ _____

6. $25.2 - 0.193 =$ _____

7. $0.58 - 0.062 =$ _____

8. $\$10.10 - \$0.62 =$ _____

9. $\$19 - \$0.09 =$ _____

10. $\$5.05 + \$0.17 + \$17.49 =$ _____

11. $4 + 1.98 + 0.42 + 0.003 =$ _____

12. $0.3 - 0.03 =$ _____

13. $16.3 - 12.15 =$ _____

14. $2.5 - 0.99 =$ _____

15. $5 + 2.5 + 0.05 + 0.15 + 2.55 =$ _____

16. $0.03 + 0.16 + 2.327 =$ _____

17. $700 - 325.65 =$ _____

18. $645.32 - 40.9 =$ _____

19. $18 + 2.35 + 7.006 + 0.093 =$ _____

20. $13.529 + 10.09 =$ _____

21. A dietitian calculates the sodium in a patient's breakfast: raisin bran cereal = 0.1 gram, 1 cup 2% milk = 0.125 gram, 6 ounces orange juice = 0.001 gram, 1 corn muffin = 0.35 gram, and butter = 0.121 gram. How many grams of sodium did the patient consume? _____

22. In a 24-hour period, an infant drank 30.5 milliliters, 45 milliliters, 60 milliliters, 15 milliliters, 15.25 milliliters, and 22.5 milliliters of formula. How many milliliters did the infant drink in 24 hours? _____

23. A patient has a hospital bill for $16,709.43. Her insurance company pays $14,651.37. What is her balance due? _____

24. A patient's hemoglobin was 14.8 grams before surgery. During surgery, the hemoglobin dropped 4.5 grams. What was the hemoglobin value after it dropped? _____

25. A home health nurse accounts for her day of work. If she spent 3 hours and 20 minutes at the office, 40 minutes traveling, $3\frac{1}{2}$ hours caring for patients, 24 minutes for lunch, and 12 minutes on break, what is her total number of hours including all of her activities? Express your answer as a decimal. (Hint: First convert each time to hours and minutes.) _____

After completing these problems, see page 503 to check your answers.

Multiplying Decimals

The procedure for multiplication of decimals is similar to that used for whole numbers. The only difference is the decimal point, which must be properly placed in the product or answer. Use the following simple rule.

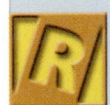

RULE

To multiply decimals:

1. Multiply the decimals without concern for decimal point placement.

2. Count off the total number of decimal places in both of the decimals multiplied.

3. Move the decimal point in the product by moving it to the left the number of places counted.

EXAMPLE 1 ■

$1.5 \times 0.5 =$ 1.5   (1 decimal place)

　　　　　 $\times\ 0.5$ (1 decimal place)
　　　　　 ‾‾‾‾‾‾
　　　　　 0.75   (The decimal point is located 2 places to the left because a total of 2 decimal places are counted in the numbers that are multiplied.)

EXAMPLE 2 ■

$1.72 \times 0.9 =$ 1.72   (2 decimal places)

　　　　　 $\times\ 0.9$ (1 decimal place)
　　　　　 ‾‾‾‾‾‾
　　　　　 1.548   (The decimal point is located 3 places to the left because a total of 3 decimal places are counted.)

EXAMPLE 3 ▪

$5.06 \times 1.3 =$ 5.06   (2 decimal places)

$\underline{\times\ 1.3}$ (1 decimal place)

1518

$\underline{506}$

6.578   (The decimal point is located 3 places to the left because a total of 3 decimal places are counted.)

EXAMPLE 4 ▪

$1.8 \times 0.05 =$ 1.8   (1 decimal place)

$\underline{\times\ 0.05}$ (2 decimal places)

0.090   (The decimal point is located 3 places to the left. Notice that a zero has to be inserted between the decimal point and the 9 to allow for enough decimal places.)

0.090   = 0.09 (Eliminate unnecessary zero.)

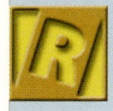

RULE

When multiplying a decimal by a power of 10, move the decimal point as many places to the right as there are zeros in the multiplier.

EXAMPLE 1 ▪

1.25×10

The multiplier 10 has 1 zero; move the decimal point 1 place to the right.

$1.25 \times 10 = 1.2.5 = 12.5$

EXAMPLE 2 ▪

2.3×100

The multiplier 100 has 2 zeros; move the decimal point 2 places to the right. (Note: Add zeros as necessary to complete the operation.)

$2.3 \times 100 = 2.30. = 230$

EXAMPLE 3 ▪

$0.001 \times 1,000$

The multiplier 1,000 has 3 zeros; move the decimal point 3 places to the right.

$0.001 \times 1,000 = 0.001. = 1$

Dividing Decimals

When dividing decimals, set up the problem the same as for the division of whole numbers. Follow the same procedure for dividing whole numbers after you apply the following rule.

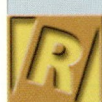

RULE

To divide decimals:

1. Move the decimal point in the *divisor* (number divided by) and the *dividend* (number divided) the number of places needed to make the *divisor* a *whole number.*

2. Place the decimal point in the *quotient* (answer) above the *new* decimal point place in the *dividend.*

EXAMPLE 1 ■

$$
\begin{array}{r}
40.3 \text{ (quotient)} \\
100.75 \div 2.5 = 2.5\overline{)100.7\,5} = 40.3 \\
\underline{100} \\
07 \\
\underline{00} \\
75 \\
\underline{75}
\end{array}
$$

(dividend)   (divisor)

EXAMPLE 2 ■

$$
\begin{array}{r}
2,825. \\
56.5 \div 0.02 = 0.02\overline{)56.50} = 2,825 \\
\underline{4} \\
16 \\
\underline{16} \\
5 \\
\underline{4} \\
10 \\
\underline{10}
\end{array}
$$

MATH TIP

Recall that adding a zero at the end of a decimal number does not change its value (56.5 = 56.50). Adding a zero was necessary in the last example to complete the operation.

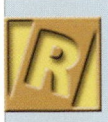

RULE

When dividing a decimal by a power of 10, move the decimal point to the left as many places as there are zeros in the divisor.

EXAMPLE 1 ■

$0.65 \div 10$

The divisor 10 has 1 zero; move the decimal point 1 place to the left.

$0.65 \div 10 = .0.65 = 0.065$

(Note: Place a zero to the left of the decimal point to avoid confusion and to emphasize that this is a decimal.)

EXAMPLE 2 ▪

7.3 ÷ 100

The divisor 100 has 2 zeros; move the decimal point 2 places to the left.

7.3 ÷ 100 = .07.3 = 0.073

(Note: Add zeros as necessary to complete the operation.)

EXAMPLE 3 ▪

0.5 ÷ 1,000

The divisor 1,000 has 3 zeros; move the decimal point 3 places to the left.

0.5 ÷ 1,000 = .000.5 = 0.0005

Rounding Decimals

For many dosage calculations, it will be necessary to compute decimal calculations to *thousandths* (*three* decimal places) and round back to *hundredths* (*two* places) for the final answer. For example, pediatric care and critical care require this degree of accuracy. At other times, you will need to round to *tenths* (*one* place). Let's look closely at this important math skill.

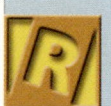

RULE

To round a decimal to hundredths, drop the number in thousandths place, and

1. Do not change the number in hundredths place, if the number in thousandths place was 4 or less.

2. Increase the number in hundredths place by 1, if the number in thousandths place was 5 or more.

When rounding for dosage calculations, unnecessary zeros can be dropped. For example, 5.20 rounded to hundredths place should be written as 5.2 because the 0 is not needed to clarify the number.

EXAMPLES ▪

	Tenths	Hundredths	Thousandths		

All rounded to hundredths (2 places)

0 . 1 2 3   = 0.12

1 . 7 4 4   = 1.74

5 . 3 2 5   = 5.33

0 . 6 6 6   = 0.67

0 . 3 0   = 0.3   (When this is rounded to hundredths, the final zero should be dropped. It is not needed to clarify the number and is potentially confusing.)

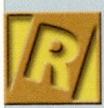

RULE

To round a decimal to tenths, drop the number in hundredths place, and

1. Do not change the number in tenths place, if the number in hundredths place was 4 or less.

2. Increase the number in tenths place by 1, if the number in hundredths place was 5 or more.

EXAMPLES ■

Tenths
Hundredths

All rounded to tenths (1 place)

0 . 1 3 = 0.1

5 . 6 4 = 5.6

0 . 7 5 = 0.8

1 . 6 6 = 1.7

0 . 9 5 = 1.0 = 1   (The zero at the end of this decimal number is dropped because it is unnecessary and potentially confusing.)

QUICK REVIEW

■ To multiply decimals, place the decimal point in the product to the left as many total decimal places as there are in the two decimals multiplied.

Example:
$0.25 \times 0.2 = 0.050 = 0.05$ (Zero at the end of the decimal is unnecessary.)

■ To divide decimals, move the decimal point in the divisor and dividend the number of decimal places that will make the divisor a whole number and align it in the quotient.

Example: $24 \div 1.2$

$$1.2 \overline{)24.0} = 20.$$

■ To multiply or divide decimals by a power of 10, move the decimal point to the right (to multiply) or to the left (to divide) the number of decimal places as there are zeros in the power of 10.

Examples:
$5.06 \times 10 = 5.0.6 = 50.6$

$2.1 \div 100 = .02.1 = 0.021$

■ When rounding decimals, add 1 to the place value considered if the next decimal place is 5 or greater.

Examples:
Rounded to hundredths: $3.054 = 3.05$; $0.566 = 0.57$

Rounded to tenths: $3.05 = 3.1$; $0.54 = 0.5$

Review Set 6

Multiply, and round your answers to two decimal places.

1. $1.16 \times 5.03 =$ _____

2. $0.314 \times 7 =$ _____

3. $1.71 \times 25 =$ _____

4. $3.002 \times 0.05 =$ _____

5. $16.1 \times 25.04 =$ _____

6. $75.1 \times 1,000.01 =$ _____

7. $16.03 \times 2.05 =$ _____

8. $55.50 \times 0.05 =$ _____

9. $23.2 \times 15.025 =$ _____

10. $1.14 \times 0.014 =$ _____

Divide, and round your answers to two decimal places.

11. $16 \div 0.04 =$ _____

12. $25.3 \div 6.76 =$ _____

13. $0.02 \div 0.004 =$ _____

14. $45.5 \div 15.25 =$ _____

15. $515 \div 0.125 =$ _____

16. $73 \div 13.40 =$ _____

17. $16.36 \div 0.06 =$ _____

18. $0.375 \div 0.25 =$ _____

19. $100.04 \div 0.002 =$ _____

20. $45 \div 0.15 =$ _____

Multiply or divide by the power of 10 indicated. Draw an arrow to demonstrate movement of the decimal point. Do not round answers.

21. $562.5 \times 100 =$ _____

22. $16 \times 10 =$ _____

23. $25 \div 1,000 =$ _____

24. $32.005 \div 1,000 =$ _____

25. $0.125 \div 100 =$ _____

26. $23.25 \times 10 =$ _____

27. $717.717 \div 10 =$ _____

28. $83.16 \times 10 =$ _____

29. $0.33 \times 100 =$ _____

30. $14.106 \times 1,000 =$ _____

After completing these problems, see page 504 to check your answers.

PRACTICE PROBLEMS—CHAPTER 1

1. Convert 0.35 to a fraction in lowest terms. _____

2. Convert $\frac{3}{8}$ to a decimal. _____

Find the least common denominator for the following pairs of fractions.

3. $\frac{5}{7}; \frac{2}{3}$ _____

4. $\frac{1}{5}; \frac{4}{11}$ _____

5. $\frac{4}{9}; \frac{5}{6}$ _____

6. $\frac{1}{3}; \frac{3}{5}$ _____

Perform the indicated operation, and reduce fractions to lowest terms.

7. $1\frac{2}{3} + \frac{9}{5} =$ _____

8. $4\frac{5}{12} + 3\frac{1}{15} =$ _____

9. $\frac{7}{9} - \frac{5}{18} =$ _____

10. $5\frac{1}{6} - 2\frac{7}{8} =$ _____

11. $\frac{4}{9} \times \frac{7}{12} =$ _____

17. $\frac{13\frac{1}{3}}{4\frac{6}{13}} =$ _____

12. $1\frac{1}{2} \times 6\frac{3}{4} =$ _____

18. $\frac{\frac{1}{10}}{\frac{2}{3}} =$ _____

13. $7\frac{1}{5} \div 1\frac{7}{10} =$ _____

19. $\frac{1}{125} \times \frac{1}{25} =$ _____

14. $\frac{3}{16} + \frac{3}{10} =$ _____

20. $\frac{\frac{7}{8}}{\frac{1}{3}} \div \frac{3\frac{1}{2}}{\frac{1}{3}} =$ _____

15. $8\frac{4}{11} \div 1\frac{2}{3} =$ _____

21. $\frac{20}{35} \times 3 =$ _____

16. $\frac{9\frac{1}{2}}{1\frac{4}{5}} =$ _____

22. $2\frac{1}{4} \times 7\frac{1}{8} =$ _____

Perform the indicated operations, and round the answers to two decimal places.

23. $11.33 + 29.16 + 19.78 =$ _____

30. $5 + 2.5 + 0.05 + 0.15 =$ _____

24. $93.712 - 26.97 =$ _____

31. $1.71 \times 25 =$ _____

25. $43.69 - 0.7083 =$ _____

32. $45 \div 0.15 =$ _____

26. $66.4 \times 72.8 =$ _____

33. $2{,}974 \div 0.23 =$ _____

27. $360 \times 0.53 =$ _____

34. $51.21 \div 0.016 =$ _____

28. $268.4 \div 14 =$ _____

35. $0.74 \div 0.37 =$ _____

29. $10.10 - 0.62 =$ _____

36. $1.5 + 146.73 + 1.9 + 0.832 =$ _____

Multiply or divide by the power of 10 indicated. Draw an arrow to demonstrate movement of the decimal point. Do not round answers.

37. $9.716 \times 1{,}000 =$ _____

40. $5.75 \times 1{,}000 =$ _____

38. $50.25 \div 100 =$ _____

41. $0.25 \div 10 =$ _____

39. $0.25 \times 100 =$ _____

42. $11.525 \times 10 =$ _____

43. A 1-month-old infant drinks $3\frac{1}{2}$ fluid ounces of formula every 4 hours day and night. How many fluid ounces will the infant drink in 1 week on this schedule? _____

44. There are 368 people employed at Riverview Clinic. If $\frac{3}{8}$ of the employees are nurses, $\frac{1}{8}$ are maintenance/cleaners, $\frac{1}{4}$ are technicians, and $\frac{1}{4}$ are all other employees, calculate the number of employees that each fraction represents. _____

45. True or false? A specific gravity of urine of $1\frac{2}{32}$ falls within the normal range of 1.01 to 1.025 for an adult patient. _____

46. Last week a nurse earning $20.43 per hour gross pay worked 40 hours plus 6.5 hours overtime, which is paid at twice the hourly rate. What is the total regular and overtime gross pay for last week? _____

47. The instructional assistant is ordering supplies for the nursing skills laboratory. A single box of 12 urinary catheters costs $98.76. A case of 12 boxes of these catheters costs $975. Calculate the savings per catheter when a case is purchased. _____

48. If each ounce of a liquid laxative contains 0.065 gram of a drug, how many grams of the drug would be contained in 4.75 ounces? (Round answer to the nearest hundredth.) _____

49. A patient is to receive 1,200 milliliters of fluid in a 24-hour period. How many milliliters should the patient drink between the hours of 7:00 AM and 7:00 PM if he is to receive $\frac{2}{3}$ of the total amount during that time? _____

50. A baby weighed 3.7 kilograms at birth. The baby now weighs 6.65 kilograms. How many kilograms did the baby gain? _____

After completing these problems, see page 504 to check your answers.

REFERENCE

The Joint Commission. (2005). *Official "do not use" list*. Retrieved September 25, 2009, from http://www.jointcommission.org/PatientSafety/DoNotUseList/

The Joint Commission. (2008). *Facts about the Official "do not use" list*. Retrieved September 25, 2009, from http://www.jointcommission.org/PatientSafety/DoNotUseList/facts_dnu.htm

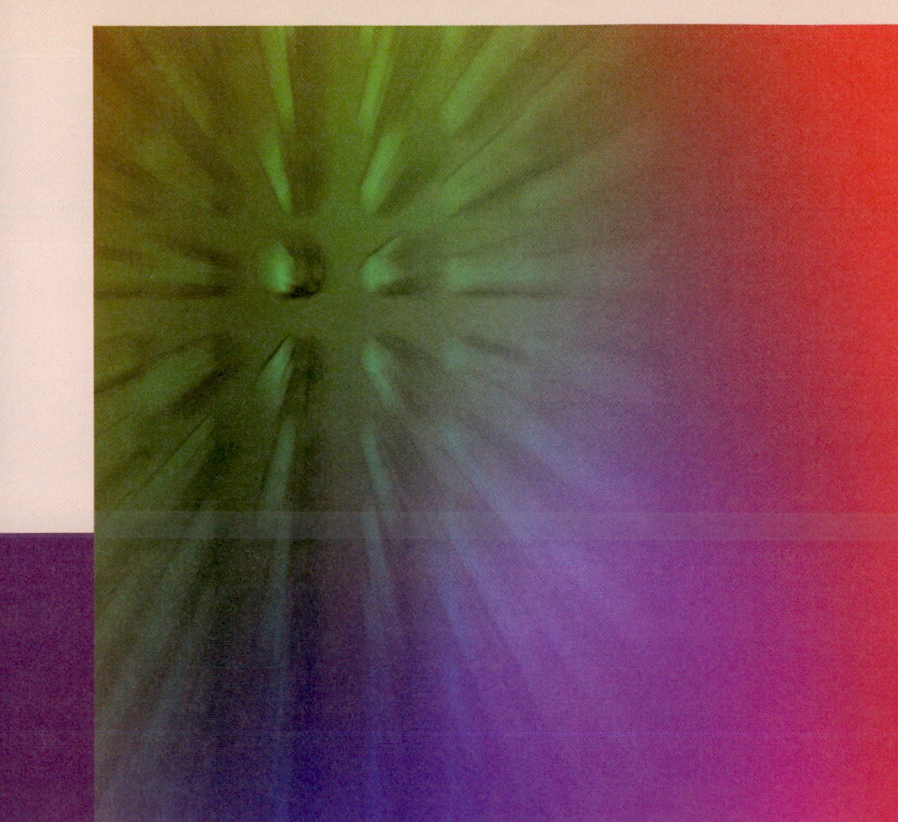
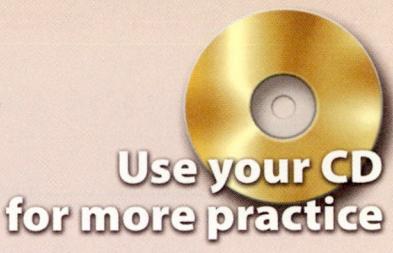

2

Ratios, Percents, Simple Equations, and Ratio-Proportion

OBJECTIVES

Upon mastery of Chapter 2, you will be able to perform basic mathematical computations that involve ratios, percents, simple equations, and proportions. Specifically, you will be able to:

- Interpret values expressed in ratios.
- Convert among fractions, decimals, ratios, and percents.
- Compare the size of fractions, decimals, ratios, and percents.
- Determine the value of X in simple equations.
- Set up proportions for solving problems.
- Cross-multiply to find the value of X in a proportion.
- Calculate the percentage of a quantity.

Health care professionals need to understand ratios and percents to be able to accurately interpret, prepare, and administer a variety of medications and treatments. Let's take a look at each of these important ways of expressing ratios and percents and how they are related to fractions and decimals. It is important for you to be able to convert equivalent ratios, percents, decimals, and fractions quickly and accurately.

RATIOS AND PERCENTS

Ratios

Like a fraction, a *ratio* is used to indicate the relationship of one part of a quantity to the whole. The two quantities are written as a fraction or separated by a colon (:). The use of the colon is a traditional way to write the division sign within a ratio.

EXAMPLE ■

On an evening shift, if there are 5 nurses and 35 patients, what is the ratio of nurses to patients? 5 nurses to 35 patients = 5 nurses per 35 patients = $\frac{5}{35} = \frac{1}{7}$. This is the same as a ratio of 5:35 or 1:7.

MATH TIP

The terms of a ratio are the numerator (always to the left of the colon) and the denominator (always to the right of the colon) of a fraction. Like fractions, ratios should be stated in lowest terms.

If you think back to the discussion of fractions and parts of a whole, it is easy to see that a ratio is actually the same as a fraction and its equivalent decimal. It is just a different way of expressing the same quantity. Recall from Chapter 1 that to convert a fraction to a decimal, you simply divide the numerator by the denominator.

EXAMPLE ■

Adrenalin 1:1,000 for injection = 1 part Adrenalin to 1,000 total parts of solution. It is a fact that 1:1,000 is the same as $\frac{1}{1,000}$.

In some drug solutions, such as Adrenalin 1:1,000, the ratio is used to indicate the drug's concentration. This will be covered in more detail later.

Percents

A type of ratio is a percent. *Percent* comes from the Latin phrase *per centum,* translated *per hundred.* This means per hundred parts or hundredth part.

MATH TIP

To remember the value of a given percent, replace the % symbol with "/" for *per* and "100" for *cent.* THINK: Percent (%) means *"/100"* or *"per hundred."*

EXAMPLE ■

$3\% = 3$ percent $= 3/100 = \frac{3}{100} = 0.03$

Converting among Ratios, Percents, Fractions, and Decimals

When you understand the relationship of ratios, percents, fractions, and decimals, you can readily convert from one to the other. Let's begin by converting a percent to a fraction.

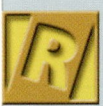

RULE

To convert a percent to a fraction:

1. Delete the % sign.

2. Write the remaining number as the numerator.

3. Write 100 as the denominator.

4. Reduce the result to lowest terms.

EXAMPLE ■

$5\% = \frac{5}{100} = \frac{1}{20}$

It is also easy to express a percent as a ratio.

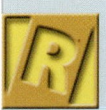

RULE

To convert a percent to a ratio:

1. Delete the % sign.

2. Write the remaining number as the numerator.

3. Write 100 as the denominator.

4. Reduce the result to lowest terms.

5. Express the fraction as a ratio.

EXAMPLE ■

$25\% = \frac{25}{100} = \frac{1}{4} = 1:4$

Because the denominator of a percent is always 100, it is easy to find the equivalent decimal. Recall that to divide by 100, you move the decimal point two places to the left, the number of places equal to the number of zeros in the denominator.

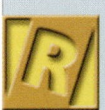

RULE

To convert a percent to a decimal:

1. Delete the % sign.

2. Divide the remaining number by 100, which is the same as moving the decimal point two places to the left.

EXAMPLE ■

$25\% = \frac{25}{100} = 25 \div 100 = .25. = 0.25$

Conversely, it is easy to change a decimal to a percent.

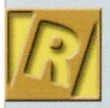

RULE

To convert a decimal to a percent:

1. Multiply the decimal number by 100, which is the same as moving the decimal point two places to the right.

2. Add the % sign.

EXAMPLE ▪

$0.25 \times 100 = 0.\underset{\smile}{25.} = 25\%$

MATH TIP

When converting a decimal to a percent, always move the decimal point two places so that the resulting percent is the larger number.

Now you know all the steps to change a ratio to the equivalent percent.

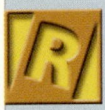

RULE

To convert a ratio to a percent:

1. Convert the ratio to a fraction.

2. Convert the fraction to a decimal.

3. Convert the decimal to a percent.

EXAMPLE ▪

Convert 1:1,000 Adrenalin solution to the equivalent concentration expressed as a percent.

1. $1:1,000 = \frac{1}{1,000}$ (ratio converted to fraction)

2. $\frac{1}{1,000} = .\underset{\smile}{001.} = 0.001$ (fraction converted to decimal)

3. $0.001 = 0.\underset{\smile}{00.}1 = 0.1\%$ (decimal converted to percent)

Thus, 1:1,000 Adrenalin solution = 0.1% Adrenalin solution.

Review the preceding example again slowly until it is clear. Ask your instructor for assistance as needed. If you go over this one step at a time, you can master these important calculations. You need never fear fractions, decimals, ratios, and percents again.

Comparing Percents and Ratios

Nurses and other health care professionals frequently administer solutions with the concentration expressed as a percent or ratio. Consider two intravenous (which means given directly into a person's vein) solutions: one that is 0.9%; the other 5%. It is important to be clear that 0.9% is *less* than 5%. A 0.9% solution means that there are 0.9 parts of the solid per 100 total parts (0.9 parts is less than one whole part, so it is less than 1%). Compare this to the 5% solution, with 5 parts of the solid (or more than five times 0.9 parts) per 100 total parts. Therefore, the 5% solution is much more concentrated, or stronger, than the 0.9% solution. A misunderstanding of these numbers and the quantities they represent can have dire consequences.

Likewise, you may see a solution concentration expressed as $\frac{1}{3}\%$ and another expressed as 0.45%. Convert these amounts to equivalent decimals to clarify values and compare concentrations.

EXAMPLES ▪

$\frac{1}{3}\% = \dfrac{\frac{1}{3}}{100} = \frac{1}{3} \div \frac{100}{1} = \frac{1}{3} \times \frac{1}{100} = \frac{1}{300} = 0.003\overline{3}$

$0.45\% = \frac{0.45}{100} = 0.0045$ (greater value, stronger concentration)

MATH TIP

In the last set of examples, the line over the last 3 in the decimal fraction $0.003\overline{3}$ indicates that the number 3 repeats itself indefinitely.

Compare solution concentrations expressed as a ratio, such as 1:1,000 and 1:100.

EXAMPLES ■

$1:1,000 = \dfrac{1}{1,000} = 0.001$

$1:100 = \dfrac{1}{100} = 0.01$ or 0.010 (add zero for comparison), 1:100 is a stronger concentration

QUICK REVIEW

■ Fractions, decimals, ratios, and percents are related equivalents.

Example: $1:2 = \dfrac{1}{2} = 0.5 = 50\%$

■ Like fractions, ratios should be reduced to lowest terms.

Example: 2:4 = 1:2

■ To express a ratio as a fraction, the number to the left of the colon becomes the numerator and the number to the right of the colon becomes the denominator. The colon in a ratio is equivalent to the division sign in a fraction.

Example: $2:3 = \dfrac{2}{3}$

■ To change a ratio to a decimal, convert the ratio to a fraction and divide the numerator by the denominator.

Example: $1:4 = \dfrac{1}{4} = 1 \div 4 = 0.25$

■ To change a percent to a fraction, drop the % sign and place the remaining number as the numerator over the denominator 100. Reduce the fraction to lowest terms. THINK: per (/) cent (100).

Example: $75\% = \dfrac{75}{100} = \dfrac{3}{4}$

■ To change a percent to a ratio, first convert the percent to a fraction in lowest terms. Then, place the numerator to the left of a colon and the denominator to the right of that colon.

Example: $35\% = \dfrac{35}{100} = \dfrac{7}{20} = 7:20$

■ To change a percent to a decimal, drop the % sign and divide by 100.

Example: 4% = .04. = 0.04

■ To change a decimal to a percent, multiply by 100, and add the % sign.

Example: 0.5 = 0.50. = 50%

■ To change a ratio to a percent, first convert the ratio to a fraction. Convert the resulting fraction to a decimal and then to a percent.

Example: $1:2 = \dfrac{1}{2} = 1 \div 2 = 0.5 = 0.50. = 50\%$

Review Set 7

Change the following ratios to fractions that are reduced to lowest terms.

1. 3:150 = _____   4. 4:7 = _____

2. 6:10 = _____   5. 6:8 = _____

3. 0.05:0.15 = _____

Change the following ratios to decimals; round to two decimal places, if needed.

6. $20:40 =$ _____   9. $0.3:4.5 =$ _____

7. $\frac{1}{1,000}:\frac{1}{150} =$ _____   10. $1\frac{1}{2}:6\frac{2}{9} =$ _____

8. $0.12:0.88 =$ _____

Change the following ratios to percents; round to two decimal places, if needed.

11. $12:48 =$ _____   14. $7:10 =$ _____

12. $2:5 =$ _____   15. $50:100 =$ _____

13. $0.08:0.64 =$ _____

Change the following percents to fractions that are reduced to lowest terms.

16. $45\% =$ _____   19. $1\% =$ _____

17. $60\% =$ _____   20. $66\frac{2}{3}\% =$ _____

18. $0.5\% =$ _____

Change the following percents to decimals; round to two decimal places, if needed.

21. $2.94\% =$ _____   24. $33\% =$ _____

22. $4.5\% =$ _____   25. $0.9\% =$ _____

23. $6.32\% =$ _____

Change the following percents to ratios that are reduced to lowest terms.

26. $16\% =$ _____   29. $45\% =$ _____

27. $25\% =$ _____   30. $6\% =$ _____

28. $50\% =$ _____

Which of the following is largest? Circle your answer.

31. 0.9% 0.9 $1:9$ $\frac{1}{90}$ 34. $\frac{1}{150}$ $\frac{1}{300}$ 0.5 $\frac{2}{3}\%$

32. 0.05 $\frac{1}{5}$ 0.025 $1:25$ 35. $1:1,000$ 0.0001 $\frac{1}{100}$ 0.1%

33. 0.0125% 0.25% 0.1% 0.02%

After completing these problems, see pages 504–505 to check your answers.

SOLVING SIMPLE EQUATIONS FOR X

You can set up and solve dosage calculations in different ways. One way is to use a simple equation form. The following examples demonstrate the various forms of this equation. Learn to express your answers in decimal form because decimals will be used most often in dosage calculations and administration. Round decimals to hundredths or to two places. For most dosage calculations you will round to no more than two decimal places.

MATH TIP

The unknown quantity is represented by X.

EXAMPLE 1 ■

$\frac{100}{200} \times 1 = X$

MATH TIP
You can drop the 1 because a number multiplied by 1 is the same number.

$$\frac{100}{200} \times 1 = X \text{ is the same as } \frac{100}{200} = X.$$

1. Reduce to lowest terms: $\frac{100}{200} = \frac{\overset{1}{\cancel{100}}}{\underset{2}{\cancel{200}}} = \frac{1}{2} = X$

2. Convert to decimal form: $\frac{1}{2} = 0.5 = X$

3. You have your answer. $X = 0.5$

EXAMPLE 2 ■

$$\frac{3}{5} \times 2 = X$$

MATH TIP
Dividing a number by 1 does not change its value.

1. Convert: Express 2 as a fraction: $\frac{3}{5} \times \frac{2}{1} = X$

2. Multiply fractions: $\frac{3}{5} \times \frac{2}{1} = \frac{6}{5} = X$

3. Convert to a mixed number: $\frac{6}{5} = 1\frac{1}{5} = X$

4. Convert to decimal form: $1\frac{1}{5} = 1.2 = X$

5. You have your answer. $X = 1.2$

EXAMPLE 3 ■

$$\frac{\frac{1}{6}}{\frac{1}{4}} \times 5 = X$$

1. Convert: Express 5 as a fraction: $\frac{\frac{1}{6}}{\frac{1}{4}} \times \frac{5}{1} = X$

2. Divide fractions: $\frac{1}{6} \div \frac{1}{4} \times \frac{5}{1} = X$

3. Invert the divisor, and multiply: $\frac{1}{6} \times \frac{4}{1} \times \frac{5}{1} = X$

4. Cancel terms: $\frac{1}{\underset{3}{\cancel{6}}} \times \frac{\overset{2}{\cancel{4}}}{1} \times \frac{5}{1} = \frac{1}{3} \times \frac{2}{1} \times \frac{5}{1} = \frac{10}{3} = X$

5. Convert to a mixed number: $\frac{10}{3} = 3\frac{1}{3} = X$

6. Convert to decimal form: $3\frac{1}{3} = 3.33\overline{3} = X$

7. Round to hundredths place: $3.33\overline{3} = 3.33 = X$

8. It is easy, when you take it one step at a time. $X = 3.33$

EXAMPLE 4 ▪

$$\frac{\frac{1}{10}}{\frac{1}{15}} \times 2.2 = X$$

1. Convert: Express 2.2 in fraction form: $\dfrac{\frac{1}{10}}{\frac{1}{15}} \times \dfrac{2.2}{1} = X$

2. Divide fractions: $\dfrac{1}{10} \div \dfrac{1}{15} \times \dfrac{2.2}{1} = X$

3. Invert the divisor, and multiply: $\dfrac{1}{10} \times \dfrac{15}{1} \times \dfrac{2.2}{1} = X$

4. Cancel terms: $\dfrac{1}{\cancel{10}_2} \times \dfrac{\cancel{15}^3}{1} \times \dfrac{2.2}{1} = \dfrac{1}{\cancel{2}_1} \times \dfrac{3}{1} \times \dfrac{\cancel{2.2}^{1.1}}{1} = \dfrac{1}{1} \times \dfrac{3}{1} \times \dfrac{1.1}{1} = X$

5. Multiply: $\dfrac{1}{1} \times \dfrac{3}{1} \times \dfrac{1.1}{1} = \dfrac{3.3}{1} = 3.3 = X$

6. That's it! X = 3.3

EXAMPLE 5 ▪

$$\frac{0.125}{0.25} \times 1.5 = X$$

1. Convert: Express 1.5 in fraction form: $\dfrac{0.125}{0.25} \times \dfrac{1.5}{1} = X$

2. Convert: Add a zero to thousandths place for 0.25 for easier comparison: $\dfrac{0.125}{0.250} \times \dfrac{1.5}{1} = X$

3. Cancel terms: $\dfrac{\cancel{0.125}^1}{\cancel{0.250}_2} \times \dfrac{1.5}{1} = \dfrac{1}{2} \times \dfrac{1.5}{1} = X$

4. Multiply: $\dfrac{1}{2} \times \dfrac{1.5}{1} = \dfrac{1.5}{2} = X$

5. Divide: $\dfrac{1.5}{2} = 0.75 = X$

6. You've got it! X = 0.75

MATH TIP

It may be easier to work with whole numbers than decimals. If you had difficulty with Step 3, try multiplying the numerator and denominator by 1,000 to eliminate the decimal fractions.

$$\frac{0.125}{0.250} \times \frac{1,000}{1,000} = \frac{125}{250} = \frac{1}{2}$$

Example 5 can also be solved by computing with fractions instead of decimals.

Try this: $\dfrac{0.125}{0.25} \times 1.5 = X$

1. Convert: Express 1.5 in fraction form: $\dfrac{0.125}{0.25} \times \dfrac{1.5}{1} = X$

2. Convert: Add zeros for easier comparison, making *both* decimals of equal length:

$$\frac{0.125}{0.250} \times \frac{1.5}{1.0} = X$$

3. Cancel terms: $\dfrac{\overset{1}{\cancel{0.125}}}{\underset{2}{\cancel{0.250}}} \times \dfrac{\overset{3}{\cancel{1.5}}}{\underset{2}{\cancel{1.0}}} = \dfrac{1}{2} \times \dfrac{3}{2} = X$ (It is easier to work with whole numbers.)

4. Multiply: $\dfrac{1}{2} \times \dfrac{3}{2} = \dfrac{3}{4} = X$

5. Convert: $\dfrac{3}{4} = 0.75 = X$

6. You've got it again! $X = 0.75$

Which way do you find easier?

EXAMPLE 6 ■

$\dfrac{3}{4} \times 45\% = X$

1. Convert: Express 45% as a fraction reduced to lowest terms: $45\% = \dfrac{45}{100} = \dfrac{9}{20}$

2. Multiply fractions: $\dfrac{3}{4} \times \dfrac{9}{20} = X$

   $\dfrac{27}{80} = X$

3. Divide: $\dfrac{27}{80} = 0.337 = X$

4. Round to hundredths place: $0.34 = X$

5. You have your answer. $X = 0.34$

QUICK REVIEW

■ To solve simple equations, perform the mathematical operations indicated to find the value of the unknown X.

■ Express the result (value of X) in decimal form.

Review Set 8

Solve the following problems for X. Express answers as decimals rounded to two places.

1. $\dfrac{75}{125} \times 5 = X$ _____

8. $\dfrac{1{,}200{,}000}{400{,}000} \times 4.2 = X$ _____

2. $\dfrac{\frac{3}{4}}{\frac{1}{2}} \times 2.2 = X$ _____

9. $\dfrac{\frac{2}{3}}{\frac{1}{6}} \times 10 = X$ _____

3. $\dfrac{150}{300} \times 2.5 = X$ _____

10. $\dfrac{30}{50} \times 0.8 = X$ _____

4. $\dfrac{40\%}{60\%} \times 8 = X$ _____

11. $\dfrac{200{,}000}{300{,}000} \times 1.5 = X$ _____

5. $\dfrac{0.35}{2.5} \times 4 = X$ _____

12. $\dfrac{0.08}{0.1} \times 1.2 = X$ _____

6. $\dfrac{0.15}{0.1} \times 1.2 = X$ _____

13. $\dfrac{7.5}{5} \times 3 = X$ _____

7. $\dfrac{0.4}{2.5} \times 4 = X$ _____

14. $\dfrac{250{,}000}{2{,}000{,}000} \times 7.5 = X$ _____

15. $\dfrac{600}{150} \times 2.5 = X$ _____

16. $\dfrac{600,000}{750,000} \times 0.5 = X$ _____

17. $\dfrac{75\%}{60\%} \times 1.2 = X$ _____

18. $\dfrac{0.25}{0.125} \times 5 = X$ _____

19. $\dfrac{1,000,000}{250,000} \times 5 = X$ _____

20. $\dfrac{\frac{1}{100}}{\frac{1}{150}} \times 1.2 = X$ _____

After completing these problems, see page 505 to check your answers.

RATIO-PROPORTION: CROSS-MULTIPLYING TO SOLVE FOR X

A *proportion* is two ratios that are equal or an equation between two equal ratios.

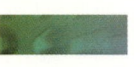

MATH TIP

A proportion is written as two ratios separated by an equal sign, such as 5:10 = 10:20. The two ratios in a proportion may also be separated by a double colon sign, such as 5:10::10:20.

Some of the calculations you will perform will have the unknown X as a different term in the equation. To determine the value of the unknown X, you must apply the rule for cross-multiplying used in a proportion.

RULE

In a proportion, the product of the means (the two inside numbers) equals the product of the extremes (the two outside numbers). Finding the product of the means and the extremes is called cross-multiplying.

EXAMPLE ■

Extremes

5:10 = 10:20

Means

$5 \times 20 = 10 \times 10$

$100 = 100$

Because ratios are the same as fractions, the same proportion can be expressed like this: $\dfrac{5}{10} = \dfrac{10}{20}$. The fractions are *equivalent,* or equal. The numerator of the first fraction and the denominator of the second fraction are the extremes, and the denominator of the first fraction and the numerator of the second fraction are the means.

EXAMPLE ■

Extreme 5 ⟍ 10 Mean
Mean   10 ⟋ 20 Extreme

Cross-multiply to find the equal products of the means and extremes.

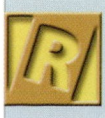

RULE

If two fractions are equivalent, or equal, their cross-products are also equal.

EXAMPLE ■

$$\frac{5}{10} \begin{array}{c} \diagdown \diagup \\ \diagup \diagdown \end{array} \frac{10}{20}$$

$5 \times 20 = 10 \times 10$

$100 = 100$

When one of the quantities in a proportion is unknown, a letter, such as X, may be substituted for this unknown quantity. You would solve the equation to find the value of X. In addition to cross-multiplying, there is one more rule you need to know to solve for X in a proportion.

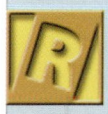

RULE

Dividing or multiplying each side (member) of an equation by the same nonzero number produces an equivalent equation.

MATH TIP

Dividing each side of an equation by the same nonzero number is the same as reducing or simplifying the equation. Multiplying each side by the same nonzero number enlarges the equation.

Let's examine how to simplify an equation.

EXAMPLE ■

$25X = 100$ (25X means $25 \times X$)

Simplify the equation to find X. Divide both sides by 25, the number before X. Reduce to lowest terms.

$$\frac{\overset{1}{\cancel{25}}X}{\underset{1}{\cancel{25}}} = \frac{\overset{4}{\cancel{100}}}{\underset{1}{\cancel{25}}}$$

$\frac{1X}{1} = \frac{4}{1}$ (Dividing or multiplying a number by 1 does not change its value. 1X is understood to be simply X.)

$X = 4$

Replace X with 4 in the same equation, and you can prove that the calculations are correct.

$25 \times \mathbf{4} = 100$

Now you are ready to apply the concepts of cross-multiplying and simplifying an equation to solve for X in a proportion.

EXAMPLE 1 ■

$$\frac{90}{2} = \frac{45}{X}$$

You have a proportion with an unknown quantity X in the denominator of the second fraction. Find the value of X.

1. Cross-multiply: $\frac{90}{2}\times\frac{45}{X}$

2. Multiply terms: $90 \times X = 2 \times 45$

    $90X = 90$ (90X means $90 \times X$)

3. Simplify the equation: Divide both sides of the equation by the number before the unknown X. You are equally reducing the terms on both sides of the equation.

    $$\frac{\overset{1}{\cancel{90}}X}{\underset{1}{\cancel{90}}} = \frac{\overset{1}{\cancel{90}}}{\underset{1}{\cancel{90}}}$$

    $X = 1$

Try another one. You will use a proportion to solve this equation.

EXAMPLE 2 ■

$$\frac{80}{X} \times 60 = 20$$

1. Convert: Express 60 as a fraction.

    $$\frac{80}{X} \times \frac{60}{1} = 20$$

2. Multiply fractions: $\frac{80}{X} \times \frac{60}{1} = 20$

    $$\frac{4,800}{X} = 20$$

3. Convert: Express 20 as a fraction.

    $$\frac{4,800}{X} = \frac{20}{1}$$

    You now have a proportion.

4. Cross-multiply: $\frac{4,800}{X}\times\frac{20}{1}$

    $20X = 4,800$

5. Simplify: Divide both sides of the equation by the number before the unknown X.

    $$\frac{\overset{1}{\cancel{20}}X}{\underset{1}{\cancel{20}}} = \frac{\overset{240}{\cancel{4,800}}}{\underset{1}{\cancel{20}}}$$

    $X = 240$

EXAMPLE 3 ■

$$\frac{X}{160} = \frac{2.5}{80}$$

1. Cross-multiply: $\frac{X}{160}\times\frac{2.5}{80}$

    $80 \times X = 2.5 \times 160$

    $80X = 400$

2. Simplify: $\dfrac{\cancel{80}^{1}X}{\cancel{80}_{1}} = \dfrac{\cancel{400}^{5}}{\cancel{80}_{1}}$

$$X = 5$$

EXAMPLE 4 ■

$$\frac{40}{100} = \frac{X}{2}$$

1. Cross-multiply: $\dfrac{40}{100} \diagdown\!\!\!\!\diagup \dfrac{X}{2}$

2. Multiply terms: $100 \times X = 40 \times 2$

$$100X = 80$$

3. Simplify the equation: $\dfrac{\cancel{100}^{1}X}{\cancel{100}_{1}} = \dfrac{80}{100}$

$$X = 0.8$$

Calculations that result in an amount less than 1 should be expressed as a decimal. Most medications are ordered and supplied in metric measure. Metric measure is a decimal-based system.

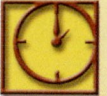

QUICK REVIEW

■ A *proportion* is an equation of two equal ratios. The ratios may be expressed as fractions.

■ Example: 1:4 = X:8 or $\dfrac{1}{4} = \dfrac{X}{8}$

■ In a proportion, the product of the means equals the product of the extremes.

Extremes

■ Example: 1:4 = X:8   Therefore, $4 \times X = 1 \times 8$

Means

■ If two fractions are equal, their cross-products are equal. This operation is referred to as cross-multiplying.

■ Example: $\dfrac{1}{4} \diagdown\!\!\!\!\diagup \dfrac{X}{8}$ Therefore, $4 \times X = 1 \times 8$ or $4X = 8$

■ Dividing each side of an equation by the same number produces an equivalent equation. This operation is referred to as *simplifying the equation*.

■ Example: If $4X = 8$, then $\dfrac{4X}{4} = \dfrac{8}{4}$, and $X = 2$

Review Set 9

Find the value of X. Express answers as decimals rounded to two places.

1. $\dfrac{1,000}{2} = \dfrac{125}{X}$ _____

2. $\dfrac{500}{2} = \dfrac{250}{X}$ _____

3. $\dfrac{500}{1} = \dfrac{280}{X}$ _____

4. $\dfrac{0.5}{2} = \dfrac{250}{X}$ _____

5. $\dfrac{75}{1.5} = \dfrac{35}{X}$ _____

6. $\dfrac{40}{X} \times 12 = 60$ _____

7. $\dfrac{10}{X} \times 60 = 28$ _____

8. $\dfrac{2}{2,000} \times X = 0.5$ _____

9. $\frac{15}{500} \times X = 6$ _____

10. $\frac{5}{X} = \frac{10}{21}$ _____

11. $\frac{250}{1} = \frac{750}{X}$ _____

12. $\frac{80}{5} = \frac{10}{X}$ _____

13. $\frac{5}{20} = \frac{X}{40}$ _____

14. $\frac{\frac{1}{100}}{1} = \frac{\frac{1}{150}}{X}$ _____

15. $\frac{2.2}{X} = \frac{8.8}{5}$ _____

16. $\frac{60}{15} = \frac{125}{X}$ _____

17. $\frac{60}{10} = \frac{100}{X}$ _____

18. $\frac{80}{X} \times 60 = 20$ _____

19. $\frac{X}{0.5} = \frac{6}{4}$ _____

20. $\frac{5}{2.2} = \frac{X}{1}$ _____

21. $\frac{\frac{1}{4}}{15} = \frac{X}{60}$ _____

22. $\frac{25\%}{30\%} = \frac{5}{X}$ _____

23. In any group of 100 nurses, you would expect to find 45 nurses who will specialize in a particular field of nursing. In a class of 240 graduating nurses, how many would you expect to specialize? _____

24. Low-fat cheese has 48 calories per ounce. A client who is having his caloric intake measured has eaten $1\frac{1}{2}$ ounces of low-fat cheese. How many calories has he eaten? _____

25. If a patient receives 450 milligrams of a medication given evenly over 5.5 hours, how many milligrams did the patient receive per hour? _____

After completing these problems, see page 506 to check your answers.

FINDING THE PERCENTAGE OF A QUANTITY

An important computation that health care professionals use for dosage calculations is to find a given percentage or part of a quantity. *Percentage* is a term that describes a *part* of a whole quantity. A *known percent* determines the part in question. Said another way, the percentage (or part in question) is equal to some known percent multiplied by the whole quantity.

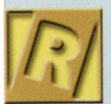

RULE

Percentage (Part) = Percent × Whole Quantity
To find a percentage or part of a whole quantity:

1. Change the percent to a decimal.

2. Multiply the decimal by the whole quantity.

EXAMPLE ■

A patient reports that he drank 75% of his 8 fluid ounce cup of coffee for breakfast. To record the amount he actually drank in his chart, you must determine what amount is 75% of 8 fluid ounces.

MATH TIP

In a mathematical expression, the word *"of"* means *"times"* and indicates that you should multiply.

To continue with the example:

Percentage (Part) = Percent × Whole Quantity

Let X represent the unknown.

1. Change 75% to a decimal: $75\% = \frac{75}{100} = .75. = 0.75$

2. Multiply 0.75 × 8 fluid ounces: X = 0.75 × 8 fluid ounces = 6 fluid ounces

Therefore, 75% of 8 fluid ounces is 6 fluid ounces.

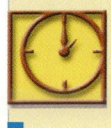

QUICK REVIEW

■ Percentage (Part) = Percent × Whole Quantity

Example What is 12% of 48? X = 12% × 48 = 0.12 × 48 = 5.76

Review Set 10

Perform the indicated operation; round decimals to hundredths place.

1. What is 0.25% of 520? _____
2. What is 5% of 95? _____
3. What is 40% of 140? _____
4. What is 0.7% of 62? _____
5. What is 3% of 889? _____

6. What is 20% of 75? _____
7. What is 4% of 20? _____
8. What is 7% of 34? _____
9. What is 15% of 250? _____
10. What is 75% of 150? _____

11. A patient has an order for an anti-infective in the amount of 500 milligrams by mouth twice a day for 10 days to treat pneumonia. He received a bottle of 20 pills. How many pills has this patient taken if he has used 40% of the 20 pills? _____

12. The patient is on oral fluid restrictions of 1,200 milliliters for a 24-hour period. For breakfast and lunch he has consumed 60% of the total fluid allowance. How many milliliters has he had? _____

13. A patient's hospital bill for surgery is $17,651.07. Her insurance company pays 80%. How much will the patient owe? _____

14. Table salt (sodium chloride) is 40% sodium by weight. If a box of salt weighs 18 ounces, how much sodium is in the box of salt? _____

15. A patient has an average daily intake of 3,500 calories. At breakfast she eats 20% of the total daily caloric allowance. How many calories did she ingest? _____

After completing these problems, see page 506 to check your answers.

PRACTICE PROBLEMS—CHAPTER 2

Find the equivalent decimal, fraction, percent, and ratio forms. Reduce fractions and ratios to lowest terms; round decimals to hundredths and percents to the nearest whole number.

Decimal	Fraction	Percent	Ratio
1. _____	$\frac{2}{5}$	_____	_____
2. 0.05	_____	_____	_____
3. _____	_____	17%	_____
4. _____	_____	_____	1:4
5. _____	_____	6%	_____
6. _____	$\frac{1}{6}$	_____	_____
7. _____	_____	50%	_____
8. _____	_____	_____	1:100
9. 0.09	_____	_____	_____
10. _____	$\frac{3}{8}$	_____	_____
11. _____	_____	_____	2:3
12. _____	$\frac{1}{3}$	_____	_____
13. 0.52	_____	_____	_____
14. _____	_____	_____	9:20
15. _____	$\frac{6}{7}$	_____	_____
16. _____	_____	_____	3:10
17. _____	$\frac{1}{50}$	_____	_____
18. 0.6	_____	_____	_____
19. 0.04	_____	_____	_____
20. _____	_____	10%	_____

Convert as indicated.

21. 1:25 to a decimal _____   24. 17:34 to a fraction _____

22. $\frac{10}{400}$ to a ratio _____   25. 75% to a ratio _____

23. 0.075 to a percent _____

Perform the indicated operation. Round decimals to hundredths.

26. What is 35% of 750? _____   28. What is 8.2% of 24? _____

27. What is 7% of 52? _____

Identify the strongest solution in each of the following groups:

29. 1:40   1:400   1:4   _____

30. 1:10   1:200   1:50   _____

Find the value of X in the following equations. Express your answers as decimals rounded to the nearest hundredth.

31. $\frac{20}{400} = \frac{X}{1,680} =$ _____   36. $\frac{3}{9} = \frac{X}{117}$ _____

32. $\frac{75}{X} = \frac{\frac{1}{300}}{4}$ _____   37. $\frac{\frac{1}{8}}{\frac{1}{3}} \times 2 = X$ _____

33. $\frac{X}{5} = \frac{3}{15}$ _____   38. $\frac{X}{7} = \frac{12}{4}$ _____

34. $\frac{500}{250} = \frac{2.2}{X}$ _____   39. $\frac{X}{8} = \frac{9}{0.6}$ _____

35. $\frac{0.6}{1.2} = \frac{X}{200}$ _____   40. $\frac{0.4}{0.1} \times 22.5 = X$ _____

41. A portion of meat totaling 125 grams contains 20% protein and 5% fat. How many grams each of protein and fat does the meat contain? _____ protein _____ fat

42. The total points for a course in a nursing program is 308. A nursing student needs to achieve 75% of the total points to pass the semester. How many points are required to pass? _____

43. To work off 90 calories, Angie must walk for 27 minutes. How many minutes would she need to walk to work off 200 calories? _____

44. The doctor orders a record of the patient's fluid intake and output. The patient drinks 25% of a bowl of broth. How many milliliters of intake will be recorded if the bowl holds 200 milliliters? _____

45. The recommended daily allowance (RDA) of a particular vitamin is 60 milligrams. If a multivitamin tablet claims to provide 45% of the RDA, how many milligrams of the particular vitamin would a patient receive from the multivitamin tablet? _____

46. A label on a dinner roll wrapper reads, "2.7 grams of fiber per $\frac{3}{4}$ ounce serving." If you eat $1\frac{1}{2}$ ounces of dinner rolls, how many grams of fiber will you consume? _____

47. A patient received an intravenous medication at a rate of 6.75 milligrams per minute. After 42 minutes, how much medication had she received? _____

48. A person weighed 130 pounds at his last doctor's office visit. At this visit the patient has lost 5% of his weight. How many pounds has the patient lost? _____

49. The cost of a certain medication is expected to decrease by 17% next year. If the cost is $12.56 now, how much would you expect it to cost at this time next year? _____

50. A patient is to be started on 150 milligrams of a medication and then decreased by 10% of the original dose for each dose until he is receiving 75 milligrams. When he takes his 75 milligram dose, how many total doses will he have taken? HINT: Be sure to count his first (150 milligrams) and last (75 milligrams) doses. _____

After completing these problems, see pages 506–507 to check your answers.

SECTION 1 SELF-EVALUATION

Directions

1. Round decimals to two places, as needed.

2. Express fractions in lowest terms.

Section 1 Mathematics Review for Dosage Calculations

Multiply or divide by the power of 10 indicated. Draw an arrow to demonstrate movement of the decimal point.

1. $30.5 \div 10 =$ _____   3. $63 \div 100 =$ _____

2. $40.025 \times 100 =$ _____   4. $72.327 \times 10 =$ _____

Identify the least common denominator for the following sets of numbers.

5. $\dfrac{1}{6}, \dfrac{2}{3}, \dfrac{3}{4}$ _____   6. $\dfrac{2}{5}, \dfrac{3}{10}, \dfrac{3}{11}$ _____

Complete the operations indicated.

7. $\dfrac{1}{4} + \dfrac{2}{3} =$ _____   13. $80.3 - 21.06 =$ _____

8. $\dfrac{6}{7} - \dfrac{1}{9} =$ _____   14. $0.3 \times 0.3 =$ _____

9. $1\dfrac{3}{5} \times \dfrac{5}{8} =$ _____   15. $1.5 \div 0.125 =$ _____

10. $\dfrac{3}{8} \div \dfrac{3}{4} =$ _____   16. $\dfrac{1}{150} \div \dfrac{1}{100} =$ _____

11. $13.2 + 32.55 + 0.029 =$ _____   17. $\dfrac{\frac{1}{120}}{\frac{1}{60}} =$ _____

12. 20% of $0.09 =$ _____   18. $\dfrac{16\%}{\frac{1}{4}} =$ _____

Arrange in order from smallest to largest.

19. $\dfrac{1}{3}\quad \dfrac{1}{2}\quad \dfrac{1}{6}\quad \dfrac{1}{10}\quad \dfrac{1}{5}$ _____

20. $\dfrac{3}{4}\quad \dfrac{7}{8}\quad \dfrac{5}{6}\quad \dfrac{2}{3}\quad \dfrac{9}{10}$ _____

21. $0.25\quad 0.125\quad 0.3\quad 0.009\quad 0.1909$ _____

22. $0.9\%\quad \dfrac{1}{2}\%\quad 50\%\quad 500\%\quad 100\%$ _____

23. Identify the strongest solution of the following: 1:3, 1:60, 1:6. _____

24. Identify the weakest solution of the following: 1:75, 1:600, 1:60. _____

Convert as indicated.

25. 1:100 to a decimal _____   27. 0.009 to a percent _____

26. $\dfrac{6}{150}$ to a decimal _____   28. $33\dfrac{1}{3}\%$ to a fraction _____

29. $\frac{5}{9}$ to a ratio   _____

30. 0.05 to a fraction   _____

31. $\frac{1}{2}\%$ to a ratio   _____

32. 2:3 to a fraction   _____

33. 3:4 to a percent   _____

34. $\frac{2}{5}$ to a percent   _____

35. $\frac{1}{6}$ to a decimal   _____

Find the value of X in the following equations. Express your answers as decimals; round to the nearest hundredth.

36. $\frac{0.35}{1.3} \times 4.5 = X$ _____

37. $\frac{0.3}{2.6} = \frac{0.15}{X}$ _____

38. $\frac{1,500,000}{500,000} \times X = 7.5$ _____

39. $\frac{\frac{1}{6}}{\frac{1}{4}} \times 1 = X$ _____

40. $\frac{1:100}{1:4} \times 2,500 = X$ _____

41. $\frac{0.25}{0.125} \times 2 = X$ _____

42. $\frac{10\%}{\frac{1}{2}\%} \times 1,000 = X$ _____

43. $\frac{\frac{1}{100}}{\frac{1}{150}} \times 2.2 = X$ _____

44. X:15 = 150:7.5   _____

45. $\frac{1,000,000}{600,000} \times 5 = X$ _____

46. In a drug study, it was determined that 4% of the participants developed the headache side effect. If there were 600 participants in the study, how many developed headaches?   _____

47. You are employed in a health care clinic where each employee must work 25% of 8 major holidays. How many holidays will you expect to work?   _____

48. If the cost of 1 roll of gauze is $0.69, what is the cost of $3\frac{1}{2}$ rolls?   _____

49. To prepare a nutritional formula from frozen concentrate, you mix 3 cans of water to every 1 can of concentrate. How many cans of water will you need to prepare formula from 4 cans of concentrate?   _____

50. If 1 centimeter equals $\frac{3}{8}$ inch, how many centimeters is a laceration that measures 3 inches?   _____

After completing these problems, see pages 507–508 to check your answers. Give yourself 2 points for each correct answer.

Perfect score = 100   My score = _____

Minimum mastery score = 86 (43 correct)

For more practice, go back to the beginning of this section and repeat the Mathematics Diagnostic Evaluation.

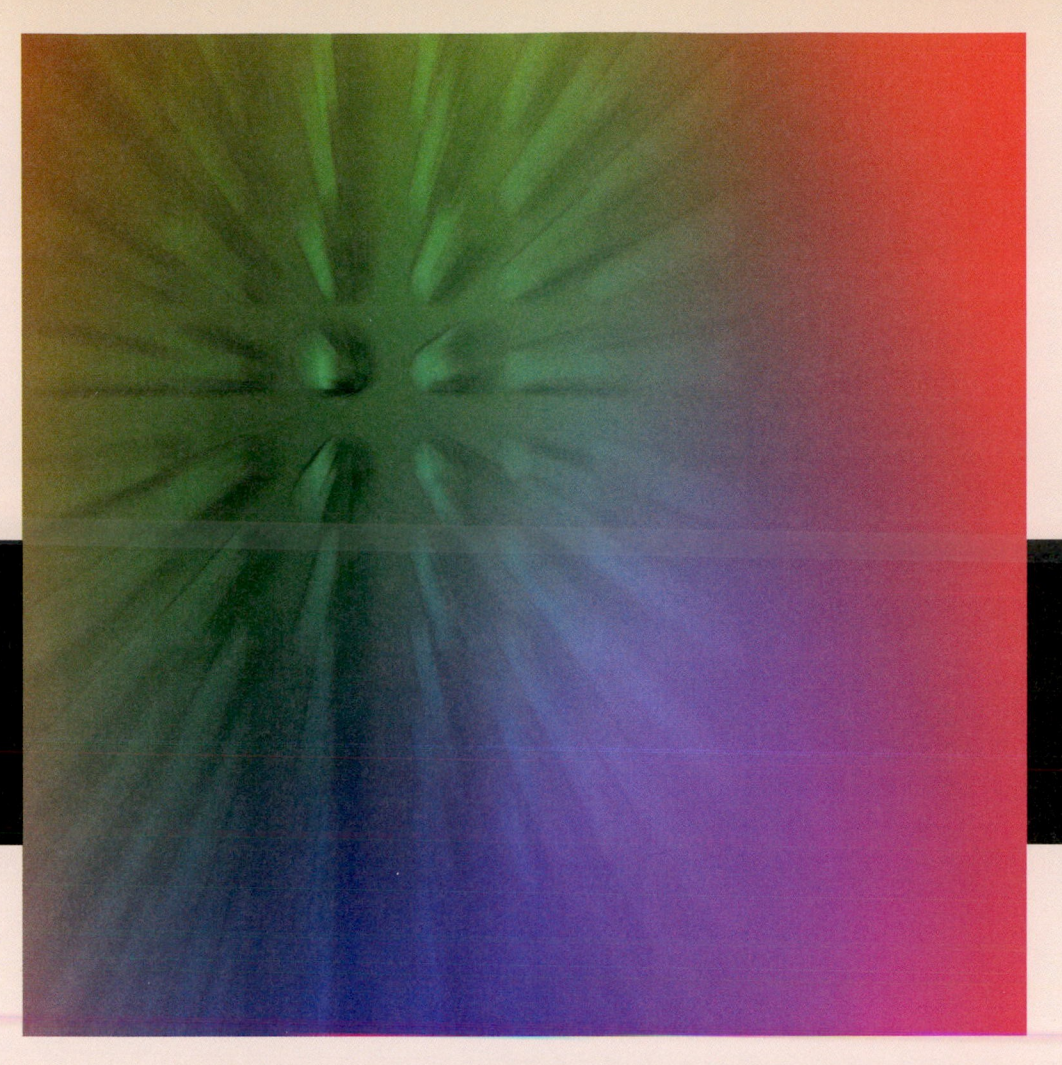

Measurement Systems, Drug Orders, and Drug Labels

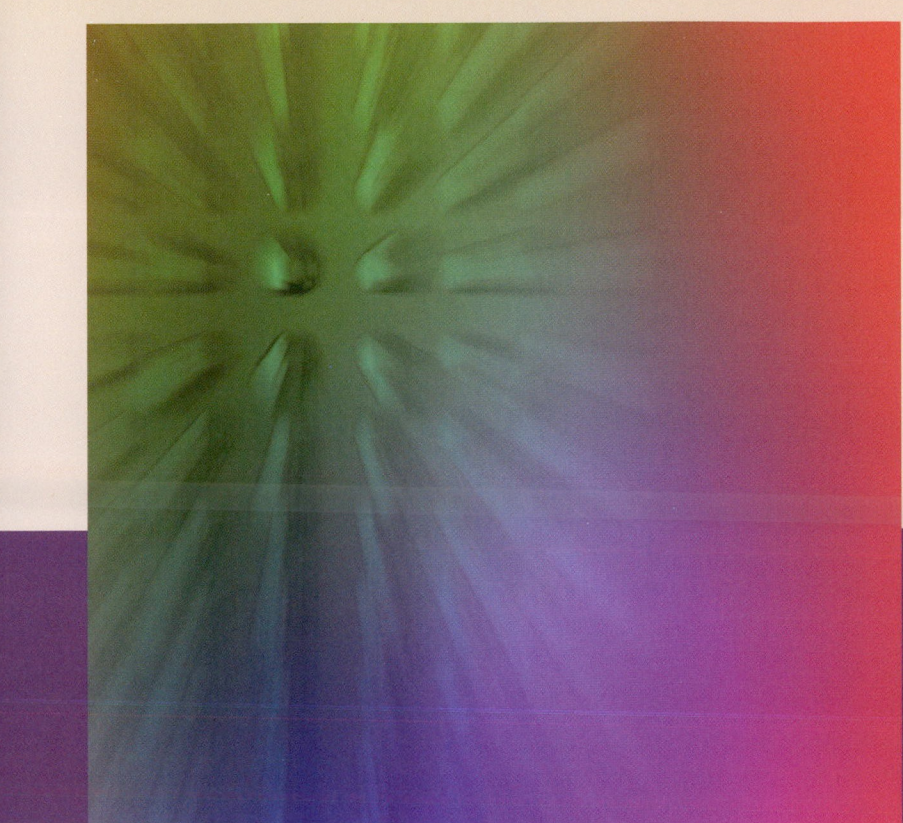

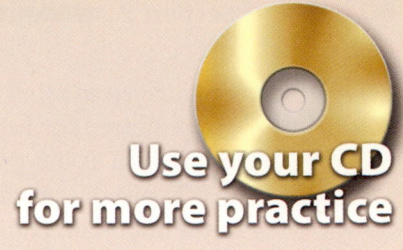
Use your CD
for more practice

3

Systems of Measurement

OBJECTIVES

Upon mastery of Chapter 3, you will be able to recognize and express the basic systems of measurement used to calculate dosages. To accomplish this you will also be able to:

- Interpret and properly express metric, apothecary, and household notation.
- Recall metric, apothecary, and household equivalents.
- Explain the use of milliequivalent (mEq), international unit, unit, and milliunit in dosage calculation.

To administer the correct amount of the prescribed medication to the patient, you must have a thorough knowledge of the weights and measures used in the prescription and administration of medications. The three systems used by health professionals are the *metric,* the *apothecary,* and the *household* systems.

It is necessary for you to understand each system and how to convert from one system to another. All prescriptions should be written with the metric system, and all U.S. drug labels provide metric measurements. The household system uses measurements found in familiar containers such as *teaspoons, cups,* and *quarts.* It is helpful to understand the relationship between metric and household systems for home health care situations and discharge instructions. You may occasionally see prescriptions and medical notation using the apothecary system, usually written by physicians trained in this system. Until the metric system completely replaces the apothecary and household systems, health care professionals should be familiar with each system.

Three essential parameters of measurement are associated with the prescription and administration of drugs within each system of measurement: weight, volume, and length. *Weight* is the most utilized parameter. It is important as a dosage unit. Most drugs are ordered and supplied by the weight of the drug. Keep in mind that the metric weight units, such as *gram* and *milligram*, are the most accurate and are preferred for health care applications. Occasionally you will also use the apothecary unit of weight referred to as the *grain*.

Think of capacity, or how much a container holds, as you contemplate *volume*, which is the next most important parameter. Volume usually refers to liquids. Volume also adds two additional parameters to dosage calculations: *quantity* and *concentration*. The *milliliter* is the most common metric volume unit for dosage calculations. Much less frequently you will use household and apothecary measures, such as *teaspoon* and *ounce*.

Length is the least utilized parameter for dosage calculations, but linear measurement is still essential to learn for health care situations. A person's height, the circumference of an infant's head, body surface area, and the size of lacerations and tumors are examples of important length measurements. You are probably familiar with the household measurements of *inches* and *feet*. Typically in the health care setting, length is measured in *millimeters* and *centimeters*.

THE METRIC SYSTEM

The metric system was first adopted in 1799 in France. It is the most widely used system of measurement in the world today and is preferred for prescribing and administering medications.

The metric system is a decimal system, which means it is based on powers of 10. The base units (the primary units of measurement) of the metric system are *gram* for weight, *liter* for volume, and *meter* for length. In this system, prefixes are used to show which portion of the base unit is being considered. It is important that you learn the most commonly used prefixes.

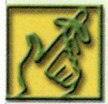

REMEMBER

Metric Prefixes

micro	=	one millionth or 0.000001 or $\frac{1}{1,000,000}$ of the base unit
milli	=	one thousandth or 0.001 or $\frac{1}{1,000}$ of the base unit
centi	=	one hundredth or 0.01 or $\frac{1}{100}$ of the base unit
deci	=	one tenth or 0.1 or $\frac{1}{10}$ of the base unit
kilo	=	one thousand or 1,000 times the base unit

Figure 3-1 demonstrates the relationship of metric units. Notice that the values of most of the common prefixes used in health care and the ones applied in this text are highlighted in red: **kilo-, base, milli-,** and **micro-.** These units are three places away from the next place. Often you can either multiply or divide by 1,000 to calculate an equivalent quantity. The only exception is **centi-,** which is also highlighted. Centi- is easy to remember, though, if you think of the relationship between one cent and

FIGURE 3-1   Relationship and value of metric units, with comparison of common metric units used in health care

Prefix	Kilo-	Hecto-	Deca-	BASE	Deci-	Centi-	Milli-	Decimilli-	Centimilli-	Micro-
Weight	kilogram			gram			milligram			microgram
Volume				liter	deciliter		milliliter			
Length				meter		centimeter	millimeter			
Value to Base	1,000	100	10	1	0.1	0.01	0.001	0.0001	0.00001	0.000001

one U.S. dollar as a clue to the relationship of centi- to the base, $\frac{1}{100}$. **Deci-** is one-tenth ($\frac{1}{10}$) of the base. See Chapter 1 to review the rules of multiplying and dividing decimals by a power of 10.

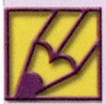

MATH TIP

Try this to remember the order of six of the metric units—**k**ilo-, **h**ecto-, **d**eca-, (BASE), **d**eci-, **c**enti-, and **m**illi-: "**K**ing **H**enry **D**ied from a **D**isease **C**alled **M**umps."

			gram			
			liter			
			meter			
kilo	hecto	deca	BASE	deci	centi	milli
K	**H**	**D**	Δ	**D**	**C**	**M**
"King	Henry	Died	from a	Disease	Called	Mumps."

The international standardization of metric units was adopted throughout much of the world in 1960 with the International System of Units or SI (from the French *Système International*). The abbreviations of this system of metric notation are the most widely accepted. The metric units of measurement and the SI abbreviations most often used for dosage calculations and measurements of health status are given in the following units of weight, volume, and length. This text uses SI standardized abbreviations throughout. Learn and practice these notations.

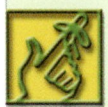

REMEMBER

SI METRIC SYSTEM

	Unit	Abbreviation	Equivalents
Weight	**gram** (base unit)	g	**1 g** = 1,000 mg = 1,000,000 mcg
	milligram	mg	0.001 g = **1 mg** = 1,000 mcg
	microgram	mcg	0.000001 g = 0.001 mg = **1 mcg**
	kilogram	kg	**1 kg** = 1,000 g
Volume	**liter** (base unit)	L	**1 L** = 1,000 mL
	milliliter	mL	0.001 L = **1 mL**
Length	**meter** (base unit)	m	**1 m** = 100 cm = 1,000 mm
	centimeter	cm	0.01 m = **1 cm** = 10 mm
	millimeter	mm	0.001 m = 0.1 cm = **1 mm**

CAUTION

You may see gram abbreviated as Gm or gm, liter as lowercase l, milliliter as ml, or microgram as μg. These abbreviations are considered obsolete or too easily misinterpreted, and should be avoided. You should only use the standardized SI abbreviations. Use g for gram, L for liter, and mL for milliliter. Further, the unit of measurement *cubic centimeter,* abbreviated cc, has been used interchangeably with mL. The use of cc for mL is now prohibited by many health care organizations because cc can be mistaken for zeros (00) or units (U). The abbreviation U is also now prohibited and must be spelled out (unit).

CAUTION

The SI abbreviations for milligram (mg) and milliliter (mL) appear to be somewhat similar, but in fact mg is a weight unit and mL is a volume unit. Confusing these two units can have dire consequences in dosage calculations. Learn to clearly differentiate them now.

In addition to learning the metric units, their equivalent values, and their abbreviations, it is important to use the following rules of metric notation.

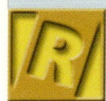

RULES

The following 10 critical rules will help to ensure that you accurately write and interpret metric notation.

1. The unit or abbreviation always follows the amount. Example: *5 g* NOT *g 5*

2. Do not put a period after the unit abbreviation because it may be mistaken for the number 1 if poorly written. Example: *20 mg* NOT *20 mg.*

3. Do not add an s to make the unit plural because it may be misread for another unit. Example: *5 mL* NOT *5 mLs*

4. Separate the amount from the unit so the number and unit of measure do not run together because the unit can be mistaken as zero or zeros, risking a 10-fold to 100-fold overdose. Example: *20 mg* NOT *20mg*

5. Place commas for amounts at or above 1,000. Example: *10,000 mcg* NOT *10000 mcg*

6. Decimals are used to designate fractional amounts. Example: *1.5 mL* NOT *1½ mL*

7. Use a leading zero to emphasize the decimal point for fractional amounts less than 1. Without the zero the amount may be interpreted as a whole number, resulting in serious overdosing. Example: *0.5 mg* NOT *.5 mg*

8. Omit unnecessary or trailing zeros that can be misread as part of the amount if the decimal point is not seen. Example: *1.5 mg* NOT *1.50 mg*

9. Do not use the abbreviation μg for microgram because it might be mistaken for mg, which is 1,000 times the intended amount. Example: *150 mcg* NOT *150 μg*

10. Do not use the abbreviation cc for mL because the unit can be mistaken for zeros. Example: *500 mL* NOT *500 cc*

Always ask the writer to clarify if you are not sure of the abbreviation or notation used. Never guess!

The metric system is the most common and the only standardized system of measurement in health care. Take a few minutes to review these essential points.

QUICK REVIEW

- The metric base units are gram (g), liter (L), and meter (m).

- Subunits are designated by the appropriate prefix and the base unit (such as milligram) and standard abbreviations (such as mg).

- There are 10 critical rules for ensuring that units and amounts are accurately interpreted. Review them again now and learn to rigorously adhere to them.

- Never guess as to the meaning of metric notation. When in doubt about the exact amount or the abbreviation used, ask the writer to clarify.

Review Set 11

1. The system of measurement most commonly used for prescribing and administering medications is the _____ system.

2. Liter and milliliter are metric units that measure _____.

3. Gram and milligram are metric units that measure _____.

4. Meter and millimeter are metric units that measure _____.

5. 1 mg is _____ of a g.

6. There are _____ mL in a liter.

7. Which is the smallest—milligram or microgram? _____

8. Which is the largest—kilogram, gram, or milligram? _____

9. Which is the smallest—kilogram, gram, or milligram? _____

10. 1 liter = _____ mL

11. 1,000 mcg = _____ mg

12. 1 kg = _____ g

13. 1 cm = _____ mm

Select the correctly written metric notation.

14. .3 g, 0.3 Gm, 0.3 g, .3 Gm, 0.30 g   _____

15. $1\frac{1}{3}$ ml, 1.33 mL, 1.33 ML, $1\frac{1}{3}$ ML, 1.330 mL   _____

16. 5 Kg, 5.0 kg, kg 05, 5 kg, 5 kG   _____

17. 1.5 mm, $1\frac{1}{2}$ mm, 1.5 Mm, 1.50 MM, $1\frac{1}{2}$ MM   _____

18. mg 10, 10 mG, 10.0 mg, 10 mg, 10 MG   _____

Interpret these metric abbreviations.

19. mcg   _____   23. mm   _____

20. mL   _____   24. kg   _____

21. mg   _____   25. cm   _____

22. g   _____

After completing these problems, see page 508 to check your answers.

THE APOTHECARY AND HOUSEHOLD SYSTEMS

The Joint Commission recommends that the metric system be used exclusively for the ordering, measuring, and reporting of medications. However, some apothecary notations—such as lowercase Roman numerals, ounces, and grains—are still in use. Likewise, the household system persists, and nurses and other health care providers need to be familiar with the equivalent measurements that patients or clients use at home.

The historic interconnection between the apothecary and household systems is interesting. The apothecary system was the first system of medication measurement used by pharmacists (apothecaries) and physicians. It originated in Greece and made its way to Europe via Rome and France. The English used it during the late 1600s, and the colonists brought it to America. A modified system of measurement for everyday use evolved; it is now recognized as the household system. Large liquid volumes were based on familiar trading measurements, such as *pints, quarts,* and *gallons,* which originated as apothecary measurements. Vessels to accommodate each measurement were made by craftspersons and widely circulated in colonial America.

Units of weight, such as the *grain, ounce,* and *pound,* also are rooted in the apothecary system. The grain originated as the standard weight of a single grain of wheat, which is approximately 60 milligrams. This one equivalency of weight (1 grain = 60 milligrams) is recognized in drug orders. After more than 100 years as the world's most popular pill, aspirin may still be prescribed in grains.

The Apothecary System

Apothecary notation is unusual. Exercise caution when using this system. The apothecary system utilizes Roman numerals. The ability to interpret Roman numerals is therefore essential. The letters **I, V,** and **X** are the basic symbols of this system that you will use in dosage calculations. In medical notation, lowercase letters are typically used to designate Roman numerals (**i, v,** and **x**).

In addition to Roman numerals, apothecary notation also uses common fractions, special symbols, and units of measure that typically precede numeric values. The common units are *grain* and *ounce.*

CAUTION

In 2004, The Joint Commission (2005) first published its *Official "Do Not Use" List* for medical abbreviations and notation. This was followed later that year with another list of abbreviations, acronyms, and symbols recommended not to use (and for **possible** future inclusion on the official list), including apothecary ones. Although The Joint Commission does not prohibit the use of apothecary abbreviations at this time, it does discourage their use because they can be easily misinterpreted. This can be confusing because rules and guidelines are regularly updated to best ensure patient safety; but it is prudent for you to be familiar with notations that you may find in practice. It is important that all health care practitioners be diligent in their efforts to stay current with The Joint Commission's and their local health care organizations' requirements regarding medical abbreviations and notation and to rigorously follow those guidelines. You will learn more about medical abbreviations in Chapter 7, and you will find the *Official "Do Not Use" List* in Chapter 9, as we consider the prevention of medication errors.

The style of apothecary notation includes:

1. The unit or abbreviation typically precedes the amount. Example: gr v

2. Lowercase Roman numerals are often used to express whole numbers: i, v, x

3. Fractions are used to designate amounts less than 1. Examples: gr $\frac{1}{2}$, gr $\frac{1}{4}$

4. You may see the symbol *ss* used to designate the fraction $\frac{1}{2}$. Because this symbol can be easily misinterpreted, it is provided here for recognition purposes only. We will not use this symbol.

MATH TIP

To decrease errors in interpretation of medical notation, a line may be drawn over the lowercase Roman numerals to distinguish them from other letters in a word or phrase. The lowercase i is dotted above, not below, the line.

EXAMPLE ■

3 = iii or i̅i̅i̅

Learn the following common Roman numerals and their Arabic equivalents. These are the values that you may see.

REMEMBER

Arabic Number	Roman Numeral	Apothecary Notation	Arabic Number	Roman Numeral	Apothecary Notation
1	I	i, ī	5	V	v, v̄
2	II	ii, īi	10	X	x, x̄
3	III	iii, īii	15	XV	xv, x̄v̄
4	IV	iv, īv	20	XX	xx, x̄x̄

The essential apothecary unit of measurement to learn is given in the following Remember box. There are no essential equivalents of weight or length to learn for this system.

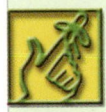

REMEMBER

The one apothecary unit you may still see in use is grain. It is abbreviated *gr.*

CAUTION

Notice that the abbreviations for the apothecary grain **(gr)** and the metric gram **(g)** can be confusing. The style indicating the abbreviation or symbol before the quantity in apothecary notation further distinguishes it from the metric system. If you are ever doubtful about the meaning that is intended, be sure to ask the writer for clarification.

CAUTION

The following apothecary units and symbols may appear on some syringes and medicine cups. Do not use these measurements, and be careful to differentiate them from acceptable units of measure.

minim (ɱ)   fluid dram (ʒ)   fluid ounce (ʒ̄)

QUICK REVIEW

In the apothecary system:

- A unit for dosage calculation is grain (gr).

- The quantity is often expressed in lowercase Roman numerals. Amounts greater than 10 may be expressed in Arabic numbers, except 15 (xv), 20 (xx), and 30 (xxx).

- Quantities of less than 1 are expressed as fractions.

- The abbreviation is typically written before the quantity, especially for grains.

- If you are unsure about the exact meaning of any medical notation, do not guess or assume. Ask the writer for clarification.

- Be sure to check with your health care facility regarding the acceptable use of apothecary notation.

The Household System

Household units are likely to be used by the patient at home where hospital measuring devices are not usually available. You should be familiar with the household system of measurement so that you can explain take-home prescriptions to your patient at the time of discharge. There is no standardized system of notation, but it is preferred to express the quantity in Arabic numbers and common fractions with the abbreviation following the amount. The common household units and abbreviations are given in the following table (Remember box).

CAUTION

Some units are used in both the apothecary and household systems (such as ounce, pint, and quart). The ounce household unit is used for both volume (fluid ounce) and weight (ounce). These similarities can be confusing. In apothecary, the amount technically follows the unit with Roman numerals used to designate the amount (such as oz ii). In the household system, the unit follows the amount (2 oz). However, either notation is acceptable.

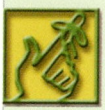

REMEMBER

HOUSEHOLD		
Unit	Abbreviation	Equivalents
drop	gtt	
teaspoon	t (or tsp)	3 t = 1 T
tablespoon	T (or tbs)	1 T = 3 t
ounce (fluid)	fl oz	2 T = 1 fl oz
cup	cup	1 cup = 8 fl oz
pint	pt	1 pt = 2 cups = 16 fl oz
quart	qt	1 qt = 2 pt = 4 cups = 32 fl oz
ounce (weight)	oz	1 lb = 16 oz
pound	lb	

Note: The *drop (gtt)* unit is given only for the purpose of recognition. There are no standard equivalents for *drop* to learn. The amount of each drop varies according to the diameter of the utensil used for measurement. (See Figure 6-2, calibrated dropper, and Figure 15-16, intravenous drip chambers.)

MATH TIP

Tablespoon is the larger unit, and the abbreviation is expressed with a capital or "large" T. Teaspoon is the smaller unit, and the abbreviation is expressed with a lowercase or "small" t.

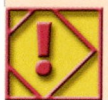

CAUTION

Although some households may use metric measure, many do not. There can be a wide variation in household measuring devices, such as in tableware teaspoons, which can constitute a safety risk. Talking to your patients and their families about administering medications at home is an excellent teaching opportunity. Determine their familiarity with metric units, such as milliliters, and ask what kind of medicine measuring devices they use at home. It is best to advise your patients and their families to use the measuring devices packaged with the medication or provided by the pharmacy.

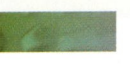

OTHER COMMON DRUG MEASUREMENTS: UNITS AND MILLIEQUIVALENTS

Four other measurements may be used to indicate the quantity of medicine prescribed: international unit, unit, milliunit, and milliequivalent (mEq). The quantity is expressed in Arabic numbers with the unit of measure following. The *international unit* represents a unit of potency used to measure such things as vitamins and chemicals. The *unit* is a standardized amount needed to produce a desired effect. Medications such as penicillin, heparin, and insulin have their own meaning and numeric value related to the type of unit. One thousandth ($\frac{1}{1,000}$) of a unit is a *milliunit*. The equivalent of 1 unit is 1,000 milliunits. Oxytocin is a drug measured in milliunits. The *milliequivalent* (mEq) is one thousandth ($\frac{1}{1,000}$) of an equivalent weight of a chemical. The mEq is the unit used when referring to the concentration of serum electrolytes, such as calcium, magnesium, potassium, and sodium.

CAUTION

The obsolete abbreviations *U* and *IU* are included on the *Official "Do Not Use" List* published by The Joint Commission (2005). The written words *unit* and *international unit* should be used instead. See Chapter 9 for the full list.

It is not necessary to learn conversions for the international unit, unit, or milliequivalent because medications prescribed in these measurements are also prepared and administered in the same system.

EXAMPLE 1 ■

Heparin 800 units is ordered, and *heparin 1,000 units per 1 mL* is the stock drug.
Because there is no standard equivalent for units, when a medication is ordered in units, such as heparin, the stock drug should be supplied in units.

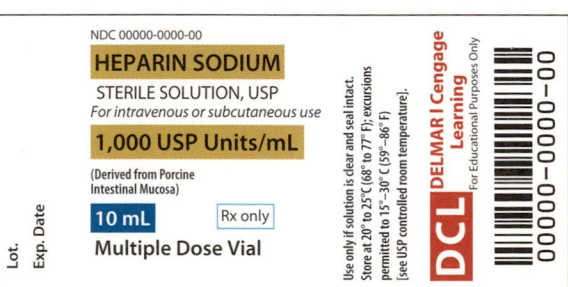

EXAMPLE 2 ■

Potassium chloride 10 mEq is ordered, and *potassium chloride 20 mEq per 15 mL* is the stock drug.
Because there is no standard equivalent for mEq, when a medication is ordered in mEq, such as potassium chloride, the stock drug should be supplied in mEq.

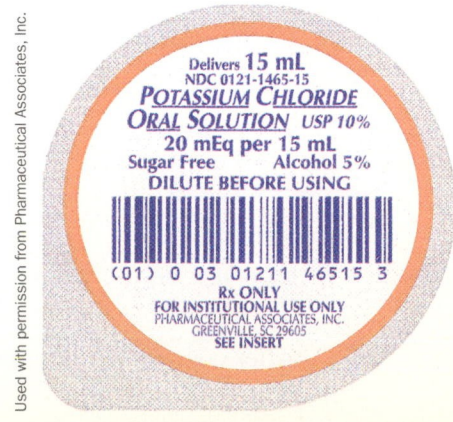

EXAMPLE 3 ■

Oxytocin 2 milliunits (0.002 international units) intravenous **per minute** is ordered and *oxytocin 10 international units per 1 mL* to be added to 1,000 mL intravenous solution is available. Very small doses of a medication, such as oxytocin, may be ordered in milliunits. Remember the prefix milli means one thousandth. Sometimes converting from units to milliunits is necessary.

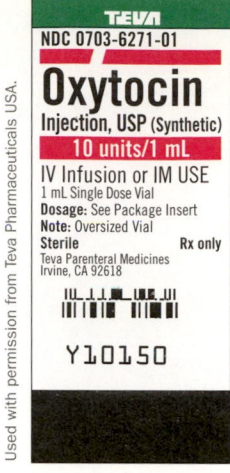

Used with permission from Teva Pharmaceuticals USA.

QUICK REVIEW

- The international unit, unit, milliunit, and milliequivalent (mEq) are special measured quantities expressed in Arabic numbers.

- No conversion is necessary for unit, international unit, and mEq because the ordered dosage and supply dosage are in the same system.

- 1 unit = 1,000 milliunits

Review Set 12

Interpret the following notations.

1. 20 gtt _____

2. 10 lb _____

3. 10 mEq _____

4. gr iv _____

5. 10 T _____

Express the following using medical notation.

6. four drops _____

7. thirty milliequivalents _____

8. five tablespoons _____

9. one-and-one-half teaspoons _____

10. ten grains _____

11. True or False? The household system of measurement is commonly used in hospital dosage calculations. _____

12. True or False? The drop is a standardized unit of measure. _____

13. True or False? Fluid ounce is equivalent to the ounce that measures weight. _____

14. Drugs such as heparin and insulin are commonly measured in _____.

15. 1 T = _____ t

16. 1 fl oz = _____ T

17. 16 oz = _____ lb

18. 2 T = _____ fl oz

19. 8 fl oz = _____ cup

20. The unit used to measure the concentration of serum electrolytes, such as calcium, magnesium, potassium, and sodium is the _____ and is abbreviated _____.

After completing these problems, see page 508 to check your answers.

CRITICAL THINKING SKILLS

The importance of the placement of the decimal point cannot be overemphasized. Let's look at some examples of potential medication errors related to placement of the decimal point.

ERROR 1

Not placing a zero before a decimal point in medication orders.

Possible Scenario

An emergency room physician wrote an order for the bronchodilator terbutaline for a patient with asthma. The order was written as follows.

Incorrectly Written
___

Terbutaline .5 mg subcutaneously now, repeat dose in 30 minutes if no improvement

Suppose the nurse, not noticing the faint decimal point, administered 5 mg of terbutaline subcutaneously instead of 0.5 mg. The patient would receive ten times the dose intended by the physician.

Potential Outcome

Within minutes of receiving the injection the patient would likely complain of headache and develop tachycardia, nausea, and vomiting. The patient's hospital stay would be lengthened because of the need to recover from the overdose.

Prevention

This type of medication error is avoided by remembering the rule to place a 0 in front of a decimal to avoid confusion regarding the dosage: 0.5 mg. Further, remember to question orders that are unclear or seem impractical.

Correctly Written
___

Terbutaline 0.5 mg subcutaneously now, repeat dose in 30 minutes if no improvement

CRITICAL THINKING SKILLS

Many medication errors occur by confusing mg and mL. Remember that mg is the weight of the medication, and mL is the volume of the medication preparation.

ERROR 2

Confusing mg and mL.

Possible Scenario

Suppose a physician ordered the steroid Prelone (prednisolone) 15 mg by mouth twice a day for a patient with cancer. Prelone syrup is supplied in a concentration of 15 mg in 5 mL. The pharmacist supplied a bottle of Prelone containing a total volume of 240 mL with 15 mg of Prelone in every 5 mL. The nurse, in a rush to give her medications on time, misread the order as 15 mL and gave the patient 15 mL of Prelone instead of 5 mL. Therefore, the patient received 45 mg of Prelone, or three times the correct dosage.

Potential Outcome

The patient could develop a number of complications related to a high dosage of steroids: gastrointestinal bleeding, hyperglycemia, hypertension, agitation, and severe mood disturbances, to name a few.

Prevention

The mg is the weight of a medication, and mL is the volume you prepare. Do not allow yourself to get rushed or distracted so that you confuse milligrams with milliliters. When you know you are distracted or stressed, have another nurse double-check the calculation of the dose.

PRACTICE PROBLEMS—CHAPTER 3

Give the metric prefix for the following parts of the base units.

1. 0.001 _____   3. 0.01 _____

2. 0.000001 _____   4. 1,000 _____

Identify the equivalent unit with a value of 1 that is indicated by the following amounts (such as 1 unit = 1,000 milliunits).

5. 0.001 gram _____   7. 0.001 milligram _____

6. 1,000 grams _____   8. 0.01 meter _____

Identify the metric base unit for the following.

9. length _____   11. volume _____

10. weight _____

Interpret the following notations.

12. gtt _____   22. mL _____

13. fl oz _____   23. pt _____

14. oz _____   24. T _____

15. gr _____   25. mm _____

16. mg _____   26. g _____

17. mcg _____   27. cm _____

18. lb _____   28. L _____

19. mEq _____   29. m _____

20. t _____   30. kg _____

21. qt _____   31. ℁ _____

Express the following amounts in proper notation.

32. three hundred and twenty-five micrograms _____

33. one-half grain _____

34. two teaspoons _____

35. one-third fluid ounce _____

36. five million units _____

37. one-half liter _____

38. one-fourth grain _____

39. one two hundredths of a grain _____

40. five hundredths of a milligram _____

Express the following numeric amounts in words.

41. $8\frac{1}{4}$ oz _____

42. 375 g _____

43. gr $\frac{1}{4}$ _____

44. 2.6 mL _____

45. 20 mEq _____

46. 0.4 L _____

47. gr $\frac{1}{400}$ _____

48. 0.17 mg _____

49. Describe the strategy that would prevent the medication error.

Possible Scenario

Suppose a physician ordered oral Coumadin (an anticoagulant) for a patient with a history of deep vein thrombosis. The physician wrote an order for 10 mg but while writing the order placed a decimal point after the 10 and added a 0:

Incorrectly Written
_____

Coumadin 10.0 mg orally once per day
_____

Coumadin 10.0 mg was transcribed on the medication record as Coumadin 100 mg. The patient received ten times the correct dosage.

Potential Outcome

The patient would likely begin hemorrhaging. An antidote, such as vitamin K, would be necessary to reverse the effects of the overdose. However, it is important to remember that not all drugs have antidotes.

Prevention

_____

_____

50. Describe the strategy that would prevent a medication error or the need to notify the prescribing practitioner.

Possible Scenario

Suppose a physician ordered oral codeine (a mild narcotic analgesic) for an adult patient recovering from nasal surgery. The physician wrote the following order for 1 grain (equivalent to about 60 mg) but while writing the order placed the 1 before the abbreviation gr. The gr smeared and the abbreviation gr is unclear. Is it *grains* or *grams?*

Incorrectly Written
_____

Codeine 1 gr orally every 4 hours as needed for pain
_____

Codeine 1 gram was transcribed on the medication record. Because 1 gram is equivalent to 1,000 mg or about 15 grains, this erroneous dosage is about 15 times more than the intended amount.

Potential Outcome

Even though the nurse was in a rush to help ease the patient's pain, she realized that the available codeine pills would not be dispensable in this amount. She would have to give the patient 15 tablets to equal the 1 gram amount. The nurse saw the questionable order and called the physician for clarification. The nurse correctly concluded it was unlikely that the physician would have ordered such an excessive number of pills or dosage.

Prevention

_____

_____

After completing these problems, see page 508 to check your answers.

REFERENCE

The Joint Commission. (2005). *Official "do not use" list*. Retrieved September 25, 2009, from http://www.jointcommission.org/PatientSafety/DoNotUseList/

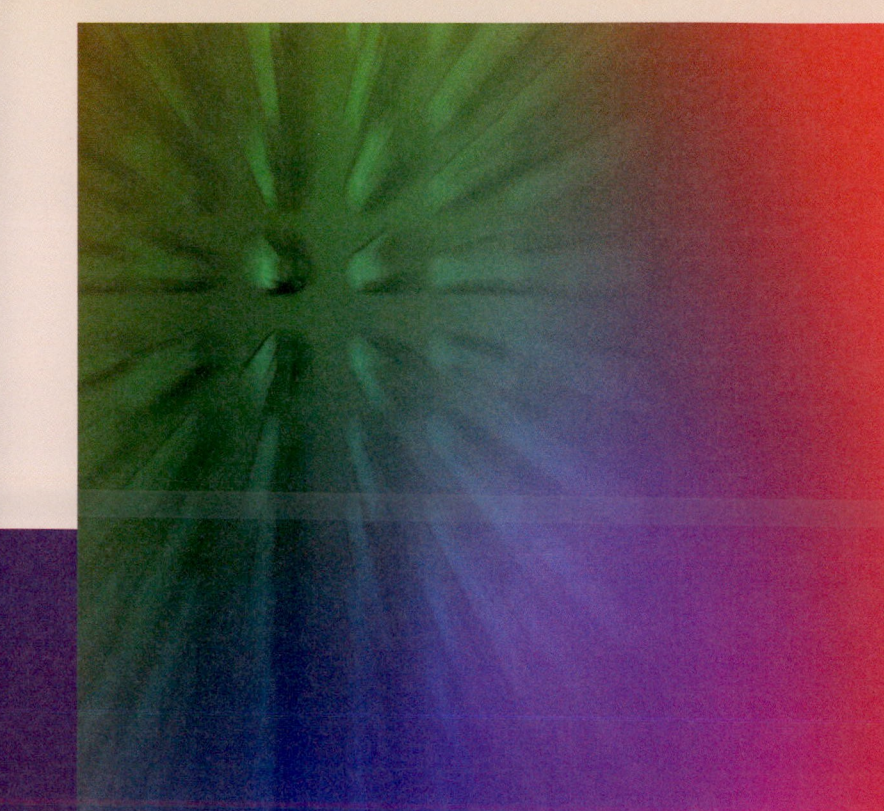

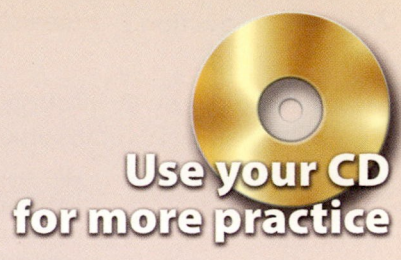
4

Conversions: Metric, Apothecary, and Household Systems

OBJECTIVES

Upon mastery of Chapter 4, you will be able to complete Step 1, Conversion, in the three-step process of dosage calculations. To accomplish this, you will also be able to:

- Recall from memory the metric, apothecary, and household approximate equivalents.
- Convert among units of measurement within the same system.
- Convert units of measurement from one system to another.

Medications are usually prescribed or ordered in a unit of weight measurement such as grams or milligrams. The nurse must interpret this order and administer the correct number of tablets, capsules, teaspoons, milliliters, or some other unit of volume or capacity measurement to deliver the prescribed amount of medication.

EXAMPLE 1 ■

A prescription notation may read:

_____

Aldactone 100 mg to be given orally twice a day

_____

The nurse has on hand a 100 tablet bottle of *Aldactone labeled 50 mg in each tablet.* To administer the correct amount of the drug, the nurse must convert the prescribed weight of 100 mg to the correct number of tablets. In this case, the nurse gives the patient two of the 50 mg tablets, which equals *100 mg of Aldactone.*

To give the prescribed dosage, the nurse must be able to calculate the order in weight to the correct amount of tablets of the drug on hand or in stock. THINK: If one tablet equals 50 mg, then two tablets equal 100 mg.

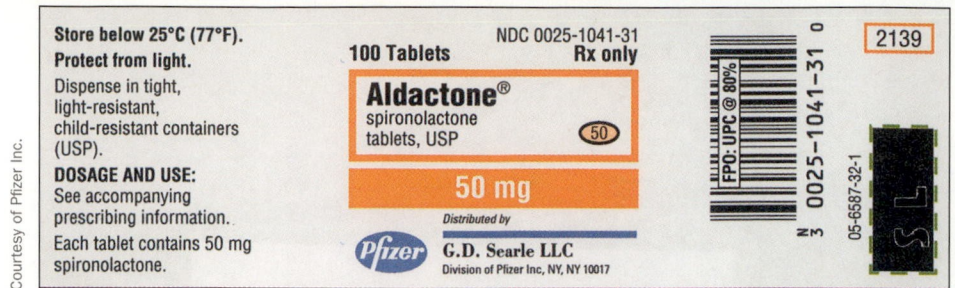

Courtesy of Pfizer Inc.

EXAMPLE 2 ■

A prescription notation may read:

midazolam HCl 2.5 mg by intravenous injection immediately

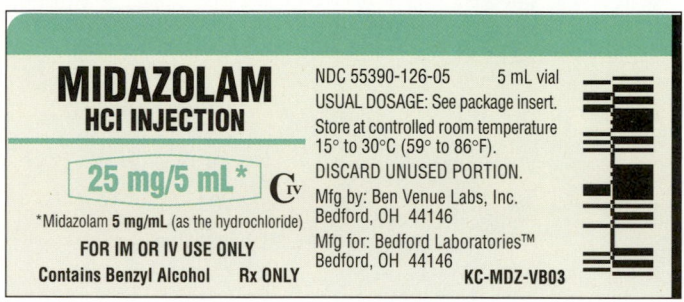

Used with permission from Bedford Laboratories, A Division of Ben Venue Laboratories. A Division of Boehringer-Ingelheim Company.

The nurse has on hand a vial of *midazolam HCl* labeled *25 mg per 5 mL* or *5 mg/mL*. To administer the correct amount of the drug, the nurse must be able to fill the injection syringe with the correct number of milliliters. As the nurse, how many milliliters would you give? THINK: If 5 mg = 1 mL, then 2.5 mg = 0.5 mL. Therefore, 0.5 mL should be administered.

Sometimes a drug order may be written in a unit of measurement that is different from the supply of drugs the nurse has on hand. Usually this will be an order for a medicine that is written in one size of metric unit (such as milligrams), but the medicine is supplied in another metric unit (such as grams). You will occasionally encounter a medicine ordered in apothecary measure (such as grains) by an older physician originally trained in that system of measurement. However, the drug will be supplied in metric measure (such as grams or milligrams). Even though apothecary medicine orders are rare, they are good practice for learning to convert between systems of measurement. The Joint Commission (2005) discourages the use of apothecary measure; but until it is prohibited, you may still see it in use. Therefore, we will consider examples of conversion within the metric system and between other systems, such as apothecary and household measure. Let's look at examples of medicines ordered and supplied in both different size units and different systems of measurement.

EXAMPLE 1 ■

Medication order: triazolam 250 mcg orally at bedtime

Supply on hand: Halcion 0.25 mg tablets

The drug order is written in micrograms, but the drug is supplied in milligrams.

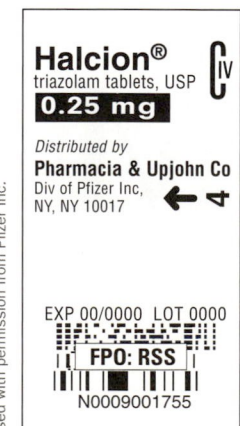

Used with permission from Pfizer Inc.

EXAMPLE 2 ■

Medication order: *codeine sulfate gr $\frac{1}{2}$ orally every 4 hours as needed for pain*

Supply on hand: codeine sulfate 30 mg tablets

The drug order is written in grains (apothecary measurement), but the drug is supplied in milligrams (metric measurement).

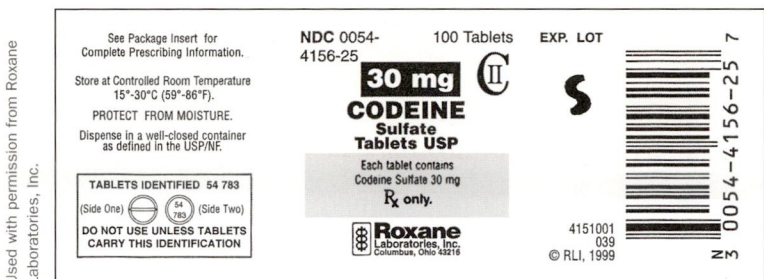

In such cases, the prescribed quantities must be converted into the units as supplied. The nurse or health care professional can then calculate the correct dosage to prepare and administer to the patient. Thus, determining the need for and calculating unit conversion is the first step in the calculation of dosages.

CONVERTING USING RATIO-PROPORTION

After learning the systems of measurement common for dosage calculations and their equivalents (Chapter 3), the next step is to learn how to use them. First, you must be able to convert, or change, from one unit to another within the same measurement system and between systems of measurement. A method of performing conversions is to set up a proportion of two ratios expressed as fractions. Refer to Chapter 2 to review ratio-proportion, if needed.

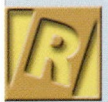

RULE

In a proportion, the ratio for a known equivalent equals the ratio for an unknown equivalent. To use ratio-proportion to convert from one unit to another, you need to follow these three steps.

1. Recall the equivalents.

2. Set up a proportion of two equivalent ratios.

3. Cross-multiply to solve for an unknown quantity, X.

Each ratio in a proportion must have the same relationship and follow the same sequence. A proportion compares like things to like things. Be sure the units in the numerators match and the units in the denominators match. Label the units in each ratio.

Let's start by converting units within the same measurement system and with common household units.

EXAMPLE 1 ■

How many cups are equivalent to 3 quarts?

1. What is the known equivalent that applies to this problem? You know it is 1 qt = 4 cups.

2. Now you are ready to set up a proportion of two equivalent ratios. The first ratio of the proportion contains the *known equivalent*, that is 1 quart : 4 cups. The second ratio contains the *desired unit*

of measure and the *unknown equivalent* expressed as X, that is 3 quarts : X cups. Express the ratios as fractions. The proportion now looks like this.

$$\frac{1 \text{ qt}}{4 \text{ cups}} = \frac{3 \text{ qt}}{X \text{ cups}}$$

CAUTION

Notice that the ratios follow the same sequence. **THIS IS ESSENTIAL.** The proportion is set up so that like units are across from each other. The units in the numerators match (qt) and the units in the denominators match (cups).

3. Cross-multiply to solve the proportion for X. Refer to Chapter 2 to review this skill, if needed.

$$\frac{1 \text{ qt}}{4 \text{ cups}} \times \frac{3 \text{ qt}}{X \text{ cups}} \quad \text{Cross-multiply}$$

$$1 \times X = 4 \times 3$$

$$1X = 12$$

$$\frac{1X}{1} = \frac{12}{1} \quad \text{Simplify: Divide both sides of the equation by the number before the unknown X}$$

$$X = 12 \text{ cups} \quad \text{Label the units to match the unknown X}$$

You know the answer is in cups, because cups is the unknown equivalent. Therefore, 3 qt = 12 cups.

MATH TIP

Multiplying or dividing a number by 1 does not change its value. It is the same number.

Therefore in the previous example, it is not necessary to simplify, because 1X = X. You can shorten the calculation. Look again at the math.

$$\frac{1 \text{ qt}}{4 \text{ cups}} \times \frac{3 \text{ qt}}{X \text{ cups}} \quad \text{Cross-multiply}$$

$$X = 4 \times 3$$

$$X = 12 \text{ cups}$$

In the next example the unknown X is in the numerator. It does not matter, as long as the sequence is the same (numerator units match and denominator units match). Remember, a proportion must compare like things to like things. In the first example, the unknown was cups. In the second example the unknown is quarts.

EXAMPLE 2 ■

How many quarts are in 8 cups?

To solve this you also use the ratio-proportion rule.

1. Recall the known equivalent (1 qt = 4 cups).

2. Set up a proportion of two equivalent ratios.

3. Cross-multiply to solve for X.

$$\frac{1 \text{ qt}}{4 \text{ cups}} = \frac{X \text{ qt}}{8 \text{ cups}}$$

$$\frac{1 \text{ qt}}{4 \text{ cups}} \quad\Large\times\quad \frac{X \text{ qt}}{8 \text{ cups}}$$ Cross-multiply

$$4X \quad = \quad 8$$

$$\frac{4X}{4} \quad = \quad \frac{8}{4}$$ Simplify: Divide both sides of the equation by the number before the unknown X

$$X \quad = \quad 2 \text{ qt}$$ Label the units to match the unknown X

CONVERTING WITHIN THE METRIC SYSTEM

The most common conversions in dosage calculations and health care are within the metric system. As you recall from Chapter 3, most metric conversions are simply derived by multiplying or dividing by 1,000. Recall from Chapter 1 that multiplying by 1,000 is the same as moving the decimal point three places to the right.

EXAMPLE 1 ■

Convert 2 grams to the equivalent number of milligrams.

1. Recall the known equivalent: 1 g = 1,000 mg.

2. Set up a proportion of two equivalent ratios.

3. Cross-multiply to solve for X.

Notice that in this and the following examples you are asked to find the equivalent amount of the smaller unit. It makes sense that the resulting number of smaller units would be greater than the original number of larger units. In this first example you are converting grams to milligrams.

$$\frac{1 \text{ g}}{1,000 \text{ mg}} \quad = \quad \frac{2 \text{ g}}{X \text{ mg}}$$

$$\frac{1 \text{ g}}{1,000 \text{ mg}} \quad\Large\times\quad \frac{2 \text{ g}}{X \text{ mg}}$$ Cross-multiply

$$X = 1,000 \times 2$$

$$X = 2,000 \text{ mg}$$ Label the units to match the unknown X

Thus, you know that a medicine container labeled 2 grams per tablet is the same as 2,000 milligrams per tablet.

MATH TIP

Notice that to multiply 2 by 1,000, you are moving the decimal three places to the right. This is a shortcut. Sometimes to complete this operaton, you add zeros to hold the places equal to the number of zeros in the equivalent. In this case 1 g = 1,000 mg, so you add three zeros: 2 × 1,000 = 2.000. = 2,000

EXAMPLE 2 ■

Convert: 0.3 g to mg

Equivalent: 1 g = 1,000 mg

$$\frac{1 \text{ g}}{1,000 \text{ mg}} \quad = \quad \frac{0.3 \text{ g}}{X \text{ mg}}$$

$$\frac{1 \text{ g}}{1,000 \text{ mg}} \quad\Large\times\quad \frac{0.3 \text{ g}}{X \text{ mg}}$$ Cross-multiply

X = 1,000 × 0.3

0.300. Move the decimal 3 places to the right to multiply by 1,000. Add zeros to complete the operation.

X = 300 mg

Label the units to match the unknown X

EXAMPLE 3 ■

Convert: 2.5 g to mg

Equivalent: 1 g = 1,000 mg

$$\frac{1\ g}{1,000\ mg} = \frac{2.5\ g}{X\ mg}$$

$$\frac{1\ g}{1,000\ mg} \diagdown\!\!\!\!\diagup \frac{2.5\ g}{X\ mg} \quad \text{Cross-multiply}$$

X = 1,000 × 2.5

2.500. Move the decimal 3 places to the right to multiply by 1,000. Add zeros to complete the operation.

X = 2,500 mg

Label the units to match the unknown X

EXAMPLE 4 ■

Convert: 0.15 kg to g

Equivalent: 1 kg = 1,000 g

$$\frac{1\ kg}{1,000\ g} = \frac{0.15\ kg}{X\ g}$$

$$\frac{1\ kg}{1,000\ g} \diagdown\!\!\!\!\diagup \frac{0.15\ kg}{X\ g} \quad \text{Cross-multiply}$$

X = 1,000 × 0.15

0.150. Move the decimal 3 places to the right to multiply by 1,000. Add a zero to complete the operation.

X = 150 g

Label the units to match the unknown X

EXAMPLE 5 ■

Convert: 0.004 L to mL

Equivalent: 1 L = 1,000 mL

$$\frac{1\ L}{1,000\ mL} = \frac{0.004\ L}{X\ mL}$$

$$\frac{1\ L}{1,000\ mL} \diagdown\!\!\!\!\diagup \frac{0.004\ L}{X\ mL} \quad \text{Cross-multiply}$$

X = 1,000 × 0.004

0.004. Move the decimal 3 places to the right to multiply by 1,000. (There are already enough places, so you do not need to add a zero to complete the operation.)

X = 4 mL

Label the units to match the unknown X

EXAMPLE 6 ■

An infant's head circumference is 40.5 cm. How many millimeters is that?

Convert: 40.5 cm to mm

Equivalent: 1 cm = 10 mm

Notice the ratio is now 1:10, not 1:1,000. In this example you are multiplying by 10 (not 1,000), so you will move the decimal point one place to the right.

$$\frac{1\ cm}{10\ mm} = \frac{40.5\ cm}{X\ mm}$$

$$\frac{1\ cm}{10\ mm} \bowtie \frac{40.5\ cm}{X\ mm}$$ Cross-multiply

$X = 10 \times 40.5$ 40.5. Move the decimal 1 place to the right to multiply by 10.

$X = 405\ mm$ Label the units to match the unknown X

Now let's consider conversions that go the opposite way—from a smaller unit (such as mL) to a larger unit (such as L). It makes sense that the resulting number of larger units will now be less than the original number of smaller units. In the next set of examples notice that the unknown X is in the numerator and you must divide to solve for X.

EXAMPLE 1 ▪

Convert: 5,000 mL to L

Equivalent: 1 L = 1,000 mL

$$\frac{1\ L}{1,000\ mL} = \frac{X\ L}{5,000\ mL}$$

$$\frac{1\ L}{1,000\ mL} \bowtie \frac{X\ L}{5,000\ mL}$$ Cross-multiply

$1,000X = 5,000$

$$\frac{1,000X}{1,000} = \frac{5,000}{1,000}$$ Simplify: Divide both sides of the equation by the number before the unknown X. The zeros cancel.

$X = 5\ L$ Label the units to match the unknown X

MATH TIP

Let's look at the shortcut for dividing 5,000 by 1,000. Now you are moving the decimal three places to the left, and then eliminating unnecessary zeros. 5,000 ÷ 1,000 = 5.000. = 5

CAUTION

Leaving unnecessary zeros may lead to confusion and misinterpretation. For safety the unnecessary zeros must be eliminated. Likewise, use a leading zero for emphasis of a decimal point when a decimal number is less than 1. Both of these cautions are demonstrated in the next example.

EXAMPLE 2 ▪

Convert: 500 mL to L

Equivalent: 1 L = 1,000 mL

$$\frac{1\ L}{1,000\ mL} = \frac{X\ L}{500\ mL}$$

$$\frac{1\ L}{1,000\ mL} \bowtie \frac{X\ L}{500\ mL}$$ Cross-multiply

$1,000X = 500$

$$\frac{1,000X}{1,000} = \frac{500}{1,000}$$ Simplify: Divide both sides of the equation by the number before the unknown X

$X = 0.5$ 0.500. Move the decimal 3 places to the left to divide by 1,000. Eliminate unnecessary zeros. As the amount is less than 1, use a leading zero for emphasis of the decimal point.

$X = 0.5\ L$ Label the units to match the unknown X

MATH TIP

Sometimes to complete the operation, you must add zeros to hold the places equal to the number of zeros in the equivalent, as shown in Examples 3 and 4.

EXAMPLE 3 ■

Convert: 50 mL to L

Equivalent: 1 L = 1,000 mL

$$\frac{1\text{ L}}{1{,}000\text{ mL}} = \frac{X\text{ L}}{50\text{ mL}}$$

$$\frac{1\text{ L}}{1{,}000\text{ mL}} \diagdown\!\!\!\!\!\diagup \frac{X\text{ L}}{50\text{ mL}} \qquad \text{Cross-multiply}$$

$$1{,}000X = 50$$

$$\frac{1{,}000X}{1{,}000} = \frac{50}{1{,}000} \qquad \text{Simplify: Divide both sides of the equation by the number before the unknown X}$$

$$X = 0.05 \qquad\qquad 0.\underset{\smile}{050}.\text{ Move the decimal 3 places to the left to divide by 1,000. First you must add a zero to complete the operation. Then eliminate unnecessary zero and use a leading zero for emphasis in your final answer.}$$

$$X = 0.05\text{ L} \qquad\qquad \text{Label the units to match the unknown X}$$

EXAMPLE 4 ■

Convert: 5 mL to L

Equivalent: 1 L = 1,000 mL

$$\frac{1\text{ L}}{1{,}000\text{ mL}} = \frac{X\text{ L}}{5\text{ mL}}$$

$$\frac{1\text{ L}}{1{,}000\text{ mL}} \diagdown\!\!\!\!\!\diagup \frac{X\text{ L}}{5\text{ mL}} \qquad \text{Cross-multiply}$$

$$1{,}000X = 5$$

$$\frac{1{,}000X}{1{,}000} = \frac{5}{1{,}000} \qquad \text{Simplify: Divide both sides of the equation by the number before the unknown X}$$

$$X = 0.005 \qquad\qquad 0.\underset{\smile}{005}.\text{ Move the decimal 3 places to the left after adding zeros to complete the operation. Use a leading zero for emphasis.}$$

$$X = 0.005\text{ L} \qquad\qquad \text{Label the units to match the unknown X}$$

EXAMPLE 5 ■

A patient's wound measures 31 millimeters. How many centimeters is that?

Convert: 31 mm to cm

Equivalent: 1 cm = 10 mm

Notice the ratio is now 1:10, not 1:1,000. In this example you are dividing by 10 (not 1,000), so you will move the decimal point one place to the left.

$$\frac{1\text{ cm}}{10\text{ mm}} = \frac{X\text{ cm}}{31\text{ mm}}$$

$$\frac{1\text{ cm}}{10\text{ mm}} \diagdown\!\!\!\!\!\diagup \frac{X\text{ cm}}{31\text{ mm}} \qquad \text{Cross-multiply}$$

$$10X = 31$$

$$\frac{10X}{10} = \frac{31}{10}$$

X = 3.1   3.1. Move the decimal 1 place to the left to divide by 10.

X = 3.1 cm   Label the units to match the unknown X

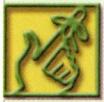

REMEMBER

When converting from a larger to a smaller unit of measure, the resulting number of smaller units should be greater than the original number of larger units. Conversely, when converting from a smaller to a larger unit of measure the resulting number of larger units should be less than the original number of smaller units. After all calculations ask yourself, "Does this answer make sense?" If it does not, stop, and check for your mistake.

MATH TIP

Remember this diagram when converting dosages within the metric system.

Move decimal point three places to the left for each step.

$$\longleftarrow$$

| kg | g | mg | mcg |

Move decimal point three places to the right for each step.

EXAMPLES ■

1 mcg = 0.001 mg (moved decimal point to the left 3 places)

2 g = 2,000 mg (moved decimal point to the right 3 places)

2 g = 2,000,000 mcg (moved decimal point to the right 6 places, as the conversion required two steps)

In time you will probably do these calculations in your head with little difficulty. If you feel you do not understand the concept of conversions within the metric system, review the decimal section in Chapter 1 and the metric section in Chapter 3 again. Get help from your instructor before proceeding further.

QUICK REVIEW

To use the ratio-proportion method to convert between units in the metric system:

1. Recall the metric equivalents.

2. Set up a proportion of two equivalent ratios.

3. Cross-multiply to solve for an unknown quantity, X.

Example: 3L = X mL
Equivalent: 1L = 1,000 mL

$$\frac{1\ L}{1,000\ mL} \quad\times\quad \frac{3\ L}{X\ mL}$$

X = 1,000 × 3
X = 3,000 mL   3.000. Move the decimal 3 places to the right to multiply by 1,000.

Example: 400 mg = X g
Equivalent: 1 g = 1,000 mg

$$\frac{1\ g}{1,000\ mg} \quad\times\quad \frac{X\ g}{400\ mg}$$

1,000X = 400

$$\frac{1,000X}{1,000} = \frac{400}{1,000}$$

X = 0.4 g   0.400. Move the decimal 3 places to the left to divide by 1,000.

Review Set 13

Convert each of the following to the equivalent unit indicated.

1. 500 mL =	_____ L	16. 0.75 L =	_____ mL
2. 0.015 g =	_____ mg	17. 5,000 mL =	_____ L
3. 8 mg =	_____ g	18. 1 L =	_____ mL
4. 10 mg =	_____ g	19. 1 g =	_____ mg
5. 60 mg =	_____ g	20. 3,000 mL =	_____ L
6. 300 mg =	_____ g	21. 23 mcg =	_____ mg
7. 0.2 g =	_____ mg	22. 1.05 g =	_____ kg
8. 1.2 g =	_____ mg	23. 18 mcg =	_____ mg
9. 0.0025 kg =	_____ g	24. 0.4 mg =	_____ mcg
10. 0.065 g =	_____ mg	25. 2,625 g =	_____ kg
11. 0.005 L =	_____ mL	26. 50 cm =	_____ m
12. 1.5 L =	_____ mL	27. 10 L =	_____ mL
13. 100 mcg =	_____ mg	28. 450 mL =	_____ L
14. 250 mL =	_____ L	29. 5 mL =	_____ L
15. 2 kg =	_____ g	30. 30 mg =	_____ mcg

After completing these problems, see page 509 to check your answers.

Approximate Equivalents

Fortunately, the use of the apothecary and household systems is becoming less and less frequent. However, the nurse must be familiar with conversions among the metric, apothecary, and household systems of measurement until they are obsolete.

Approximate equivalents are used for conversions from one system to another. More exact equivalents are not practical and, therefore, rarely used by health care workers. For example, the more exact equivalent of 1 gram as measured in grains is 1 gram = 15.432 grains. This is rounded to give the approximate equivalent of 1 g = gr 15 (xv). The more exact equivalent of one grain is 64.8 milligrams. This is rounded to give the approximate equivalent of gr i = 60 mg. This is the conversion most frequently used; however, there will be a few instances in calculations of some common oral medications (such as aspirin and iron) where gr i = 65 mg will be more convenient. This points out the true meaning of approximate equivalents.

Approximate equivalents that are used for dosage calculations are listed in the following Remember box. Learn the equivalents so that you can change from one system to another quickly and accurately. Commit the equivalents to memory. Review them often. When you learn these essential equivalents in addition to the other equivalents you learned in Chapter 3, you are on your way to mastering the skill of dosage calculations.

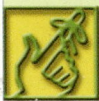

REMEMBER

Approximate Equivalents

1 g = gr xv

gr i = 60 mg or gr i = 65 mg (in select instances)

1 t = 5 mL

$1 T = 3 t = 15 mL = \frac{1}{2} fl oz$

1 fl oz = 30 mL = 6 t

1 L = 1 qt = 32 fl oz = 2 pt = 4 cups

1 pt = 500 mL = 16 fl oz = 2 cups

1 cup = 250 mL = 8 fl oz

1 kg = 2.2 lb

1 in = 2.5 cm

Look at the "Conversion Clock" (Figure 4-1) for an easy-to-remember method for converting between common metric and apothecary weight measures. It is based on the approximate equivalent of gr i = 60 mg, with 15 mg increments around the clock (similar to the 15 minute, 30 minute, 45 minute, and 60 minute increments equivalent to $\frac{1}{4}, \frac{1}{2}, \frac{3}{4}$, and 1 hour).

Figures 4-2 and 4-3 are visual aids that associate most of the base equivalents. You may find these diagrams easier to remember than the tables.

Look at the first triangle of weight equivalents (Figure 4-2). Beginning at the top of the triangle, use your finger to trace the arrow from g (gram) down to gr (grain). The arrow indicates that 1 g = gr xv (15). On the other side, trace down from g (gram) to mg (milligram). This arrow indicates that 1 g = 1,000 mg. Likewise, the bottom arrow goes from gr to mg to remind you that gr i = 60 mg. In summary, the triangle simply says:

1 g = gr xv, 1 g = 1,000 mg, and gr i = 60 mg

Look at the second triangle of volume equivalents (Figure 4-3). Beginning at the top of the triangle, use your finger to trace the arrow from fl oz (fluid ounce) down to t (teaspoon). The arrow indicates that 1 fl oz = 6 t. On the other side, trace down from fl oz (fluid ounce) to mL (milliliter). This arrow reminds you that 1 fl oz = 30 mL. Likewise, the bottom arrow goes from t (teaspoon) to mL (milliliter). This arrow reminds you that 1 t = 5 mL. In summary this triangle simply says:

1 fl oz = 6 t, 1 fl oz = 30 mL, and 1 t = 5 mL

FIGURE 4-1

Metric–Apothecary approximate equivalent "Conversion Clock"

DELMAR | Cengage Learning

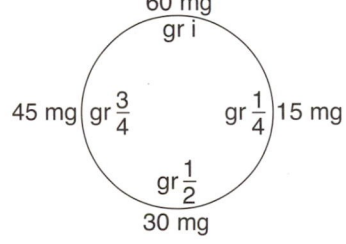

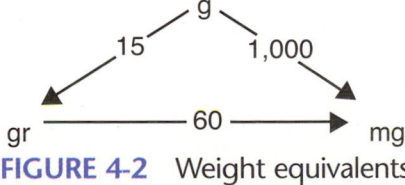

FIGURE 4-2 Weight equivalents

DELMAR | Cengage Learning

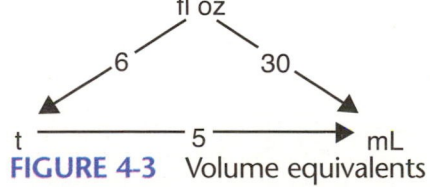

FIGURE 4-3 Volume equivalents

DELMAR | Cengage Learning

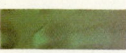

CONVERTING BETWEEN SYSTEMS OF MEASUREMENT

Now let's convert between systems of measurement using approximate equivalents. In the first four examples we will convert from a larger to a smaller unit of measure. Remember, the resulting number of smaller units should be greater than the original number of larger units.

EXAMPLE 1 ■

Convert 0.5 g to gr

Approximate equivalent: 1 g = gr xv = gr 15 (Let's use Arabic numbers for calculations.)

$$\frac{1\ g}{gr\ 15} \times \frac{0.5\ g}{gr\ X}$$

X = 15 × 0.5

X = gr 7.5

gr 7.5 = gr vii $\frac{1}{2}$

CAUTION

As is customary, the capital letter X is consistently used in this text to denote the unknown quantity in an equation and proportion. It is important that you do not confuse the unknown X with the value of gr x, which designates 10 grains.

EXAMPLE 2 ■

Convert: 2 fl oz to mL

Approximate equivalent: 1 fl oz = 30 mL

$$\frac{1\ fl\ oz}{30\ mL} \times \frac{2\ fl\ oz}{X\ mL}$$

X = 30 × 2

X = 60 mL

EXAMPLE 3 ■

Convert: gr $\frac{1}{300}$ to mg

Approximate equivalent: gr i = gr 1 = 60 mg

$$\frac{gr\ 1}{60\ mg} \times \frac{gr\ \frac{1}{300}}{X\ mg}$$

$$X = \frac{60}{1} \times \frac{1}{300} = \frac{60}{300} = \frac{1}{5} = 0.2$$

X = 0.2 mg   The answer must be a decimal fraction, because the unit of measure is the metric system.

EXAMPLE 4 ■

The scale weighs a child at 40 kilograms. The mother wants to know her child's weight in pounds.

Convert 40 kg to lb

Approximate equivalent: 1 kg = 2.2 lb

$$\frac{1\ kg}{2.2\ lb} \times \frac{40\ kg}{X\ lb}$$

X = 2.2 × 40

X = 88 lb

Use the same method to convert from a smaller to a larger unit of measure. Now the resulting number of larger units will be less than the original number of smaller units. Notice that the unknown is in the numerator. Remember to keep like units across from each other.

EXAMPLE 1 ■

Convert 120 mg to gr

Approximate equivalent: gr i = gr 1 = 60 mg

$$\frac{\text{gr } 1}{60 \text{ mg}} \quad \times \quad \frac{\text{gr } X}{120 \text{ mg}}$$

$$60 X = 120$$

$$\frac{60 X}{60} = \frac{120}{60}$$

$$X = \text{gr } 2 = \text{gr ii}$$

The final answer is written in lower case Roman numerals, because the unit of measure is apothecary.

EXAMPLE 2 ■

Convert 45 mL to t

Approximate equivalent: 1 t = 5 mL

$$\frac{1 \text{ t}}{5 \text{ mL}} \quad \times \quad \frac{X \text{ t}}{45 \text{ mL}}$$

$$5X = 45$$

$$\frac{5X}{5} = \frac{45}{5}$$

$$X = 9 \text{ t}$$

EXAMPLE 3 ■

Convert 66 lb to kg

Approximate equivalent: 1 kg = 2.2 lb

$$\frac{1 \text{ kg}}{2.2 \text{ lb}} \quad \times \quad \frac{X \text{ kg}}{66 \text{ lb}}$$

$$2.2 X = 66$$

$$\frac{2.2 X}{2.2} = \frac{66}{2.2}$$

$$X = 30 \text{ kg}$$

EXAMPLE 4 ■

Convert 40 cm to in (inches)

Approximate equivalent: 1 in = 2.5 cm

$$\frac{1 \text{ in}}{2.5 \text{ cm}} \quad \times \quad \frac{X \text{ in}}{40 \text{ cm}}$$

$$2.5 X = 40$$

$$\frac{2.5 X}{2.5} = \frac{40}{2.5}$$

$$X = 16 \text{ in}$$

MATH TIP

A clue to remember the approximate equivalent 1 kg = 2.2 lb is to realize that there are about 2 pounds for every kilogram, so the number of kilograms you weigh is about half the number of pounds you weigh. (This could almost make getting on a metric scale pleasant.)

Try this: Convert your weight in pounds to kilograms rounded to hundredths or two decimal places.

QUICK REVIEW

To use the ratio-proportion method to convert from one unit to another or between systems of measurement:

- Recall the equivalent.

- Set up a proportion: Ratio for known equivalent equals ratio for unknown equivalent.

- Label the units and match the units in the numerators and denominators.

- Cross-multiply to find the value of the unknown X equivalent.

- Label the units in the answer to match the unknown X.

Review Set 14

Convert each of the following amounts to the unit indicated. Indicate the approximate equivalent(s) used in the conversion. If rounding is necessary, round decimals to two places (hundredths).

		Approximate Equivalent				Approximate Equivalent
1. gr $\frac{1}{2}$ =		_____ mg _____		21. gr v =		_____ mg _____
2. gr $\frac{3}{4}$ =		_____ mg _____		22. 30 mg =	gr _____	_____
3. 3 g =		_____ kg _____		23. 1 pt =		_____ mL _____
4. gr $\frac{1}{150}$ =		_____ mg _____		24. gr x =		_____ mg _____
5. gr x =		_____ mg _____		25. 300 mg =	gr _____	_____
6. 15 mg =	gr _____	_____		26. 30 cm =		_____ in _____
7. 13 t =		_____ mL _____		27. 90 mg =	gr _____	_____
8. 15 mL =		_____ fl oz _____		28. 60 mL =		_____ fl oz _____
9. 2$\frac{1}{2}$ fl oz =		_____ mL _____		29. gr $\frac{1}{6}$ =		_____ mg _____
10. 750 mL =		_____ pt _____		30. 65 mg =	gr _____	_____
11. 20 mL =		_____ t _____		31. 32 in =		_____ cm _____
12. 4 T =		_____ mL _____		32. 350 mm =		_____ in _____
13. 9 kg =		_____ lb _____		33. 7.5 cm =		_____ in _____
14. 250 lb =		_____ kg _____		34. 2 in =		_____ mm _____
15. 3 L =		_____ fl oz _____		35. 40 kg =		_____ lb _____
16. 55 kg =		_____ lb _____		36. 7.16 kg =		_____ g _____
17. 12 in =		_____ cm _____		37. 110 lb =		_____ kg _____
18. 2 qt =		_____ L _____		38. 3.5 kg =		_____ lb _____
19. 3 t =		_____ mL _____		39. 63 lb =		_____ kg _____
20. 99 lb =		_____ kg _____				

40. A newborn infant is 21$\frac{1}{2}$ inches long. Her length is _____ cm.

41. The label for a granular medicine recommends mixing it with at least 120 mL of water or juice. At the time of discharge, the nurse should advise the patient to mix the medicine with _____ fluid ounce(s) or _____ cup(s) of water or juice.

42. A patient who weighs 250 lb starts a weight loss program with a goal of losing 10 lb before the next doctor's appointment. At the next office visit the patient is weighed at 108 kg. Has the patient met the weight loss goal? _____

43. Calculate the total fluid intake in mL for 24 hours.

Breakfast	8 fluid ounces milk
	6 fluid ounces orange juice
	4 fluid ounces water with medication
Lunch	8 fluid ounces iced tea
Snack	10 fluid ounces coffee
	4 fluid ounces gelatin dessert
Dinner	8 fluid ounces water
	6 fluid ounces tomato juice
	6 fluid ounces beef broth
Snack	5 fluid ounces pudding
	12 fluid ounces diet soda
	4 fluid ounces water with medication

Total = _____ mL

44. A child who weighs 55 lb is to receive 0.05 mg of a drug per kg of body weight per dose. How much of the drug should the child receive for each dose? _____ mg

45. A child is taking 12 mL of a medication 4 times per day. If the full bottle contains 16 fluid ounces of the medication, how many days will the bottle last? _____ day(s)

46. The doctor prescribes 10 mL of Betadine concentrate in 500 mL of warm water as a soak for a finger infection. Using measures commonly found in the home, how would you instruct the patient to prepare the solution? _____

47. The patient is to receive 10 mL of a drug. How many teaspoonsful should the patient take? _____ t

48. An infant is taking a ready-to-feed formula. The formula comes in quart containers. If the infant usually takes 4 fluid ounces of formula every 3 hours during the day and night, how many quarts of formula should the mother buy for a 3 day supply? _____ qt

49. An infant's head circumference is 40 cm. The parents ask for the equivalent in inches. You tell the parents their infant's head circumference is _____ in.

50. The patient tells you he was weighed in the doctor's office and was told he is 206 pounds. What is his weight in kilograms? _____ kg

After completing these problems, see pages 509–511 to check your answers.

SUMMARY

At this point, you should be quite familiar with the equivalents for converting within the metric, apothecary, and household systems and from one system to another. From memory, you should be able to recall quickly and accurately the equivalents for conversions. If you are having difficulty understanding the concept of converting from one unit of measurement to another, review this chapter and seek additional help from your instructor.

Consider the two Critical Thinking Skills scenarios and work the practice problems for Chapter 4. Concentrate on accuracy. One error can be a serious mistake when calculating the dosages of medicines or performing critical measurements of health status.

CRITICAL THINKING SKILLS

ERROR
Incorrectly interpreting grains as grams.

Possible Scenario

A physician ordered a single dose of **15 grains of aspirin** for a patient complaining of a severe headache. Aspirin was available in *500 mg aspirin tablets*. While preparing the medication, the nurse was distracted by a visitor who fell by the nurses' station. The nurse returned to read the order as *1.5 grams* and calculated the dose this way:

If: 1 g = 1,000 mg and 0.5 g = 0.5 g̸ × 1,000 mg/g̸ = 500 mg
then: 1.5 g = 1,000 mg + 500 mg = 1,500 mg, so the patient was given 3 tablets.   **INCORRECT**

You know that 15 grains is equivalent to 1 g or 1,000 mg. By misreading the dose, the nurse gave 500 mg more than ordered, overdosing the patient.

Potential Outcome

The patient received $1\frac{1}{2}$ times, or 150%, of the dosage ordered. This larger dose, 1,500 mg, could cause nausea, heartburn, and gastrointestinal upset. In aspirin-sensitive patients it could result in gastrointestinal bleeding.

Prevention

This type of medication error is avoided by carefully checking the drug order at least three times: before preparing a medication, once the dose is prepared, and prior to giving the patient the medication. Also, the nurse should recognize that the ordered dose is in apothecary measurement, whereas the supply dosage is in metric measurement, and carefully convert between systems.

PRACTICE PROBLEMS—CHAPTER 4

Give the following equivalents without consulting conversion tables. If rounding is necessary, round decimals to two places (hundredths).

1. 0.5 g = _____ mg

2. 0.01 g = _____ mg

3. 7.5 mL = _____ L

4. 3 qt = _____ L

5. 4 mg = _____ mcg

6. 500 mL = _____ L

7. 250 mL = _____ pt

8. 300 g = _____ kg

9. 28 in = _____ cm

10. 68 kg = _____ lb

11. gr iii = _____ mg

12. $3\frac{1}{2}$ fl oz = _____ mL

13. gr $\frac{1}{200}$ = _____ mg

14. gr $\frac{1}{4}$ = _____ mg

15. gr $\frac{1}{10}$ = _____ mg

16. gr i $\frac{1}{2}$ = _____ mg

17. $70\frac{1}{2}$ lb = _____ kg

18. 3,634 g = _____ lb

19. 8 mL = _____ L

20. 450 mg = _____ g

21. 237.5 cm = _____ in

22. 0.5 g = _____ mg

23. 0.6 mg = _____ mcg

24. gr x = _____ g

CRITICAL THINKING SKILLS

ERROR

Not moving the correct amount of decimal spaces when using the shortcut method to divide by a power of 10.

Possible Scenario

A physician ordered **125 mcg of digoxin** to be administered daily for a patient treated for congestive heart failure. Supplied were scored tablets in individual packages labeled 0.25 mg per tablet. The conversion needed was mg to mcg, a larger unit to a smaller unit. The nurse remembered that to convert from a larger unit to a smaller unit you multiply by the conversion factor. The nurse also knew that 1,000 mcg = 1 mg and that the conversion factor was 1,000 mcg/mg. But in a hurry, the nurse forgot to add a zero to create the correct amount of decimal spaces and incorrectly figured the problem this way:

$$0.25 \times 1,000 = 0.25. = 25 \text{ mcg} \qquad \textbf{INCORRECT}$$

The nurse then reasoned, "If the physician's order was 125 mcg, then with 25 mcg tablets on hand, the patient must need 5 tablets because 5 tablets of 25 mcg each equal 125 mcg." The nurse started to administer the 5 tablets but hesitated because it seemed like a large number of tablets. The nurse asked a fellow nurse to double-check the calculations. The second nurse found the error.

The **correct** conversion is:

$$0.25 \times 1,000 = 0.250. = 250 \text{ mcg}$$

The patient should receive $\frac{1}{2}$ tablet, not 5 tablets.

Potential Outcome

Digoxin is a high-alert cardiac medication that may lead to serious adverse reactions at toxic levels. If this nurse proceeded with the incorrect amount, the patient would have received 10 times the normal dose and very likely would have had serious complications, such as severe bradycardia or cardiac arrhythmias.

Prevention

Fortunately the error was caught and the patient was given the correct amount, which was $\frac{1}{2}$ tablet. An error was prevented because the nurse stopped to consider, "Does this make sense?" After every dosage calculation, ask if the answer makes sense. If still in doubt, especially with high-alert medications, ask another nurse to double-check your thinking and the calculation.

25. 150 lb =	_____ kg		36. 1.5 g =	_____ mg
26. 60 mg =	gr _____		37. $1\frac{1}{2}$ fl oz =	_____ mL
27. 22 lb =	_____ kg		38. 1,500 mL =	_____ qt
28. 2 cups =	_____ mL		39. 10 mg =	gr _____
29. 6 t =	_____ T		40. 25 mg =	_____ g
30. 90 mL =	_____ fl oz		41. 4.3 kg =	_____ g
31. 375 mcg =	_____ mg		42. 60 mg =	_____ g
32. 2 T =	_____ mL		43. 0.015 g =	_____ mg
33. 2.2 lb =	_____ kg		44. 45 mL =	_____ T
34. 5 mL =	_____ t		45. 0.25 mg =	_____ mcg
35. 1,000 mL =	_____ L			

46. As a camp nurse for 9- to 12-year-old children, you are administering $2\frac{1}{2}$ teaspoons of oral liquid Children's Tylenol to 6 feverish campers every 4 hours for oral temperatures above 100°F. You have on hand a 4 fluid ounce bottle of liquid Children's Tylenol. How many complete or full doses are available from this bottle? _____ full doses

47. At this same camp, the standard dosage of Pepto-Bismol for 9- to 12-year-old children is 1 tablespoon. How many full doses are available in a 120 mL bottle? _____ full doses

48. Calculate the total fluid intake in mL of this clear liquid lunch:

apple juice	4 fluid ounces
chicken broth	8 fluid ounces
gelatin dessert	6 fluid ounces
hot tea	10 fluid ounces
TOTAL =	_____ mL

49. An ampule contains 10 mg of morphine. The doctor orders **morphine gr $\frac{1}{6}$ intravenously every 4 hours as needed for pain**. How much of the solution in the ampule should the patient receive for 1 dose? _____

50. Describe the strategy to prevent this medication error.

    Possible Scenario

    An attending physician ordered **Claforan 2 g intravenously immediately** for a patient with a leg abscess. The supply dosage available is *1,000 mg per 10 mL*. The nurse was in a rush to give the medication and calculated the dose this way:

            If: 1 g = 1,000 mg

            then: 2 g = 1,000 ÷ 2 = 500 mg per 5 mL

    Then the nurse administered 5 mL of the available Claforan.

    Potential Outcome

    The patient received only $\frac{1}{4}$, or 25%, of the dosage ordered. The patient should have received 2,000 mg, or 20 mL, of Claforan. The leg abscess could progress to osteomyelitis (a severe bone infection) or septicemia (a blood infection) because of underdosage.

    Prevention

    _____

    _____

    After completing these problems, see page 511 to check your answers.

REFERENCE

The Joint Commission. (2005). *Additional abbreviations, acronyms and symbols (for possible future inclusion in the official "do not use" list).* Retrieved September 25, 2009, from http://www.jointcommission.org/PatientSafety/DoNotUseList/

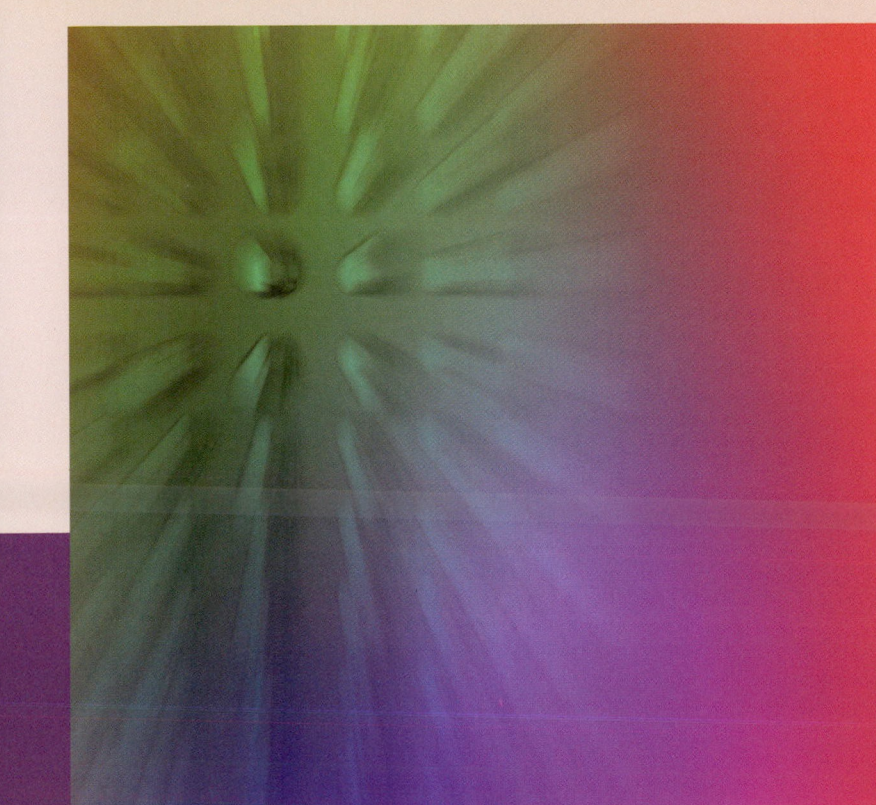
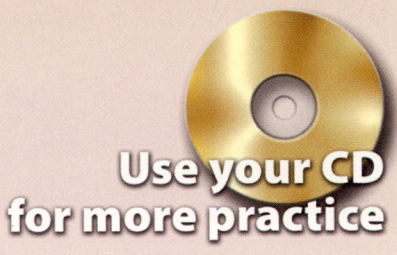

Use your CD for more practice

5

Conversions for Other Clinical Applications: Time and Temperature

OBJECTIVES

Upon mastery of Chapter 5, you will be able to:

- Convert between traditional and international time.
- Convert between Celsius and Fahrenheit temperature.

This chapter focuses on two other conversions applied in health care. *Time* is an essential part of the drug order. *Temperature* is an important measurement of health status.

CONVERTING BETWEEN TRADITIONAL AND INTERNATIONAL TIME

It is becoming increasingly popular in health care settings to keep time with a more straightforward system using the 24-hour clock. In use around the world and in the U.S. military for many years, this system is known as *international time* or *military time*.

Look at the 24-hour clock (Figure 5-1). Each time designation is comprised of a unique four-digit number. Notice there is an inner and outer circle of numbers that identify the hours from 0100 to 2400. The inside numbers correlate to traditional AM time (midnight to 11:59 AM)—time periods

FIGURE 5-1 24-hour clock depicting 0015 (12:15 AM) and 1215 (12:15 PM)

DELMAR | Cengage Learning

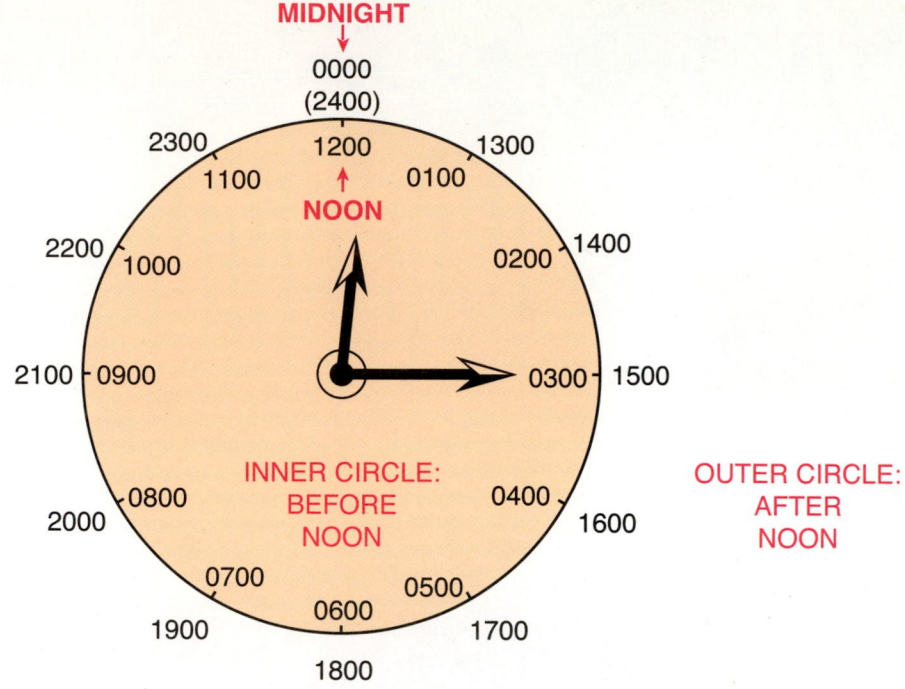

that are ante meridian or before noon. The outside numbers correlate to traditional PM time (noon to 11:59 PM)—time periods that are post meridian or after noon.

Hours on the 24-hour clock after 0059 minutes (zero-zero fifty-nine) are stated in hundreds. The word *zero* precedes single-digit hours.

EXAMPLE 1 ■

0400 is stated as *zero four hundred*.

EXAMPLE 2 ■

1600 is stated as *sixteen hundred*.

Between each hour, the time is read simply as the hour and the number of minutes, preceded by zero as needed.

EXAMPLE 1 ■

0421 is stated as *zero four twenty-one*.

EXAMPLE 2 ■

1659 is stated as *sixteen fifty-nine*.

The minutes between 2400 (midnight) and 0100 (1:00 AM) are written as 0001, 0002, 0003 . . . 0058, 0059. Each zero is stated before stating the number of minutes.

EXAMPLE 1 ■

0009 is stated as *zero-zero-zero nine*.

EXAMPLE 2 ■

0014 is stated as *zero-zero fourteen*.

Midnight can be written two different ways in international time:

■ 2400 and read as *twenty-four hundred*, or

■ 0000 (used by the military) and read as *zero hundred*.

Use of the 24-hour clock decreases the possibility for error in administering medications and documenting time because no two times are expressed by the same number. There is less chance for misinterpreting time using the 24-hour clock.

EXAMPLE 1 ■

13 minutes after 1 AM is written *0113*.

EXAMPLE 2 ■

13 minutes after 1 PM is written *1313*.

FIGURE 5-2 Comparison of traditional and international time

DELMAR | Cengage Learning

AM	Int'l. Time		PM	Int'l. Time
12:00 midnight	2400		12:00 noon	1200
1:00	0100		1:00	1300
2:00	0200		2:00	1400
3:00	0300		3:00	1500
4:00	0400		4:00	1600
5:00	0500		5:00	1700
6:00	0600		6:00	1800
7:00	0700		7:00	1900
8:00	0800		8:00	2000
9:00	0900		9:00	2100
10:00	1000		10:00	2200
11:00	1100		11:00	2300

The same cannot be said for traditional time. The AM or PM notations are the only things that differentiate traditional times.

EXAMPLE 1 ■

13 minutes after 1 AM is written *1:13 AM*

EXAMPLE 2 ■

13 minutes after 1 PM is written *1:13 PM*

Careless notation in a medical order or in patient records can create misinterpretation about when a therapy is due or actually occurred. Figure 5-2 shows the comparison of traditional and international time. Notice that international time is less ambiguous.

RULES

1. Traditional time and international time are the same hours starting with 1:00 AM (0100) through 12:59 PM (1259).

2. Minutes after 12:00 AM (midnight) and before 1:00 AM are 0001 through 0059 in international time.

3. Hours starting with 1:00 PM through 12:00 AM (midnight) are 12:00 hours greater in international time (1300 through 2400).

4. International time is designated by a unique four-digit number.

5. The hour(s) and minute(s) are separated by a colon in traditional time, but no colon is typically used in international time. However, you may see international time represented with a colon, such as 14:00 for 1400 (for 2:00 PM) and so forth.

MATH TIP

Between the hours of 1:00 PM (1300) and 12:00 AM (2400), add 1200 to traditional time to find equivalent international time; subtract 1200 from international time to convert to equivalent traditional time.

Let's apply these rules to convert between the two time systems.

EXAMPLE 1 ■

3:00 PM = 3:00 + 12:00 = 1500

EXAMPLE 2 ■

2212 = 2212 − 1200 = 10:12 PM

EXAMPLE 3 ■

12:45 AM = 0045

EXAMPLE 4 ■

0004 = 12:04 AM

EXAMPLE 5 ■

0130 = 1:30 AM

EXAMPLE 6 ■

11:00 AM = 1100

QUICK REVIEW

■ International time is designated by 0001 through 1259 for 12:01 AM through 12:59 PM and 1300 through 2400 for 1:00 PM through 12:00 midnight.

■ The hours from 1:00 PM through 12:00 midnight are 12:00 hours greater in international time (1300 through 2400).

Review Set 15

Convert international time to traditional AM/PM time.

1. 0032 = _____

2. 0730 = _____

3. 1640 = _____

4. 2121 = _____

5. 2359 = _____

6. 1215 = _____

7. 0220 = _____

8. 1010 = _____

9. 1315 = _____

10. 1825 = _____

Convert traditional to international time.

11. 1:30 PM = _____

12. 12:04 AM = _____

13. 9:45 PM = _____

14. 12:00 noon = _____

15. 11:15 PM = _____

16. 3:45 AM = _____

17. 12:00 midnight = _____

18. 3:30 PM = _____

19. 6:20 AM = _____

20. 5:45 PM = _____

Fill in the blanks by writing out the words as indicated.

21. 24-hour time 0623 is stated _____.

22. 24-hour time 0041 is stated _____.

23. 24-hour time 1903 is stated _____.

24. 24-hour time 2311 is stated _____.

25. 24-hour time 0300 is stated _____.

After completing these problems, see page 512 to check your answers.

CONVERTING BETWEEN CELSIUS AND FAHRENHEIT TEMPERATURE

Another important conversion in health care involves Celsius and Fahrenheit temperatures. Simple formulas are used for converting between the two temperature scales. It is easier to remember the formulas when you understand how they were developed.

The Fahrenheit (F) scale establishes the freezing point of pure water at 32° and the boiling point of pure water at 212°. The Celsius (C) scale establishes the freezing point of pure water at 0° and the boiling point of pure water at 100°.

FIGURE 5-3 Comparison of Celsius and Fahrenheit temperature scales

DELMAR | Cengage Learning

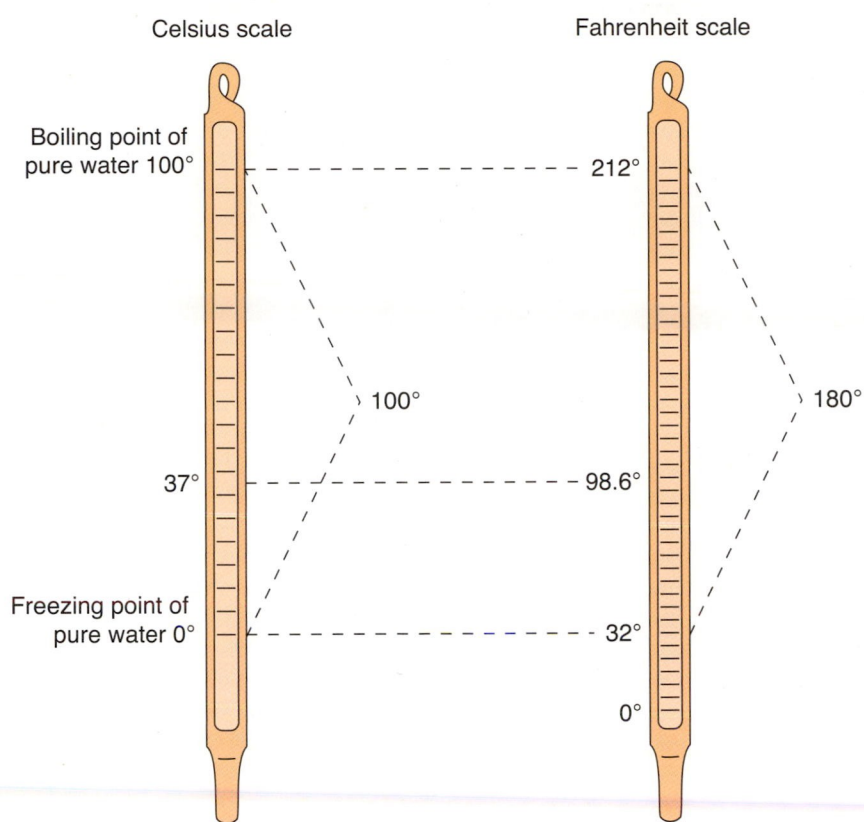

°C	°F
40.6	105.1
40.4	104.7
40.2	104.4
40.0	104.0
39.8	103.6
39.6	103.3
39.4	102.9
39.2	102.6
39.0	102.2
38.8	101.8
38.6	101.5
38.4	101.1
38.2	100.8
38.0	100.4
37.8	100.0
37.6	99.7
37.4	99.3
37.2	99.0
37.0	**98.6**
36.0	96.8
35.0	95.0
34.0	93.2
33.0	91.4

NOTE: Glass thermometers pictured in Figure 5-3 are for demonstration purposes. Electronic digital temperature devices are more commonly used in health care settings. Most electronic devices can instantly convert between the two scales, freeing the health care provider from doing the actual calculations. However, the health care provider's ability to understand the difference between Celsius and Fahrenheit remains important.

Look at Figure 5-3. Note that there is 180° difference between the boiling and freezing points on the Fahrenheit thermometer and 100° between the boiling and freezing points on the Celsius thermometer. The ratio of the difference between the Fahrenheit and Celsius scales can be expressed as 180:100 or $\frac{180}{100}$. When reduced, this ratio is equivalent to 1.8. You will use this constant in temperature conversions.

The range of body temperatures seen in health care situations is usually limited to those that are compatible with life, so it is practical to keep a chart handy that lists potential equivalent temperatures (Figure 5-4). You will find it helpful to memorize Celsius and Fahrenheit normal body temperature

Normal body temperature

FIGURE 5-4 Comparison of Celsius and Fahrenheit body temperature scales

DELMAR | Cengage Learning

and some other commonly reported ones (as highlighted on the body temperature chart) for quick conversions.

To convert between Fahrenheit and Celsius temperature, formulas have been developed based on the differences between the freezing and boiling points on each scale.

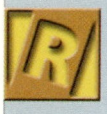

RULE

To convert a given Fahrenheit temperature to Celsius, first subtract 32 and then divide the result by 1.8.

$$°C = \frac{°F - 32}{1.8}$$

EXAMPLE ■

Convert 98.6°F to °C

$$°C = \frac{98.6 - 32}{1.8}$$

$$°C = \frac{66.6}{1.8}$$

$$°C = 37°$$

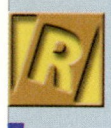

RULE

To convert Celsius temperature to Fahrenheit, multiply by 1.8 and add 32.
$$°F = 1.8°C + 32$$

EXAMPLE ■

Convert 35°C to °F

$$°F = 1.8 \times 35 + 32$$

$$°F = 63 + 32$$

$$°F = 95°$$

QUICK REVIEW

Use these formulas to convert between Fahrenheit and Celsius temperatures:

■ $°C = \frac{°F - 32}{1.8}$

■ $°F = 1.8°C + 32$

Review Set 16

Convert these temperatures as indicated. Round your answers to tenths.

1. 100.4°F = _____ °C   3. 36.2°C = _____ °F

2. 38.4°C = _____ °F   4. 32°C = _____ °F

5. 98.6°F = _____ °C   11. 100°F = _____ °C

6. 99°F = _____ °C   12. 39°C = _____ °F

7. 103.6°F = _____ °C   13. 37.4°C = _____ °F

8. 40°C = _____ °F   14. 94.2°F = _____ °C

9. 38.9°C = _____ °F   15. 102.8°F = _____ °C

10. 36.4°C = _____ °F

For each of the following statements, convert the given temperature in °F or °C to its corresponding equivalent in °C or °F.

16. An infant has a body temperature of 95.5°F.   _____ °C

17. Store the vaccine serum at 7°C.   _____ °F

18. Do not expose medication to temperatures greater than 88°F.   _____ °C

19. Normal body temperature is 37°C.   _____ °F

20. If Mr. Rose's temperature is greater than 103.5°F, call MD.   _____ °C

After completing these problems, see page 512 to check your answers.

CRITICAL THINKING SKILLS

ERROR

Incorrect interpretation of an order because of a misunderstanding of traditional time.

Possible Scenario

A physician ordered a mild sedative for an anxious patient who is scheduled for a sigmoidoscopy in the morning. The order read *Valium 5 mg orally at 6:00 X 1 dose.* The evening nurse interpreted that single-dose order to be scheduled for 6 o'clock PM along with the enema and other preparations to be given to the patient. The doctor meant for the Valium to be given at 6 o'clock AM to help the patient relax prior to the actual test.

Potential Outcome

Valium would help the patient relax during the enema and make the patient sleepy. But it is not desirable for the patient to be drowsy or sedated during the evening preparations. Because of the omission of the AM designation, the patient would not benefit from this mild sedative at the intended time, just before the test. The patient would have likely experienced unnecessary anxiety both before and during the test.

Prevention

This scenario emphasizes the benefit of the 24-hour clock. If international time had been in use at this facility, the order would have been written as *Valium 5 mg orally at 0600 X 1 dose* clearly indicating the exact time of administration. *Be careful to verify AM and PM times if your facility uses traditional time.*

PRACTICE PROBLEMS—CHAPTER 5

Give the following time equivalents as indicated.

AM/PM Clock	24-Hour Clock	AM/PM Clock	24-Hour Clock
1. _____	0257	11. 7:31 PM	_____
2. 3:10 AM	_____	12. 12:00 midnight	_____
3. 4:22 PM	_____	13. 6:45 AM	_____
4. _____	2001	14. _____	0915
5. _____	1102	15. _____	2107
6. 12:33 AM	_____	16. _____	1823
7. 2:16 AM	_____	17. _____	0540
8. _____	1642	18. 11:55 AM	_____
9. _____	2356	19. 10:12 PM	_____
10. 4:20 AM	_____	20. 9:06 PM	_____

Find the length of each time interval for questions 21 through 30.

21. 0200 to 0600	_____	26. 2316 to 0328	_____
22. 1100 to 1800	_____	27. 8:22 AM to 1:10 PM	_____
23. 1500 to 2330	_____	28. 4:35 PM to 8:16 PM	_____
24. 0935 to 2150	_____	29. 1:00 AM to 7:30 AM	_____
25. 0003 to 1453	_____		

30. 10:05 AM Friday to 2:43 AM Saturday _____

31. True or False? The 24-hour clock is imprecise and not suited to health care. _____

32. Indicate whether these international times would be AM or PM when converted to traditional time.

    a. 1030 _____   c. 0158 _____

    b. 1920 _____   d. 1230 _____

Give the following temperature equivalents as indicated.

33. 99.6°F	_____ °C	41. 97.8°F	_____ °C
34. 36.5°C	_____ °F	42. 35.4°C	_____ °F
35. 39.2°C	_____ °F	43. 103.5°F	_____ °C
36. 100.2°F	_____ °C	44. 39°C	_____ °F
37. 98°F	_____ °C	45. 36.9°C	_____ °F
38. 37.4°C	_____ °F	46. 101.4°F	_____ °C
39. 38.2°C	_____ °F	47. 97.2°F	_____ °C
40. 104°F	_____ °C		

48. Four temperature readings in °C for Mrs. Baskin are 37.6, 35.5, 38.1, and 37.6. Find her average (or mean) °C temperature and convert it to °F. _____ °C _____ °F

49. True or False? The freezing and boiling points of pure water on the Fahrenheit and Celsius temperature scales were used to develop the conversion formulas. _____

50. Describe the strategy you would implement to prevent this conversion error.

Possible Scenario

A student nurse takes a child's temperature and finds that it is 38.2°C. The child's mother asks what that equates to in Fahrenheit temperature. The student nurse does a quick calculation in her head and multiplies 38° by 2 and adds 32 because she recalls the conversion constant is 1.8 and 2 is close enough. The student nurse tells the mother, "Well, about 108°." The mother replies, "I hope not" and smiles.

Potential Outcome

The student nurse immediately recognizes that she made an error and feels embarrassed. The mother could have become alarmed and experienced undue anxiety and a loss of confidence in the student nurse. The correct temperature measurement is 100.8°F. Fever-reducing medical orders often vary the dosage depending on the severity of the elevated temperature. An incorrect conversion could result in over- or under-medication of the child.

Prevention

_____

_____

After completing these problems, see page 512 to check your answers.

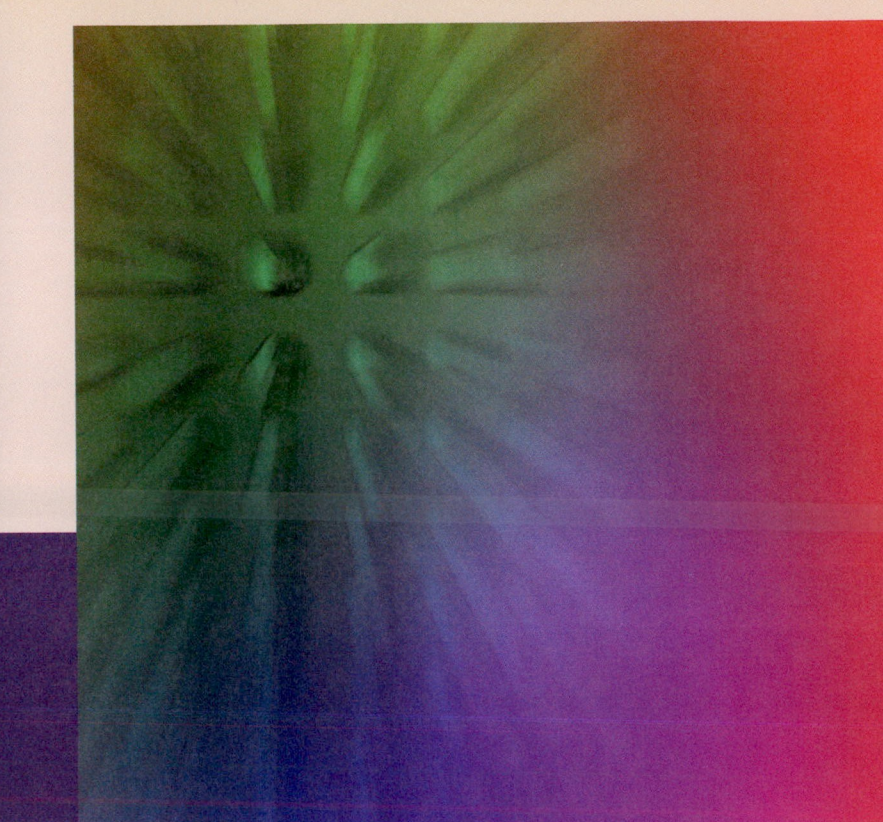
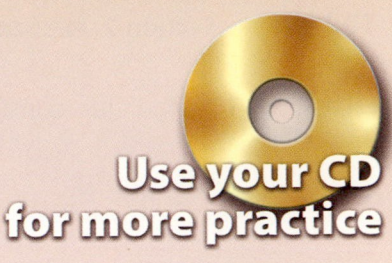

6

Equipment Used in Dosage Measurement

OBJECTIVES

Upon mastery of Chapter 6, you will be able to correctly measure the prescribed dosages that you calculate. To accomplish this, you will also be able to:

- Recognize and select the appropriate equipment for the medication, dosage, and method of administration ordered.
- Read and interpret the calibrations of each utensil presented.

N ow that you are familiar with the systems of measurement used in the calculation of dosages, let's take a look at the common measuring utensils. In this chapter you will learn to recognize and read the calibrations of devices used in both oral and parenteral (other than gastrointestinal) administration. The oral utensils include the medicine cup, pediatric oral devices, and calibrated droppers. The parenteral devices include the 3 mL syringe, prefilled syringe, a variety of insulin syringes, 1 mL syringe, and special safety and intravenous syringes.

ORAL ADMINISTRATION

Medicine Cup

Figure 6-1 shows three views of the 30 milliliter or 1 fluid ounce medicine cup that is used to measure most liquids for oral administration. Two views are presented to show all of the scales. Notice that the approximate equivalents of the metric, apothecary, and household systems of measurement are indicated

FIGURE 6-1   Medicine cup (three views) with approximate equivalent measures

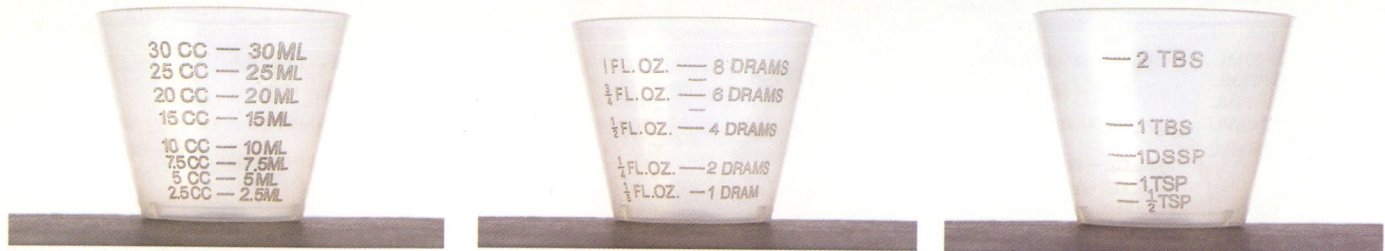

DELMAR | Cengage Learning

on the cup. The medicine cup can serve as a great study aid to help you learn the volume equivalents of the three systems of measurement. Look at the calibrations for milliliters, cubic centimeters, teaspoons, tablespoons, fluid ounces, and drams. As you fill the cup, you can see that 30 milliliters equal 1 fluid ounce, 5 milliliters equal 1 teaspoon, and so forth. Dram, a unit of measurement in the apothecary system, is no longer used but may still appear on medicine cups. For volumes less than 2.5 mL, a smaller, more accurate device should be used (see Figures 6-2, 6-3, and 6-4).

Calibrated Dropper

Figure 6-2 shows the calibrated dropper, which is used to administer some small quantities. A dropper is used when giving medicine to children and the elderly and when adding small amounts of liquid to water or juice. Eye and ear medications are also dispensed from a medicine dropper or squeeze drop bottle.

The amount of the drop varies according to the diameter of the hole at the tip of the dropper. For this reason, a properly calibrated dropper usually accompanies the medicine (Figure 6-3). It is calibrated according to the way that drug is prescribed. The calibrations are usually given in milliliters or drops.

FIGURE 6-2   Calibrated dropper

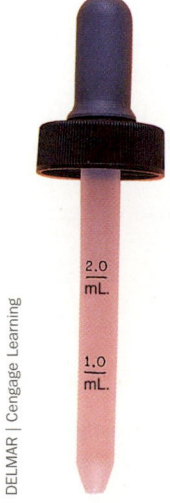

DELMAR | Cengage Learning

FIGURE 6-3   Furosemide Oral Solution label

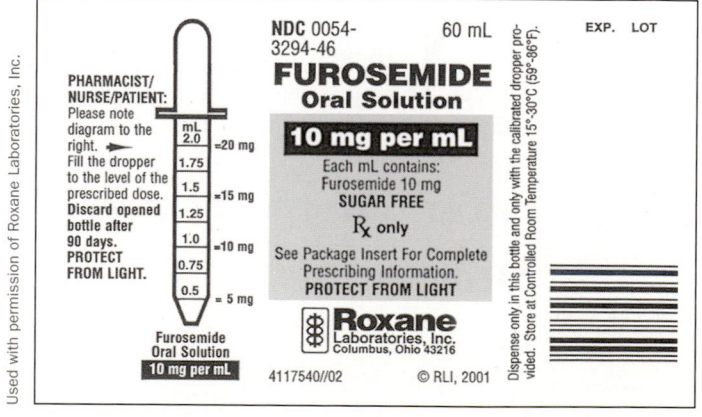

Used with permission of Roxane Laboratories, Inc.

CAUTION
To be safe, never exchange packaged droppers between medications because drop size varies from one dropper to another.

FIGURE 6-4 Devices for administering oral medications to children

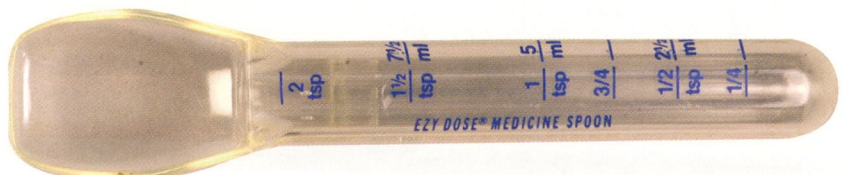

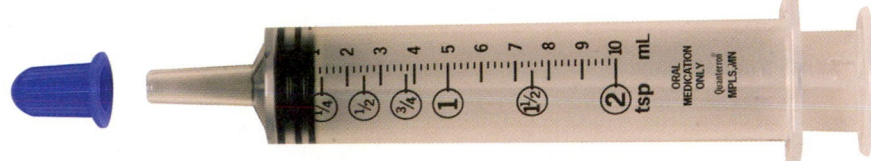

DELMAR | Cengage Learning

Pediatric Oral Devices

Various types of calibrated equipment are available to administer oral medications to children. Two devices intended only for oral use are shown in Figure 6-4. Parents and child caregivers should be taught to always use calibrated devices when administering medications to children. Household spoons vary in size and are not reliable for accurate dosing.

CAUTION
To be safe, do not use syringes intended for injections in the administration of oral medications. Confusion about the route of administration may occur.

You can distinguish oral from parenteral syringes in two ways. Syringes intended for oral use typically do not have a luerlock hub (see Figure 6-6). They also usually have a cap on the tip that must be removed before administering the medication. Syringes intended for parenteral use have a luerlock hub that allows a needle to be secured tightly.

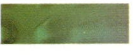

PARENTERAL ADMINISTRATION

The term *parenteral* is used to designate routes of administration other than gastrointestinal. However, in this text, parenteral always means injection routes.

3 mL Syringe

Figure 6-5 shows a 3 mL syringe assembled with needle unit. The parts of the syringe are identified in Figure 6-6. Notice that the black rubber tip of the suction plunger is visible. The nurse pulls back on the plunger to withdraw the medicine from the storage container. *The calibrations are read from the top black ring, NOT the raised middle section and NOT the bottom ring.* Look closely at the metric scale in

Figure 6-5, which is calibrated in milliliters (mL) for each tenth (0.1) of a milliliter. Each $\frac{1}{2}$ (or 0.5) milliliter is marked up to the maximum volume of 3 milliliters.

Standardized to the syringe calibrations, standard drug dosages of 1 mL or greater can be rounded to the nearest tenth (0.1) of a mL and measured on the mL scale. Refer to Chapter 1 to review the rules of decimal rounding. For example, 1.45 mL is rounded to 1.5 mL. Notice that the colored liquid in Figure 6-5 identifies 1.5 mL.

FIGURE 6-5   3 mL syringe with needle unit measuring 1.5 mL

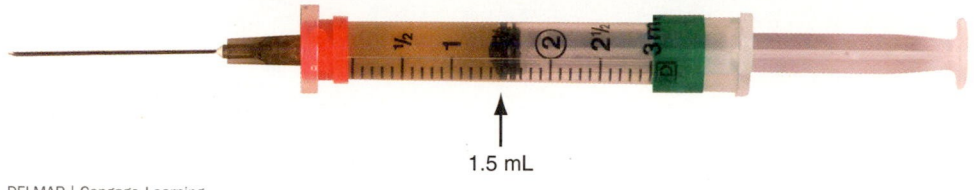

1.5 mL

DELMAR | Cengage Learning

FIGURE 6-6   3 mL syringe with needle unit measuring 2 mL

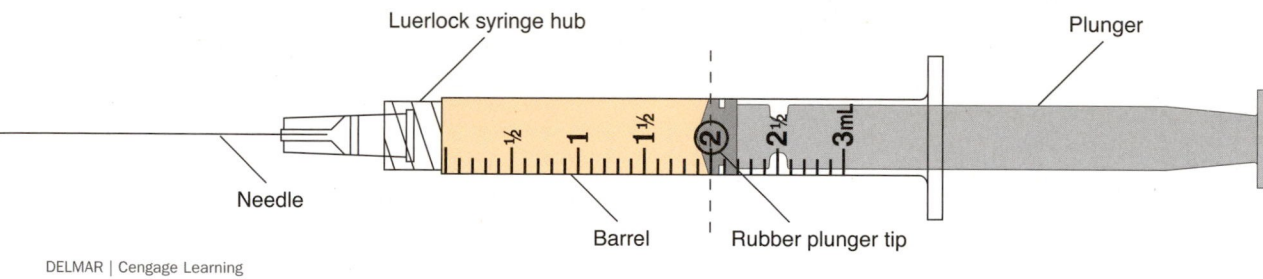

Luerlock syringe hub

Plunger

Needle

Barrel

Rubber plunger tip

DELMAR | Cengage Learning

Prefilled, Single-Dose Syringe

Figure 6-7 is an example of a *prefilled, single-dose syringe.* Such syringes contain the usual single dose of a medication and are to be used only once. The syringe is discarded after the single use.

If you are to give *less* than the full single dose of a drug provided in a prefilled, single-dose syringe, you should discard the extra amount *before* injecting the patient.

EXAMPLE ■

The drug order prescribes 100 mg of medroxyprogesterone acetate to be administered to a patient. You have a prefilled, single-dose syringe containing 150 mg per mL of solution (as in Figure 6-7). You would discard 50 mg of the drug solution; then 100 mg would remain in the syringe. You will learn more about calculating drug dosages beginning in Chapter 10. (Some medications, such as controlled substances, require another nurse to observe discarding the unused portion.)

FIGURE 6-7   Prefilled, single-dose syringe

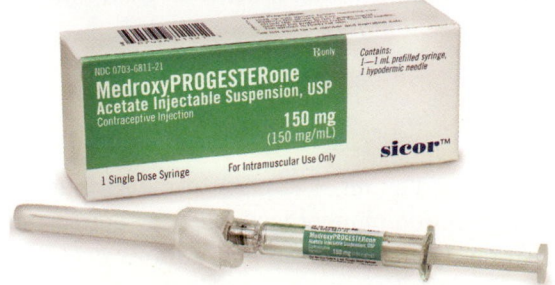

Courtesy of Roche Laboratories, Inc.

Insulin Syringe

Figure 6-8(a) shows both sides of a standard U-100 insulin syringe. This syringe is to be used for the measurement and administration of U-100 insulin *only*. It must not be used to measure other medications that are measured in units.

CAUTION

U-100 insulin should only be measured in a U-100 insulin syringe. U-100 insulin concentration is 100 units of insulin per mL.

Notice that Figure 6-8(a) pictures one side of the insulin syringe calibrated in odd-number two-unit increments and the other side calibrated in even-number two-unit increments. The plunger in Figure 6-9(a) simulates the measurement of 70 units of U-100 insulin. It is important to note that for U-100 insulin, 100 units equal 1 mL.

FIGURE 6-8 Insulin syringes (a) front and reverse of a standard U-100 insulin syringe; (b) Lo-Dose U-100 insulin syringes, 50 and 30 units

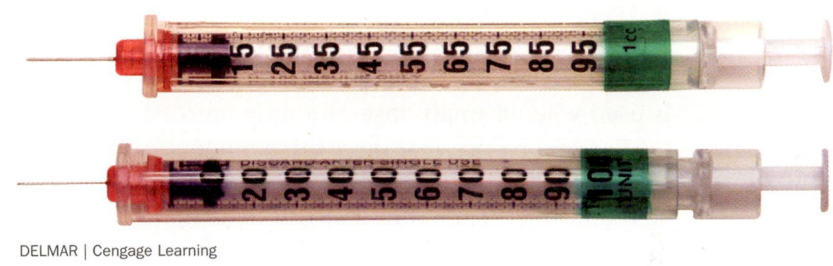

DELMAR | Cengage Learning

(a)

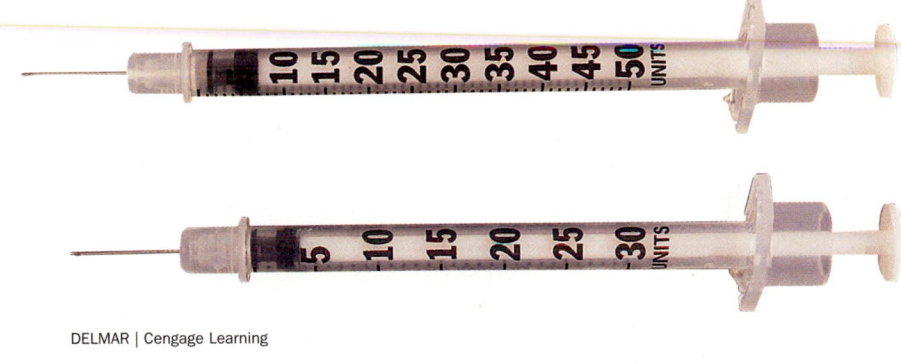

DELMAR | Cengage Learning

(b)

FIGURE 6-9 (a) Standard U-100 insulin syringe measuring 70 units of U-100 insulin; (b) Lo-Dose U-100 insulin syringe measuring 19 units of U-100 insulin

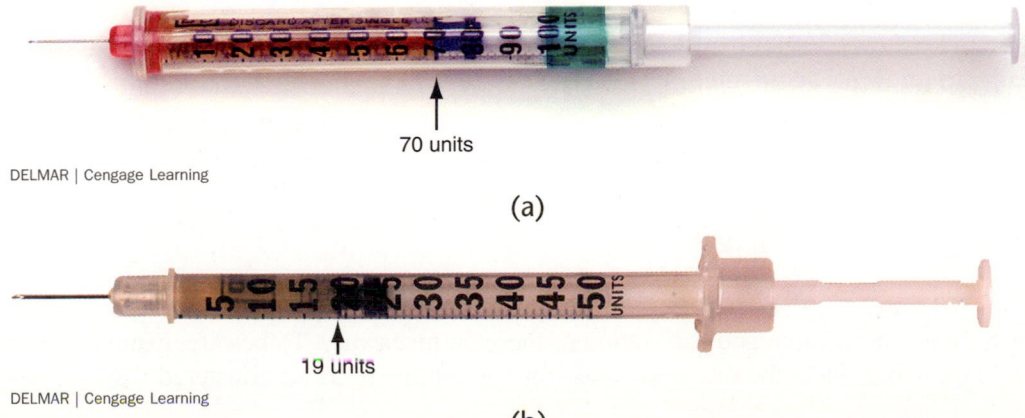

70 units

DELMAR | Cengage Learning

(a)

19 units

DELMAR | Cengage Learning

(b)

Figure 6-8(b) shows two Lo-Dose U-100 insulin syringes. The enlarged scale is easier to read and is calibrated for each 1 unit up to 50 units per 0.5 mL or 30 units per 0.3 mL. Every 5 units are labeled. The 30-unit syringe is commonly used for pediatric administration of insulin. The plunger in Figure 6-9(b) simulates the measurement of 19 units of U-100 insulin.

CAUTION

Be careful to measure the insulin dose by reading the units at the top of the black rubber stopper at the end of the plunger, not the bottom. A common error is to incorrectly read the dose by looking at the bottom of the stopper. Look again at Figure 6-9 to see that the insulin syringes demonstrate doses of 70 and 19 units respectively.

All insulin doses should be double-checked by another nurse before administration to the patient.

1 mL Syringe

Figure 6-10 shows the 1 mL syringe. This syringe is also referred to as the *tuberculin* or *TB syringe*. It is used when a small dose of a drug must be measured, such as an allergen extract, vaccine, or child's medication. Notice that the 1 mL syringe is calibrated in hundredths (0.01) of a milliliter, with each one tenth (0.1) milliliter labeled on the metric scale. Pediatric and critical care doses of less than 1 mL can be rounded to hundredths and measured in the 1 mL syringe. It is preferable to measure all amounts less than 0.5 mL in a 1 mL syringe.

EXAMPLE ■

The amount 0.366 mL would be rounded to 0.37 mL and measured in the 1 mL syringe (Figure 6-10).

FIGURE 6-10   1 mL syringe

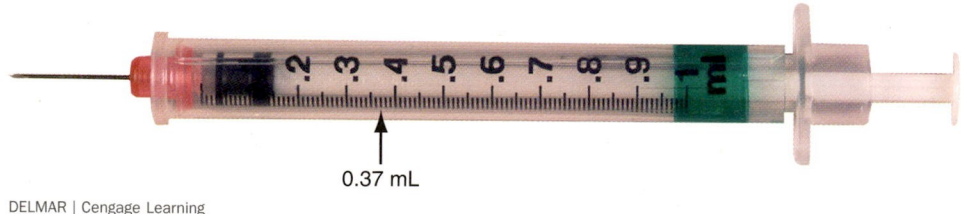

0.37 mL

DELMAR | Cengage Learning

Safety Syringe

Figure 6-11 shows 3 mL, 1 mL, and insulin safety syringes. Notice that the needles are protected by shields to prevent accidental needlestick injury to the nurse after administering an injectable medication.

Intravenous Syringe

Figures 6-12 and 6-13 show large syringes commonly used to prepare medications for intravenous administration. The volume and calibration of these syringes vary. To be safe, examine the calibrations of the syringes, and select the one best suited for the volume to be administered.

FIGURE 6-11 Safety syringes (a) 3 mL; (b) 1 mL; (c) Lo-Dose U-100 insulin; (d) standard U-100 insulin

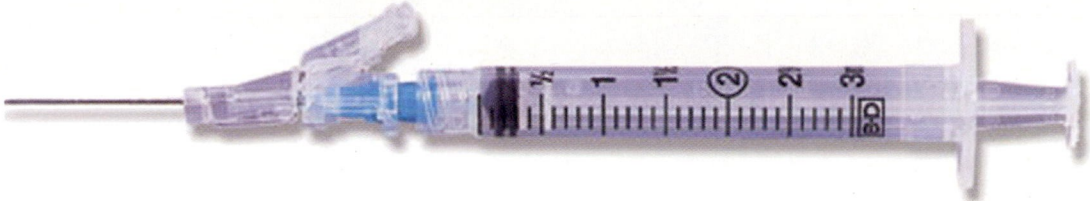

Courtesy of Becton, Dickinson and Company.

(a)

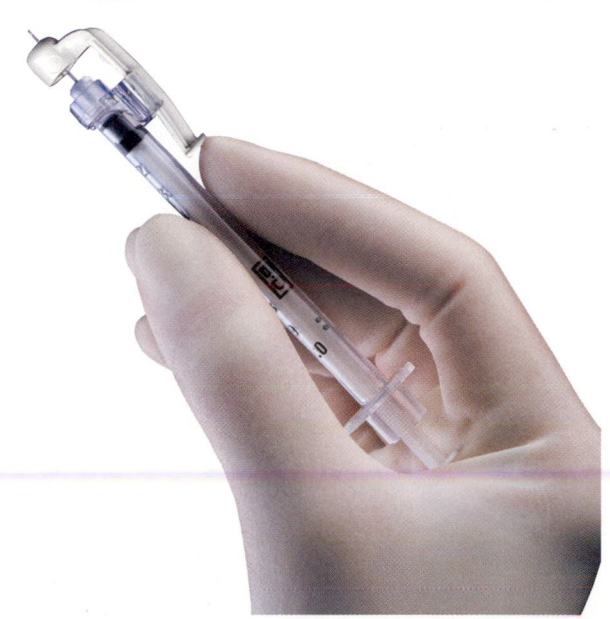

Courtesy of Becton, Dickinson and Company.

(b)

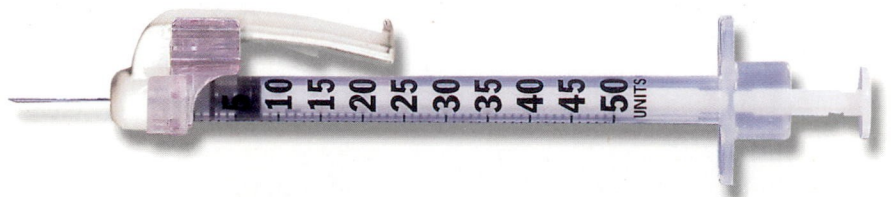

Courtesy of Becton, Dickinson and Company.

(c)

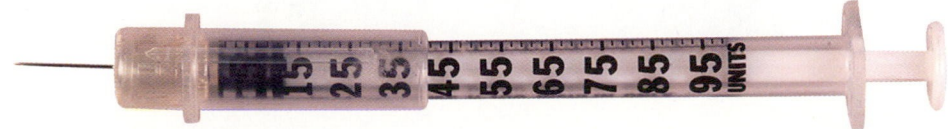

Courtesy of Becton, Dickinson and Company.

(d)

FIGURE 6-12 Intravenous syringes (a) 5 mL; (b) 10 mL

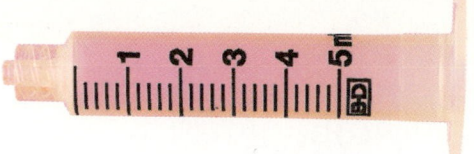

DELMAR | Cengage Learning

(a)

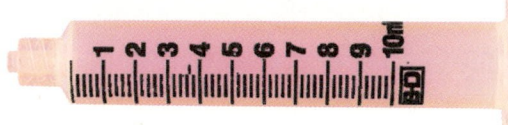

DELMAR | Cengage Learning

(b)

FIGURE 6-13 Intravenous syringes (a) front and reverse of a 30 mL or 1 fl oz syringe; (b) front and reverse of a 60 mL or 2 fl oz syringe

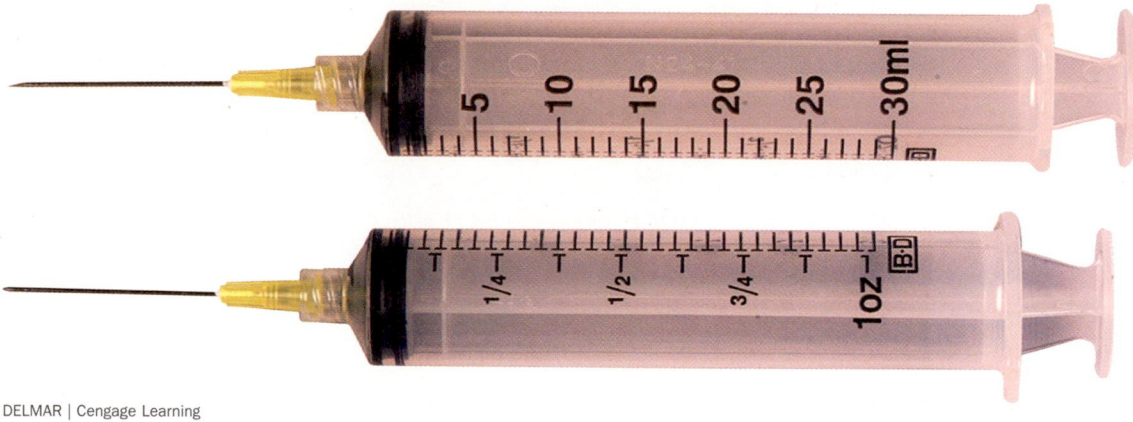

DELMAR | Cengage Learning

(a)

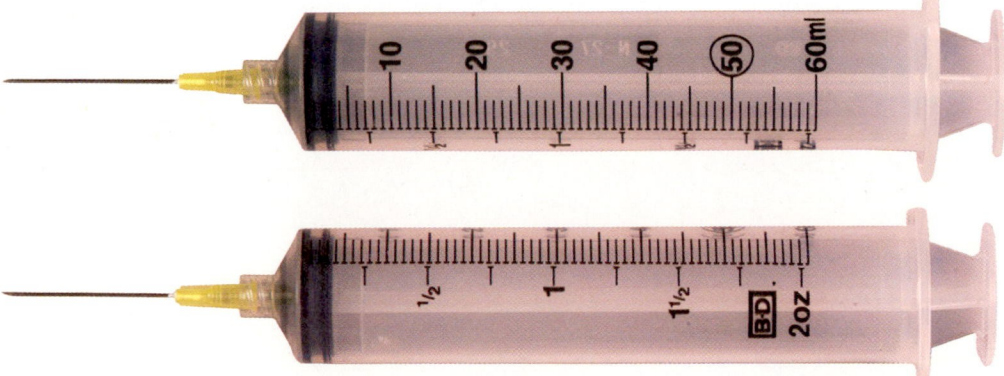

DELMAR | Cengage Learning

(b)

Needleless Syringe

Figure 6-14 pictures a needleless syringe system designed to prevent accidental needlesticks during intravenous administration.

FIGURE 6-14 Example of a needleless syringe system

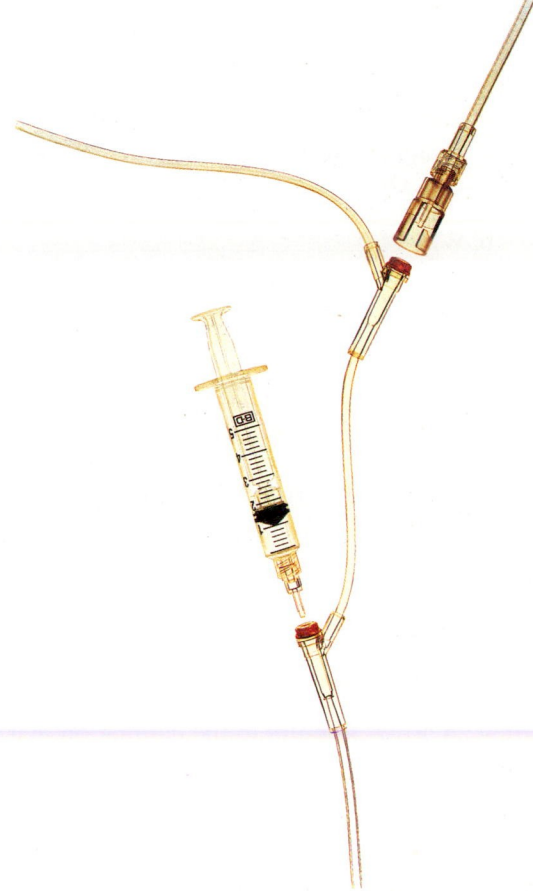

Courtesy of Becton, Dickinson and Company.

QUICK REVIEW

- The medicine cup has a 1 fluid ounce or 30 milliliter capacity for oral liquids. It is also calibrated to measure teaspoons, tablespoons, and drams. The apothecary measurement, dram, is no longer used. Amounts less than 2.5 milliliters should be measured in a smaller device, such as an oral syringe.

- The calibrated dropper measures small amounts of oral liquids. The size of the drop varies according to the diameter of the tip of the dropper.

- The standard 3 mL syringe is used to measure most injectable drugs. It is calibrated in tenths of a mL.

- The prefilled, single-dose syringe cartridge is to be used once and then discarded.

- The Standard U-100 insulin syringe is only used to measure U-100 insulin. It is calibrated for a total of 100 units per 1 mL.

- The Lo-Dose U-100 insulin syringe is used for measuring small amounts of U-100 insulin. It is calibrated for a total of 50 units per 0.5 mL or 30 units per 0.3 mL. The smaller syringe is commonly used for administering small amounts of insulin.

- The 1 mL syringe is used to measure small or critical amounts of injectable drugs. It is calibrated in hundredths of a mL.

- Safety and needleless syringes prevent needlestick injuries.

- Syringes intended for injections should never be used to measure or administer oral medications.

Review Set 17

1. In which syringe should 0.25 mL of a drug solution be measured? _____

2. How can 1.25 mL be measured in the regular 3 mL syringe? _____

   _____

3. Should insulin be measured in a 1 mL syringe? _____

4. Fifty (50) units of U-100 insulin equals how many milliliters? _____

5. a. True or False? The gtt is considered a consistent quantity for comparisons between different droppers. _____

   b. Why? _____

6. Can you measure 3 mL in a medicine cup? _____

7. How would you measure 3 mL of oral liquid to be administered to a child? _____

   _____

8. The medicine cup indicates that each teaspoon is the equivalent of _____ mL.

9. Describe your action if you are to administer less than the full amount of a drug supplied in a pre-filled, single-dose syringe. _____

   _____

10. What is the primary purpose of the safety and needleless syringes? _____

   _____

Draw an arrow to point to the calibration that corresponds to the dose to be administered.

11. Administer 0.75 mL

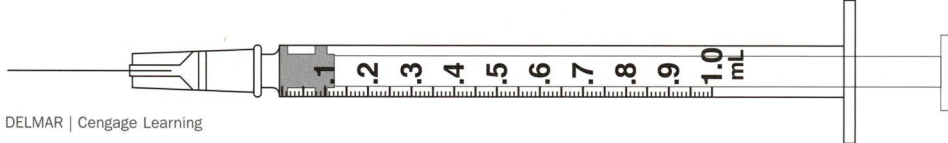

DELMAR | Cengage Learning

12. Administer 1.33 mL

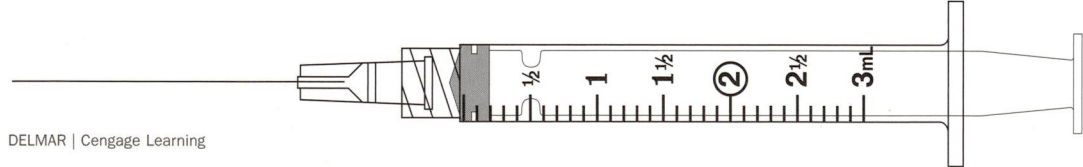

DELMAR | Cengage Learning

13. Administer 2.2 mL

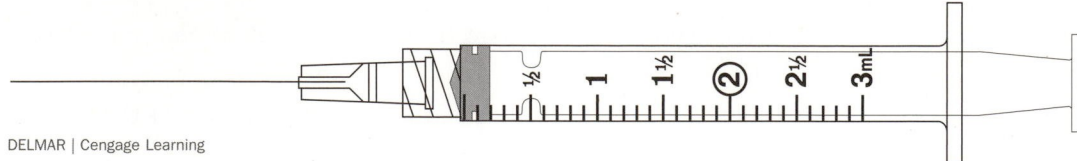

DELMAR | Cengage Learning

14. Administer 1.3 mL

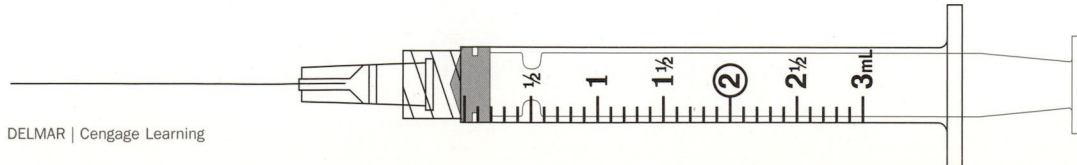

DELMAR | Cengage Learning

15. Administer 0.33 mL

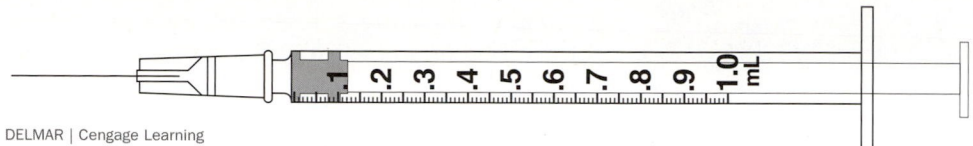

DELMAR | Cengage Learning

16. Administer 65 units of U-100 insulin

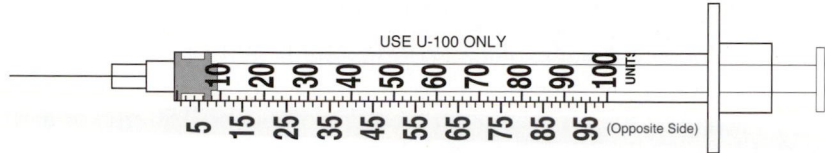

DELMAR | Cengage Learning

17. Administer 27 units of U-100 insulin

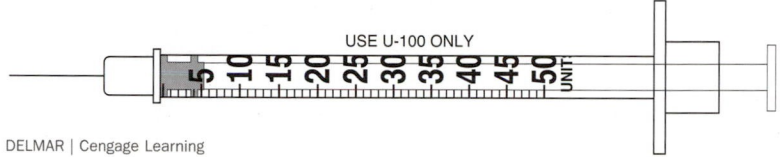

DELMAR | Cengage Learning

18. Administer 75 units of U-100 insulin

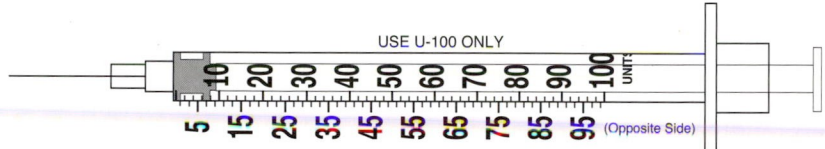

DELMAR | Cengage Learning

19. Administer 4.4 mL

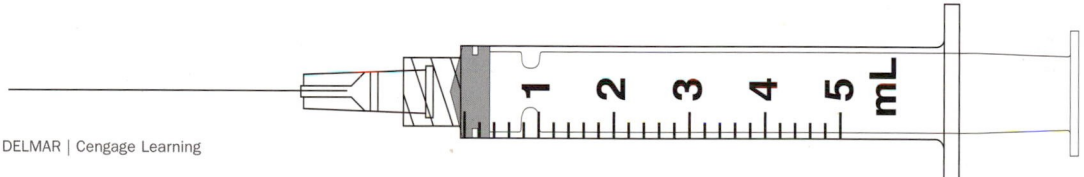

DELMAR | Cengage Learning

20. Administer 16 mL

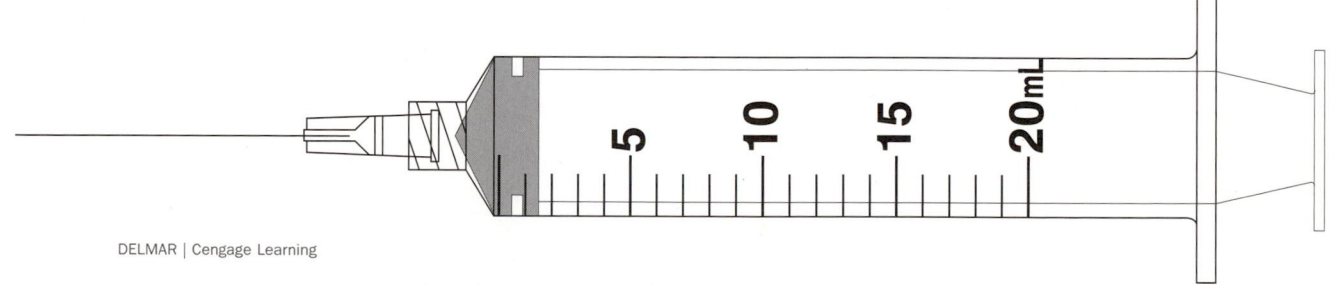

DELMAR | Cengage Learning

21. On the 5 mL syringe, each calibration is equal to _____. (Express the answer as a decimal.)

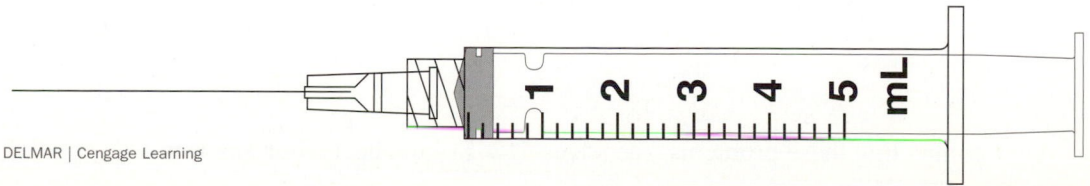

DELMAR | Cengage Learning

CRITICAL THINKING SKILLS   Select correct equipment to prepare medications. In the following situation, the correct dosage was not given because an incorrect measuring device was used.

ERROR

Using an inaccurate measuring device for oral medications.

Possible Scenario

Suppose a pediatrician ordered *Amoxil suspension (250 mg per 5 mL) 1 teaspoon every 8 hours* to be given to a child. The child should receive the medication for 10 days for otitis media, an ear infection. The pharmacy dispensed the medication in a bottle containing 150 mL, or a 10-day supply. The nurse did not clarify for the mother how to measure and administer the medication. The child returned to the clinic in 10 days for routine follow-up. The nurse asked whether the child had taken all the prescribed Amoxil. The child's mother stated, "No, we have almost half of the bottle left." When the nurse asked how the medication had been given, the mother described small plastic disposable teaspoons she had obtained from the grocery store. The nurse measured the spoon's capacity and found it to be less than 3 mL. (Remember, 1 t = 5 mL.) The child would have received only $\frac{3}{5}$, or 60%, of the correct dose.

Potential Outcome

The child did not receive a therapeutic dosage of the medication and was actually underdosed. The child could develop a resistant infection, which could lead to a more severe illness such as meningitis.

Prevention

Teach family members (and patients, as appropriate) to use calibrated measuring spoons or specially designed oral syringes to measure the correct dosage of medication. The volumes of serving spoons may vary considerably, as this situation illustrates.

22. On the 20 mL syringe, each calibration is equal to _____.

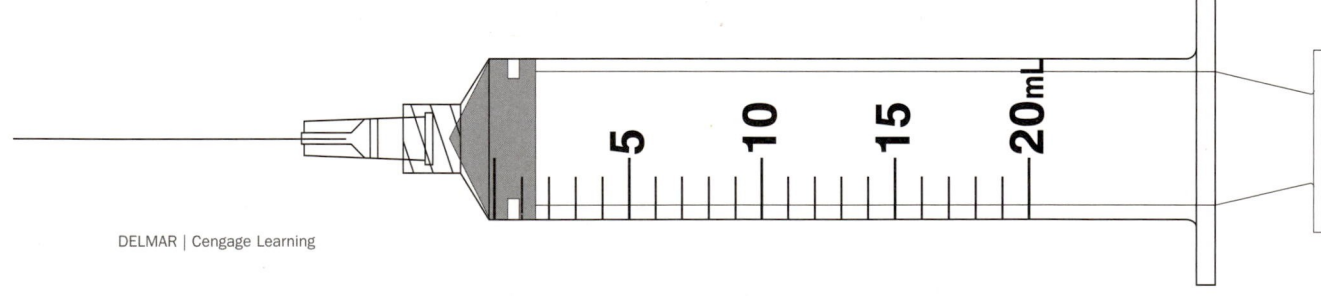

DELMAR | Cengage Learning

23. On the 10 mL syringe, each calibration is equal to _____. (Express the answer as a decimal.)

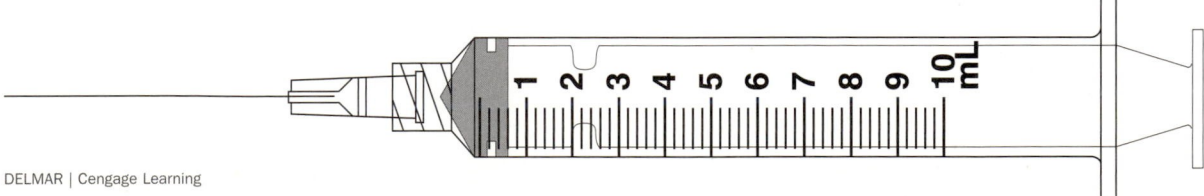

DELMAR | Cengage Learning

After completing these problems, see pages 512–514 to check your answers.

CRITICAL THINKING SKILLS

Recognize variations in syringes used to measure insulin. In the following situation, the nurse administered the incorrect dose of insulin because the nurse did not understand the design of the insulin syringe and the relationship of the rubber stopper at the end of the plunger as the measuring device for the insulin dose.

ERROR

Incorrectly reading the dose of insulin in an insulin syringe.

Possible Scenario

The physician ordered 25 units of U-100 Regular Humulin insulin for a patient with diabetes. In a hurry the nurse prepared and administered the incorrect insulin dose as shown.

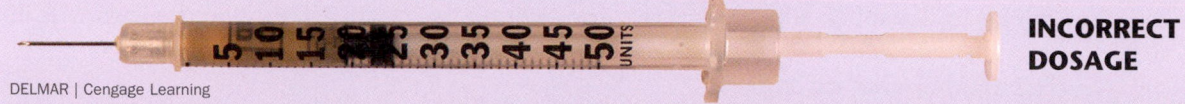

INCORRECT DOSAGE

DELMAR | Cengage Learning

Potential Outcome

The patient received only 19 units of insulin, which is a significant underdosage of almost 20 percent less than the prescribed dosage. The patient would likely develop symptoms of hyperglycemia. If the nurse continued to incorrectly measure each insulin dosage, the patient could progress into a diabetic coma.

Prevention

The nurse needs to review the proper measurement of injectable medications in syringes. Inaccurate measurement of insulin is a common and extremely serious medication error with dire consequences. The insulin syringe demonstrated above measures 19 units of insulin. The top of the rubber stopper is the correct part of the syringe for determining the amount of insulin and the proper dose. Further, each insulin dose should be double-checked by another nurse before administration.

PRACTICE PROBLEMS—CHAPTER 6

1. In the U-100 insulin syringe, 100 units = _____ mL.

2. The 1 mL syringe is calibrated in _____ of a mL.

3. Can you measure 1.25 mL in a single tuberculin syringe? _____ Explain. _____
   _____
   _____

4. How would you measure 1.33 mL in a 3 mL syringe? _____

5. The medicine cup has a _____ mL or _____ fl oz capacity.

6. To administer exactly 0.52 mL to a child, select a _____ syringe.

7. Seventy-five (75) units of U-100 insulin equals _____ mL.

8. True or False? All droppers are calibrated to deliver standardized drops of equal amounts regardless of the dropper used. _____

CRITICAL THINKING SKILLS

Precise measurement of doses in 1 mL and 3 mL syringes. In the following situation an incorrect dose was administered because the computed volume was not rounded properly.

ERROR

Rounding more decimal places than are necessary and selecting the wrong size syringe.

Possible Scenario

A newborn infant was ordered to receive *gentamicin sulfate 7.5 mg intravenously every 24 hours.* Using the 2 mL vial supplied with 10 mg/mL of gentamicin, the nurse calculated the volume needed as 0.75 mL. This volume may be administered precisely using a 1 mL syringe. No rounding is needed. In this case the nurse rounded 0.75 to the whole number 1 and administered 1 mL of medication using a 3 mL syringe. The infant was given 0.25 mL or 2.5 mg additional medication. If the nurse continued to care for this infant on subsequent days, the error might continue with serious overdosage implications.

Potential Outcome

Gentamicin sulfate, an aminoglycoside, is a high-alert drug with serious potential adverse effects. One adverse effect associated with high doses is ototoxicity, leading to irreversible hearing loss. Blood levels are monitored during therapy to assure that safe doses are ordered. By administering this higher dose the nurse may have placed this infant at an increased risk for ototoxicity.

Prevention

It is important to know the correct size of syringe to use and the number of decimal places to round for computed dose volumes. Syringes with a total volume of 1 mL are calibrated in hundredths (2 decimal places), and 3 mL syringes are calibrated in tenths (1 decimal place). Volumes of less than 1 mL should be measured as precisely as possible in a 1 mL syringe, especially when administering high-alert medications.

9. True or False? The prefilled syringe is a multiple-dose system. _____

10. True or False? Insulin should only be measured in an insulin syringe. _____

11. The purpose of needleless syringes is _____.

12. Medications are measured in syringes by aligning the calibrations with the _____ of the black rubber tip of the plunger (top ring, raised middle, or bottom ring).

13. The medicine cup calibrations indicate that 2 teaspoons are approximately _____ milliliters.

14. True or False? Safety syringes are designed to protect the patient. _____

15. The _____ syringe(s) is (are) intended to measure parenteral doses of medications. (3 mL, 1 mL, or insulin)

Draw an arrow to indicate the calibration that corresponds to the dose to be administered.

16. Administer 0.45 mL

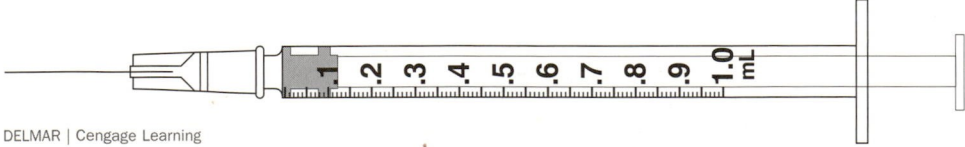

17. Administer 80 units of U-100 insulin

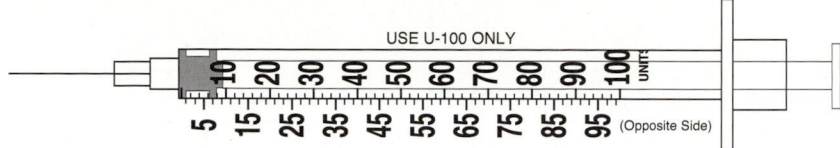

USE U-100 ONLY

(Opposite Side)

DELMAR | Cengage Learning

18. Administer $\frac{1}{2}$ fluid ounce

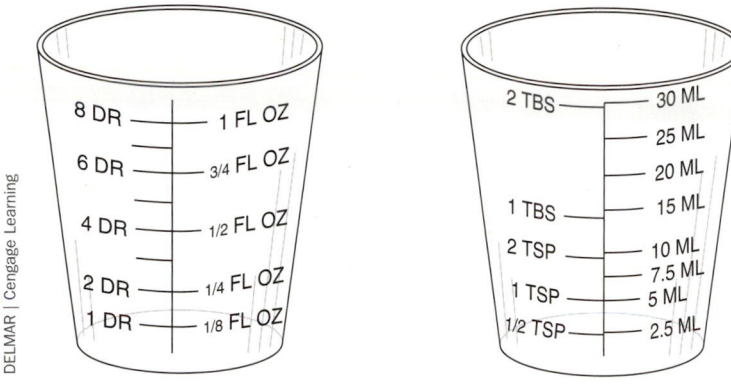

DELMAR | Cengage Learning

19. Administer 2.4 mL

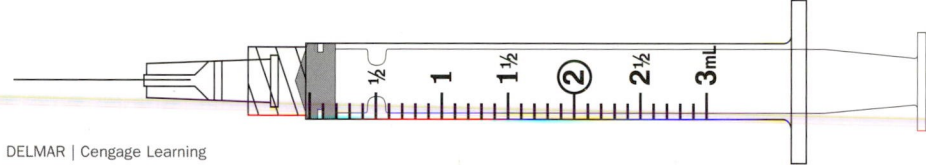

DELMAR | Cengage Learning

20. Administer 1.1 mL

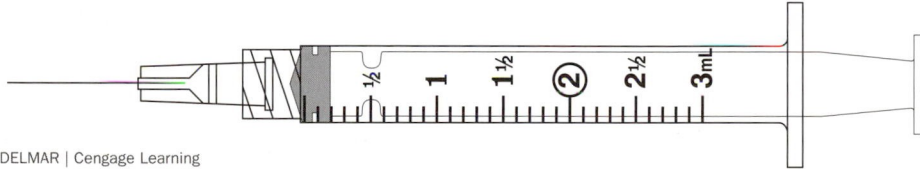

DELMAR | Cengage Learning

21. Administer 6.2 mL

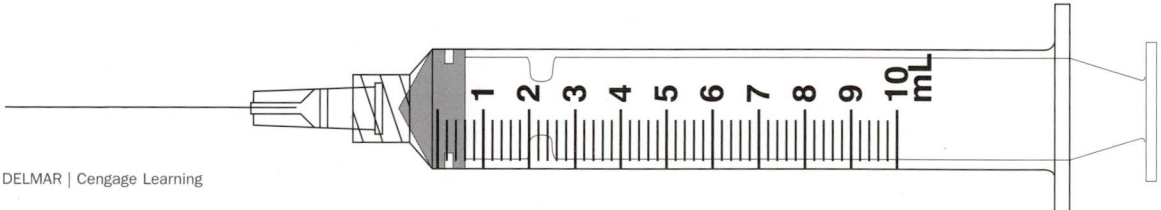

DELMAR | Cengage Learning

22. Administer 3.6 mL

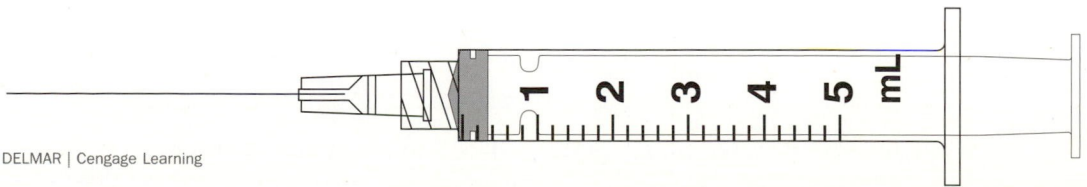

DELMAR | Cengage Learning

23. Administer 4.8 mL

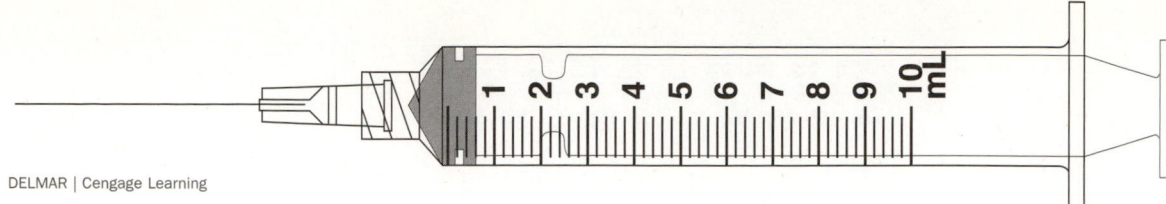

DELMAR | Cengage Learning

24. Administer 12 mL

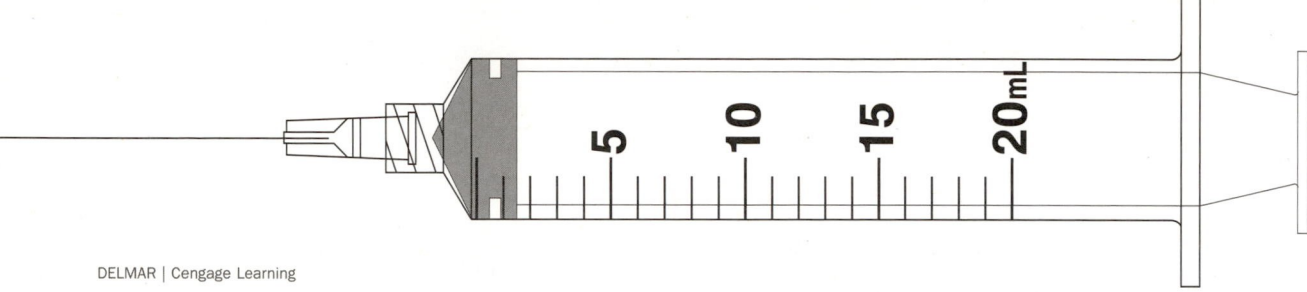

DELMAR | Cengage Learning

25. Describe the strategy that would prevent this medication error.

Possible Scenario
Suppose a patient with cancer has oral Compazine (prochlorperazine) liquid ordered for nausea. Because the patient has had difficulty taking the medication, the nurse decided to draw up the medication in a syringe without a needle to facilitate giving the medication. The nurse found this to be quite helpful and prepared several doses in syringes without the needles. A nurse from another unit covered for the nurse during lunch, and when the patient complained of nausea, the nurse assumed that the Compazine prepared in an injection syringe was to be given via injection. The nurse attached a needle and injected the oral medication.

Potential Outcome
The oral preparation may not be sterile and if absorbed systemically could lead to a bloodstream infection. Also, oral preparations have different preparative agents that likely should not be injected (such as glucose, which is traumatic to veins).

Prevention

_____

_____

26. Describe the strategy that would prevent this medication administration error.

Possible Scenario
A child with ear infections is to receive cefaclor oral liquid as an anti-infective. The medication is received in oral syringes for administration. The nurse fails to remove the cap on the tip of the syringe and attempts to administer the medication.

Potential Outcome
The nurse would exert enough pressure on the syringe plunger that the protective cap could pop off in the child's mouth and possibly cause the child to choke.

Prevention

_____

_____

After completing these problems, see pages 514–515 to check your answers.

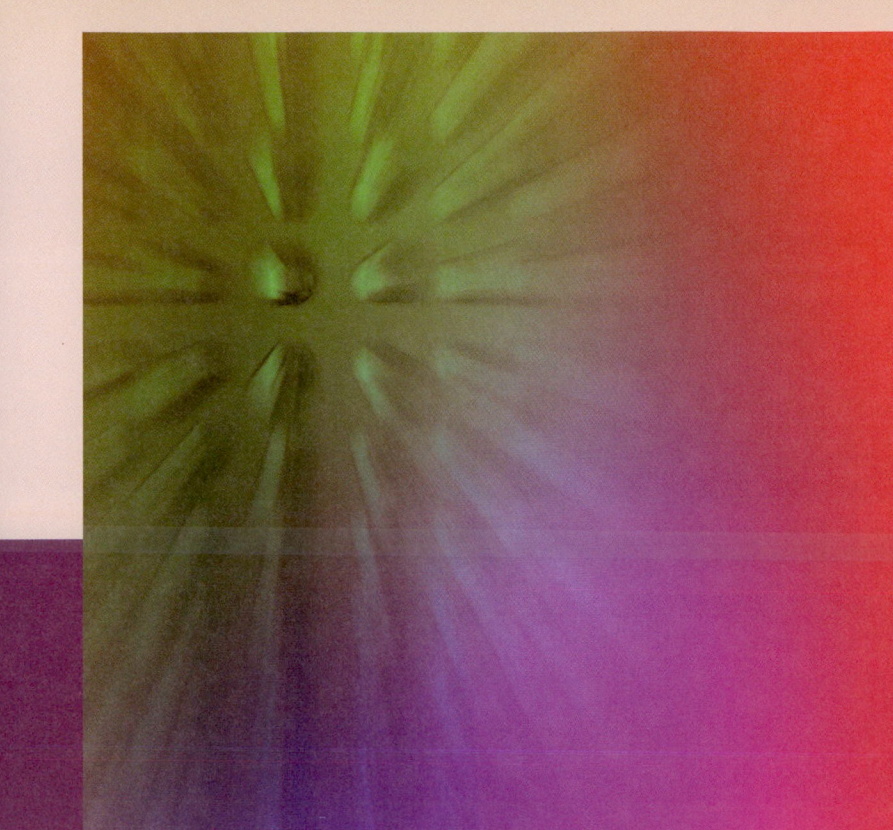

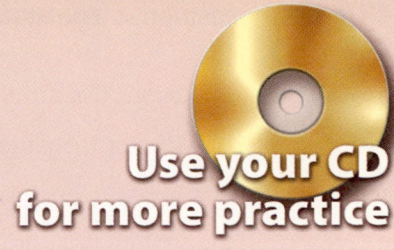

7

Interpreting Drug Orders

OBJECTIVES

Upon mastery of Chapter 7, you will be able to interpret the drug order. To accomplish this you will also be able to:

- Read and write correct medical notation.
- Write the standard medical abbreviation from a list of common terminology.
- Classify the notation that specifies the dosage, route, and frequency of the medication to be administered.
- Interpret physician and other prescribing practitioner orders and medication administration records.

The prescription or medication order conveys the therapeutic drug plan for the patient. It is the responsibility of the nurse to:

- Interpret the order.
- Prepare the exact dosage of the prescribed drug.
- Identify the patient.
- Administer the proper dosage by the prescribed route, at the prescribed time intervals.
- Educate the patient regarding the medication.

117

- Record the administration of the prescribed drug.

- Monitor the patient's response for desired (therapeutic) and adverse effects.

Before you can prepare the correct dosage of the prescribed drug, you must learn to interpret or read the written drug order. For brevity and speed, the health care professions have adopted certain standards and common abbreviations for use in notation. You should learn to recognize and interpret the abbreviations from memory. As you practice reading drug orders, you will find that this skill becomes second nature to you.

An example of a typical written drug order is:

9/4/XX 0730 Amoxil 500 mg p.o. q.i.d. (p.c. et bedtime)

J. Physician, M.D.

This order means the patient should receive 500 milligrams of an antibiotic named Amoxil (or amoxicillin) orally four times a day (after meals and at bedtime). You can see that the medical notation shortens the written-out order considerably.

MEDICAL ABBREVIATIONS

The following table lists common medical abbreviations used in writing drug orders. The abbreviations are grouped according to those that refer to the route (or method) of administration, the frequency (time interval), and other general terms. Commit these to memory, along with the other abbreviations related to systems of measurement presented in Chapter 3.

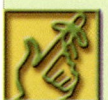

REMEMBER
Common Medical Abbreviations

Abbreviation	Interpretation	Abbreviation	Interpretation
Route:		**Frequency:**	
IM	intramuscular	h	hour
IV	intravenous	q.h	every hour
IV PB	intravenous piggyback	q.2h	every two hours
subcut	subcutaneous	q.3h	every three hours
SL	sublingual, under the tongue	q.4h	every four hours
ID	intradermal	q.6h	every six hours
GT	gastrostomy tube	q.8h	every eight hours
NG	nasogastric tube	q.12h	every twelve hours
NJ	nasojejunal tube	**General:**	
p.o.	by mouth, orally	$\bar{a}$	before
p.r.	per rectum, rectally	$\bar{p}$	after
Frequency:		$\bar{c}$	with
a.c.	before meals	$\bar{s}$	without
p.c.	after meals	q	every
ad. lib.	as desired, freely	qs	quantity sufficient
p.r.n.	when necessary	aq	water
stat	immediately, at once	NPO	nothing by mouth
b.i.d.	twice a day	gtt	drop
t.i.d.	three times a day	tab	tablet
q.i.d.	four times a day	cap	capsule
min	minute	et	and
		noct	night

THE DRUG ORDER

The drug order consists of seven parts:

1. Name of the *patient*.

2. Name of the *drug* to be administered.

3. *Dosage* of the drug.

4. *Route* by which the drug is to be administered.

5. *Frequency*, time, and special instructions related to administration.

6. *Date and time* when the order was written.

7. *Signature and licensure* of the person writing the order.

CAUTION

If any of the seven parts is missing or unclear, the order is considered incomplete and is, therefore, not a legal drug order.

Parts one through five of the drug order are known as the original Five Rights of safe medication administration. They are essential and each one must be faithfully checked every time a medication is prepared and administered. After safe administration of the medication, the nurse or health care practitioner must accurately document the drug administration. Combining accurate documentation with the original Five Rights, the patient is entitled to *Six Rights* of safe and accurate medication administration and documentation with each and every dose.

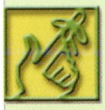

REMEMBER

The Six Rights of safe and accurate medication administration are as follows:

The *right patient* must receive the *right drug* in the *right amount* by the *right route* at the *right time*, followed by the *right documentation*.

Each drug order should follow a specific sequence. The name of the drug is written first, followed by the dosage, route, and frequency. When correctly written, the brand (or trade) name of the drug begins with a capital or uppercase letter. The generic name begins with a lowercase letter.

EXAMPLE ■

Procanbid 500 mg p.o. b.i.d.

1. **Procanbid** is the brand name of the drug.

2. **500 mg** is the dosage.

3. **p.o.** is the route.

4. **b.i.d.** is the frequency.

This order means: *Give 500 milligrams of Procanbid orally twice a day.*

CAUTION

If the nurse has difficulty understanding and interpreting the drug order, the nurse must clarify the order with the writer. Usually this person is the physician or another authorized practitioner, such as an advanced registered nurse practitioner.

Let's practice reading and interpreting drug orders.

EXAMPLE 1 ■

phenytoin 100 mg p.o. t.i.d.

This order means: *Give 100 milligrams of phenytoin orally 3 times a day.*

EXAMPLE 2 ■

procaine penicillin G 400,000 units IV q.6h

This order means: *Give 400,000 units of procaine penicillin G intravenously every 6 hours.*

EXAMPLE 3 ■

hydromorphone 2 mg IM q.4h p.r.n., moderate to severe pain

This order means: *Give 2 milligrams of hydromorphone intramuscularly every 4 hours when necessary for moderate to severe pain.*

CAUTION

The p.r.n. frequency designates the minimum time allowed between doses. There is no maximum time other than automatic stops as defined by hospital or agency policy.

EXAMPLE 4 ■

Humulin R Regular U-100 insulin 5 units subcut stat

This order means: *Give 5 units of Humulin R Regular U-100 insulin subcutaneously immediately.*

EXAMPLE 5 ■

cefazolin 1 g IV PB q.6h

This order means: *Give 1 gram of cefazolin by intravenous piggyback every 6 hours.*

The administration times are designated by hospital policy. For example, t.i.d. administration times may be 0900 or 9 AM, 1300 or 1 PM, and 1700 or 5 PM. This is different than q.8h times which may be 0600, 1400, and 2200.

QUICK REVIEW

- The *right patient* must receive the *right drug* in the *right amount* by the *right route* at the *right time* followed by the *right documentation*.

- Understanding drug orders requires interpreting common medical abbreviations.

- The drug order must contain (in this sequence): drug name, dosage, route, and frequency.

- All parts of the drug order must be stated clearly for accurate, exact interpretation.

- If you are ever in doubt as to the meaning of any part of a drug order, ask the writer to clarify before proceeding.

Review Set 18

Interpret the following medication (drug) orders:

1. naproxen 250 mg p.o. b.i.d. _____

_____

2. Humulin N NPH U-100 insulin 30 units subcut daily 30 min ā breakfast _____
_____

3. cefaclor 500 mg p.o. stat, then 250 mg q.8h _____
_____

4. Synthroid 25 mcg p.o. daily _____
_____

5. Ativan 10 mg IM q.4h p.r.n., agitation _____
_____

6. furosemide 20 mg IV stat (slowly) _____
_____

7. Mylanta 10 mL p.o. p.c. et bedtime _____
_____

8. atropine sulfate ophthalmic 1% 2 gtt right eye q.15 min × 4 _____
_____

9. morphine sulfate gr $\frac{1}{4}$ IM q.3h p.r.n., pain _____
_____

10. digoxin 0.25 mg p.o. daily _____
_____

11. tetracycline 250 mg p.o. q.i.d. _____
_____

12. nitroglycerin gr $\frac{1}{400}$ SL stat _____
_____

13. Cortisporin otic suspension 2 gtt each ear t.i.d. et bedtime _____
_____

14. Compare and contrast *t.i.d.* and *q.8h* administration times. Include sample administration times for each in your explanation. _____
_____

15. Describe your action if no method of administration is written. _____
_____

16. Do q.i.d. and q.4h have the same meaning? _____ Explain. _____
_____

17. Who determines the medication administration times? _____
_____

18. Name the seven parts of a written medication prescription. _____
_____

19. Which parts of the written medication prescription/order are included in the original Five Rights of medication administration? _____
_____

20. State the Six Rights of safe and accurate medication administration. _____
_____

After completing these problems, see page 516 to check your answers.

Medication Order and Administration Forms

Hospitals have a special form for recording drug orders. Figure 7-1 shows a sample physician's order form. Find and name each of the seven parts of the drug orders listed. Notice that the nurse or other health care professional must verify and initial each order, ensuring that each of the seven parts is accurate. In some facilities, the pharmacist may be responsible for verifying the order as part of the computerized record.

FIGURE 7-1 Physician's order form

			ENTERED	FILLED	CHECKED	VERIFIED

NOTE: A NON-PROPRIETARY DRUG OF EQUAL QUALITY MAY BE DISPENSED - IF THIS COLUMN IS NOT CHECKED!

DATE	TIME WRITTEN	PLEASE USE BALL POINT - PRESS FIRMLY	✓	TIME NOTED	NURSES SIGNATURE
11/3/xx	0815	cephalexin 250 mg p.o. q.6h	✓		
		Humulin N NPH U-100 Insulin 40 units subcut ā breakfast	✓	0830	
		hydromorphone 2 mg IV q. 3h p.r.n. severe pain	✓		G. Pickar, R.N.
		codeine 30 mg p.o. q.4h p.r.n. mild–mod pain	✓		
		Tylenol 650 mg p.o. q.4h p.r.n., fever greater than 101° F	✓		
		furosemide 40 mg p.o. daily	✓		
		K-Dur 10 mEq p.o. b.i.d.	✓		
		J. Physician, M.D.			
11/3/xx	2200	furosemide 80 mg IV stat	✓		
		J. Physician, M.D.		2210	M. Smith, R.N.

AUTO STOP ORDERS: UNLESS REORDERED, FOLLOWING WILL BE D/C'D AT 0800 ON:

DATE	ORDER		
		☐ CONT	PHYSICIAN SIGNATURE
		☐ D/C	
		☐ CONT	PHYSICIAN SIGNATURE
		☐ D/C	
		☐ CONT	PHYSICIAN SIGNATURE
		☐ D/C	

CHECK WHEN ANTIBIOTICS ORDERED   ☐ Prophylactic   ☐ Empiric   ☐ Therapeutic

Allergies: None Known

PATIENT DIAGNOSIS   Diabetes

HEIGHT   5' 5"   WEIGHT   130 lb

FORM 959-706 (8-XX)   **PHYSICIANS ORDER**   Reynolds+Reynolds LITHO IN U.S.A. K41814 (7:xx) D339380

Patient, Mary Q.
#3-11316-7

①

The drug orders from the physician's order form are transcribed to a medication administration record (MAR) (Figure 7-2). The nurse or other health care professional uses this record as a guide to:

- Check the drug order.
- Prepare the correct dosage.
- Record the drug administered and time.

These three checkpoints help to ensure accurate medication administration.

FIGURE 7-2 Medication administration record

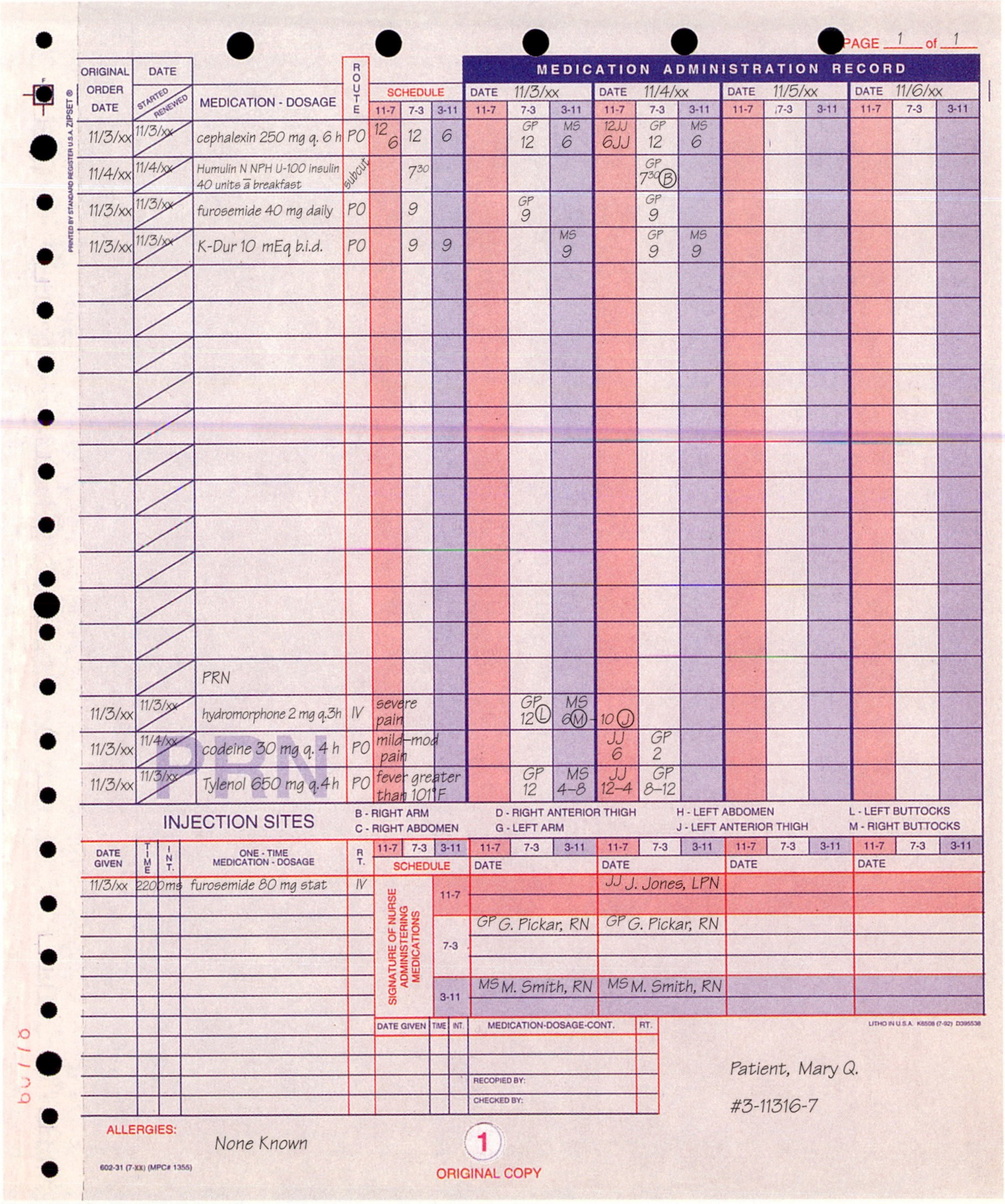

MEDICATION ADMINISTRATION RECORD

PAGE 1 of 1

ORIGINAL ORDER DATE	DATE STARTED / RENEWED	MEDICATION - DOSAGE	ROUTE	SCHEDULE 11-7 / 7-3 / 3-11	DATE 11/3/xx 11-7 / 7-3 / 3-11	DATE 11/4/xx 11-7 / 7-3 / 3-11	DATE 11/5/xx 11-7 / 7-3 / 3-11	DATE 11/6/xx 11-7 / 7-3 / 3-11
11/3/xx	11/3/xx	cephalexin 250 mg q. 6 h	PO	12 6 / 12 / 6	/ GP 12 / MS 6	12JJ 6JJ / GP 12 / MS 6		
11/4/xx	11/4/xx	Humulin N NPH U-100 insulin 40 units ā breakfast	subcut	7³⁰		7³⁰ (B)		
11/3/xx	11/3/xx	furosemide 40 mg daily	PO	9	GP 9	GP 9		
11/3/xx	11/3/xx	K-Dur 10 mEq b.i.d.	PO	9 / 9		MS 9	GP 9 / MS 9	

PRN

ORIGINAL ORDER DATE	DATE STARTED / RENEWED	MEDICATION - DOSAGE	ROUTE	SCHEDULE	11-7 / 7-3 / 3-11	11-7 / 7-3 / 3-11		
11/3/xx	11/3/xx	hydromorphone 2 mg q.3h	IV	severe pain	GP 12 (L) / MS 6 (M) / 10 (J)			
11/3/xx	11/4/xx	codeine 30 mg q. 4 h	PO	mild–mod pain	JJ 6 / GP 2			
11/3/xx	11/3/xx	Tylenol 650 mg q.4h	PO	fever greater than 101°F	GP 12 / MS 4–8	JJ 12–4 / GP 8–12		

INJECTION SITES

B - RIGHT ARM	D - RIGHT ANTERIOR THIGH	H - LEFT ABDOMEN	L - LEFT BUTTOCKS
C - RIGHT ABDOMEN	G - LEFT ARM	J - LEFT ANTERIOR THIGH	M - RIGHT BUTTOCKS

DATE GIVEN	TIME	INT.	ONE - TIME MEDICATION - DOSAGE	RT.	SCHEDULE	11-7 / 7-3 / 3-11 DATE	11-7 / 7-3 / 3-11 DATE	11-7 / 7-3 / 3-11 DATE	11-7 / 7-3 / 3-11 DATE
11/3/xx	2200	ms	furosemide 80 mg stat	IV					

SIGNATURE OF NURSE ADMINISTERING MEDICATIONS

11-7		JJ J. Jones, LPN	
7-3	GP G. Pickar, RN	GP G. Pickar, RN	
3-11	MS M. Smith, RN	MS M. Smith, RN	

DATE GIVEN	TIME	INT.	MEDICATION-DOSAGE-CONT.	RT.

LITHO IN U.S.A. K8508 (7-92) D395538

RECOPIED BY:

CHECKED BY:

Patient, Mary Q.

#3-11316-7

ALLERGIES: None Known

(1) ORIGINAL COPY

602-31 (7-XX) (MPC# 1355)

PRINTED BY STANDARD REGISTER U.S.A. ZIPSET ®

COMPUTERIZED MEDICATION ADMINISTRATION SYSTEMS

Many health care facilities now use computers for processing drug orders. Drug orders are either electronically transmitted or manually entered into the computer from an order form, such as Figure 7-3. Through the computer, the nurse or other health care professional can transmit the order within seconds

FIGURE 7-3 Physician's order form

			ENTERED	FILLED	CHECKED	VERIFIED

NOTE: A NON-PROPRIETARY DRUG OF EQUAL QUALITY MAY BE DISPENSED - IF THIS COLUMN IS NOT CHECKED!

DATE	TIME WRITTEN	PLEASE USE BALL POINT - PRESS FIRMLY	✓	TIME NOTED	NURSES SIGNATURE
8/31/XX	1500	Procanbid 500 mg p.o. b.i.d.	✓		
		J. Physician, M.D.		1515	M. Smith, R.N.
9/3/XX	0715	digoxin 0.125 mg p.o. every other day	✓		
		Lasix 40 mg p.o. daily	✓		
		Reglan 10 mg p.o. stat a.c. and bedtime	✓		
		Micro-K 16 mEq p.o. b.i.d.-start 9/4/XX	✓	0730	G. Pickar, R.N.
		nitroglycerin gr $^1/_{150}$ SL p.r.n. mild-moderate chest pain	✓		
		Darvocet-N 100 tab. 1 p.o. q.4h p.r.n. mild-moderate pain	✓		
		ketoralac 30 mg IM q.6h p.r.n., severe pain	✓		
		J. Physician, M.D.			

AUTO STOP ORDERS: UNLESS REORDERED, FOLLOWING WILL BE D/C'D AT 0800 ON:

DATE	ORDER		
		☐ CONT	PHYSICIAN SIGNATURE
		☐ D/C	
		☐ CONT	PHYSICIAN SIGNATURE
		☐ D/C	
		☐ CONT	PHYSICIAN SIGNATURE
		☐ D/C	

CHECK WHEN ANTIBIOTICS ORDERED ☐ Prophylactic ☐ Empiric ☐ Therapeutic

Allergies:
No known allergies

Patient, John D.
#3-81512-3

PATIENT DIAGNOSIS
congestive heart failure

HEIGHT 5' 10" WEIGHT 165 lb

FORM 959-708 (8-XX) **PHYSICIANS ORDER** Reynolds + Reynolds LITHO IN U.S.A. K41814 (7-2.0) D339360

①

DELMAR | Cengage Learning

to the pharmacy for filling. The computer can keep track of drug stock and usage patterns and even notify the business office to post charges to the patient's account. Most importantly, it can scan for information previously entered, such as drug incompatibilities, drug allergies, safe dosage ranges, doses already given, or recommended administration times. The health care staff can be readily alerted to potential problems or inconsistencies. The corresponding medication administration record may also be printed directly from the computer as in Figure 7-4. Such computerized records reduce the risk of misinterpreting handwriting.

The computerized MAR may be viewed from a printed copy as in Figure 7-4a or at the computer as in Figure 7-4b. The nurse may be able to look back at the patient's cumulative medication administration record, document administration times and comments at the computer terminal, and then keep a printed copy of the information obtained and entered. The data analysis, storage, and retrieval abilities of computers are making them essential tools for safe and accurate medication administration.

FIGURE 7-4(a)   Printed computerized medication administration record

PHARMACY MAR

START	STOP	MEDICATION	SCHEDULED TIMES	OK'D BY	0001 HRS. TO 1200 HRS.	1201 HRS. TO 2400 HRS.
08/31/xx 1800 SCH		PROCANBID 500 MG TAB-SR / 500 MG b.i.d. PO	0900 / 2100	JD	0900GP	2100 MS
09/03/xx 0900 SCH		DIGOXIN (LANOXIN) 0.125 MG TAB / 1 TAB EVERY PO OTHER DAY / ODD DAYS-SEPT	0900	JD	0900 GP	
09/03/xx 0900 SCH		FUROSEMIDE (LASIX) 40 MG TAB / 1 TAB DAILY PO	0900	JD	0900 GP	
09/03/xx 0730 SCH		REGLAN 10 MG TAB / 10 MG AC AND HS PO / GIVE ONE NOW!!	0730 1130 1630 2100	JD	0730 GP 1130 GP	1630 MS 2100 MS
09/04/xx 0900 SCH		MICRO-K 16 MEQ CAP / 16 mEq BID PO / START 09/04/XX	0900 2100	JD	0900 GP	2100 MS
09/03/xx 1507 PRN		NITROGLYCERIN $\frac{1}{150}$ GR 0.4 MG TAB-SL / 1 TABLET PRN* SL / PRN CHEST PAIN		JD		
09/03/xx 1700 PRN		DARVOCET-N 100* CAP / 1 TAB Q4H PO / PRN MILD–MODERATE PAIN		JD		
09/03/xx 2100 PRN		KETOROLAC INJ / 30 MG Q6H IM / PRN SEVERE PAIN		JD		2200 Ⓗ MS

Gluteus	Thigh
A. Right	H. Right
B. Left	I. Left
Ventro Gluteal	
C. Right	J. Right
D. Left	K. Left
E. Abdomen $\frac{1}{3}\,\frac{2}{4}$	

730-13 (12/xx)

	NURSE'S SIGNATURE	INITIAL
7–3	G. Pickar, R.N.	GP
3–11	M. Smith, R.N.	MS
11–7	J. Doe, R.N.	JD

ALLERGIES: **NKA**

DIAGNOSIS: **CHF**

FROM: 09/05/xx 0701

Patient:	Patient, John D.
Patient #	3-81512-3
Admitted:	08/31/xx
Physician:	J. Physician, MD
Room:	PCU-14 PCU

TO: 09/06/xx 0700

DELMAR | Cengage Learning

FIGURE 7-4(b) Sample of medication administration record used for computerized charting. Complete medication record is viewed using the scroll bar.

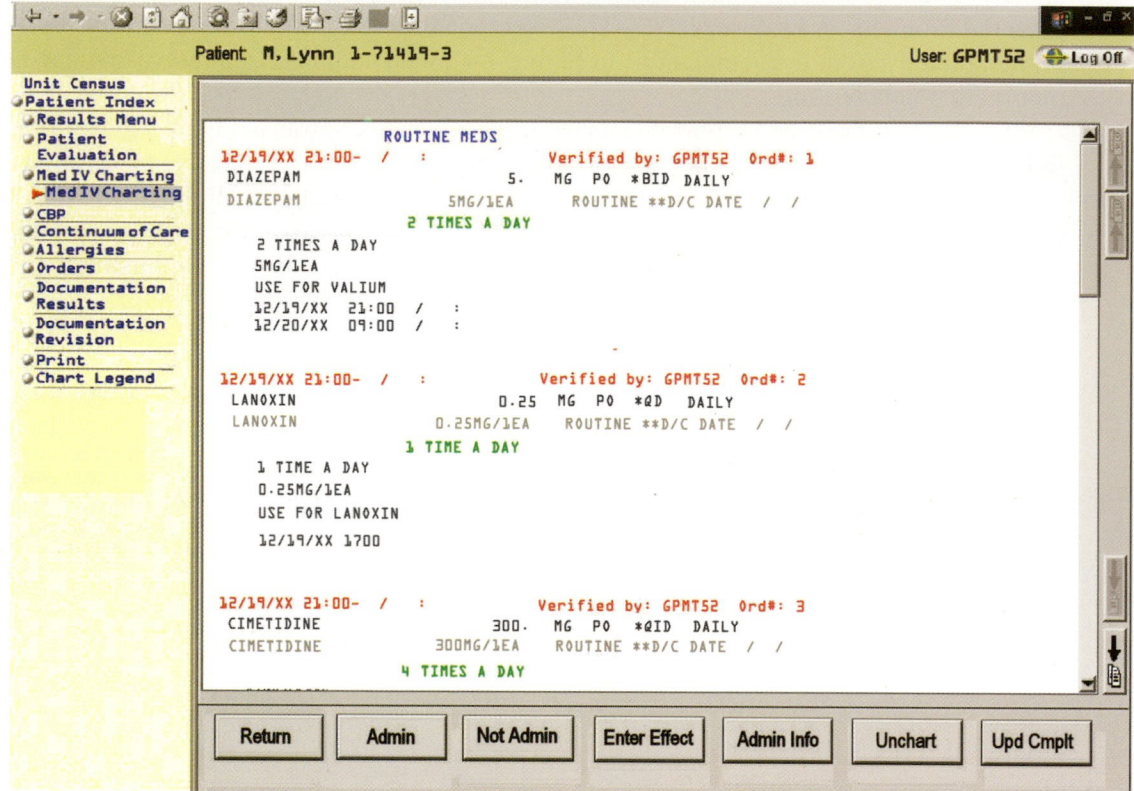

DELMAR | Cengage Learning

QUICK REVIEW

- Drug orders are prescribed on the physician's order form.

- The person who administers a drug records it on the medication administration record (MAR). This record may be handwritten or computerized.

- All parts of the drug order must be stated clearly for accurate, exact interpretation. If you are ever in doubt as to the meaning of any part of a drug order, ask the writer to clarify.

Review Set 19

Refer to the computerized MAR (Figure 7-4(a)) on page 125 to answer questions 1 through 10. Convert the scheduled international time to traditional AM/PM time.

1. Scheduled times for administering Procanbid. _____

2. Scheduled times for administering Lanoxin and Lasix. _____

3. Scheduled times for administering Reglan. _____

4. Scheduled times for administering Micro-K. _____

5. How often can the ketoralac be given? _____

6. If the Lanoxin was last given on 9/5/xx at 0900, when is the next date and time it will be given? _____

7. What is the ordered route of administration for the nitroglycerin? _____

8. How many times a day is furosemide ordered? _____

9. The equivalent dosage of Lanoxin is _____ mcg.

10. Which drugs are ordered to be administered "as necessary"? _____

Refer to the MAR (Figure 7-2) on page 123 to answer questions 11 through 20.

11. What is the route of administration for the insulin? _____

12. How many times in a 24-hour period will furosemide be administered? _____

13. What is the only medication ordered to be given routinely at noon? _____

14. What time of day is the insulin to be administered? _____

15. A dosage of 10 mEq of K-Dur is ordered. What does mEq mean? _____

16. You work 3 to 11 PM on November 5. Which routine medications will you administer to Mary Q. Patient during your shift? _____

17. Mary Q. Patient has a fever of 101.4°F. What medication should you administer? _____

18. How many times in a 24-hour period will K-Dur be administered? _____

19. What is the equivalent of the scheduled administration time(s) for the K-Dur as converted to international time? _____

20. What is the equivalent of the scheduled administration time(s) for the cephalexin as converted to international time? _____

21. Identify the place on the MAR where the stat IV furosemide was charted.

_____

After completing these problems, see page 516 to check your answers.

CRITICAL THINKING SKILLS

It is the responsibility of the nurse to clarify any drug order that is incomplete—that is, an order that does not contain the essential seven parts discussed in this chapter. Let's look at an example in which this error occurred.

ERROR

Failing to clarify incomplete orders.

Possible Scenario

Suppose a physician ordered *omeprazole capsules p.o. at bedtime* for a patient with an active duodenal ulcer. You will note there is no dosage listed. The nurse thought the medication came in only one dosage strength, added 20 mg to the order, and sent it to the pharmacy. The pharmacist prepared the dosage written on the physician's order sheet. Two days later, during rounds, the physician noted that the patient had not responded well to the medication. When asked about this, the nurse explained that the patient had received 20 mg at bedtime. The physician informed the nurse that the patient should have received the 40 mg dosage for high acid suppression.

Potential Outcome

Potentially, the delay in correct dosage could result in gastrointestinal bleeding or delayed healing of the ulcer.

Prevention

This medication error could have been avoided simply by the physician writing the strength of the medication. Because it was omitted, the nurse should have checked the dosage before sending the order to the pharmacy. When you fill in an incomplete order, you are essentially practicing medicine without a license, which is illegal and potentially dangerous.

CRITICAL THINKING SKILLS

Read the entire medication record to assure the planned administration times are scheduled correctly according to the medication order. In the following situation two doses of a medication were omitted each day until an observant nurse picked up on the transcription error.

ERROR

Omitting medication due to incorrect scheduling of doses.

Possible Scenario

An order was written for **ampicillin 500 mg IV PB q.4h**, which was handwritten on the medication administration record (MAR). The registered nurse was distracted while verifying the order and writing in the scheduled times of administration. The nurse saw the number 4 and instead of scheduling the medication every 4 hours, scheduled the medication to be given four times a day at 0600, 1200, 1800, and 2400. For 2 days, the shift nurses each checked to see what medications needed to be given on their scheduled shifts but did not take the time to compare the ordered frequency to the scheduled times. Eventually a nurse did look over the entire medication record and noticed the error. The medication times were corrected and the doctor was notified. A medication variance form was completed, documenting the error, and it was submitted to the hospital risk management department.

Potential Outcome

Over the course of 2 days the patient missed 4 doses for a total of 2 grams of ampicillin. This could have led to a prolonged illness as a result of the persistent infection, increased patient discomfort, and a prolonged hospitalization.

Prevention

At the beginning of each shift, read the entire medication administration record. Verify that the times scheduled for medications to be administered on your shift comply with the ordered frequency. Also review medications scheduled for other shifts to consider any potential drug interactions or inconsistencies. This practice might prevent others from also making a medication error.

PRACTICE PROBLEMS—CHAPTER 7

Interpret the following abbreviations and symbols without consulting another source.

1. b.i.d.	_____	9. IV	_____
2. p.r.	_____	10. q.i.d.	_____
3. a.c.	_____	11. stat	_____
4. $\bar{p}$	_____	12. ad.lib.	_____
5. t.i.d.	_____	13. p.c.	_____
6. q.4h	_____	14. IM	_____
7. p.r.n.	_____	15. $\bar{s}$	_____
8. p.o.	_____		

Give the abbreviation or symbol for the following terms without consulting another source.

16. night	_____	23. subcutaneous	_____
17. drop	_____	24. teaspoon	_____
18. milliliter	_____	25. twice daily	_____
19. grain	_____	26. every 3 hours	_____
20. gram	_____	27. after meals	_____
21. four times a day	_____	28. before	_____
22. with	_____	29. kilogram	_____

Interpret the following physician's drug orders without consulting another source.

30. Toradol 60 mg IV stat et q.6h p.r.n., pain _____

31. procaine penicillin G 300,000 units IV q.i.d. _____

32. Mylanta 5 mL p.o. 1 h a.c., 1 h p.c., bedtime, et q.2h p.r.n. at noct, gastric upset _____

_____

33. Librium 25 mg p.o. q.6h p.r.n., agitation _____

34. heparin 5,000 units subcut stat _____

35. morphine sulfate 5 mg IV q.4h p.r.n., moderate to severe pain _____

36. digoxin 0.25 mg p.o. daily _____

37. Neo-Synephrine ophthalmic 10% 2 gtt left eye q.30 min X 2 _____

_____

38. Lasix 40 mg IM stat _____

39. Decadron 4 mg IV b.i.d. _____

Refer to the MAR in Figure 7-5 on page 130 to answer questions 40 through 44.

40. Convert the scheduled times for isosorbide SR to traditional AM/PM time.

_____ _____ _____

41. How many units of heparin will be used to flush the central line at 2200? _____

42. What route is ordered for the Humulin R Regular insulin? _____

43. Interpret the order for Cipro. _____

44. If the administration times for the sliding scale insulin are accurate (30 minutes before meals), what times will meals be served? (Use traditional AM/PM time.) _____

Refer to the Computerized Pharmacy MAR in Figure 7-6 on page 131 to answer questions 45 through 49.

45. The physician visited about 5:00 PM on 8/8/xx. What order did the physician write? _____

_____

46. Using the time as a clue, interpret the symbol "w/" in the Zantac order and give the proper medical abbreviation. _____

_____

47. Interpret the order for ranitidine. _____

FIGURE 7-5 Medication administration record for Chapter 7 Practice Problems (questions 40–44)

ORIGINAL ORDER DATE	DATE STARTED / RENEWED	MEDICATION - DOSAGE	ROUTE	SCHEDULE 11-7	7-3	3-11	DATE 11/3/xx 11-7	7-3	3-11	DATE 11/4/xx 11-7	7-3	3-11	DATE 11/5/xx 11-7	7-3	3-11	DATE 11/6/xx 11-7	7-3	3-11
11/3/xx	11/3/xx	heparin lock central line flush (10 units per mL solution) 2 mL b.i.d.	IV		1000	2200												
11/3/xx	11/3/xx	isosorbide SR 40 mg q.8h	PO	2400	0800	1600												
11/3/xx	11/3/xx	Cipro 500 mg q.12h	PO		1000	2200												
11/3/xx	11/3/xx	Humulin N NPH U-100 insulin 15 units q.am	subcut	0700														
11/3/xx	11/3/xx	Humulin R Regular U-100 insulin 30 min. ac and bedtime per sliding scale Blood glucose 0-150 3 units 151-250 8 units 251-350 13 units 351-400 18 units greater than 400 call Dr.	subcut		0730 1130	1730 2200												
11/3/xx	11/3/xx	**PRN** Tylenol 1,000 mg q.4h prn headache	PO															

PRN

INJECTION SITES

B - RIGHT ARM	D - RIGHT ANTERIOR THIGH	H - LEFT ABDOMEN	L - LEFT BUTTOCKS
C - RIGHT ABDOMEN	G - LEFT ARM	J - LEFT ANTERIOR THIGH	M - RIGHT BUTTOCKS

DATE GIVEN	TIME	INT.	ONE - TIME MEDICATION - DOSAGE	RT.	11-7	7-3	3-11	11-7	7-3	3-11	11-7	7-3	3-11	11-7	7-3	3-11	11-7	7-3	3-11
					SCHEDULE			DATE			DATE			DATE			DATE		
				SIGNATURE OF NURSE ADMINISTERING MEDICATIONS	11-7														
					7-3														
					3-11														

DATE GIVEN	TIME	INT.	MEDICATION-DOSAGE-CONT.	RT.

RECOPIED BY:

CHECKED BY:

Patient, Pat H.
#6-33725-4

LITHO IN U.S.A. K6508 (7-92) D395538

ALLERGIES:
None Known

602-31 (7-XX) (MPC# 1355)

① **ORIGINAL COPY**

PRINTED BY STANDARD REGISTER U.S.A. ZIPSET ®

FIGURE 7-6 Computerized pharmacy MAR for Chapter 7 Practice Problems (questions 45–49)

START	STOP	MEDICATION		SCHEDULED TIMES	OK'D BY	0701 TO 1500	1501 TO 2300	2301 TO 0700
21:00 8/17/xx SCH		MEGESTROL ACETATE (MEGACE) 40 MG TAB 2 TABS PO BID		0900 2100				
12:00 8/17/xx SCH		VANCOMYCIN 250 MG CAP 1 CAPSULE PO QID		0800 1200 1800 2200				
9:00 8/13/xx SCH		FLUCONAZOLE (DIFLUCAN) 100 MG TAB 100 MG PO DAILY		0900				
21:00 8/11/xx SCH		PERIDEX ORAL RINSE 480 ML 30 ML ORAL RINSE BID SWISH AND SPIT		0900 2100				
17:00 8/10/xx SCH		RANITIDINE (ZANTAC) 150 MG TAB 1 TABLET PO BID W/BREAKFAST AND SUPPER		0800 1700				
17:00 8/08/xx SCH		DIGOXIN (LANOXIN) 0.125 MG TAB 1 TAB PO daily at 1700 CHECK PULSE RATE		1700				
0:01 8/27/xx PRN		LIDOCAINE 5% OINT 35 GM TUBE APPLY TOPICAL PRN* TO RECTAL AREA						
14:00 8/22/xx PRN		SODIUM CHLORIDE INJ 10 ML AS DIR IV TID DILUENT FOR ATIVAN IV						
14:00 8/22/xx PRN		LORAZEPAM (ATIVAN)*2 MG INJ 1 MG IV TID PRN ANXIETY						
9:30 8/21/xx PRN		TUCKS 40 PADS APPLY APPLY TOPICAL Q4H TO RECTUM PRN						
9:30 8/21/xx PRN		ANUSOL SUPP 1 SUPP 1 SUPP PR Q4H						
16:00 8/18/xx PRN		OXYCODONE 5 MG TAB 5 MG PO Q4H PRN PAIN						

Gluteus	Thigh
A. Right	H. Right
B. Left	I. Left
Ventro Gluteal	Deltoid
C. Right	J. Right
D. Left	K. Left
E. Abdomen	1	2
	3	4
Page **1** of 2	DAILY

STANDARD TIMES
DAILY= 0900
BID = Q12H = 0900 & 2100
TID = 0800, 1400, 2200
Q8H = 0800, 1600, 2400
QID = 0800, 1200, 1800, 2200
Q6H = 0600, 1200, 1800, 2400
Q4H = 0400, 0800, 1200. . .
DAILY DIGOXIN = 1700
DAILY WARFARIN = 1600

NURSE'S SIGNATURE	INITIAL
0701-	
1500 _____	
1501-	
2300 _____	
2301-	
0700 _____	
Ok'd	
by _____	

ALLERGIES: NAFCILLIN
                       BACTRIM
                       SULFA
                       TRIMETHOPRIM
                       CIPROFLOXACIN HCL

Patient   Smith, John
Patient #   3-90301-4
Physician: J. Physician, M.D.
Room: 407-4 South

FROM: 08/30/xx   0701   TO: 08/31/xx   0700

48. Which of the routine medications is (are) ordered for 6:00 PM? _____

49. How many hours are between the scheduled administration times for Megace? _____

50. Describe the strategy that would prevent this medication error.

Possible Scenario

Suppose a physician wrote an order for **gentamicin 100 mg IV q.8h** for a patient hospitalized with meningitis. The unit secretary transcribed the order as:

gentamicin 100 mg IV q.8h

(12 AM–6 AM–12 PM–6 PM)

The medication nurse checked the order without noticing the discrepancy in the administration times. Suppose the patient received the medication every 6 hours for 3 days before the error was noticed.

Potential Outcome

The patient would have received one extra dose each day, which is equivalent to one third more medication daily. Most likely, the physician would be notified of the error, and the medication would be discontinued with serum gentamicin levels drawn. The levels would likely be in the toxic range, and the patient's gentamicin levels would be monitored until the levels returned to normal. This patient would be at risk of developing ototoxicity or nephrotoxicity from the overdose of gentamicin.

Prevention

_____

_____

After completing these problems, see page 516 to check your answers.

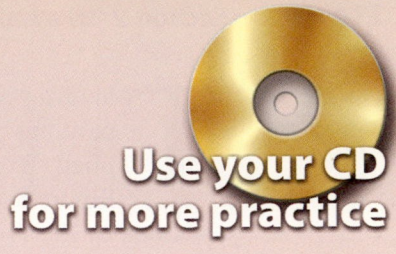
Use your CD for more practice

8

Understanding Drug Labels

OBJECTIVES

Upon mastery of Chapter 8, you will be able to read and understand the labels of the medications you have available. To accomplish this you will also be able to:

- Find and differentiate the brand and generic names of drugs.
- Determine the dosage strength.
- Determine the form in which the drug is supplied.
- Determine the supply dosage or concentration.
- Identify the total volume of the drug container.
- Differentiate the total volume of the container from the supply dosage.
- Find the directions for mixing or preparing the supply dosage of drugs, as needed.
- Recognize and follow drug alerts.
- Identify the administration route.
- Check the expiration date.
- Identify the lot or control number, National Drug Code, bar code symbols, and controlled substance classifications.
- Recognize the manufacturer's name.
- Differentiate labels for multidose and unit dose containers.
- Identify combination drugs.
- Describe supply dosage expressed as a ratio or percent.

The drug order prescribes how much of a drug the patient is to receive. The nurse must prepare the order from the drugs on hand. The drug label tells how the available drug is supplied. Examine the various preparations, labels, and dosage strengths of Valium injection, Figure 8-1.

Look at the following common drug labels to learn to recognize pertinent information about the drugs supplied.

FIGURE 8-1   Various Valium preparations

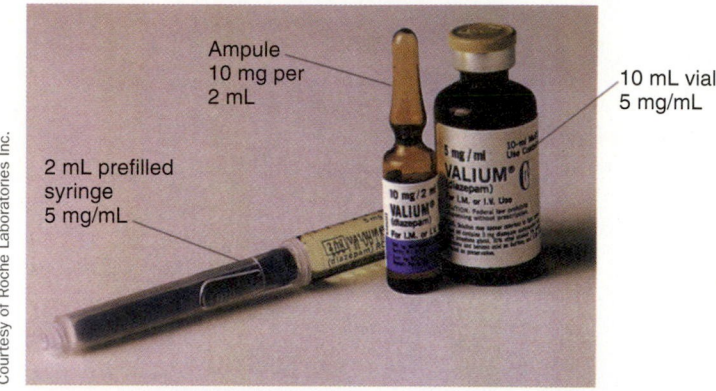

BRAND AND GENERIC NAMES

The brand, trade, or proprietary name is the manufacturer's name for a drug. Notice that the brand name is usually the most prominent word on the drug label—large type and boldly visible to easily identify and promote the product. It is often followed by the registered sign (®) meaning that both the name and formulation are so designated. The generic, or established, nonproprietary name appears directly under the brand name. Sometimes the generic name is placed inside parentheses. By law, the generic name must be identified on all drug labels.

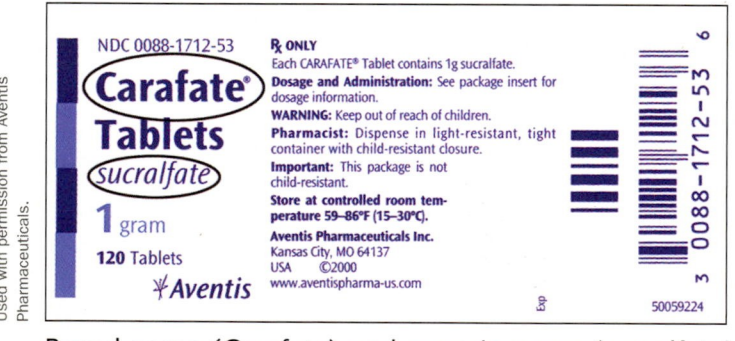

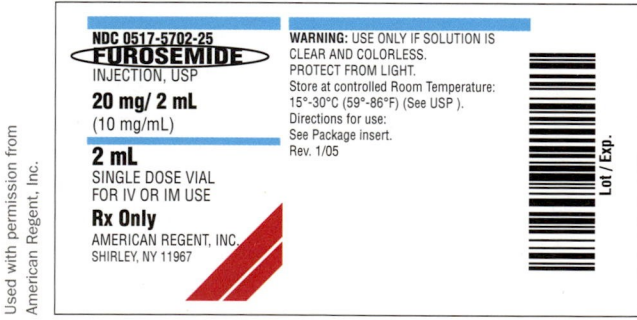

Brand name (Carafate) and generic name (sucralfate)   Generic drug (furosemide)

Generic equivalents of many brand name drugs are ordered as substitutes or allowed by the prescribing practitioner. Because only the generic name appears on these labels, nurses need to carefully cross-check all medications. Failure to do so could cause inaccurate drug identification.

DOSAGE STRENGTH

The dosage strength refers to the dosage *weight* or amount of drug provided in a specific unit of measurement. The dosage strength of Lopid tablets is 600 milligrams (the weight and specific unit of measurement) per tablet. Some drugs, such as penicillin V potassium, have two different but equivalent dosage strengths. Penicillin V potassium has a dosage strength of 250 milligrams (per tablet) or 400,000 units (per tablet). This allows prescribers to order the drug using either unit of measurement.

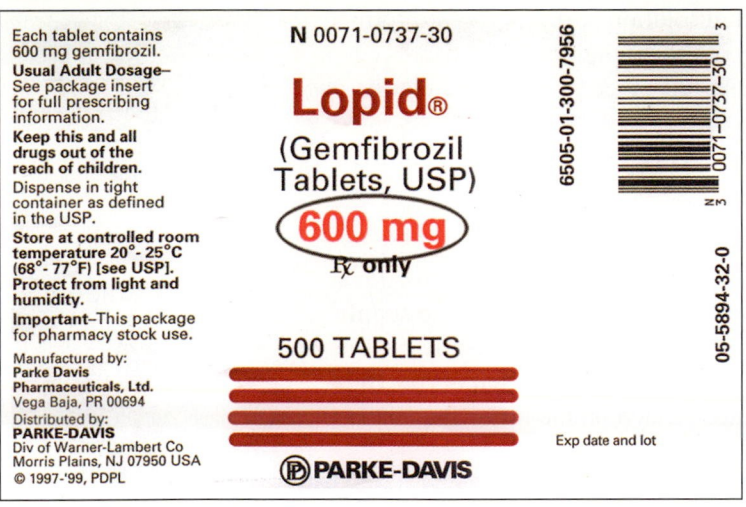

600 milligrams (per tablet)

250 milligrams (400,000 units) (per tablet)

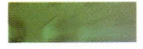

FORM

The form identifies the *structure* and *composition* of the drug. Solid dosage forms for oral use include tablets and capsules. Some powdered or granular medications that are not manufactured in tablet or capsule form can be directly combined with food or beverages and administered. Others must be reconstituted (liquefied) and measured in a precise liquid volume, such as milliliters, drops, or ounces. They may be a crystalloid (clear solution) or a suspension (solid particles in liquid that separate when held in a container).

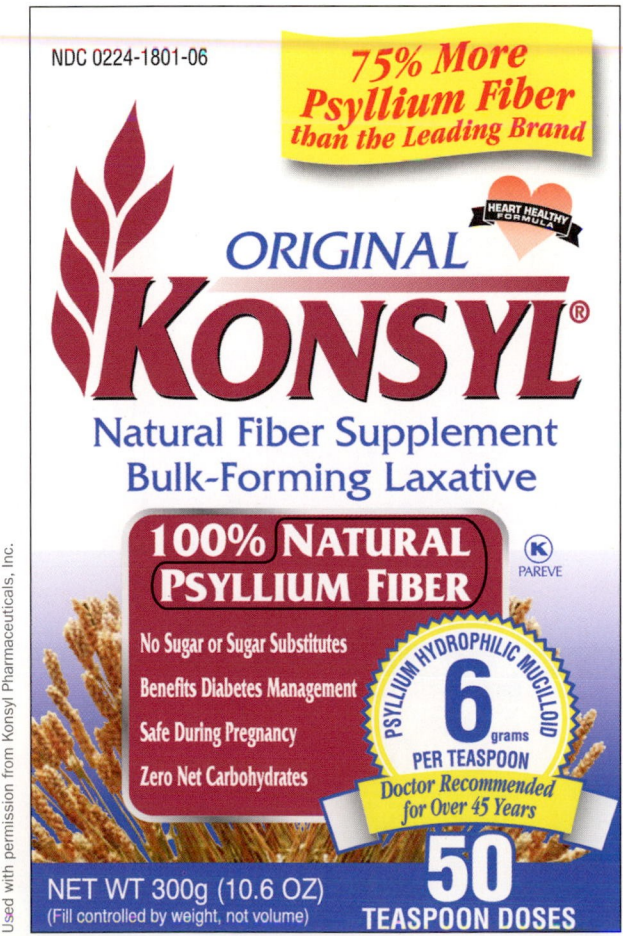

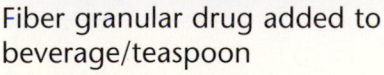

Fiber granular drug added to beverage/teaspoon

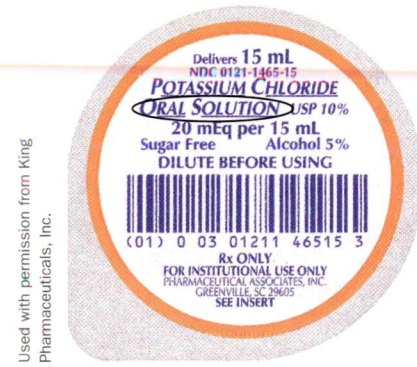

Oral solution

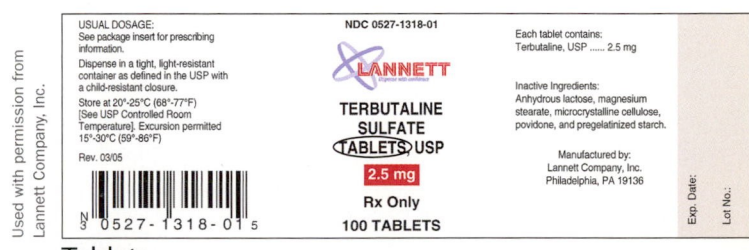

Tablets

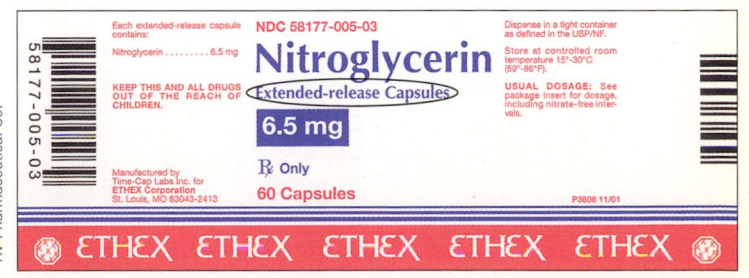

Extended-release capsules

Injectable medications may be supplied in solution or dry powdered form to be reconstituted. Once reconstituted, they are measured in milliliters.

Medications are also supplied in a variety of other forms, such as suppositories, creams, and patches.

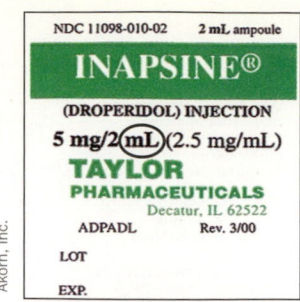

Injectable solution

SUPPLY DOSAGE

The supply dosage refers to both *dosage strength* and *form*. It is read *X measured units per some quantity*. For solid-form medications, such as tablets, the supply dosage is X measured units per tablet. For liquid medications, the supply dosage is the same as the medication's concentration, such as X measured units per milliliter. Take a minute to read the supply dosage printed on the following labels.

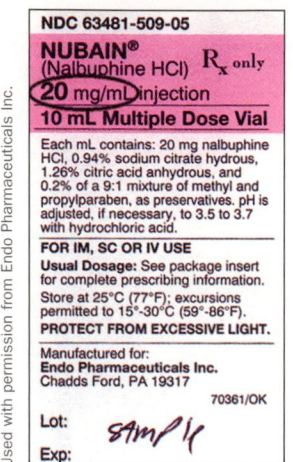

20 milligrams per milliliter

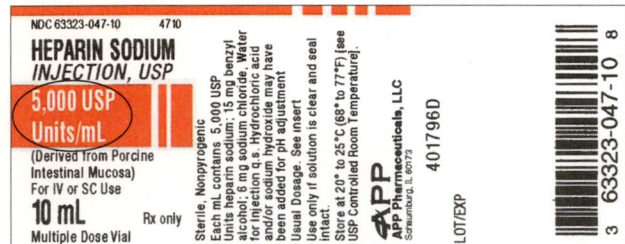

5,000 USP Units per milliliter

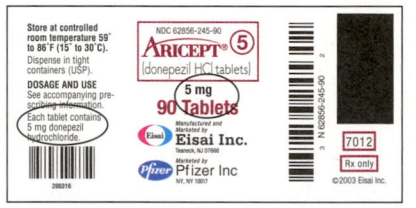

5 milligrams per tablet

TOTAL VOLUME

The total volume refers to the *full quantity* contained in a package, bottle, or vial. For tablets and other solid medications, it is the total number of individual items. For liquids, it is the total fluid volume.

All too frequently, dosage strength and total volume are misinterpreted resulting in medication errors. Beginning February 1, 2009, a new Food and Drug Administration (FDA) requirement became official that calls for the strength per total volume to be the prominent expression on single and multiple dose injectable product labels, followed in close proximity by the strength per mL enclosed in parentheses (Cohen, 2008). Notice the Inapsine (droperidol injection) label on this page that complies with this new rule: 2 mL ampule size, **5 mg/2 mL** (2.5 mg/mL). Clearly providing all of this information lowers the risk of misinterpretation and medication error.

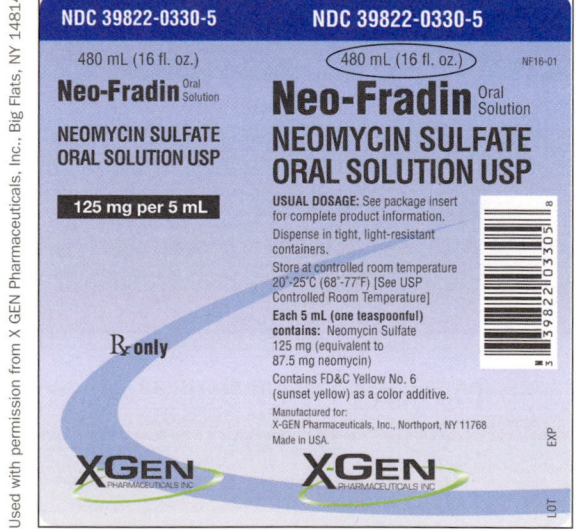

480 milliliters (16 fluid ounces)

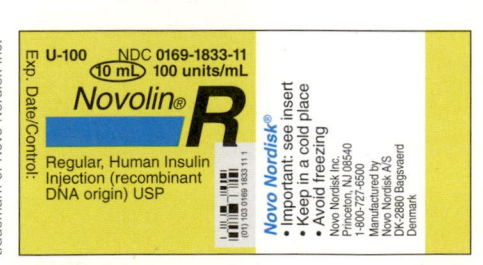

10 milliliters

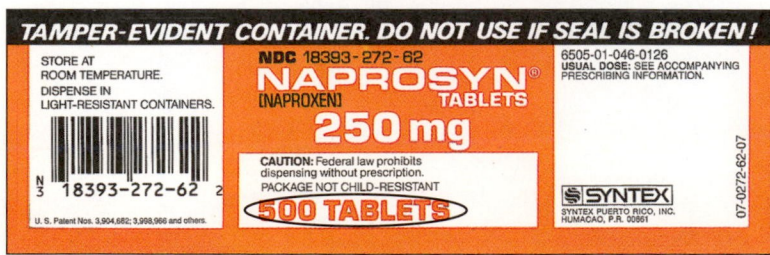

500 tablets

ADMINISTRATION ROUTE

The administration route refers to the *site* of the body or *method of drug delivery* into the patient. Examples of routes of administration include oral, enteral (into the gastrointestinal tract through a tube), sublingual, injection (IV, IM, subcut), otic, optic, topical, rectal, vaginal, and others. Unless specified otherwise, tablets, capsules, and caplets are intended for oral use.

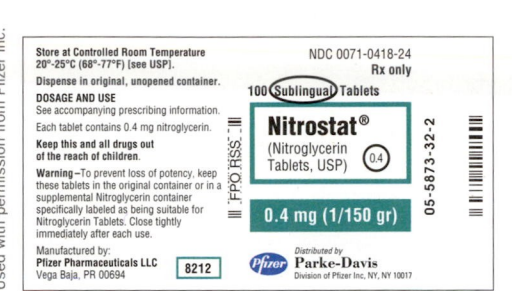

Sublingual

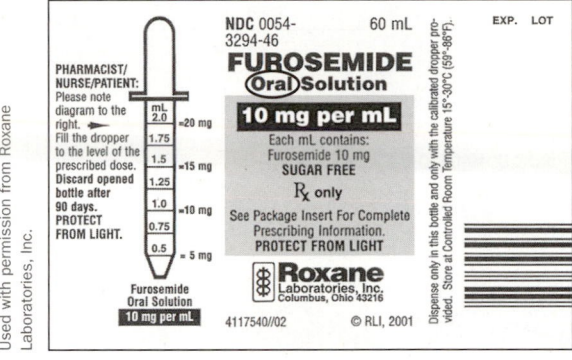

Oral

Intramuscular (IM), subcutaneous (subcut), or intravenous (IV)

DIRECTIONS FOR MIXING OR RECONSTITUTING

Some drugs are dispensed in *powder* form and must be *reconstituted for use*. (Reconstitution is discussed further in Chapters 10 and 12.)

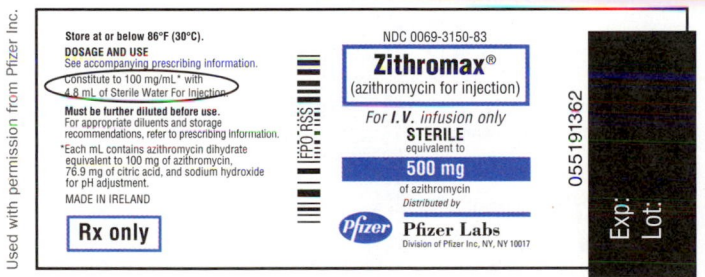

See directions

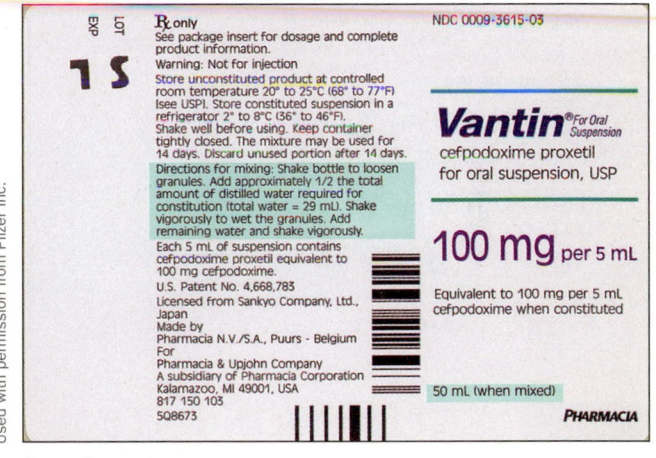

See directions

LABEL ALERTS

Manufacturers may print warnings on the packaging or special alerts may be added by the pharmacy before dispensing. Look for special storage alerts such as "refrigerate at all times," "keep in a dry place," "replace cap and close tightly before storing," or "protect from light." Reconstituted suspensions may be dispensed already prepared for use, and directions may instruct the health care professional to "shake well before using" as a reminder to remix the components. Read and follow all label instructions carefully.

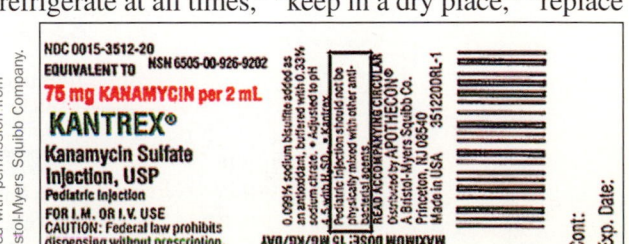

See alert

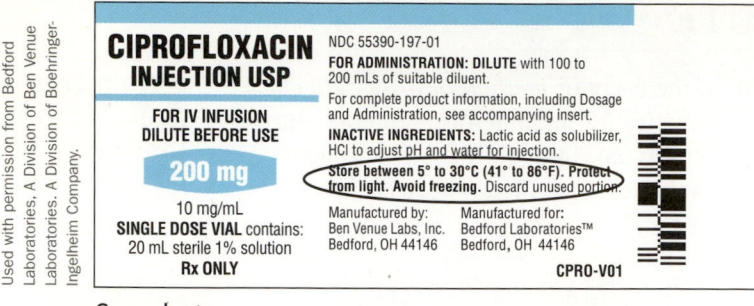

See alert

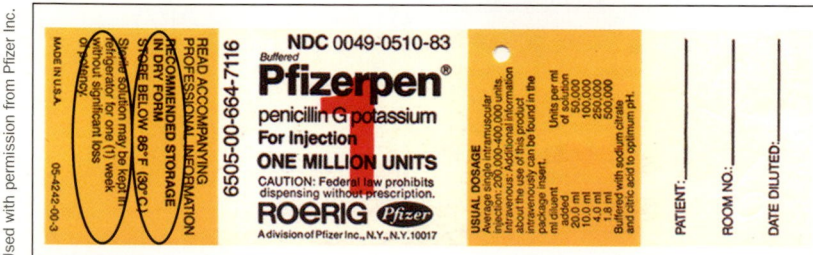

See alerts

NAME OF THE MANUFACTURER

The name of the manufacturer is circled on the following labels.

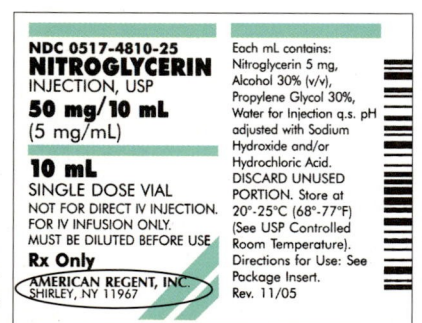

American Regent, Inc.

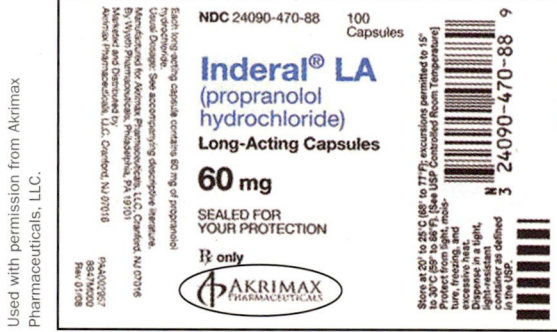

Akrimax Pharmaceuticals, Inc.

EXPIRATION DATE

The medication should be used, discarded, or returned to the pharmacy by the expiration date. Further, note the special expiration instructions given on labels for reconstituted medications. Refer to the Vantin label on page 137.

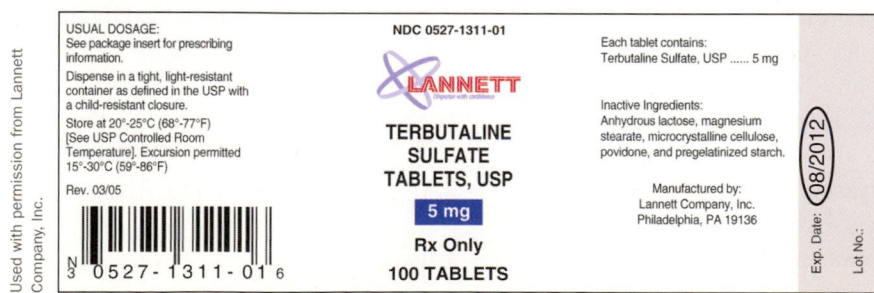

Expiration date: 08/2012

LOT OR CONTROL NUMBERS

Federal law requires all medication packages to be identified with a lot or control number. If a drug is recalled, for reasons such as damage or tampering, the lot number quickly identifies the particular group of medication packages to be removed from shelves. This number has been invaluable for vaccine and over-the-counter medication recalls.

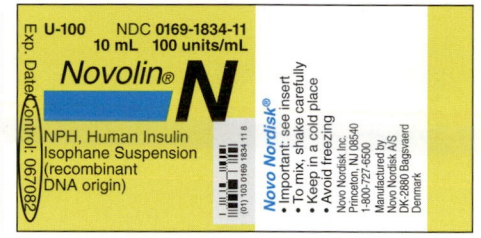

Control number: 067082

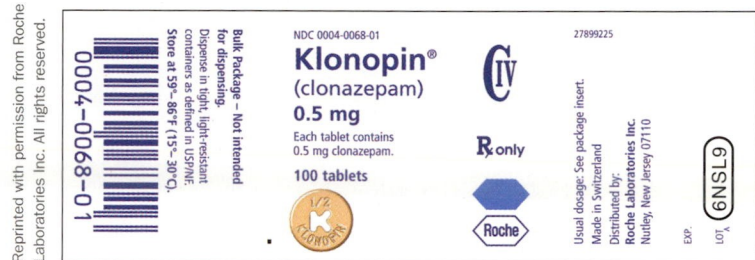

Lot number: 6NSL9

NATIONAL DRUG CODE (NDC)

Federal law requires every prescription medication to have a unique identifying number, much like every U.S. citizen has a unique Social Security number. This number must appear on every manufacturer's label and is printed with the letters "NDC" followed by three discrete groups of numbers.

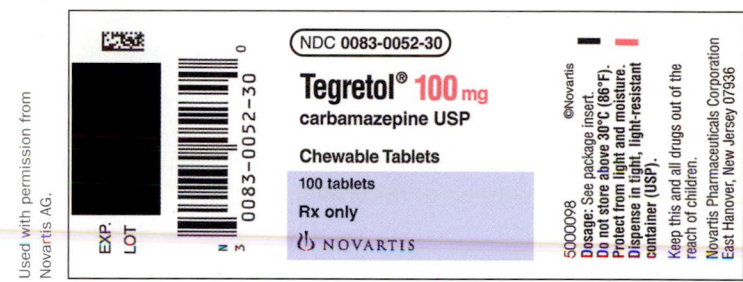

NDC: 0083-0052-30

CONTROLLED SUBSTANCE SCHEDULE

The Controlled Substances Act was passed in May 1971. One of its purposes was to improve the administration and regulation of the production, distribution, and dispensing of controlled substances. Drugs considered controlled substances are classified according to their potential for use and abuse.

Drugs are classified into numbered levels or schedules from Schedule I to Schedule V. Drugs that have the highest potential for abuse are Schedule I drugs and those with the lowest potential for abuse are Schedule V drugs. The schedule number of controlled substances is indicated on the drug label.

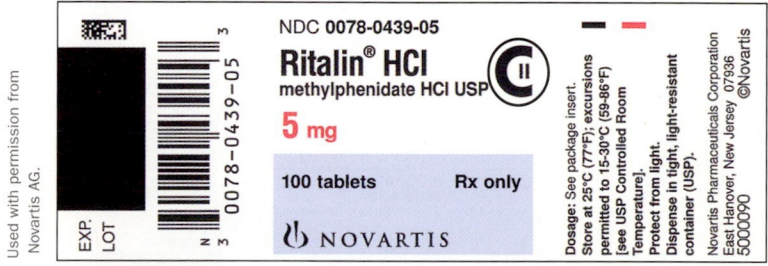

Schedule II

BAR CODE SYMBOLS

Bar code symbols are commonly used in retail sales. Bar code symbols also document drug dosing for recordkeeping and stock reorder and can automate medication documentation right at the patient's bedside.

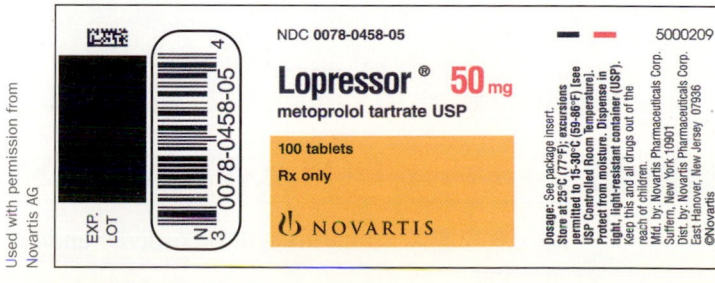

Bar code

UNITED STATES PHARMACOPEIA (USP) AND NATIONAL FORMULARY (NF)

These codes are found on many manufacturer-printed medication labels. The USP and NF are the two official national lists of approved drugs. Each manufacturer follows special guidelines that determine when to include these initials on a label. These initials are placed after the generic drug name. Be careful not to mistake these abbreviations for other initials that designate specific characteristics of a drug, such as *SR,* which means *sustained release.*

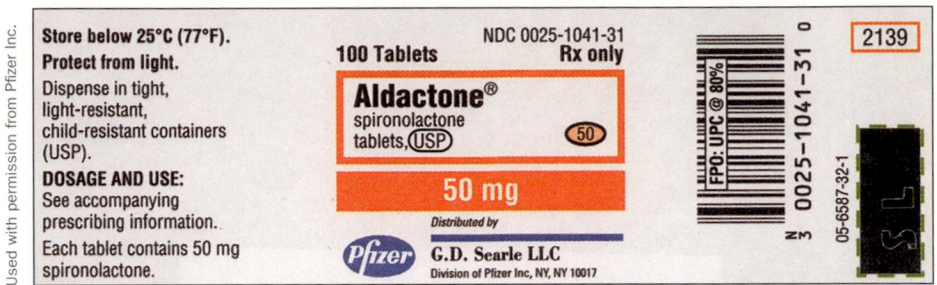

USP

UNIT- OR SINGLE-DOSE LABELS

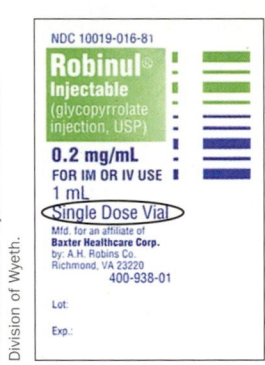

Most oral medications administered in the hospital setting are available in unit dosage, such as a single capsule or tablet packaged separately in a typical blister pack. The pharmacy provides a 24-hour supply of each drug for the patient. The only major difference in this form of labeling is that the total volume of the container is usually omitted because the volume is 1 tablet or capsule. Likewise, the dosage strength is understood as *per one.* Further, injectable medicines may be packaged in single- dose preparations.

Unit dose single-use vial

COMBINATION DRUGS

Some medications are a combination of two or more drugs in one form. Read the labels for Percocet and Lortab and notice the different substances that are combined in each tablet. Combination drugs are sometimes prescribed by the number of tablets, capsules, or milliliters to be given rather than by the dosage strength.

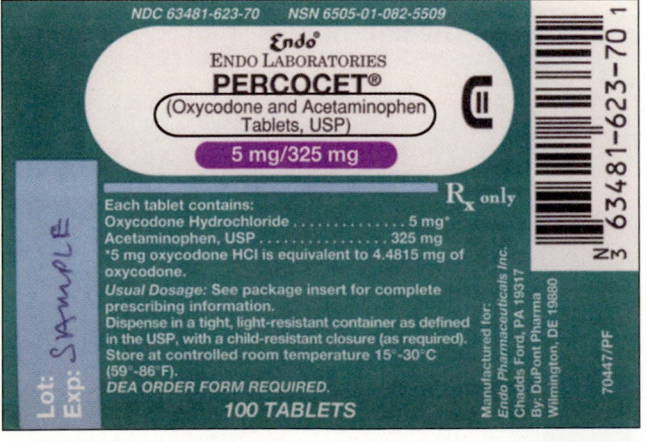
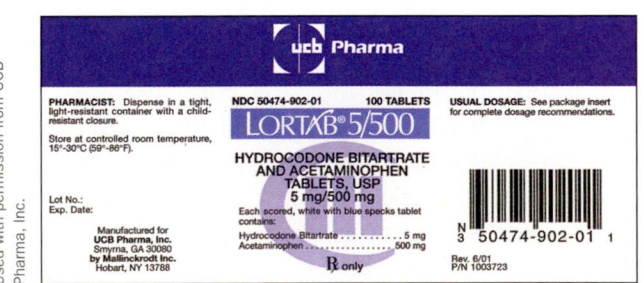

Combination drugs

SUPPLY DOSAGE EXPRESSED AS A RATIO OR PERCENT

Occasionally, solutions will be ordered and/or manufactured in a supply dosage expressed as a ratio or percent.

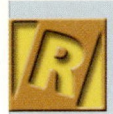

RULE

Ratio solutions express the number of grams of the drug per total milliliters of solution.

EXAMPLE ■

Epinephrine 1:1,000 contains 1 g pure drug per 1,000 mL solution, 1 g:1,000 mL = 1,000 mg:1,000 mL = 1 mg:1 mL.

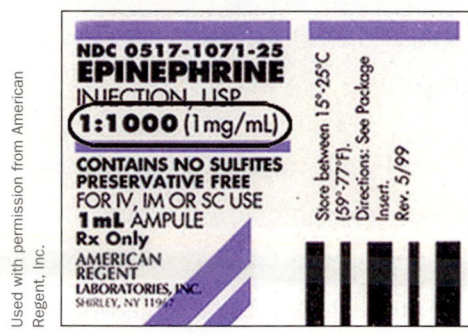

1:1,000

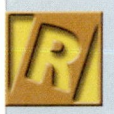

RULE

Percentage (%) solutions express the number of grams of the drug per 100 milliliters of solution.

EXAMPLE ■

Lidocaine 2% contains 2 g pure drug per 100 mL solution, 2 g per 100 mL = 2,000 mg per 100 mL = 20 mg/mL.

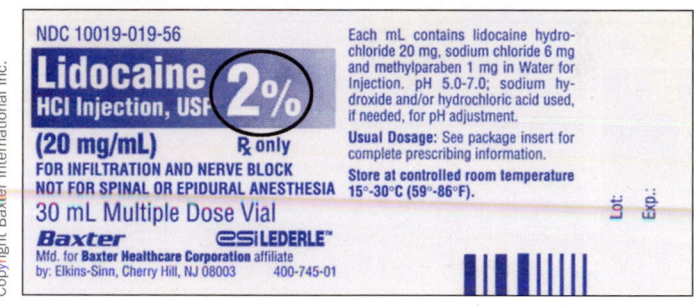

2%

Although these labels look different from many of the other labels, it is important to recognize that the supply dosage can still be determined. Many times the label will have a more commonly identified supply dosage and not just the ratio or percent. Look at the epinephrine and lidocaine labels. On the epinephrine label, the ratio is 1:1,000; the supply dosage also can be identified as 1 mg/mL. On the lidocaine label, the percentage is 2%; the supply dosage also can be identified as 20 mg/mL.

CHECKING LABELS

Recall the Six Rights of medication administration: The *right patient* must receive the *right drug* in the *right amount* by the *right route* at the *right time* followed by the *right documentation*. To be absolutely sure the patient receives the right drug, check the label three times.

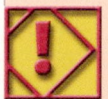

CAUTION

Before administering a medication to a patient, check the drug label three times:

1. Against the medication order or MAR.

2. Before preparing the medication.

3. After preparing the medication and before administering it.

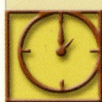

QUICK REVIEW

Read labels carefully to:

- Identify the drug and the manufacturer.

- Differentiate between brand and generic names, dosage strength, form, supply dosage, total container volume, and administration route.

- Recognize that the drug's supply dosage similarly refers to a drug's weight per unit of measure or concentration.

- Find the directions for reconstitution, as needed.

- Note expiration date and alerts.

- Describe lot or control number, NDC number, and schedule (if controlled substance).

- Identify supply dosage on labels with ratios and percents.

- Be sure you administer the right drug.

Review Set 20

Used with permission from Novartis AG.

NDC 0083-0052-30

Tegretol® **100** mg
carbamazepine USP

Chewable Tablets

100 tablets

Rx only

◊ NOVARTIS

5000098 **Dosage: See package insert.
Do not store above 30°C (86°F).
Protect from light and moisture.
Dispense in tight, light-resistant
container (USP).**

Keep this and all drugs out of the reach of children.

Novartis Pharmaceuticals Corporation
East Hanover, New Jersey 07936

©Novartis

EXP.
LOT

0083-0052-30

A

Used with permission from Bedford Laboratories, A Division of Ben Venue Laboratories. A Division of Boehringer-Ingelheim Company.

TERBUTALINE
SULFATE INJECTION USP

FOR SC INJECTION ONLY.

1 mg/mL

Rx ONLY

NDC 55390-101-10
1 mL Sterile Vial
Protect from light.
Manufactured for:
Bedford Laboratories™
Bedford, OH 44146

TBT-V01

B

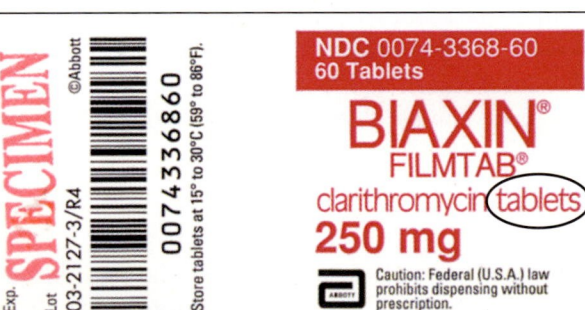

Used with permission from Abbott Laboratories.

SPECIMEN   ©Abbott

Exp.
Lot
03-2127-3/R4

Store tablets at 15° to 30°C (59° to 86°F).

0074336860

NDC 0074-3368-60
60 Tablets

BIAXIN®
FILMTAB®
clarithromycin tablets
250 mg

Caution: Federal (U.S.A.) law
prohibits dispensing without
prescription.

6505-01-354-8582
Do not accept if break-away
ring on cap is broken or missing.
Dispense in a USP tight, light-
resistant container.
Each tablet contains:
250 mg clarithromycin.
Each yellow tablet bears the ⊇
and Abbo-Code KT for product
identification.
Usual Adult Dose: One or two
tablets every twelve hours. See
enclosure for full prescribing
information.
Filmtab – Film-sealed tablets,
Abbott.
Abbott Laboratories
North Chicago, IL60064, U.S.A.

C

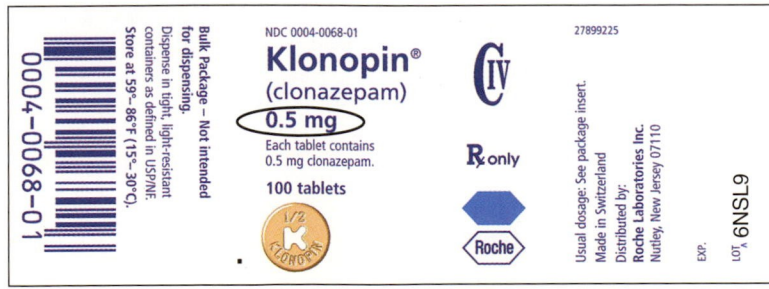

Used with permission from Abbott Laboratories.

0-0968-01

Store at 59°– 86°F (15°–30°C).

**Bulk Package – Not intended
for dispensing.**
Dispense in tight, light-resistant
containers as defined in USP/NF.

NDC 0004-0068-01

Klonopin®
(clonazepam)
0.5 mg

Each tablet contains
0.5 mg clonazepam.

100 tablets

1/2
KLONOPIN

27899225

CIV

Rx only

Roche

Usual dosage: See package insert.
Made in Switzerland
Distributed by:
Roche Laboratories Inc.
Nutley, New Jersey 07110

EXP.

LOT A 6NSL9

D

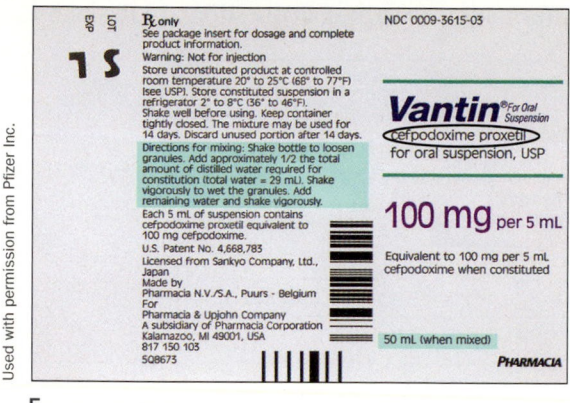

Used with permission from Pfizer Inc.

E

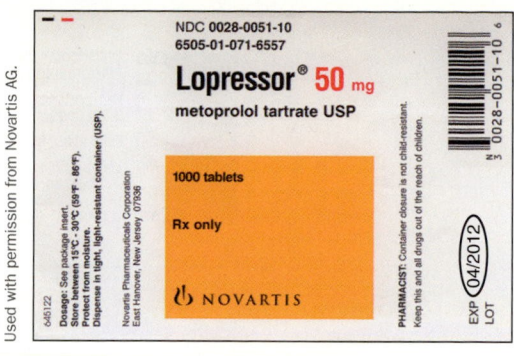

Used with permission from Novartis AG.

F

Used with permission from Aventis Pharmaceuticals.

Each CLAFORAN® STERILE vial contains 2g cefotaxime for injection, Dextrose Hydrous, USP to adjust osmolality, sodium citrate hydrous, USP to buffer injection, and hydrochloric acid to adjust pH.
℞ ONLY   Dosage and Administration: Read package insert for prescribing information and reconstitution. Shake to dissolve. **Store dry powder below 30°C. Protect from excessive light.** Mfd for: **Hoechst-Roussel Pharmaceuticals** Division of **Aventis Pharmaceuticals Inc.** Kansas City, MO 64137   ©2000 Made in United Kingdom   50053567   CND 70100

NDC 0039-0019-01
Claforan® Sterile
cefotaxime for injection, USP (formerly sterile cefotaxime sodium)
Lot (BA799)   Exp 08/2011
2g IM/IV   ✚*Aventis*

G

Use labels A through G to find the information requested in questions 1 through 15. Indicate your answer by letter (A through G).

1. The total volume of the liquid container is circled. _____

2. The dosage strength is circled. _____

3. The form of the drug is circled. _____

4. The brand name of the drug is circled. _____

5. The generic name of the drug is circled. _____

6. The expiration date is circled. _____

7. The lot number is circled. _____

8. Look at label E and determine how much of the supply drug you will administer to the patient per dose for the order *cefpodoxime 100 mg p.o. q.12h.* _____

9. Look at label A and determine the route of administration. _____

10. Indicate which labels have a visible imprinted bar code symbol. _____

11. Look at label C. What does the word *Filmtab* mean on this label? _____

12. Look at label B, and determine the supply dosage. _____

13. Look at label F, and determine how much of the supply drug you will administer to the patient per dose for the order *metoprolol 100 mg p.o. daily.* _____

14. Which drug label(s) represent controlled substance(s)? _____

15. Evaluate the potential for abuse of the controlled substance drug(s) identified in question 14.

_____

Refer to the following label to identify the specific drug information described in questions 16 through 21.

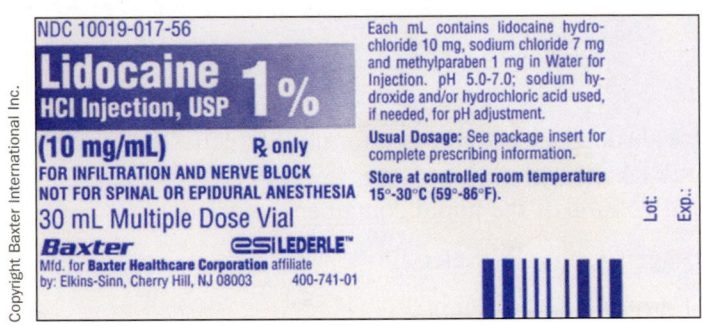

16. Generic name _____

17. Brand name _____

18. Dosage strength _____

19. Route of administration _____

20. National Drug Code _____

21. Manufacturer _____

Refer to the following label to answer questions 22 through 24.

22. The supply dosage of the drug is _____ %.

23. The supply dosage of the drug is _____ g per 1 mL.

24. The supply dosage of the drug is _____ mg per mL.

After completing these problems, see page 517 to check your answers.

CRITICAL THINKING SKILLS

Reading the labels of medications is critical. Make sure that the drug you want is what you have on hand before you prepare it. Let's look at an example of a medication error related to reading the label incorrectly.

ERROR

Not checking the label for correct dosage.

Possible Scenario

A nurse flushed a triple central venous catheter (an IV with three ports). According to hospital policy, the nurse was to flush each port with 10 mL of normal saline followed by 2 mL of heparin flush solution in the concentration of 100 units/mL. The nurse mistakenly picked up a vial of heparin containing heparin 10,000 units/mL. Without checking the label, she prepared the solution for all three ports. The patient received 60,000 units of heparin instead of 600 units.

(Continued)

Potential Outcome

The patient in this case would be at great risk for hemorrhage, leading to shock and death. Protamine sulfate would likely be ordered to counteract the action of the heparin, but a successful outcome is questionable.

Prevention

There is no substitute for checking the label before administering a medication. The nurse in this case, having drawn three different syringes of medication for the three ports, had three opportunities to catch the error.

PRACTICE PROBLEMS—CHAPTER 8

Look at labels A through G, and identify the information requested.

Label A:

1. The supply dosage of the drug in milliequivalents is _____.

2. The National Drug Code is _____.

3. The supply dosage of the drug in milligrams is _____.

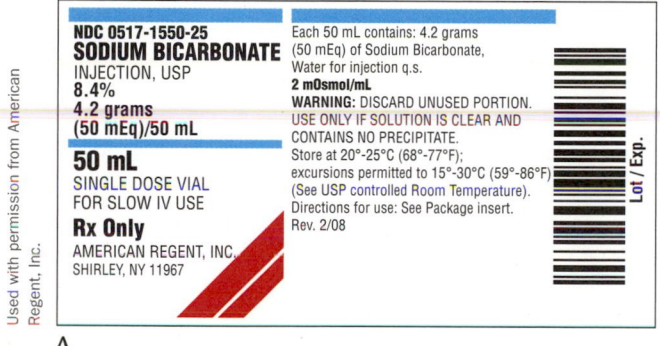

Used with permission from American Regent, Inc.

A

Label B:

4. The generic name of the drug is _____.

5. The reconstitution instruction to mix a supply dosage of 100 mg per 5 mL for oral suspension is

    _____.

6. The manufacturer of the drug is _____.

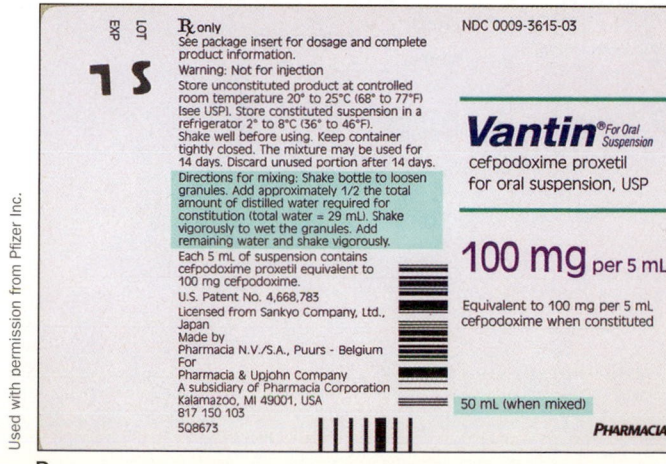

Used with permission from Pfizer Inc.

B

Label C:

7. The total volume of the medication container is _____.

8. The supply dosage is _____.

9. How much will you administer to the patient per dose for the order **methotrexate 25 mg IV stat?**

    _____.

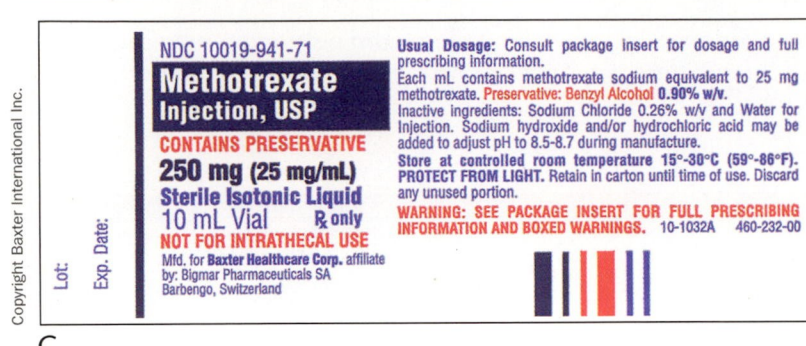

C

Label D:

10. The brand name of the drug is _____.

11. The generic name is _____.

12. The National Drug Code of the drug is _____.

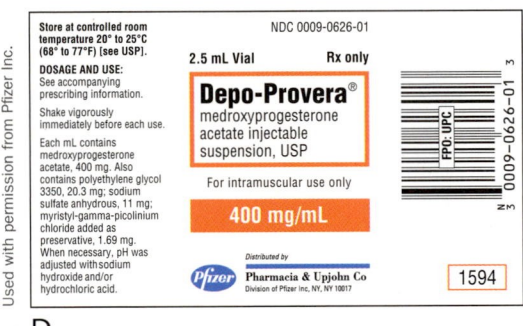

D

Label E:

13. The form of the drug is _____.

14. The total volume of the drug container is _____.

15. The administration route is _____.

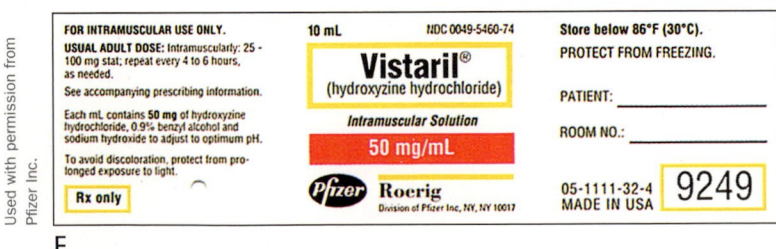

E

Label F:

16. The name of the drug manufacturer is _____.

17. The form of the drug is _____.

18. The appropriate temperature for storage of this drug is _____.

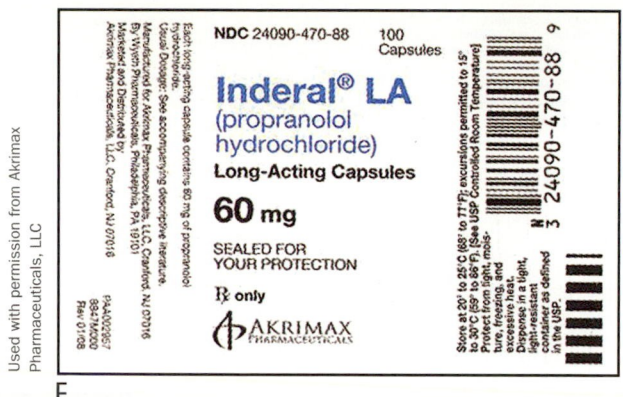

F

Used with permission from Akrimax Pharmaceuticals, LLC

Label G:

19. The supply dosage of the drug is _____.

20. The dosage strength of the drug container is _____.

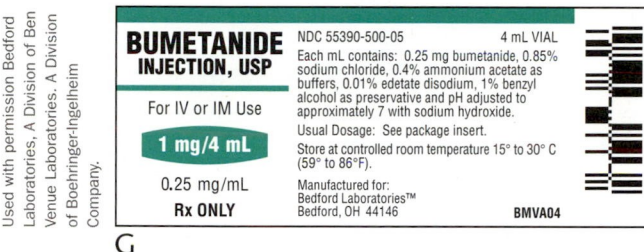

G

Used with permission Bedford Laboratories, A Division of Ben Venue Laboratories. A Division of Boehringer-Ingelheim Company.

Match label H or I with the correct descriptive statement.

21. This label represents a unit- or single-dose drug. _____

22. This label represents a combination drug. _____

23. This label represents a drug that may be ordered by the number of tablets or capsules to be administered rather than the dosage strength. _____

24. The administration route for the drug labeled H is _____.

25. The lot number for the drug labeled I is _____.

26. The controlled substance schedule for the drug labeled H is _____.

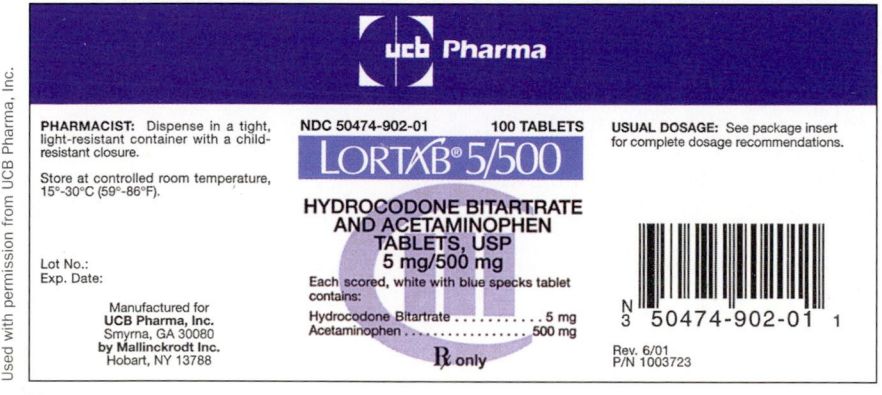

H

Used with permission from UCB Pharma, Inc.

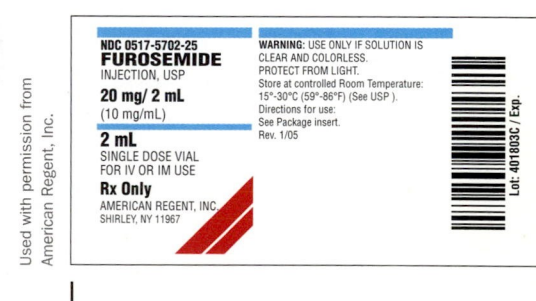

I

Used with permission from American Regent, Inc.

Label J:

27. Expressed as a percentage, the supply dosage of the drug is _____.

28. The supply dosage is equivalent to _____ g per _____ mL or _____ mg per mL.

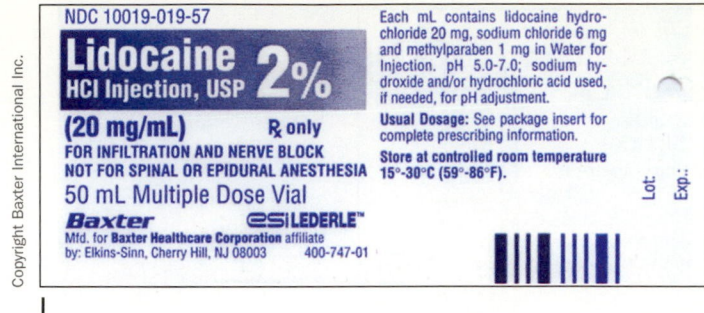

29. Describe the strategy you would implement to prevent this medication error.

Possible Scenario

Suppose a physician ordered an antibiotic **Principen .5 g p.o. q.6h.** The writing was not clear on the order, and Prinivil (an anti-hypertensive medication) 5 mg was sent up by the pharmacy. However, the order was correctly transcribed to the MAR. In preparing the medication, the nurse did not read the MAR or label carefully and administered Prinivil, the wrong medication.

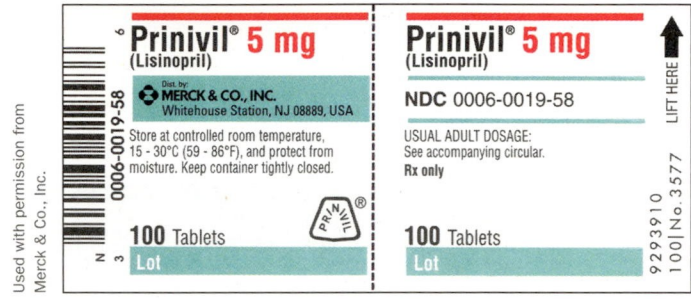

Potential Outcome

A medication error occurred because the wrong medication was given. The patient's infection treatment would be delayed. Furthermore, the erroneous blood pressure drug could have harmful effects.

Prevention

_____

_____

30. Describe the strategy you would implement to prevent this medication error.

Possible Scenario

Suppose a physician wrote the order **Celebrex 100 mg p.o. q.12h** (anti-inflammatory to treat rheumatoid arthritis pain), but the order was difficult to read. The unit secretary and pharmacy interpreted the order as *Celexa* (antidepressant), a medication with a similar spelling. Celexa was written on the MAR.

Potential Outcome

The nurse administered the Celexa for several days, and the patient began complaining of severe knee and hip pain from rheumatoid arthritis. Also, the patient experienced side effects of Celexa, including drowsiness and tremors. A medication error occurred because several health care professionals misinterpreted the order.

Prevention

a) What should have alerted the nurse that something was wrong?

_____

b) What should have been considered to prevent this error?

_____

After completing these problems, see page 517 to check your answers.

REFERENCE

Cohen, Michael R. (2008). ISMP medication error report analysis: Strength misread as total dose [Electronic version]. *Hospital Pharmacy, 43,* 7. Retrieved November 23, 2008 from http://www.factsandcomparisons.com/assets/hpdatenamed/20080701_July2008_ismp.pdf

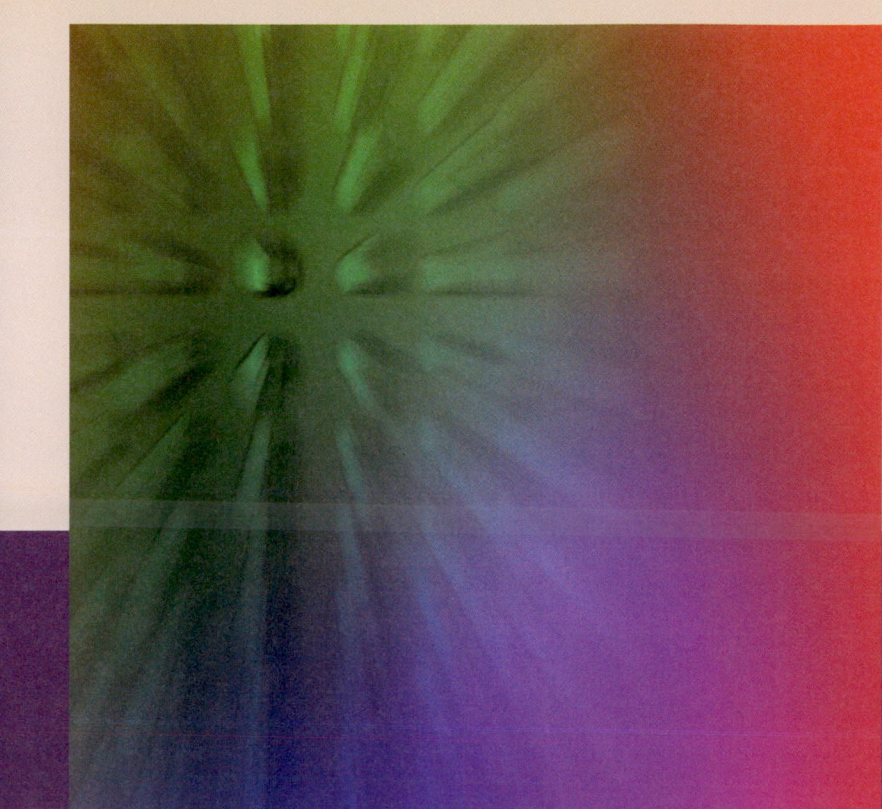
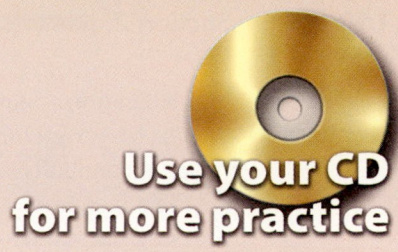

Preventing Medication Errors

OBJECTIVES

Upon mastery of Chapter 9, you will be able to identify and prevent the common situations that lead to medication administration errors. To accomplish this you will also be able to:

- Describe the consequences and costs of medication errors.
- Cite incidence of hospital injuries and deaths attributable to medication errors.
- Explore evidence and rationale for underreporting of medication errors.
- Name the steps involved in medication administration.
- Identify six common causes of medication errors.
- Identify the role of the nurse in preventing medication errors.
- Describe the role of technology and health care administration in medication error prevention.
- Recognize examples of prescription, transcription, and recording notation errors.
- Correct medical notation errors.
- Describe the requirements of The Joint Commission to prevent medication errors.
- Provide a sound rationale for the critical nature of medication administration and the importance of accurate and safe dosage calculations and medication administration.

Medication administration is one of the primary functions of the nurse and other health care practitioners in most health care settings. Unfortunately, medication administration errors are common. Any health care practitioner is potentially at risk for making an error. Several studies addressing the problem indicate there is no relationship between the incidence of medication errors and the characteristics of the nurses who usually make them (that is, years of practice and education). Statistics indicate that 10% to 18% of all hospital injuries are attributable to medication errors (Mayo & Duncan, 2004). The Institute of Medicine reports that 44,000 to 98,000 people die in U.S. hospitals annually as a result of medication errors that could have been prevented.

The incidence of medication errors by nurses is difficult to accurately determine. Several studies addressing nurses' perception of medication errors support the existence of underreporting by nurses (Mayo & Duncan, 2004; Stetina, Groves, & Pafford, 2005; Wolf & Serembus, 2004). Other research indicates confusion among nurses about what constitutes a drug error. Failure to administer a medication and administering a medication late are the most underreported errors because some nurses erroneously perceive that the patients will not be harmed in these situations (Mayo & Duncan, 2004; Stetina et al, 2005).

The frequency of medication errors made by nurses and the consequences of these errors affect not only the health of the patient but also the overall cost of health care. These medication errors and the reactions that result from them cause increased length of stay, increased cost, patient disability, and death. There are additional indirect consequences as well. These include harm to the nurse involved in regard to his or her personal and professional status, confidence, and practice (Mayo & Duncan, 2004).

The medication delivery process is complex and involves many individuals and departments. This chapter will focus on the critical role of the nurse in this process and the importance of legible medication orders, accurate transcription and interpretation, and safe medication administration.

PRESCRIPTION

The steps involved in safe medication administration begin with the *prescription,* followed by *transcription,* and then *administration.* Only those licensed health care providers who have authority by their state to write prescriptions are permitted to do so, such as a medical doctor (MD), an osteopathic doctor (DO), a podiatrist (DPM), a dentist (DDS), a physician's assistant (PA), or an advanced practice nurse (ARNP).

Although nurses are not the originator of drug prescriptions, they play an important role in preventing errors in the *prescription* step. Refer back to Chapter 7 to review the seven parts of drug orders: patient's name, date and time of the order, name of the drug, amount of the drug (including the unit of measure), route, frequency or specific administration schedule, and the prescriber's name and licensure. It is important to always remember that the practitioner who administers a drug shares the liability for patient injury, even if the medical order was incorrect. The wise nurse always verifies the safety of the drug order by consulting a reputable drug reference, such as the *Hospital Formulary, Nurse's Drug Handbook* published annually by Delmar Cengage Learning, and the *Physicians' Desk Reference* published annually by Thomson Reuters. Most hospitals and health care systems have access to electronic drug guides available online, with many accessed directly from the electronic medication administration record (MAR) by clicking on the drug name, such as the Thomson Reuters Micromedex system for point-of-care decision support.

Verbal Orders

In most health care institutions, the nurse (or other authorized individual, such as a transcriptionist) can receive verbal orders either in person or by phone from licensed physicians or other practitioners who are licensed to prescribe. As the accrediting body for health care organizations and agencies, The Joint Commission (2009) publishes Patient Safety Goals. Goal 2 is designed to improve the effectiveness of communication among caregivers. It requires that the authorized individual receiving a verbal or telephone order first **write it down** in the patient's chart or enter it into the computer record; second, **read it back** to the prescriber; and third, **get confirmation** from the prescriber that it is correct. For the nurse to only repeat back the order as heard or repeat it while writing it down is not sufficient to regularly prevent errors, and this is not allowed by The Joint Commission. The order must first be **written** and then it must be **read back** after it is written to ensure that the order is clear to the recipient and in turn **confirmed** by the prescriber giving the order. As with written orders, the nurse must also verify that all seven parts of the verbal order have been included and are accurate. If the nurse has any question or concern about the order, it should be clarified during the conversation. Of course, The Joint Commission advises that in emergency situations, such as a code in the ER, doing a formal read back would not be feasible and would compromise patient safety. In such cases a repeat back is acceptable.

> **CAUTION**
> Accepting verbal orders is a major responsibility and a situation that can readily lead to medication errors. Most health care institutions have policies concerning telephone or verbal orders, and the nurse or other authorized staff should be informed of his or her responsibility in this regard.

TRANSCRIPTION

One of the main causes of medication errors is incorrect *transcription* of the original prescriber's order. Many studies addressing the causes of medication errors identify one of the main sources to be illegible physician's handwriting (Stetina et al, 2005). During the transcription process, the transcriber must ensure that the drug order includes all seven parts. If any of the components are absent or illegible, the nurse must obtain or clarify that information prior to signing off and implementing the order.

Further, The Joint Commission (2005) and the Institute for Safe Medication Practices (ISMP, 2006) have published lists of abbreviations, acronyms, and symbols to avoid in prescriptions and patient records because they have been common sources of errors and can be easily misinterpreted. The Joint Commission published the *Official "Do Not Use" List* (Figure 9-1) in 2005 and recommended that health care organizations publish their own lists of abbreviations to not use. It suggested that there may be other abbreviations, acronyms, and symbols added to its list in the future (Figure 9-2) and referred health care organizations to the ISMP list of dangerous abbreviations relating to medication use. ISMP (2007) recommends that these abbreviations, symbols, and dose designations be strictly prohibited when communicating medical information (Figure 9-3).

FIGURE 9-1 *Official "Do Not Use" List* of medical abbreviations

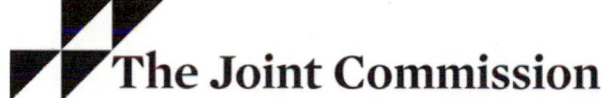

The Joint Commission

Official "Do Not Use" List[1]

Do Not Use	Potential Problem	Use Instead
U (unit)	Mistaken for "0" (zero), the number "4" (four) or "cc"	Write "unit"
IU (International Unit)	Mistaken for IV (intravenous) or the number 10 (ten)	Write "International Unit"
Q.D., QD, q.d., qd (daily)	Mistaken for each other	Write "daily"
Q.O.D., QOD, q.o.d, qod (every other day)	Period after the Q mistaken for "I" and the "O" mistaken for "I"	Write "every other day"
Trailing zero (X.0 mg)* Lack of leading zero (.X mg)	Decimal point is missed	Write X mg Write 0.X mg
MS	Can mean morphine sulfate or magnesium sulfate	Write "morphine sulfate" Write "magnesium sulfate"
MSO_4 and $MgSO_4$	Confused for one another	

[1] Applies to all orders and all medication-related documentation that is handwritten (including free-text computer entry) or on pre-printed forms.

*Exception: A "trailing zero" may be used only where required to demonstrate the level of precision of the value being reported, such as for laboratory results, imaging studies that report size of lesions, or catheter/tube sizes. It may not be used in medication orders or other medication-related documentation.

FIGURE 9-2   Additional abbreviations, acronyms, and symbols

Additional Abbreviations, Acronyms and Symbols
(For <u>possible</u> future inclusion in the Official "Do Not Use" List)

Do Not Use	Potential Problem	Use Instead
> (greater than) < (less than)	Misinterpreted as the number "7" (seven) or the letter "L" Confused for one another	Write "greater than" Write "less than"
Abbreviations for drug names	Misinterpreted due to similar abbreviations for multiple drugs	Write drug names in full
Apothecary units	Unfamiliar to many practitioners Confused with metric units	Use metric units
@	Mistaken for the number "2" (two)	Write "at"
cc	Mistaken for U (units) when poorly written	Write "mL" or "ml" or "milliliters" ("mL" is preferred)
μg	Mistaken for mg (milligrams) resulting in one thousand-fold overdose	Write "mcg" or "micrograms"

© The Joint Commission, 2009. Reprinted with permission.

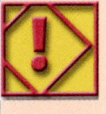

CAUTION

Stay alert to The Joint Commission, ISMP, and your own health care facility guidelines and restrictions regarding abbreviations and medical notation. Acceptable medical communication is subject to abrupt change. Check the references listed at the end of this chapter often to stay up to date.

Many health care institutions are utilizing a computerized physician order entry (CPOE) system to help eliminate transcription sources of error. Physicians choose drug orders from a menu screen (Figure 9-4) and then choose the route and dosage strength offered on the following screen (Figure 9-5). There is an option for editing (Figure 9-6), and then the physician signs the order by entering his or her assigned electronic code. These systems can also be implemented with clinical decision support systems (CDSS). The CDSS may include suggestions or default values for drug dosages, routes, and frequencies. The chance still exists that the order may be entered incorrectly, but the computer system does remove the variable of illegible writing (Hopkins, 2005).

SAFE MEDICATION ADMINISTRATION

The five rights of medication administration *(right patient, right drug, right amount, right route, and right time)* have been the cornerstones for safe and effective nursing practice in the area of medication administration. A sixth right, *right documentation,* is often added to the list. These Six Rights were introduced in Chapter 7. Thoroughly and consistently following these rights can ensure that nurses administer medications safely.

FIGURE 9-3   ISMP's List of Error-Prone Abbreviations, Symbols, and Dose Designations

 Institute for Safe Medication Practices

ISMP's List of *Error-Prone Abbreviations, Symbols,* and *Dose Designations*

The abbreviations, symbols, and dose designations found in this table have been reported to ISMP through the ISMP Medication Errors Reporting Program (MERP) as being frequently misinterpreted and involved in harmful medication errors. They should NEVER be used when communicating medical information. This includes internal communications, telephone/verbal prescriptions, computer-generated labels, labels for drug storage bins, medication administration records, as well as pharmacy and prescriber computer order entry screens.

The Joint Commission (TJC) has established a National Patient Safety Goal that specifies that certain abbreviations must appear on an accredited organization's do-not-use list; we have highlighted these items with a double asterisk (**). However, we hope that you will consider others beyond the minimum TJC requirements. By using and promoting safe practices and by educating one another about hazards, we can better protect our patients.

Abbreviations	Intended Meaning	Misinterpretation	Correction
µg	Microgram	Mistaken as "mg"	Use "mcg"
AD, AS, AU	Right ear, left ear, each ear	Mistaken as OD, OS, OU (right eye, left eye, each eye)	Use "right ear," "left ear," or "each ear"
OD, OS, OU	Right eye, left eye, each eye	Mistaken as AD, AS, AU (right ear, left ear, each ear)	Use "right eye," "left eye," or "each eye"
BT	Bedtime	Mistaken as "BID" (twice daily)	Use "bedtime"
cc	Cubic centimeters	Mistaken as "u" (units)	Use "mL"
D/C	Discharge or discontinue	Premature discontinuation of medications if D/C (intended to mean "discharge") has been misinterpreted as "discontinued" when followed by a list of discharge medications	Use "discharge" and "discontinue"
IJ	Injection	Mistaken as "IV" or "intrajugular"	Use "injection"
IN	Intranasal	Mistaken as "IM" or "IV"	Use "intranasal" or "NAS"
HS	Half-strength	Mistaken as bedtime	Use "half-strength" or "bedtime"
hs	At bedtime, hours of sleep	Mistaken as half-strength	
IU**	International unit	Mistaken as IV (intravenous) or 10 (ten)	Use "units"
o.d. or OD	Once daily	Mistaken as "right eye" (OD-oculus dexter), leading to oral liquid medications administered in the eye	Use "daily"
OJ	Orange juice	Mistaken as OD or OS (right or left eye); drugs meant to be diluted in orange juice may be given in the eye	Use "orange juice"
Per os	By mouth, orally	The "os" can be mistaken as "left eye" (OS-oculus sinister)	Use "PO," "by mouth," or "orally"
q.d. or QD**	Every day	Mistaken as q.i.d., especially if the period after the "q" or the tail of the "q" is misunderstood as an "i"	Use "daily"
qhs	Nightly at bedtime	Mistaken as "qhr" or every hour	Use "nightly"
qn	Nightly or at bedtime	Mistaken as "qh" (every hour)	Use "nightly" or "at bedtime"
q.o.d. or QOD**	Every other day	Mistaken as "q.d." (daily) or "q.i.d. (four times daily) if the "o" is poorly written	Use "every other day"
q1d	Daily	Mistaken as q.i.d. (four times daily)	Use "daily"
q6PM, etc.	Every evening at 6 PM	Mistaken as every 6 hours	Use "6 PM nightly" or "6 PM daily"
SC, SQ, sub q	Subcutaneous	SC mistaken as SL (sublingual); SQ mistaken as "5 every;" the "q" in "sub q" has been mistaken as "every" (e.g., a heparin dose ordered "sub q 2 hours before surgery" misunderstood as every 2 hours before surgery)	Use "subcut" or "subcutaneously"
ss	Sliding scale (insulin) or ½ (apothecary)	Mistaken as "55"	Spell out "sliding scale;" use "one-half" or "½"
SSRI	Sliding scale regular insulin	Mistaken as selective-serotonin reuptake inhibitor	Spell out "sliding scale (insulin)"
SSI	Sliding scale insulin	Mistaken as Strong Solution of Iodine (Lugol's)	
i/d	One daily	Mistaken as "tid"	Use "1 daily"
TIW or tiw	3 times a week	Mistaken as "3 times a day" or "twice in a week"	Use "3 times weekly"
U or u**	Unit	Mistaken as the number 0 or 4, causing a 10-fold overdose or greater (e.g., 4U seen as "40" or 4u seen as "44"); mistaken as "cc" so dose given in volume instead of units (e.g., 4u seen as 4cc)	Use "unit"

Dose Designations and Other Information	Intended Meaning	Misinterpretation	Correction
Trailing zero after decimal point (e.g., 1.0 mg)**	1 mg	Mistaken as 10 mg if the decimal point is not seen	Do not use trailing zeros for doses expressed in whole numbers"
"Naked" decimal point (e.g., .5 mg)**	0.5 mg	Mistaken as 5 mg if the decimal point is not seen	Use zero before a decimal point when the dose is less than a whole unit

FIGURE 9-3   continued

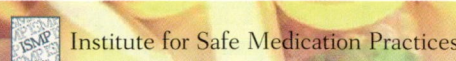
Institute for Safe Medication Practices

ISMP's List of *Error-Prone Abbreviations, Symbols,* and *Dose Designations* (continued)

Dose Designations and Other Information	Intended Meaning	Misinterpretation	Correction
Drug name and dose run together (especially problematic for drug names that end in "l" such as Inderal40 mg; Tegretol300 mg)	Inderal 40 mg Tegretol 300 mg	Mistaken as Inderal 140 mg Mistaken as Tegretol 1300 mg	Place adequate space between the drug name, dose, and unit of measure
Numerical dose and unit of measure run together (e.g., 10mg, 100mL)	10 mg 100 mL	The "m" is sometimes mistaken as a zero or two zeros, risking a 10- to 100-fold overdose	Place adequate space between the dose and unit of measure
Abbreviations such as mg. or mL. with a period following the abbreviation	mg mL	The period is unnecessary and could be mistaken as the number 1 if written poorly	Use mg, mL, etc. without a terminal period
Large doses without properly placed commas (e.g., 100000 units; 1000000 units)	100,000 units 1,000,000 units	100000 has been mistaken as 10,000 or 1,000,000; 1000000 has been mistaken as 100,000	Use commas for dosing units at or above 1,000, or use words such as 100 "thousand" or 1 "million" to improve readability

Drug Name Abbreviations	Intended Meaning	Misinterpretation	Correction
ARA A	vidarabine	Mistaken as cytarabine (ARA C)	Use complete drug name
AZT	zidovudine (Retrovir)	Mistaken as azathioprine or aztreonam	Use complete drug name
CPZ	Compazine (prochlorperazine)	Mistaken as chlorpromazine	Use complete drug name
DPT	Demerol-Phenergan-Thorazine	Mistaken as diphtheria-pertussis-tetanus (vaccine)	Use complete drug name
DTO	Diluted tincture of opium, or deodorized tincture of opium (Paregoric)	Mistaken as tincture of opium	Use complete drug name
HCl	hydrochloric acid or hydrochloride	Mistaken as potassium chloride (The "H" is misinterpreted as "K")	Use complete drug name unless expressed as a salt of a drug
HCT	hydrocortisone	Mistaken as hydrochlorothiazide	Use complete drug name
HCTZ	hydrochlorothiazide	Mistaken as hydrocortisone (seen as HCT250 mg)	Use complete drug name
MgSO4**	magnesium sulfate	Mistaken as morphine sulfate	Use complete drug name
MS, MSO4**	morphine sulfate	Mistaken as magnesium sulfate	Use complete drug name
MTX	methotrexate	Mistaken as mitoxantrone	Use complete drug name
PCA	procainamide	Mistaken as patient controlled analgesia	Use complete drug name
PTU	propylthiouracil	Mistaken as mercaptopurine	Use complete drug name
T3	Tylenol with codeine No. 3	Mistaken as liothyronine	Use complete drug name
TAC	triamcinolone	Mistaken as tetracaine, Adrenalin, cocaine	Use complete drug name
TNK	TNKase	Mistaken as "TPA"	Use complete drug name
ZnSO4	zinc sulfate	Mistaken as morphine sulfate	Use complete drug name

Stemmed Drug Names	Intended Meaning	Misinterpretation	Correction
"Nitro" drip	nitroglycerin infusion	Mistaken as sodium nitroprusside infusion	Use complete drug name
"Norflox"	norfloxacin	Mistaken as Norflex	Use complete drug name
"IV Vanc"	intravenous vancomycin	Mistaken as Invanz	Use complete drug name

Symbols	Intended Meaning	Misinterpretation	Correction
ℨ	Dram	Symbol for dram mistaken as "3"	Use the metric system
ℳ	Minim	Symbol for minim mistaken as "mL"	
x3d	For three days	Mistaken as "3 doses"	Use "for three days"
> and <	Greater than and less than	Mistaken as opposite of intended; mistakenly use incorrect symbol; "< 10" mistaken as "40"	Use "greater than" or "less than"
/ (slash mark)	Separates two doses or indicates "per"	Mistaken as the number 1 (e.g., "25 units/10 units" misread as "25 units and 110" units)	Use "per" rather than a slash mark to separate doses
@	At	Mistaken as "2"	Use "at"
&	And	Mistaken as "2"	Use "and"
+	Plus or and	Mistaken as "4"	Use "and"
°	Hour	Mistaken as a zero (e.g., q2° seen as q 20)	Use "hr," "h," or "hour"

**These abbreviations are included on TJC's "minimum list" of dangerous abbreviations, acronyms and symbols that must be included on an organization's "Do Not Use" list, effective January 1, 2004. Visit www.jointcommission.org for more information about this TJC requirement.

Permission is granted to reproduce material for internal newsletters or communications with proper attribution. Other reproduction is prohibited without written permission. Unless noted, reports were received through the ISMP Medication Errors Reporting Program (MERP). Report actual and potential medication errors to the MERP via the web at www.ismp.org or by calling 1-800-FAIL-SAF(E). ISMP guarantees confidentiality of information received and respects reporters' wishes as to the level of detail included in publications.

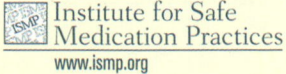
Institute for Safe Medication Practices
www.ismp.org

FIGURE 9-4 A CPOE menu screen allows the user to select a drug

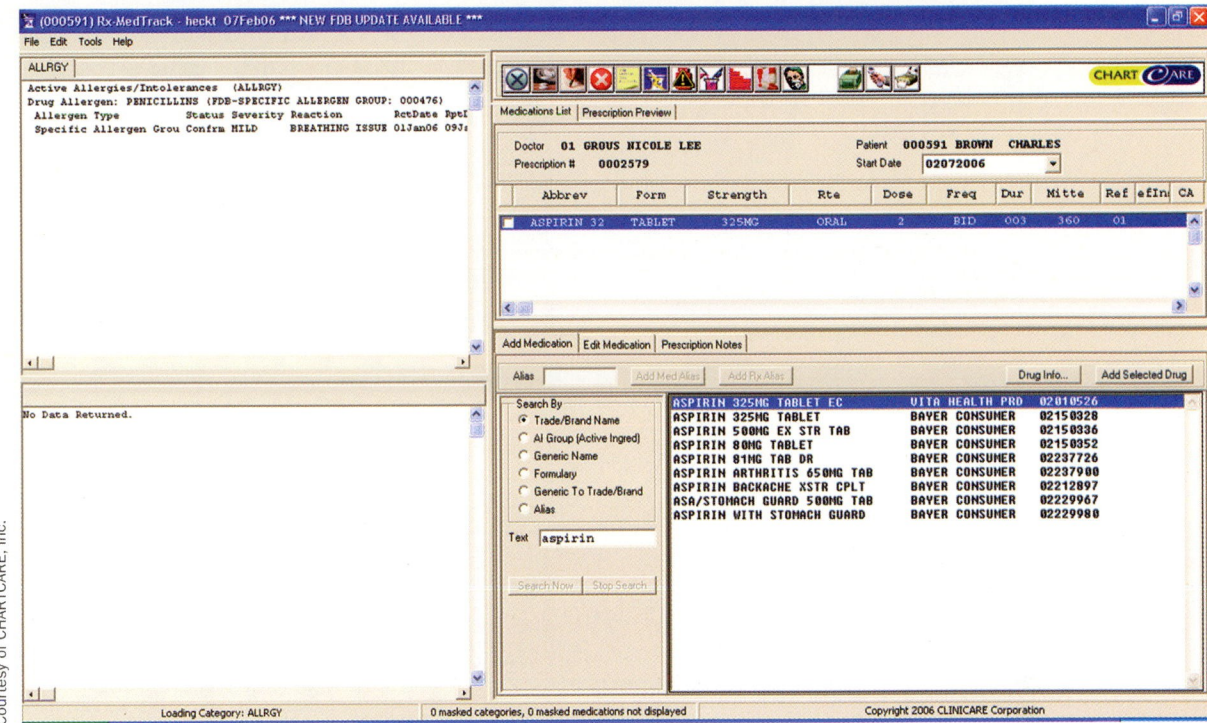

Courtesy of CHARTCARE, Inc.

FIGURE 9-5 A CPOE offers options for route and dose of the drug chosen

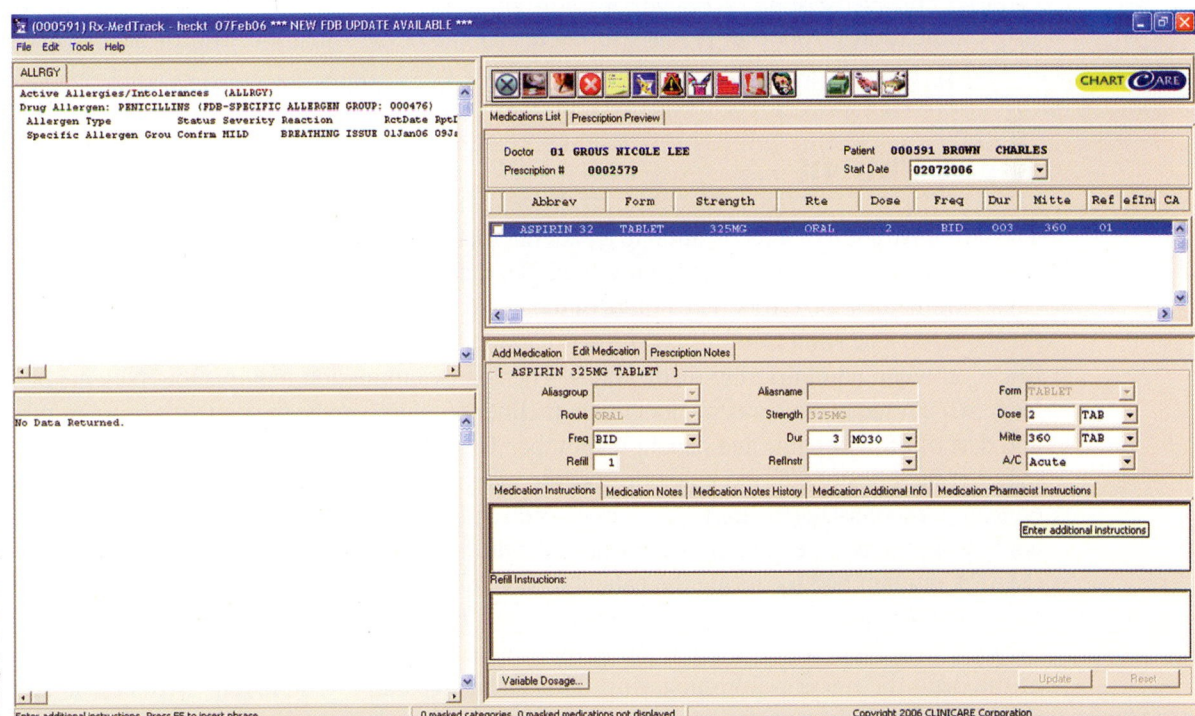

Courtesy of CHARTCARE, Inc.

FIGURE 9-6 A CPOE allows the user to edit the medication order

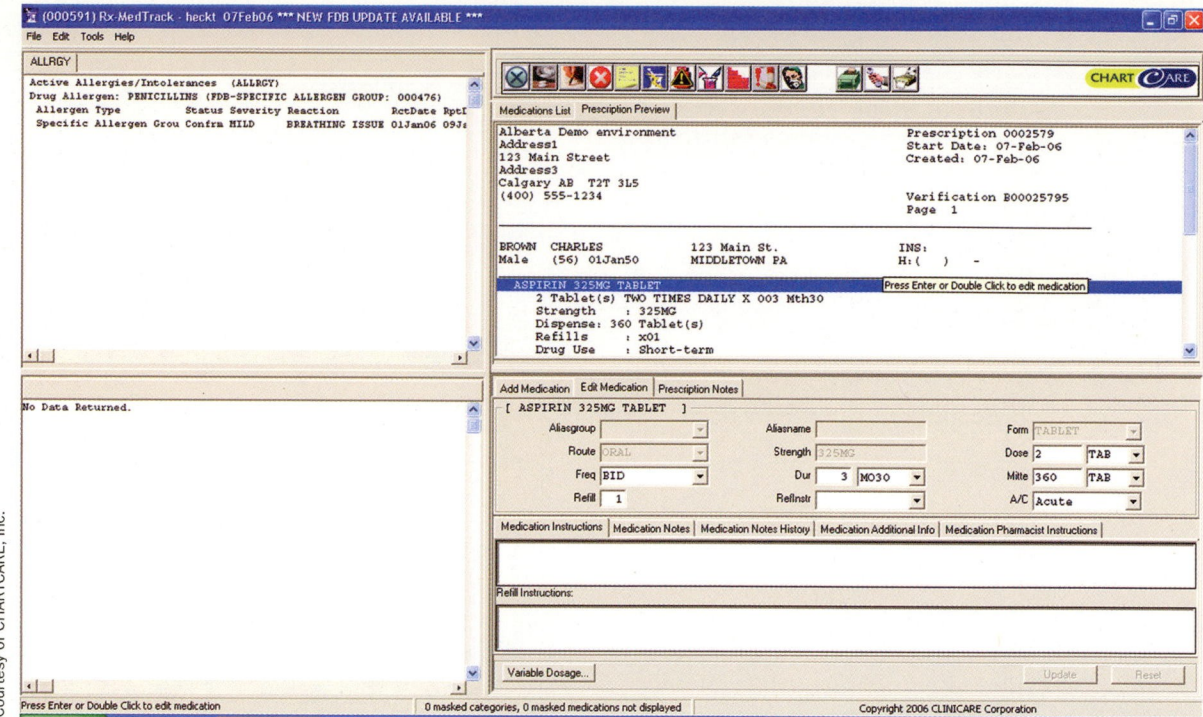

Courtesy of CHARTCARE, Inc.

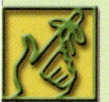

REMEMBER

Nurses should refer to reputable drug reference resources to validate the safety of the medication as ordered and transcribed. Whoever administers a medication is legally responsible for patient safety. Any medication errors that result also fall under the responsibility of the person who administered the drug, regardless of the primary source of the error.

Right Patient

The administration of a medication to a patient other than the one for whom it was ordered is clearly an error. It is also one that should be easily prevented. Yet the literature supports this as one of the three most common causes of medication errors. The failure of the nurse to accurately identify a patient is the most common cause for the error. The Joint Commission (2009) has a Patient Safety Goal to improve the accuracy of patient identification when administering medications. The Joint Commission requires that patients be identified with at least two unique person-specific identifiers (neither of which can be the patient's room number), such as name and date of birth or name and patient ID number. Electronic identification technology coding, such as bar coding, that includes two or more person-specific identifiers (not room number) will also comply. Basic nursing education emphasizes the importance of correctly identifying a patient prior to administering a medication by comparing the two person-specific identifiers with the patient's arm band, medication administration record (MAR), or chart and by asking the patient to state his or her name (as a third identifier). Both steps should be consistently implemented regardless of the nurse's familiarity with the patient or the practice arena.

It is also wise to tell the patient at the time of administration what medication and dosage strength of the drug the nurse is administering. This extra step can often prevent errors because patients who are familiar with their medications may spot an error or question a drug dosage. This is also an opportunity to engage the patient in medication teaching and learning. However, the nurse should never rely on this practice as the primary means to prevent errors. Instead, this is an extra precaution.

Technological advances in medication administration and documentation have included mechanisms to help prevent errors in this area. Computers installed at the patient's bedside and/or handheld devices that enable the nurse to scan the bar codes on the patient's identification band and on the medications serve as reinforcement to visual checks by the nurse. Few studies have been published in regard to the effectiveness of these systems in preventing errors. However, this additional mechanism to ensure correct patient identification increases the efficiency, ensuring that the right patient receives the right drug. The health care industry has invested heavily in technology to help prevent costly medication errors caused by carelessness and distraction.

Right Drug

Nurses can ensure that the right drug criterion is maintained by checking the medication label against the order or MAR at three points during the administration process:

1. On first contact with the drug (removing it from the medication cart, drawer, or shelf).

2. Prior to measuring the drug (pouring, counting, or withdrawing the drug).

3. After preparing the drug, just prior to administration.

Distraction in the workplace has been identified as a key reason for error in obtaining the right drug (Pape, Guerra, Muzquiz, & Bryant, 2005). Nurses should take measures to ensure that they are not distracted during this phase of medication administration. Optimally, the physical workplace should provide for the nurse to move to an area without distractions. However, if this is not available, the nurse should be conscious of the need to focus solely on the task at hand and avoid the temptation to multitask while dispensing medications.

In February 2004, the U.S. Food and Drug Administration (FDA) issued a regulation that requires all new pharmaceuticals to be bar coded upon launch into the market and all existing pharmaceuticals to be bar coded within 2 years of the ruling (FDA, 2004). Studies by U.S. Pharmacopeia in 2003 indicated insulin products have the highest rates of error ("Information Technology," 2005). Projections by the FDA indicate that bar coding on prescription drugs will reduce errors in the United States by 500,000 instances over the next 20 years with estimated savings of $93 billion in additional health care costs, patient pain, and lost wages (FDA, 2004). This represents a 50% reduction in the medication errors that would otherwise occur without the use of bar coding (FDA, 2004).

Bar codes on drugs are used with a bar code scanning system and computerized database. At a minimum, the code must contain the drug's National Drug Code. This number uniquely identifies the drug. The process starts as a patient enters the hospital and is given a bar coded patient identification band. The hospital has bar code scanners that are linked to the hospital's electronic medical records system. Before a health care worker administers a medication, he or she scans the patient's bar code, which allows the computer to access the patient's medical records. The health care worker then scans each drug prior to administration. This notifies the computer of each medication to be administered. This information is compared to the patient's database to ensure a match. If there is a problem, the health care worker receives an error message and investigates the problem.

Nurses are responsible for being knowledgeable about the actions, indications, and contraindications of the medications they administer. The constant changes that are occurring in health care delivery and the steady influx of new medications being released into the market have challenged the individual nurse's ability to meet this responsibility. A valid and current drug-reference system should be available in every practice setting. The nurse should not hesitate to seek information about any medication that is unfamiliar. The prescribing clinician should be contacted for clarification or confirmation for any medication order that appears inappropriate or incorrect.

Automatic Medication Dispensing Machines (AMDM) (Figure 9-7) have been utilized in many health care settings. There are many safety measures in place with the use of this technology, but the possibility still exists that the patient may receive the wrong medication. Nurses who practice in a setting utilizing this technology should continue to implement the three checks described to avoid administering the wrong drug. Review Chapter 8 about reading drug labels to ensure that all of the important information is confirmed.

A common preventable medication error is interchanging look-alike, sound-alike (LASA) medication pairs—prescribing and administering one for the other. The Joint Commission (2009) Patient Safety Goal 3

FIGURE 9-7 The Pyxis MedStation® is an example of an Automatic Medication Dispensing Machine.

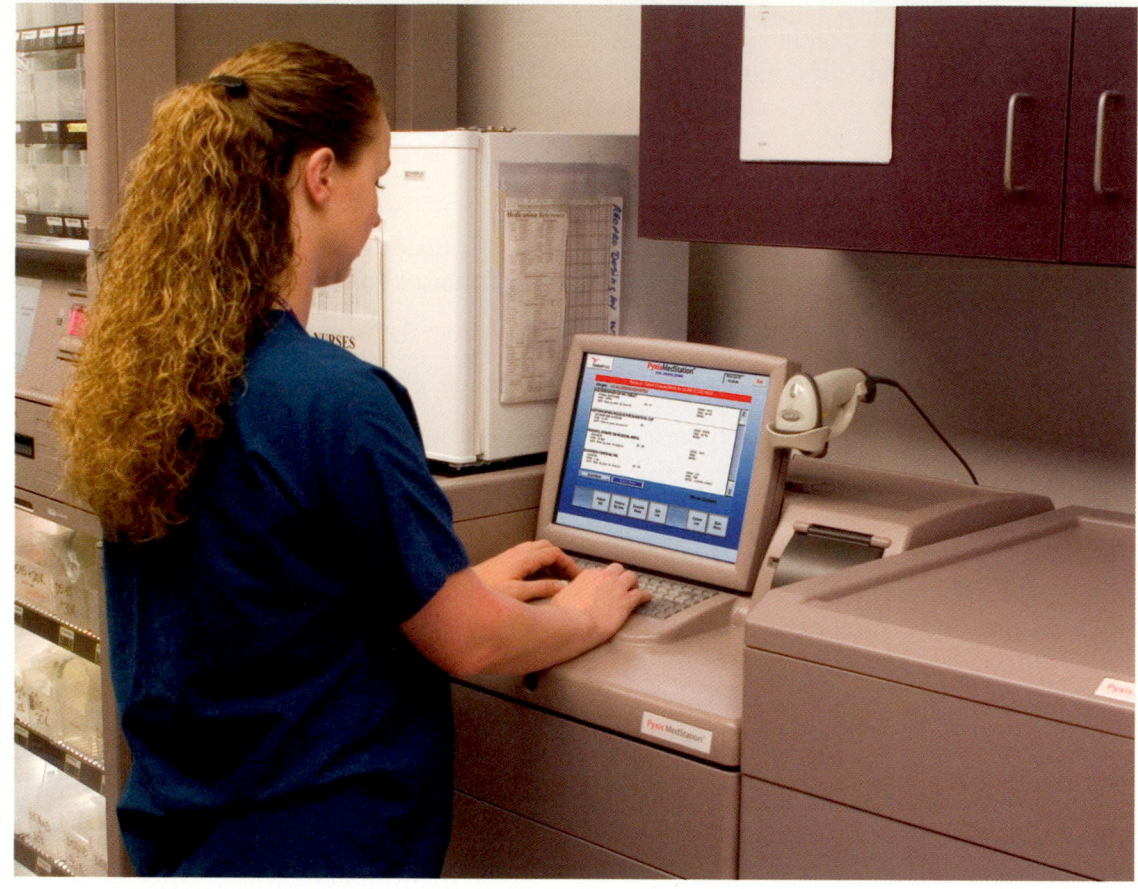

Courtesy of Cardinal Health.

addresses this issue and posts online an extensive list of look-alike, sound-alike medications that pose the greatest risk for medication errors, including LASA drugs such as ephedrine and epinephrine, hydromorphone injection and morphine injection, hydroxyzine and hydralazine, OxyContin (controlled release) and oxycodone (immediate release). Hospitals are independently required to list at least 10 look-alike, sound-alike drug pairs commonly prescribed and administered in their institution for their caregivers to monitor.

The Joint Commission (2009) Patient Safety Goal 8 addresses the practice of reconciling the right medications across the continuum of care, beginning with admission and following the patient through transfers within the health care facility (such as from a hospital intensive care unit to a medical floor) and back home or to a long term care facility. A complete list of current medications the patient is taking at home (including dose, route, and frequency) is created and documented upon admission, ideally before prescribing any new medications. The medications ordered for the patient while under care are compared to this list and discrepancies are reconciled and documented. Likewise when the patient is transferred to another unit within the hospital or to another facility, or discharged to home, the up-to-date reconciled medication list is communicated and documented. Strict adherence to these standards will prevent many medication errors of transcription, omission, duplication, and drug interactions.

Right Amount

Illegible prescriber's handwriting, a transcription error, miscalculation of the amount, or misreading the label can result in errors involving the administration of an incorrect dose of a medication. The need for each nurse to carefully read and clarify drug orders and recheck drug labels has been previously discussed. Two nurses must check some potent medications, such as insulin, which are a common source of errors. Transcription errors involving dosage can be avoided if nurses consult drug references to confirm the dosage of medications if they are in doubt. The Joint Commission's *Official "Do Not Use" List* (Figure 9-1) will also help eliminate problems of dosage for those medications ordered daily, ordered every other day, or measured in units.

Teaching effective dosage calculation methods is the main purpose of this text. The need for each nurse to estimate the correct dosage prior to calculating the exact amount is stressed throughout this book. The inclusion of this common-sense approach to calculating dosage is crucial in preventing errors in dosage calculation. Calculating, preparing, and administering the wrong dose of a drug are preventable medication errors. Full attention to accurate dosage calculations will assure that you avoid such liabilities.

Right Route

Errors involving the route of medication administration can occur for several reasons. One of the most common problems has already been addressed, that of illegible prescriber's handwriting. Another common error relates to the nurse's knowledge of medications and their dosage forms. Nurses are usually familiar with medications commonly ordered and administered in their area of practice, but the nurse should consult a drug information source to confirm that the correct route is ordered for an unfamiliar medication, particularly in regard to injectable forms of medications. Nurses should also be alert to the need to change or clarify administration forms or routes for the patient receiving medication through a feeding tube, such as nasogastric or surgically inserted tubes. Sometimes the patient may not be allowed any oral intake (NPO status) or have a nasogastric tube, but the medications are ordered for oral administration. Sometimes prescribers order time-released or enteric-coated medications to be administered via a feeding tube but do not recognize that medications must be crushed or dissolved to be administered. Such situations require the nurse to contact the prescriber for a change in the medication form or route or to seek clarification for the drug to be administered safely and correctly. It is the nurse's responsibility to be alert to potential errors of all kinds that may interfere with patient safety and rights.

Right Time

Medication orders should include the frequency that a drug is to be administered or the specific administration schedule. Computerized hospital drug administration systems automatically indicate these times on the medication administration record. The nurse is responsible for checking these records to be sure they are accurate. For example, a physician writes an order for an antibiotic to be given four times a day. The computer system might transcribe these times to 9:00 AM, 1:00 PM, 5:00 PM, and 9:00 PM. The nurse should recognize that an antibiotic should be administered at regular intervals so that the 4 doses would be 6 hours apart. The right time for the order should have been q.6h or *every 6 hours.*

The Joint Commission (2005) has recognized the frequency of misinterpretation of time and frequency in medication orders. It has taken steps to prevent common errors in regard to the time a drug is to be administered by prohibiting the use of some abbreviations related to dosing frequency. For example, the notation to give a drug q.d. has frequently been transcribed as q.i.d. with the period being mistaken for an i, resulting in a daily medication being administered four times a day instead of once daily.

Right Documentation

The last step in medication administration is correct documentation. The policy in most institutions directs nurses to administer a medication prior to documentation. Numerous studies indicate that fatigue and lack of time are factors that contribute to medication errors. Nurses who prioritize their time may find that they give medications correctly but fail to document it. This omission can result in unintentional overmedication of the patient when the follow-on nurse responds as though the drug was not given. Many of the new AMDMs document drug administration at the time the drug is removed from the machine. This ensures that administration is documented, but the error occurs if the patient does not take the medication. In that situation, the nurse must follow the institution's policy for clarifying or deleting the initial documentation. Often, this is a time-consuming process, but if omitted, it results in under-medication of the patient.

Medication Error Alerts

Throughout this text there are *Critical Thinking Skill* scenarios designed to alert you to common medication errors and to practice how to prevent them. Combating errors requires diligent adherence to safety standards prescribed by organizations like The Joint Commission, the Institute for Safe Medication Practices, and your health care agency. You can find more examples of medication error prevention by staying current with newsletters and publications devoted to this important topic like the *ISMP Medication Safety Alert! Nurse Advise–ERR* (2008) and the *Hospital Pharmacy: ISMP Medication Error Report Analysis* (Wolters Kluwer Health, 2008). Stay alert by practicing the *Six Rights of Safe Medication Administration*, regularly reading prevention publications, and spotting and reporting medication errors.

SUMMARY

In conclusion, medication administration is a critical nursing skill that can lead to costly errors, morbidity, and death if not done correctly. It is the nurse's responsibility to ensure that the right patient receives the right drug, in the right amount, by the right route, at the right time, and with the right documentation. The nurse who administers a medication is legally liable for medication errors whether the primary cause was an unsafe order, incorrect transcription, inaccurate dosage calculation, or administration error.

Review Set 21

1. What are the six patient rights of safe medication administration?

   _____

   _____

2. Correct the error(s) in the following medication order: NPH insulin 20.0 U SC qd

   _____

3. Safe medication administration requires that you check the drug against the order three times: 1) when you first make contact with the drug (such as remove it from the medication drawer), 2) when you measure it, and 3) _____

4. Give a rationale for the importance of accurate and safe dosage calculations and medication administration.

   _____

   _____

5. True or False? The nurse who administers a drug based on an incorrect or unsafe medication order shares legal liability for patient injury that results from that drug. _____

6. What is the preferred method for verifying the safety of the medication order?

   _____

7. According to the U.S. Pharmacopeia, what drug products have the highest incidence of medication errors?

_____

8. What is the purpose of bar coding?

_____

9. How much financial savings did the FDA project in 2004 that bar coding would contribute over the next 20 years? _____

10. What nursing actions should you implement following the receipt of a verbal or telephone order from a licensed prescribing practitioner to ensure accuracy of the order?

_____

After completing these problems, see page 517 to check your answers.

CRITICAL THINKING SKILLS

It is important for the nurse to check the label on each medication administered regardless of the medication dispensing mechanism.

ERROR

Failing to check the medication label.

Possible Scenario

Suppose a physician orders 40 mg of Lasix for an adult with congestive heart failure. The Lasix is supplied in 20 mg tablets. The nurse plans to administer 2 tablets and use an Automatic Medication Dispensing Machine. The nurse chooses the correct medication from the computer screen. The medication drawer, which should contain the medication, opens. The nurse removes 2 tablets without reading the label, goes to the patient's room, and administers the medication. The medication the nurse removed was Lanoxin 0.25 mg tablets. The pharmacy technician incorrectly stocked the medication drawer.

Potential Outcome

Although the patient has an order for Lanoxin 0.25 mg daily, he had already received his dose for the day. At this point, he has received three times the correct amount. He becomes nauseated, and when the nurse checks his pulse, it is 40 beats per minute. The nurse notifies the doctor of the change in the patient's condition. As the one who administered the incorrect medication, the nurse clearly shares responsibility for the medication error.

Prevention

The nurse should read the label on each medication and compare it to the order or MAR three times before administering the drug. If the nurse had checked the label as the drug was removed from the medication drawer, the error could have been prevented. And, the nurse had two more opportunities to prevent this error: prior to counting it (the amount should have been 40 mg, not 0.25 mg) and prior to administering it.

CRITICAL THINKING SKILLS   The nurse should ensure that the medication ordered can be administered by the right route.

ERROR

Opening a time-released capsule and administering it through a nasogastric tube.

Possible Scenario

Suppose a patient is hospitalized to treat a stroke. The physician's orders state to continue all of the patient's home medications. One of the medications is Theophylline 100 mg to be administered daily as a 24-hour extended-release capsule (Theo-24) for the treatment of asthma. The patient is unable to swallow as a result of the stroke, and all of his medications must be given through his nasogastric tube. The nurse opens the capsule and dissolves the contents in water and administers it via the nasogastric tube. The patient begins complaining of palpitations, and his pulse increases to 180 beats per minute. The nurse evaluates the changes in the patient's condition and realizes the error.

Potential Outcome

The physician would be notified of the error, and a peak level of Theophylline would be ordered. If the patient had a history of cardiac problems, the sympathetic stimulation caused by the Theophylline could result in anginal pain or an acute myocardial infarction. The patient would be treated symptomatically until his Theophylline blood levels returned to therapeutic range.

Prevention

The nurse should have recognized that a time-released medication could not safely be administered through a nasogastric tube. The physician should have been contacted to obtain orders for a different dosage form of the medication.

PRACTICE PROBLEMS—CHAPTER 9

1. According to the Institute of Medicine, how many hospital patients die annually because of preventable medication errors? _____

2. True or False? Studies indicate that nurses' education and years of practice are closely correlated to the incidence of medication errors. _____

3. True or False? Ten percent (10%) to 18% of patient injuries are attributable to preventable medication errors. _____

4. True or False? Administering a drug late is a frequently underreported medication error. _____

5. True or False? Illegible prescriber's handwriting is a major contributor of transcription errors. _____

6. Fill in the blanks for the following statement. "The right _____ must receive the right _____ in the right _____ by the right _____ at the right _____ followed by the right _____."

7. What are the three steps of medication administration?
   _____

8. The nurse can ensure that the patient receives the right drug by checking the drug label three times. When should the nurse perform these label checks?

_____

9. Which of the following medical notations is (are) written in the recommended format? 0.75 mg, .2 cm, q.d. _____

10. Describe a nursing action to prevent medication errors when receiving verbal drug orders.

_____

11. Cite four of the direct and/or indirect costs of medication errors.

_____

12. Describe the strategy or strategies you would implement to prevent this potential medication error.

Possible Scenario
Suppose the physician writes the following order:

_____

Dilacor XR 240 mg p.o. q.d.

_____

The order is transcribed as *Dilacor XR 240 mg p.o. q.i.d.* and the medication is scheduled for administration at 0600, 1200, 1800, and 2400 on the medication administration record.

The nurse reviews the order prior to obtaining the medication for administration. The nurse notices the XR following the name of the medication and recognizes that the letters usually indicate a sustained-release form of medication. The nurse consults the *Hospital Formulary* and finds that the drug is a sustained formula and is only to be given once daily. The nurse reviews the original orders and notes that there was a transcription error. The medication administration record is corrected, and the patient receives the correct amount of medication at the correct time.

Potential Outcome
Had the nurse administered the medication at each of the times indicated on the medication administration record, the patient would have received four times the intended dosage. The drug's therapeutic effect is a decrease in the cardiac output and decrease in blood pressure. However, the toxic effects caused by overdosing could have resulted in congestive heart failure. The patient's life would have been jeopardized.

Prevention

_____

_____

After completing these questions, see page 517 to check your answers.

REFERENCES

FDA. U.S. Food and Drug Administration. (2004). *FDA issues bar code regulation.* Retrieved May 6, 2006, from http://www.fda.gov/oc/initiatives/barcode-sadr/fs-barcode.html

Hopkins, K. (2005). CPOE: Errors can be increased with use of computerized order entry system—maybe [Electronic version]. *Hospitals and Health Networks, 4,* 2.

Information technology: Drug company announces individual bar coding on all insulin vials [Electronic version]. (2005, March 13). *Medical Letter on the CDC & FDA.*

Institute for Safe Medication Practices. (2007). *ISMP's list of error-prone abbreviations, symbols, and dose designations.* Retrieved November 23, 2008, from http://www.ismp.org/Tools/

Institute for Safe Medication Practices. (2008). *ISMP medication safety alert! Nurse advise–ERR.* Retrieved November 23, 2008, from http://www.ismp.org/Newsletters/nursing/Issues/NurseAdviseERR200805.pdf

The Joint Commission. (2005). *Official "do not use" list and additional abbreviations, acronyms, and symbols.* Retrieved January 11, 2009, from http://www.jointcommission.org/PatientSafety/DoNotUseList/

The Joint Commission. (2009). *National patient safety goals for 2009.* Retrieved January 11, 2009, from http://www.jointcommission.org/PatientSafety/NationalPatientSafetyGoals/

Mayo, A. M., & Duncan, D. (2004). Nurse perceptions of medication errors: What we need to know for patient safety [Electronic version]. *Journal of Nursing Quality Care, 19,* 3.

Pape, T. M., Guerra, D. M., Muzquiz, M., & Bryant, J. B. (2005). Innovative approaches to reducing nurses' distractions during medication administration. *The Journal of Continuing Nursing Education, 36,* 3.

Stetina, P., Groves, M., & Pafford, L. (2005). Managing medication errors—A qualitative study. *Medsurg Nursing, 14,* 3.

Wolf, Z. R., & Serembus, J. F. (2004). Medication errors: Ending the blame game. *Nursing Management, 35,* 8.

Wolters Kluwer Health. (2008). ISMP medication error report analysis [Electronic version]. *Hospital Pharmacy, 43,* 7. Retrieved November 23, 2008 from http://www.factsandcomparisons.com/assets/hpdatenamed/20080701_July2008_ismp.pdf

SECTION 2 SELF-EVALUATION

Directions

1. Round decimals to two places. Round temperatures to one decimal place.

2. Reduce fractions to lowest terms.

Chapter 3—Systems of Measurement

Express the following amounts in proper medical notation.

1. two-thirds grain   _____   4. one-half milliliter   _____

2. four teaspoons   _____   5. one-half fluid ounce   _____

3. one three-hundredths grain   _____

Interpret the following notations.

6. 4 gtt   _____   9. gr vii $\frac{1}{2}$ _____

7. 450 mg   _____   10. 0.25 L   _____

8. gr $\frac{1}{100}$ _____

Chapters 4 and 5—Conversions

Convert each of the following metric measurements.

11.   7.13 kg   =   _____ g

12.   925 mcg   =   _____ mg

13.   125 mg   =   _____ g

14.   0.165 g   =   _____ mg

Convert each of the following to the equivalent units indicated.

15. gr $\frac{1}{6}$ =   _____ mg   =   _____ g

16. 20 mg   =   _____ g   =   gr _____

17. 4 T   =   _____ t   =   _____ mL

18. 5 fl oz   =   _____ mL   =   _____ L

19. 15 in   =   _____ cm   =   _____ mm

20. 56.2 mm   =   _____ cm   =   _____ in

21. 198 lb   =   _____ kg   =   _____ g

22. 11.59 kg   =   _____ g   =   _____ lb

23. A patient is told to take 180 mg of a medication. What is the equivalent dosage in grains? gr _____

24. A patient is being treated for chronic pain with gr $\frac{3}{4}$ of morphine sulphate every 3 hours. How many milligrams will he receive in 24 hours? _____ mg

25. Your patient uses nitroglycerin for chest pain. The prescription is for gr $\frac{1}{300}$ of nitroglycerin. What is the equivalent dosage in milligrams? _____ mg

26. Most adults have about 6,000 mL of circulating blood volume. This is equivalent to _____ L.

27. Your patient drinks the following for breakfast: 3 fl oz orange juice, 8 fl oz coffee with 1 fl oz cream, and 4 fl oz of water. The total intake is _____ mL.

Convert the following times as indicated. Designate AM or PM where needed.

Traditional Time	International Time
28. 11:35 PM	_____
29. _____	1844
30. 4:17 AM	_____
31. _____	0803

Convert the following temperatures as indicated.

32. 38°C   _____ °F

33. _____ °C   101.5°F

34. 37.2°C   _____ °F

Chapter 6—Equipment Used in Dosage Measurement

Draw an arrow to demonstrate the correct measurement of the doses given.

35. 1.5 mL

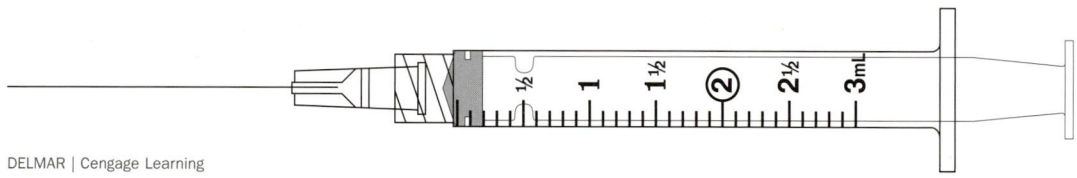

DELMAR | Cengage Learning

36. 0.33 mL

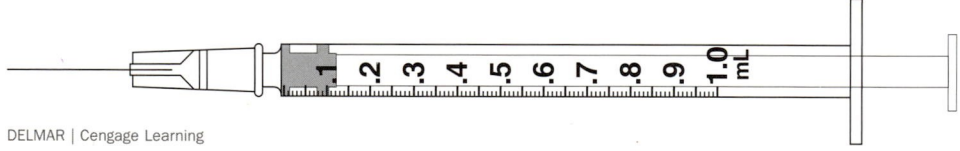

DELMAR | Cengage Learning

37. 44 units U-100 insulin

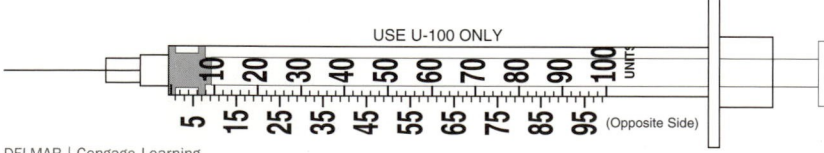

DELMAR | Cengage Learning

38. 37 units U-100 insulin

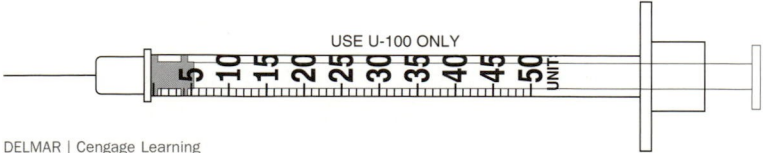

DELMAR | Cengage Learning

39. $1\frac{1}{2}$ t

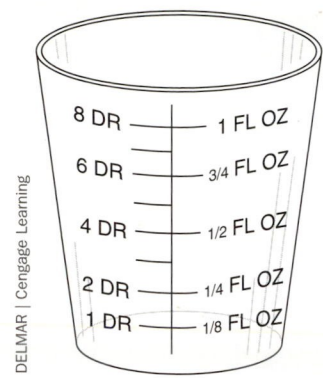 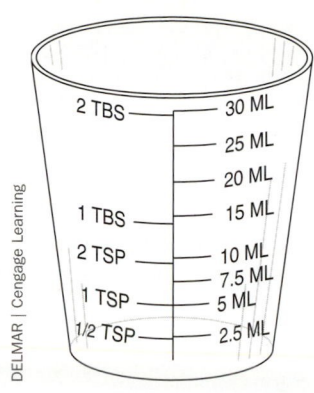

Chapters 7 and 8—Interpreting Drug Orders and Understanding Drug Labels

Use label A to identify the information requested for questions 40 through 43.

40. The generic name is _____.

41. This drug is a sublingual tablet and the route of administration is intended for _____.

42. The total volume of this container is _____.

43. Interpret this order: **nitroglycerin 400 mcg SL stat** _____.

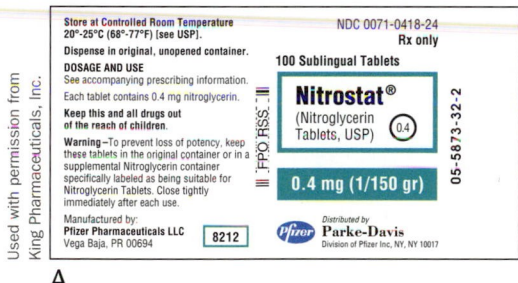

A

Use label B to identify the information requested for questions 44 through 46.

44. The supply dosage is _____

45. The National Drug Code is _____.

46. Interpret: **heparin 3,750 units subcut q.8h** _____

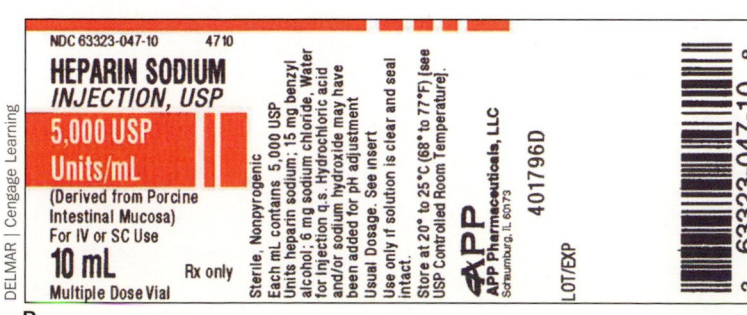

B

Use label C to identify the information requested for questions 47 and 48.

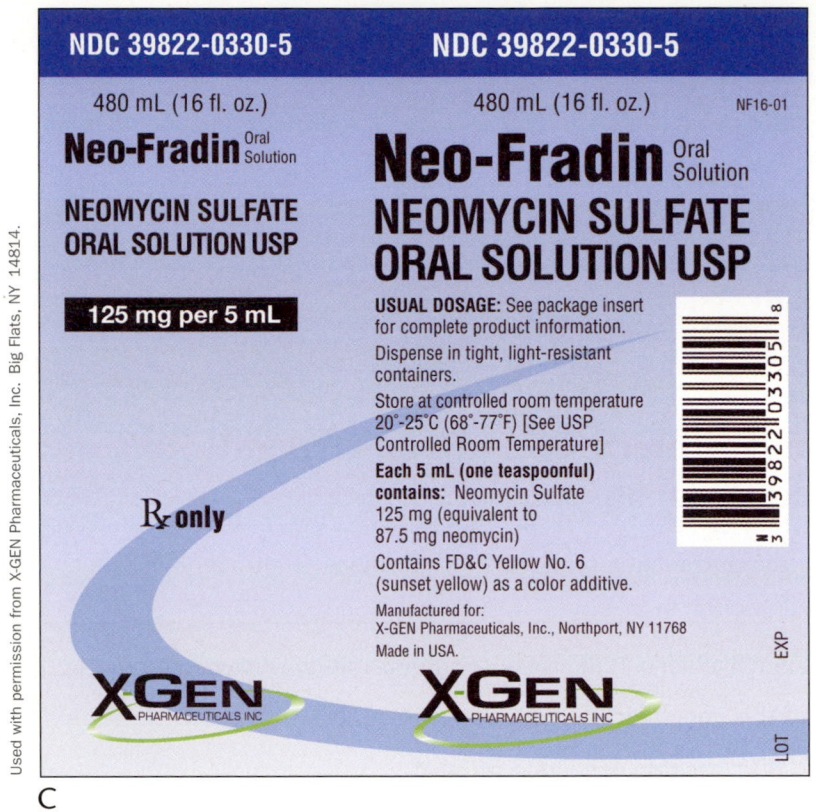

C

47. The generic name is

_____.

48. The supply dosage is _____.

Chapter 9—Preventing Medication Errors

49. Using abbreviations from both The Joint Commission and Institute for Safe Medication Practices (ISMP) sources, correct the medical notation of the following order.

    Heparin 5000 U SC qd _____

50. Complete the following statement that defines the six rights of safe medication administration.

    "The right patient must receive the right . . . _____
    _____."

After completing these problems, see pages 518–519 to check your answers. Give yourself 2 points for each correct answer.

Perfect score = 100   My score = _____

Minimum mastery score = 86 (43 correct)

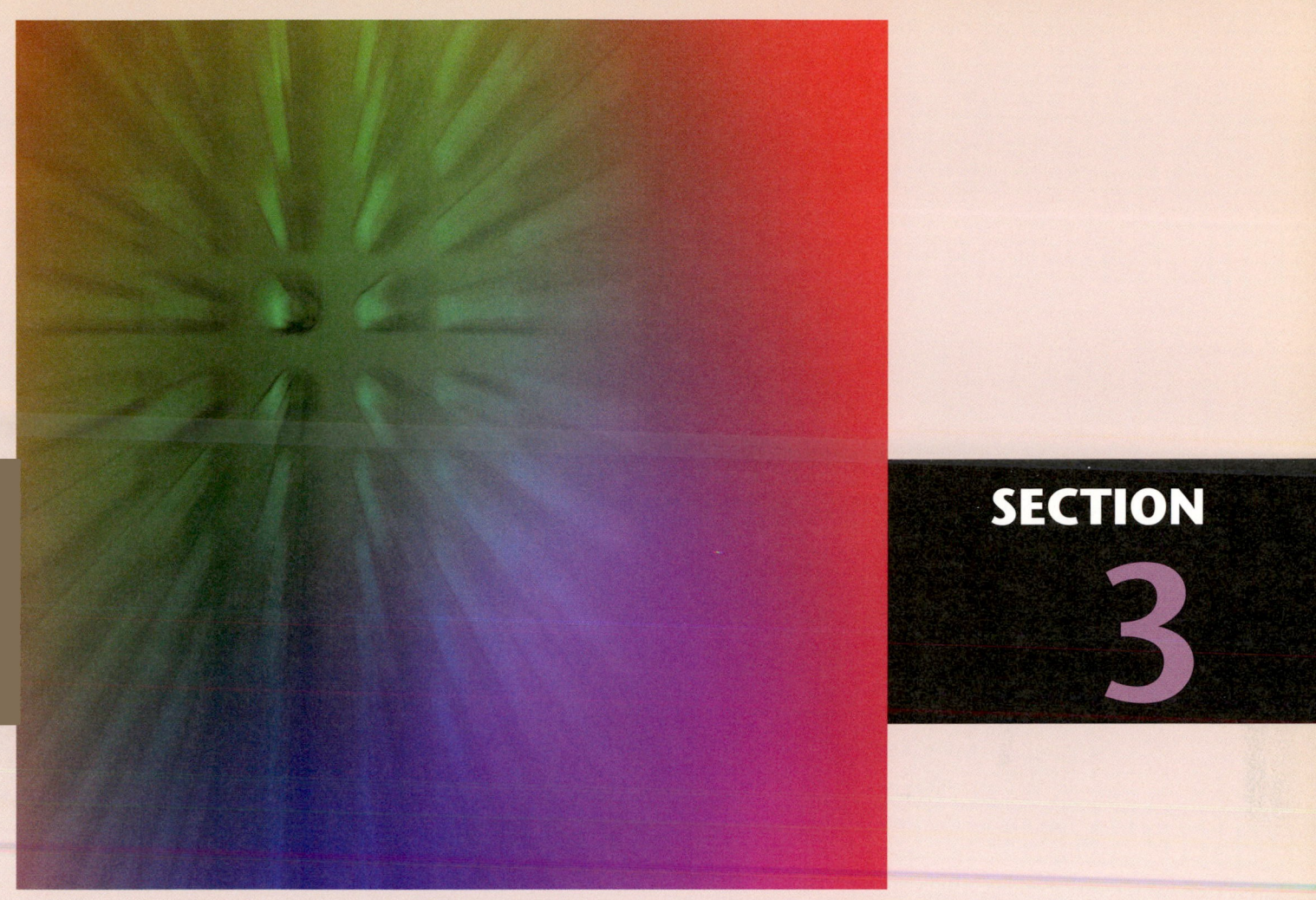

Drug Dosage Calculations

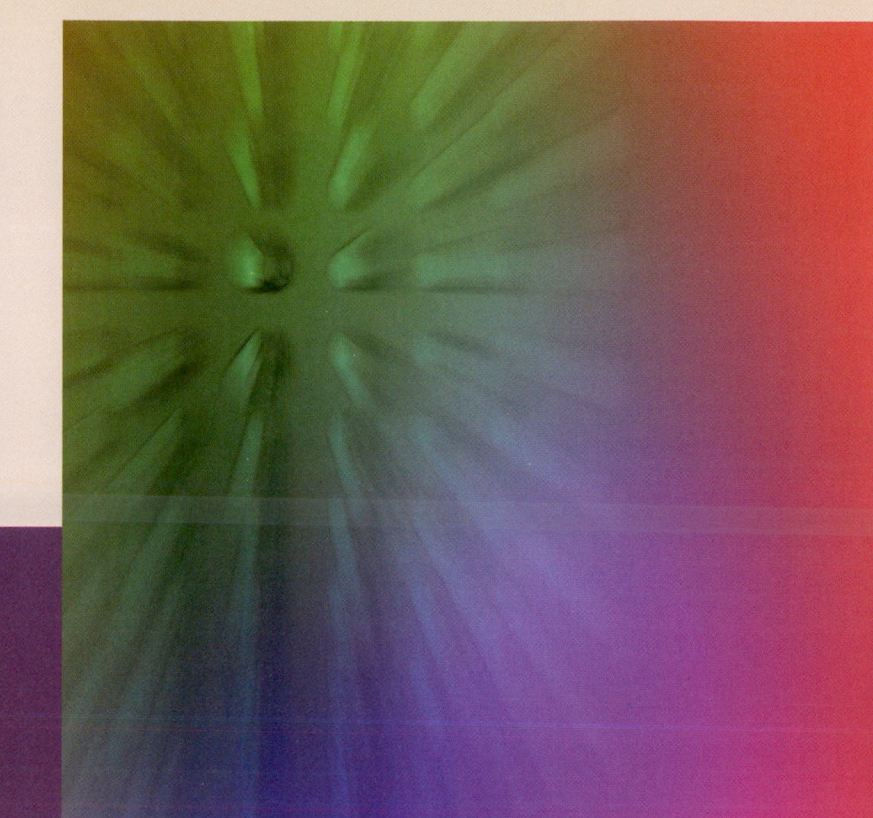

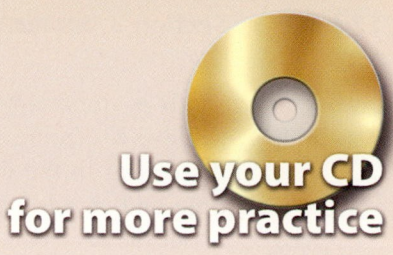

Use your CD for more practice

10

Oral Dosage of Drugs

OBJECTIVES

Upon mastery of Chapter 10, you will be able to calculate oral dosages of drugs. To accomplish this you will also be able to:

- Convert all units of measurement to the same system and same size units.
- Estimate the reasonable amount of the drug to be administered.
- Use ratio-proportion to calculate drug dosage.
- Calculate the number of tablets or capsules that are contained in prescribed dosages.
- Calculate the volume of liquid per dose when the prescribed dosage is in solution form.

Medications for oral administration are supplied in a variety of forms, such as tablets, capsules, and liquids. They are usually ordered to be administered by mouth, or *p.o.,* which is an abbreviation for the Latin phrase *per os.*

When a liquid form of a drug is unavailable, children and many elderly patients may need to have a tablet crushed or a capsule opened and mixed with a small amount of food or fluid to enable them to swallow the medication. Many of these crushed medications and oral liquids also may be ordered to be given enterally, or into the gastrointestinal tract via a specially placed tube. Such tubes and their associated enteral routes include the *nasogastric* (NG) tube from nares to stomach, the *nasojejunal* (NJ) tube from nares to jejunum, the *gastrostomy tube* (GT) placed directly through the abdomen into the stomach, the *jejunum tube* (J-tube) directly into the jejunum of the small intestines, and the *percutaneous endoscopic gastrostomy* (PEG) tube.

It is important to recognize that some solid-form medications are intended to be given whole to achieve a specific effect in the body. For example, enteric-coated medications protect the stomach by dissolving in the duodenum. Sustained-release capsules allow for gradual release of medication over time and should be swallowed whole. Consult a drug reference or the pharmacist if you are in doubt about the safety of crushing tablets or opening capsules.

TABLETS AND CAPSULES

Medications prepared in tablet and capsule form are supplied in the strengths or dosages in which they are commonly prescribed (Figure 10-1). It is desirable to obtain the drug in the same strength as the dosage ordered or in multiples of that dosage. When necessary, scored tablets (those marked for division) can be divided into halves or quarters. Only scored tablets are intended to be divided.

FIGURE 10-1   Biaxin 250 mg and 500 mg tablets

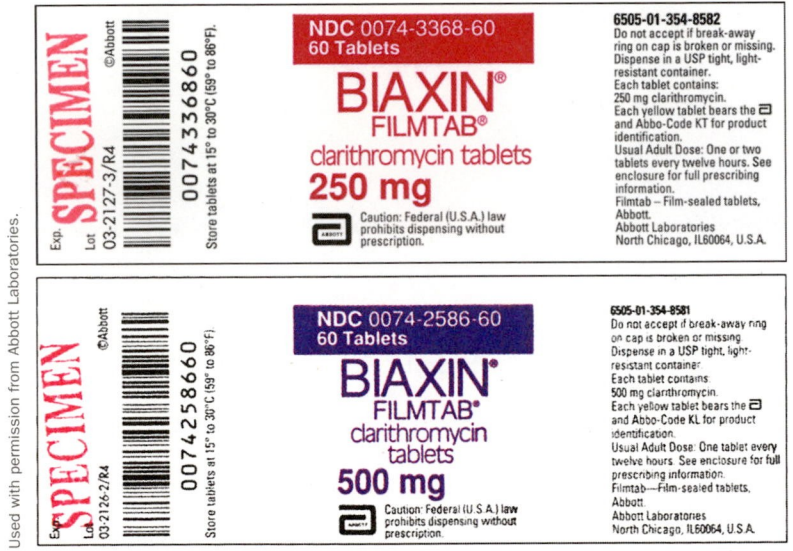

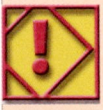 **CAUTION**
It is safest and most accurate to give the fewest number of whole, undivided tablets possible.

EXAMPLE 1 ▪

The doctor's order reads: Biaxin 500 mg p.o. q.12h

Biaxin comes in tablet strengths of 250 mg per tablet or filmtab and 500 mg per tablet. When both strengths are available, the nurse should select the 500 mg strength and give 1 whole tablet for each dose.

EXAMPLE 2 ▪

The doctor's order reads: Klonopin 1.5 mg p.o. t.i.d.

Klonopin comes in strengths of 0.5 mg, 1 mg, and 2 mg tablets (Figure 10-2). When the three strengths are available, the nurse should select one 1 mg tablet and one 0.5 mg tablet (1 mg + 0.5 mg = 1.5 mg). This provides the ordered dosage of 1.5 mg and is the least number of tablets (2 tablets total) for the patient to swallow.

You might want to halve the 2 mg tablet to obtain two 1 mg parts and pair one-half with a 0.5 mg tablet. This would also equal 1.5 mg and give you $1\frac{1}{2}$ tablets. However, cutting any tablet in half may produce slightly unequal halves. Your patient may not get the ordered dose as a result. It is preferable to give whole, undivided tablets, when they are available.

FIGURE 10-2 Klonopin 0.5 mg, 1 mg, and 2 mg tablets

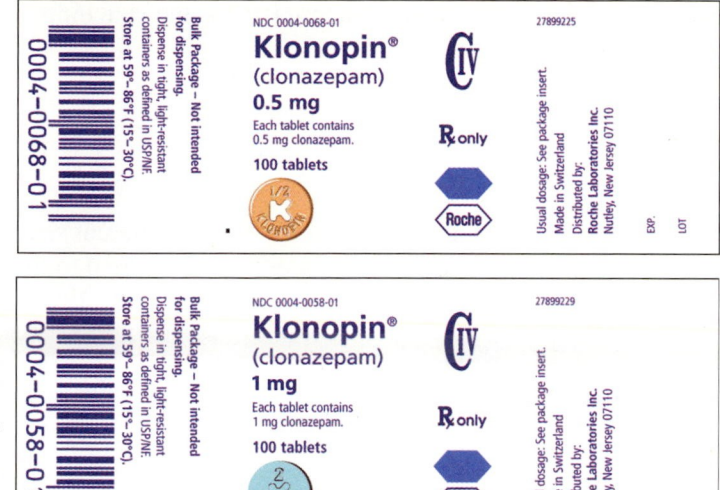

THREE-STEP APPROACH TO DOSAGE CALCULATIONS

Now you are ready to learn to solve dosage problems. The following simple three-step method has been proven to reduce anxiety about calculations and ensure that your results are accurate. Take notice that you will be asked to think or estimate before you attempt to calculate the dosage. Learn and memorize this simple three-step approach, and use it for every dosage calculation every time.

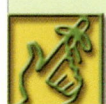

REMEMBER

Three-Step Approach to Dosage Calculations

Step 1	**Convert**	Ensure that all measurements are in the same system of measurement and the same size unit of measurement. If not, convert before proceeding.
Step 2	**Think**	Estimate what is a *reasonable amount* of the drug to administer.
Step 3	**Calculate**	Set up a proportion to calculate the drug dosage. The ratio for the drug you have on hand is equivalent to the ratio for the desired drug.

$$\frac{\text{Dosage on hand}}{\text{Amount on hand}} = \frac{\text{Dosage desired}}{\text{X Amount desired}}$$

Let's carefully examine each of the three steps as essential and consecutive rules of accurate dosage calculation.

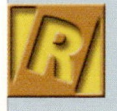

RULE

Step 1	**Convert**	Be sure that all measurements are in the same system and all units are in the same size, converting when necessary.

Many medications are both ordered and supplied in the same system of measurement and the same size unit of measurement. This makes dosage calculation easy because no conversion is necessary. When this is not the case, then you must convert to the same system or the same size units. Let's look at two examples where conversion is a necessary first step in dosage calculation.

EXAMPLE 1 ■

The drug order reads: Keflex 0.5 g p.o. q.6h

The supply dosage (what is available on hand) is labeled *Keflex 500 mg per capsule.* This is an example of a medication order written and supplied in the same system (metric) but in different size units (g and mg). A drug order written in grams but supplied in milligrams will have to be converted to the same size unit f.

MATH TIP

In most cases, it is more practical to convert to the smaller unit (such as g to mg). This usually eliminates the decimal or fraction, keeping the calculation in whole numbers.

To continue with Example 1, you should convert 0.5 gram to milligrams. Notice that milligrams is the smaller unit and converting eliminates the decimal fraction. Use ratio-proportion to convert.

Equivalent: 1 g = 1,000 mg

$$\frac{1\text{ g}}{1{,}000\text{ mg}} \diagdown \frac{0.5\text{ g}}{X\text{ mg}} \qquad \text{Cross-multiply}$$

$$X = 1{,}000 \times 0.5 \qquad 0.500. \text{ Move the decimal three places to the right. Add zeros to complete the operation.}$$

$$X = 500\text{ mg} \qquad \text{Label the units to match the unknown X.}$$

Now you can see that the order and the supply drug you have on hand are the same amount: *500 mg.*

Order: Keflex 500 mg p.o. q.6h

Supply: Keflex 500 mg per capsule

You would give the patient 1 Keflex 500 mg capsule by mouth every 6 hours.

MATH TIP

Convert apothecary and household measurements to their metric equivalents. This will be helpful for your calculations even if the conversion is to a larger unit. The metric system is the predominant system of measurement for drugs.

EXAMPLE 2 ■

The drug order reads: phenobarbital gr $\frac{1}{2}$ p.o. q.12h

The supply dosage (what you have available on hand) is labeled *phenobarbital 15 mg per tablet.* This is an example of the medication ordered in one system but supplied in a different system. The medication order is written in the apothecary system, and the medication is supplied in the metric system. You must recall the approximate equivalents and convert both amounts to the same system. You should convert the apothecary measure to metric.

Approximate equivalent: gr i = 60 mg

Recall that a proportion is a relationship comparing two ratios. Keep the *known* information on the left side of the proportion and the *unknown* on the right. Refer back to Chapter 4 about using ratio-proportion to convert between systems of measurement, as needed.

$$\frac{\text{gr } 1}{60 \text{ mg}} \diagdown \frac{\text{gr } \frac{1}{2}}{\text{X mg}} \qquad \text{Cross-multiply}$$

$$X \quad = \quad 60 \times \frac{1}{2}$$

$$X \quad = \quad 30 \text{ mg} \qquad \text{Label the units to match the unknown X}$$

$$\text{gr } \frac{1}{2} \quad = \quad 30 \text{ mg}$$

Now the problem looks like this:

Order: **phenobarbital 30 mg p.o. q.12h**

Supply: phenobarbital 15 mg per tablet

Now you can probably solve this problem in your head. That's what Step 2 is about.

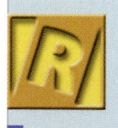

RULE

Step 2   **Think**   Carefully consider what is the reasonable amount of the drug that should be administered.

Once you have converted all units to the same system and size, Step 2 asks you to logically conclude what amount should be given. Before you go on to Step 3, you may be able to picture in your mind a reasonable amount of medication to be administered, as was demonstrated in the previous two examples. At least you should be able to estimate, such as more or less than 1 tablet (or capsule or milliliter). Basically, Step 2 asks you to *stop and think before you go any further.*

In the last example, you estimate that the patient should receive more than 1 phenobarbital tablet. In fact, you realize that you would administer 2 of the 15 mg tablets to fill the order for gr $\frac{1}{2}$ or 30 mg.

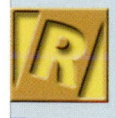

RULE

Step 3   **Calculate**   Ratio for the dosage you have on hand equals the ratio for the desired dosage.

Always double-check your estimated amount from Step 2 with the ratio-proportion method. When setting up the first ratio to calculate a drug dosage, use the supply dosage or the drug concentration information available on the drug label. This is the drug you *have on hand.* Set up the second ratio using the drug order or the *dosage desired* and the amount or volume you will give the patient. This is the unknown or X. Keep the *known* information on the left side of the proportion and the *unknown* on the right.

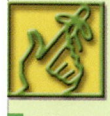

REMEMBER

$$\frac{\text{Dosage on hand}}{\text{Amount on hand}} = \frac{\text{Dosage desired}}{\text{X Amount desired}}$$

MATH TIP

When solving dosage problems for drugs supplied in tablets or capsules, the amount on hand is always 1, because the supply dosage is per 1 tablet or capsule.

Let's use ratio-proportion to double-check our thinking and calculate the dosages for the previous phenobarbital example.

Order: **phenobarbital gr $\frac{1}{2}$ p.o. q.12h**, converted to phenobarbital 30 mg

Supply: phenobarbital 15 mg per tablet

$$\frac{\text{Dosage on hand}}{\text{Amount on hand}} = \frac{\text{Dosage desired}}{\text{X Amount desired}}$$

$$\frac{15 \text{ mg}}{1 \text{ tablet}} \bowtie \frac{30 \text{ mg}}{\text{X tablets}} \qquad \text{Cross-multiply}$$

$$15\text{X} = 30$$

$$\frac{15\text{X}}{15} = \frac{30}{15} \qquad \text{Simplify: Divide both sides of the equation by the number before the unknown X}$$

$$\text{X} = 2 \text{ tablets} \qquad \text{Label the units to match the unknown X}$$

Give two of the phenobarbital 15 mg tablets orally every 12 hours. The calculations verify your estimate from Step 2.

Remember that proportions compare like things. Therefore, you must first convert all units to the same system and to the same size. As pointed out in Chapter 4, the ratio must follow the same sequence. The proportion is set up so that like units are across from each other. The numerators of each represent the weight of the dosage, and denominators represent the amount. It is important to keep like units in order, such as mg as the numerators (on top) and tablets as the denominator (on bottom). And, it is important to keep the known on the left side of the proportion and the unknown (X) on the right. Labeling units also helps you to recognize if you have set up the equation in the proper sequence.

Let's look at two more examples to reinforce this concept.

EXAMPLE 3 ■

Order: Lasix 10 mg p.o. b.i.d.

Supply: Lasix 20 mg per tablet

$$\frac{\text{Dosage on hand}}{\text{Amount on hand}} = \frac{\text{Dosage desired}}{\text{X Amount desired}}$$

$$\frac{20 \text{ mg}}{1 \text{ tablet}} \bowtie \frac{10 \text{ mg}}{\text{X tablets}} \qquad \text{Cross-multiply}$$

$$20\text{X} = 10$$

$$\frac{20\text{X}}{20} = \frac{10}{20} \qquad \text{Simplify: Divide both sides of the equation by the number before the unknown X}$$

$$\text{X} = \frac{1}{2} \text{ tablet} \qquad \text{Label the units to match the unknown X}$$

Notice that you want to give $\frac{1}{2}$ of the dosage you have on hand which in this case is $\frac{1}{2}$ of 1 tablet. Therefore, you want to give $\frac{1}{2}$ tablet of Lasix 20 mg tablets orally twice daily.

EXAMPLE 4 ■

Order: Tylenol gr x p.o. q.4h p.r.n., headache

Supply: Tylenol 325 mg per tablet

First convert to the same unit of measure.

Approximate equivalent: gr i = 60 mg

Remember: gr x = gr 10

$$\frac{\text{gr } 1}{60 \text{ mg}} \bowtie \frac{\text{gr } 10}{\text{X mg}} \qquad \text{Cross-multiply}$$

$$\text{X} = 60 \times 10$$

$$\text{X} = 600 \text{ mg} \qquad \text{Label the units to match the unknown X}$$

Then calculate the dosage.

$$\frac{\text{Dosage on hand}}{\text{Amount on hand}} = \frac{\text{Dosage desired}}{\text{X Amount desired}}$$

$$\frac{325 \text{ mg}}{1 \text{ tablet}} \bowtie \frac{600 \text{ mg}}{\text{X tablets}} \qquad \text{Cross-multiply}$$

$$325\ X\ =\ 600$$

$$\frac{325X}{325} = \frac{600}{325}$$ Simplify: Divide both sides of the equation by the number before the unknown X

$$X\ =\ 1.8\ \text{tablets}$$ Label the units to match the unknown X

An amount of 1.8 tablets is not appropriate. Remember that gr i = 60 mg, but in some instances gr i = 65 mg is more relevant. This is true because it is an *approximate* equivalent. In this case, gr i = 65 mg is more accurate.

Order: Tylenol gr x p.o. q.4h p.r.n., headache

Supply: Tylenol 325 mg per tablet

Approximate equivalent: gr i = 65 mg

Remember: gr x = gr 10

Convert gr to mg.

$$\frac{\text{gr } 1}{65\text{ mg}} \times \frac{\text{gr } 10}{X\text{ mg}}$$ Cross-multiply

$$X\ =\ 65 \times 10$$

$$X\ =\ 650\text{ mg}$$ Label the units to match the unknown X

Calculate the amount to give.

$$\frac{\text{Dosage on hand}}{\text{Amount on hand}} = \frac{\text{Dosage desired}}{\text{X Amount desired}}$$

$$\frac{325\text{ mg}}{1\text{ tablet}} \times \frac{650\text{ mg}}{X\text{ tablets}}$$ Cross-multiply

$$325\ X\ =\ 650$$

$$\frac{325X}{325} = \frac{650}{325}$$ Simplify: Divide both sides of the equation by the number before the unknown X

$$X\ =\ 2\ \text{tablets}$$ Label the units to match the unknown X

Notice that you want to give two times the amount of the dosage on hand; that is, you want to give two of the Tylenol 325 mg tablets orally every 4 hours as needed for headache.

Now you are ready to apply all three steps of this logical approach to dosage calculations. The same three steps will be used to solve both oral and parenteral dosage calculation problems. It is most important that you develop the ability to reason for the answer or estimate before you calculate the amount to give.

Note to Learner

Health care professionals can unknowingly make errors if they rely solely on a calculation method rather than first asking themselves what the answer should be. As a nurse or allied health professional, you are expected to be able to reason sensibly, solve problems, and justify your judgments rationally. With these same skills you gained admission to your educational program and to your profession. While you sharpen your math skills, your ability to think and estimate are your best resources for avoiding errors. Use ratio-proportion as a calculation tool to validate the dose amount you anticipate should be given, rather than the reverse. If your reasoning is sound, you will find the dosages you compute make sense and are accurate. For example, you would question any calculation that directs you to administer 5 tablets of any medication.

 **CAUTION**
The maximum number of tablets or capsules for a single dose is usually 3. Stop, think, and recheck your calculation if a single dose requires more.

Let's examine more examples of oral dosages supplied in capsules and tablets to reinforce the three basic steps. Then you will be ready to solve problems like these on your own.

EXAMPLE 1 ■

The drug order reads: **Lopressor 100 mg p.o. b.i.d.** The medicine container is labeled *Lopressor 50 mg per tablet*. Calculate 1 dose.

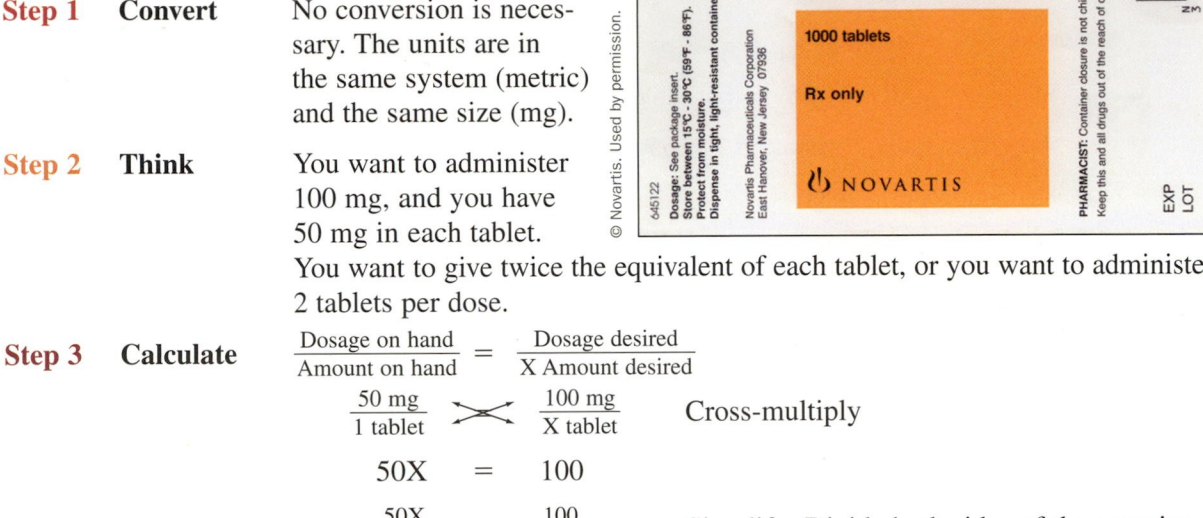

Step 1	**Convert**	No conversion is necessary. The units are in the same system (metric) and the same size (mg).
Step 2	**Think**	You want to administer 100 mg, and you have 50 mg in each tablet. You want to give twice the equivalent of each tablet, or you want to administer 2 tablets per dose.

Step 3 **Calculate**

$$\frac{\text{Dosage on hand}}{\text{Amount on hand}} = \frac{\text{Dosage desired}}{\text{X Amount desired}}$$

$$\frac{50 \text{ mg}}{1 \text{ tablet}} \diagdown \frac{100 \text{ mg}}{\text{X tablet}} \qquad \text{Cross-multiply}$$

$$50\text{X} = 100$$

$$\frac{50\text{X}}{50} = \frac{100}{50} \qquad \text{Simplify: Divide both sides of the equation by the number before the unknown X}$$

$$\text{X} = 2 \text{ tablets} \qquad \text{Label the units to match the unknown X}$$

Give 2 tablets of Lopressor orally twice daily.

Double-check to be sure your calculated dosage matches your *reasonable* dosage from Step 2. If, for example, you had calculated to give more or less than 2 tablets of Lopressor, you would suspect a calculation error.

EXAMPLE 2 ■

The physician prescribes:

    Flagyl 0.75 g p.o. t.i.d.

The dosage available is Flagyl 500 mg per tablet. How many tablets should the nurse give to the patient per dose?

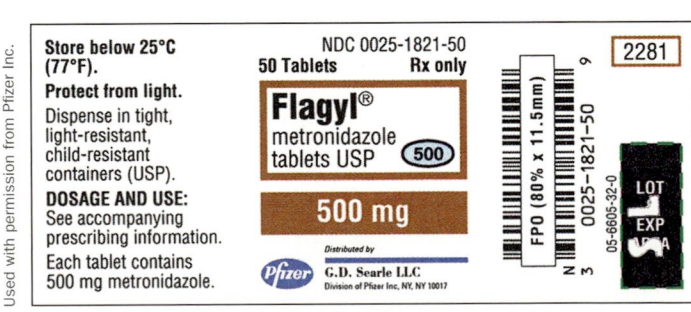

Step 1 **Convert**   To the same size units. Convert 0.75 g to mg. Remember the math tip: Convert larger unit (g) to the smaller unit (mg), which will eliminate the decimal fraction.

$$\text{Equivalent: } 1 \text{ g} = 1,000 \text{ mg}$$

$$\frac{1 \text{ g}}{1,000 \text{ mg}} \diagdown \frac{0.75 \text{ g}}{\text{X mg}} \qquad \text{Cross-multiply}$$

$$\text{X} = 1,000 \times 0.75 \qquad 0.750. \text{ Move the decimal three places to the right. Add zero to complete the operation.}$$

$$\text{X} = 750 \text{ mg} \qquad \text{Label the units to match the unknown X}$$

Now you have the order and supply measured in the same size units.

Order: Flagyl 0.75 g = 750 mg

Supply: Flagyl 500 mg tablets

By now you probably can do conversions like this from memory.

Step 2 **Think**   750 mg is more than 500 mg. You want to give more than 1 tablet but not as much as 2 tablets. Actually you want to give $1\frac{1}{2}$ tablets. Now calculate to verify your estimate.

Step 3 **Calculate**

$$\frac{\text{Dosage on hand}}{\text{Amount on hand}} = \frac{\text{Dosage desired}}{\text{X Amount desired}}$$

$$\frac{500\text{ mg}}{1\text{ tablet}} \diagup\!\!\!\!\diagdown \frac{750\text{ mg}}{\text{X tablets}}$$ Cross-multiply

$$500X = 750$$

$$\frac{500X}{500} = \frac{750}{500}$$ Simplify: Divide both sides of the equation by the number before the unknown X

$$X = 1\frac{1}{2}\text{ tablets}$$ Label the units to match the unknown X

Give $1\frac{1}{2}$ tablets of Flagyl orally three times daily.

EXAMPLE 3 ■

The drug order reads: *codeine sulfate gr $\frac{3}{4}$ p.o. q.4h p.r.n., pain.*

The drug supplied is codeine sulfate 30 mg per tablet. Calculate 1 dose.

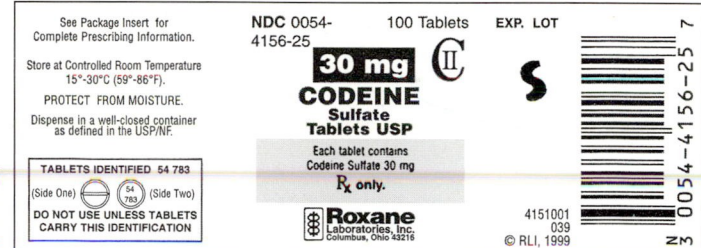

Step 1 **Convert**   To equivalent units in the same system of measurement. Convert gr to mg and you will eliminate the fraction.
Approximate equivalent: gr i = 60 mg

$$\frac{\text{gr }1}{60\text{ mg}} \diagup\!\!\!\!\diagdown \frac{\text{gr }\frac{3}{4}}{\text{X mg}}$$ Cross-multiply

$$X = 60 \times \frac{3}{4}$$

$$X = 45\text{ mg}$$ Label the units to match the unknown X

Order: codeine gr $\frac{3}{4}$ = 45 mg

Supply: codeine 30 mg tablets

Step 2 **Think**   You estimate that you want to give more than 1 tablet but less than 2 tablets.

Step 3 **Calculate**

$$\frac{\text{Dosage on hand}}{\text{Amount on hand}} = \frac{\text{Dosage desired}}{\text{X Amount desired}}$$

$$\frac{30\text{ mg}}{1\text{ tablet}} \diagup\!\!\!\!\diagdown \frac{45\text{ mg}}{\text{X tablets}}$$ Cross-multiply

$$30X = 45$$

$$\frac{30X}{30} = \frac{45}{30}$$ Simplify: Divide both sides of the equation by the number before the unknown X

$$X = 1\frac{1}{2}\text{ tablets}$$ Label the units to match the unknown X

Give $1\frac{1}{2}$ tablets codeine orally every 4 hours as needed for pain.

Now you can see that a dosage problem that may have seemed difficult on first reading is actually simple. Approach every dosage calculation just like this: one step at a time.

EXAMPLE 4 ■

The order is **Synthroid 0.05 mg p.o. daily.**

Synthroid 25 mcg tablets are available. How many tablets will you give?

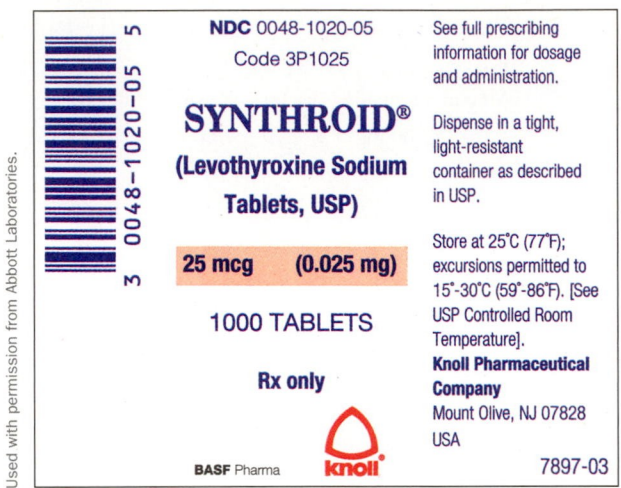

| Step 1 | Convert | To the same size units. Remember the math tip: Convert larger unit (mg) to smaller unit (mcg) and you will eliminate the decimal fraction. |

Approximate equivalent: 1 mg = 1,000 mcg

$$\frac{1 \text{ mg}}{1,000 \text{ mcg}} \bowtie \frac{0.05 \text{ mg}}{X \text{ mcg}}$$ Cross-multiply

$$X \quad = \quad 1,000 \times 0.05 \qquad 0.050. \text{ Move the decimal three places to the right. Add zero to complete the operation.}$$

$$X \quad = \quad 50 \text{ mcg} \qquad \text{Label the units to match the unknown X}$$

Order: **Synthroid 0.05 mg = 50 mcg**

Supply: Synthroid 25 mcg tablets

| Step 2 | Think | As soon as you convert the ordered dosage of *Synthroid 0.05 mg* to *Synthroid 50 mcg,* you realize that you want to give more than 1 tablet for each dose. In fact, you want to give twice the supply dosage, which is the same as 2 tablets. |

Avoid getting confused by the way the original problem is presented. Be sure that you recognize which is the dosage ordered or desired and which is the supply dosage per the amount on hand. A common error is to misread the information and mix up the ratios in Step 3. This demonstrates the importance of thinking (Step 2) before you calculate.

| Step 3 | Calculate | $$\frac{\text{Dosage on hand}}{\text{Amount on hand}} = \frac{\text{Dosage desired}}{X \text{ Amount desired}}$$ |

$$\frac{25 \text{ mcg}}{1 \text{ tablet}} \bowtie \frac{50 \text{ mcg}}{X \text{ tablets}}$$ Cross-multiply

$$25 X \quad = \quad 50$$

$$\frac{25X}{25} \quad = \quad \frac{50}{25} \qquad \text{Simplify: Divide both sides of the equation by the number before the unknown X}$$

$$X \quad = \quad 2 \text{ tablets} \qquad \text{Label the units to match the unknown X}$$

Give 2 tablets of Synthroid orally daily.

EXAMPLE 5 ■

Your client is to receive **Nitrostat gr $\frac{1}{400}$ SL p.r.n., angina.**

The label on the available Nitrostat bottle tells you that each tablet provides 0.3 mg (gr $\frac{1}{200}$). How much will you give your client?

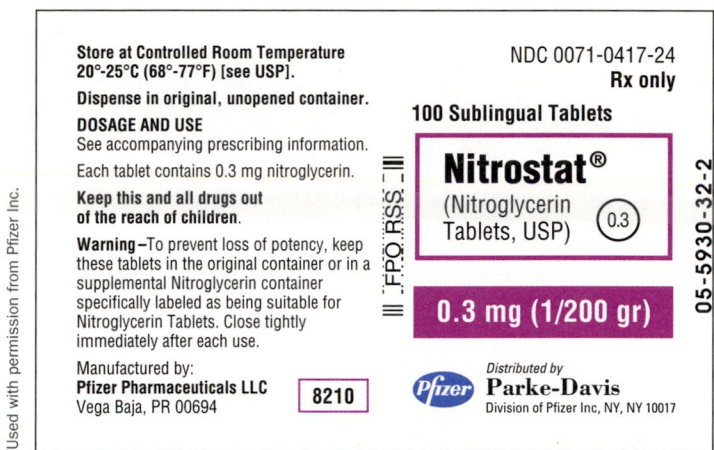

Step 1 Convert	To equivalent units in the same system of measurement. Remember the math tip: Convert apothecary measurement to metric units. Convert the order in grains to milligrams, and you will eliminate the fraction.

Approximate equivalent: gr i = 60 mg

$$\frac{\text{gr } 1}{60 \text{ mg}} \quad \bowtie \quad \frac{\text{gr } \frac{1}{400}}{X \text{ mg}} \qquad \text{Cross-multiply}$$

$$X = 60 \times \frac{1}{400}$$

$$X = 0.15 \text{ mg} \qquad \text{Label the units to match the unknown X}$$

Order: **Nitrostat gr $\frac{1}{400}$ = 0.15 mg**

Supply: Nitrostat 0.3 mg tablets

Step 2 Think Look at the supply dosage and add a zero at the end of the decimal number: 0.3 mg = 0.30 mg. Now you can compare the ordered dosage of 0.15 mg with the supply dosage of 0.30 mg per tablet. You can reason that you want to give less than 1 tablet. Further, you can see that 0.15 is $\frac{1}{2}$ of 0.30, and you know that you want to give $\frac{1}{2}$ tablet. Check your reasoning in Step 3.

Step 3 Calculate

$$\frac{\text{Dosage on hand}}{\text{Amount on hand}} = \frac{\text{Dosage desired}}{\text{X Amount desired}}$$

$$\frac{0.3 \text{ mg}}{1 \text{ tablet}} \quad \bowtie \quad \frac{0.15 \text{ mg}}{X \text{ tablets}} \qquad \text{Cross-multiply}$$

$$0.3X = 0.15$$

$$\frac{0.3X}{0.3} = \frac{0.15}{0.3} \qquad \text{Simplify: Divide both sides of the equation by the number before the unknown X}$$

$$X = \frac{1}{2} \text{ tablet} \qquad \text{Label the units to match the unknown X}$$

Give $\frac{1}{2}$ tablet Nitrostat sublingually as needed for angina.

QUICK REVIEW

Simple Three-Step Approach to Dosage Calculations

Step 1	**Convert**	To units of the same system and the same size.
Step 2	**Think**	Estimate for a reasonable amount to give.
Step 3	**Calculate**	The ratio for the dosage you have on hand equals the ratio for the dosage desired.

$$\frac{\text{Dosage on hand}}{\text{Amount on hand}} = \frac{\text{Dosage desired}}{\text{X Amount desired}}$$

■ For most dosage calculation problems:
  - convert to smaller size unit. Example: g → mg
  - convert from the apothecary or household system to the metric system. Example: gr → mg

■ Consider the reasonableness of the calculated amount to give. Example: You would question giving more than 3 tablets or capsules per dose for oral administration.

Review Set 22

Calculate the correct number of tablets or capsules to be administered per dose. Tablets are scored.

1. Order: Diabinese 0.1 g p.o. daily

   Supply: Diabinese 100 mg tablets

   Give: _____ tablet(s)

2. Order: cefadroxil 0.5 g p.o. b.i.d.

   Supply: cefadroxil 500 mg tablets

   Give: _____ tablet(s)

3. Order: Urecholine 15 mg p.o. t.i.d.

   Supply: Urecholine 10 mg tablets

   Give: _____ tablet(s)

4. Order: hydrochlorothiazide 12.5 mg p.o. t.i.d.

   Supply: hydrochlorothiazide 25 mg tablets

   Give: _____ tablet(s)

5. Order: digoxin 0.125 mg p.o. daily

   Supply: digoxin 0.25 mg tablets

   Give: _____ tablet(s)

6. Order: Motrin 600 mg p.o. b.i.d.

   Supply: Motrin 200 mg tablets

   Give: _____ tablet(s)

7. Order: Micro-K 16 mEq p.o. stat

   Supply: Micro-K 8 mEq capsules

   Give: _____ capsule(s)

8. Order: **Cytoxan 50 mg p.o. daily**

   Supply: Cytoxan 25 mg tablets

   Give: _____ tablet(s)

9. Order: **Zaroxolyn 10 mg p.o. daily**

   Supply: Zaroxolyn 5 mg tablets

   Give: _____ tablet(s)

10. Order: **Coumadin 5 mg p.o. daily**

    Supply: Coumadin 2.5 mg tablets

    Give: _____ tablet(s)

11. Order: **Levaquin 0.5 g p.o. daily**

    Supply: Levaquin 500 mg tablets

    Give: _____ tablet(s)

12. Order: **Trandate 150 mg p.o. b.i.d.**

    Supply: Trandate 300 mg tablets

    Give: _____ tablet(s)

13. Order: **Duricef 1 g p.o. b.i.d.**

    Supply: Duricef 500 mg capsules

    Give: _____ capsule(s)

14. Order: **Synthroid 0.1 mg p.o. daily**

    Supply: Synthroid 50 mcg tablets

    Give: _____ tablet(s)

15. Order: **Tranxene 7.5 mg p.o. q.i.d.**

    Supply: Tranxene 3.75 mg capsules

    Give: _____ capsule(s)

16. Order: **Inderal 15 mg p.o. t.i.d.**

    Supply: Inderal 10 mg tablets

    Give: _____ tablets(s)

17. The doctor orders **Loniten 5 mg p.o. stat** and you have available Loniten 10 mg and 2.5 mg scored tablets. Select _____ mg tablets and give _____ tablet(s).

18. Order: **Reglan 15 mg p.o. 1 h a.c. et bedtime.** You have available Reglan 10 mg and Reglan 5 mg scored tablets. Select _____ mg tablets and give _____ tablet(s). How many doses of Reglan should you anticipate the patient will receive in 24 hours? _____ dose(s)

19. Order: **phenobarbital gr $\frac{1}{4}$ p.o. daily**

    Supply: phenobarbital 15 mg, 30 mg, and 60 mg scored tablets

    Select _____ mg tablets and give _____ tablet(s).

20. Order: **Tylenol $\bar{c}$ codeine gr i̇ p.o. q.4h p.r.n., pain**

    Supply: Tylenol with codeine 7.5 mg, 15 mg, 30 mg, and 60 mg tablets

    Select _____ mg tablets and give _____ tablet(s).

Calculate 1 dose for each of the medication orders 21 through 30. The labels lettered A through I are the drugs you have available. Indicate the letter corresponding to the label you select.

21. Order: verapamil sustained-release 240 mg p.o. daily

    Select: _____

    Give: _____

22. Order: carbamazepine 0.2 g p.o. t.i.d.

    Select: _____

    Give: _____

23. Order: Lopressor 50 mg p.o. b.i.d.

    Select: _____

    Give: _____

24. Order: potassium chloride 20 mEq p.o. daily

    Select: _____

    Give: _____

25. Order: digoxin 375 mcg p.o. daily

    Select: _____

    Give: _____

26. Order: sulfasalazine 1 g p.o. b.i.d.

    Select: _____

    Give: _____

27. Order: levothyroxine sodium 0.2 mg p.o. daily

    Select: _____

    Give: _____

28. Order: digoxin 0.5 mg p.o. daily

    Select: _____

    Give: _____

29. Order: Neurontin 0.1 g p.o. t.i.d.

    Select: _____

    Give: _____

30. Order: Lopid 0.6 g p.o. daily

    Select: _____

    Give: _____

After completing these problems, see pages 519–520 to check your answers.

Store at controlled room temperature 15º- 30ºC (59º- 86ºF).

DOSAGE AND USE
See package insert for full prescribing information.

Each capsule contains 100 mg of gabapentin.

Manufactured by:
Pfizer Pharmaceuticals Ltd.
Vega Baja, PR 00694

NDC 0071-0803-24
100 Capsules   **Rx only**

Neurontin® ⟨ 100 ⟩
(gabapentin) capsules

100 mg

Distributed by
Pfizer **Parke-Davis**
Division of Pfizer Inc, NY, NY 10017

7700

FPO UPC : 80% x 11.5mm
N 3   0071-0803-24   4
05-5810-32-4

A

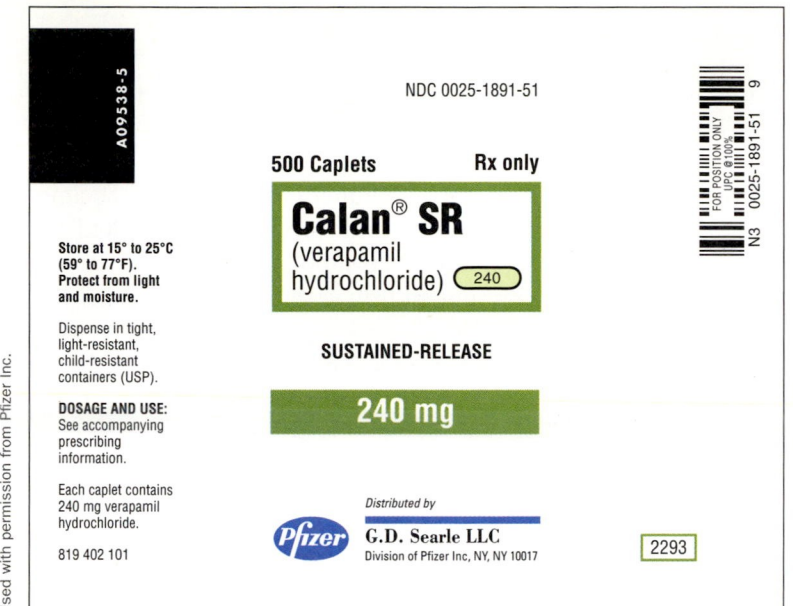

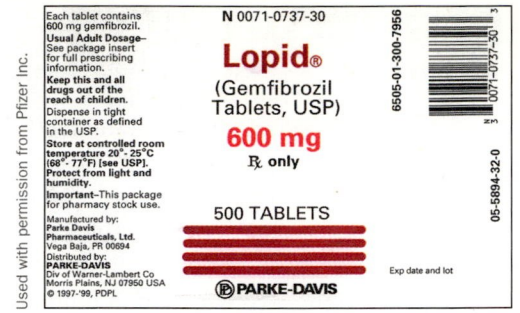

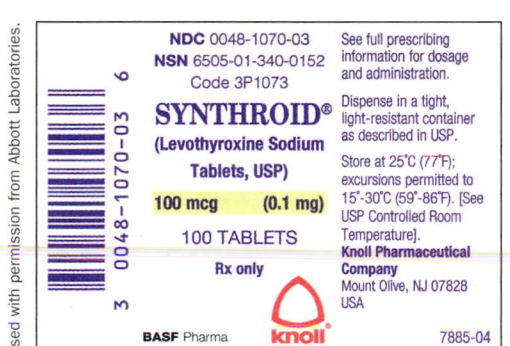

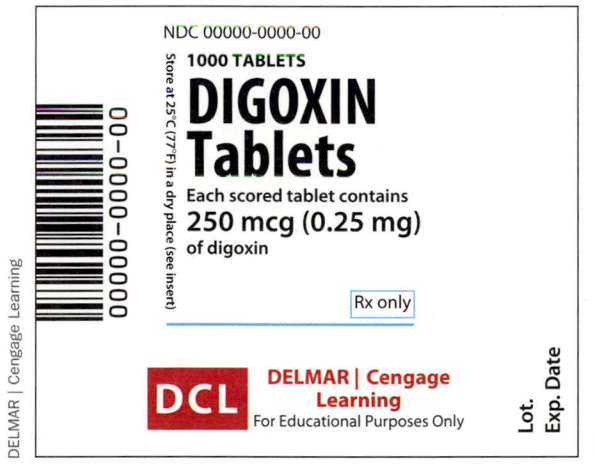

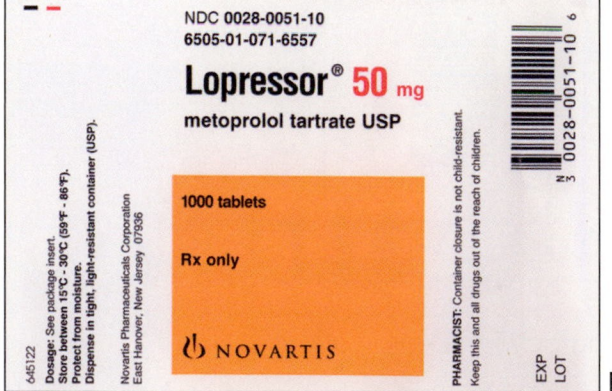

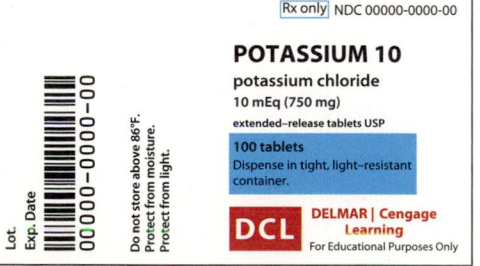

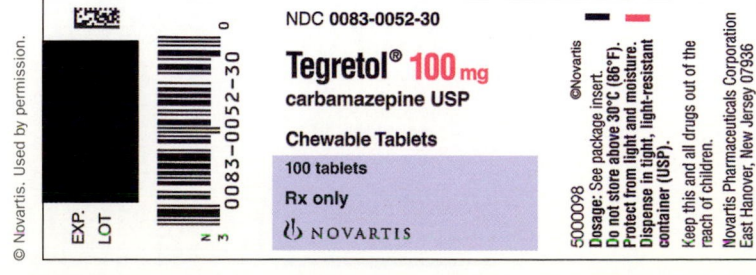

ORAL LIQUIDS

Oral liquids are supplied in solution form and contain a specific amount of drug in a given amount of solution as stated on the label (Figures 10-3a through 10-3d).

In solving dosage problems when the drug is supplied in solid form, you calculated the number of tablets or capsules that contained the prescribed dosage. The supply container label indicates the amount of medication per 1 tablet or 1 capsule. For medications supplied in liquid form, you must calculate the volume of the liquid that contains the prescribed dosage of the drug. The supply dosage noted on the label may indicate the amount of drug per 1 milliliter or per multiple milliliters of solution, such as 10 mg per 2 mL, 125 mg per 5 mL, or 1.2 g per 30 mL.

Steps 1, 2, and 3 can be used to solve liquid oral dosage calculations in the same way that solid-form oral dosages are calculated. Let's apply the three steps to dosage calculations in a few examples.

FIGURE 10-3(a)   Oral liquid: Cefaclor 125 mg per 5 mL

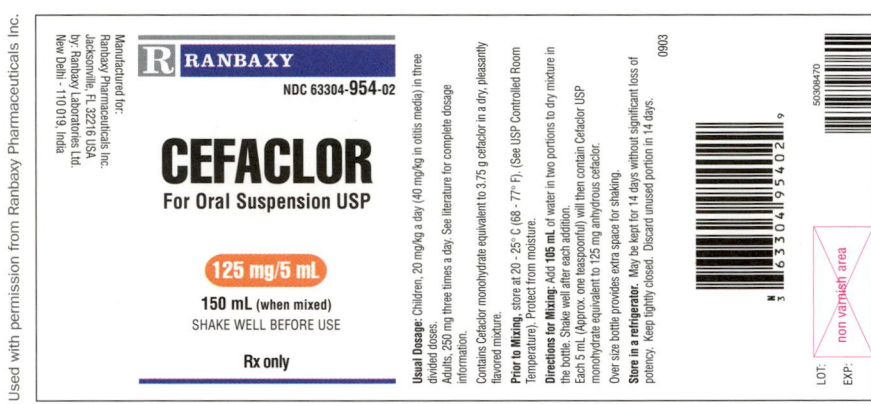

FIGURE 10-3(b)   Oral liquid: Cefaclor 187 mg per 5 mL

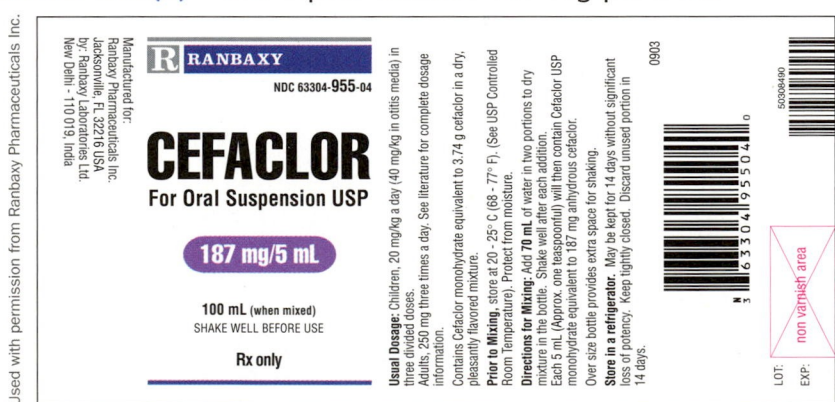

FIGURE 10-3(c)   Oral liquid: Cefaclor 250 mg per 5 mL

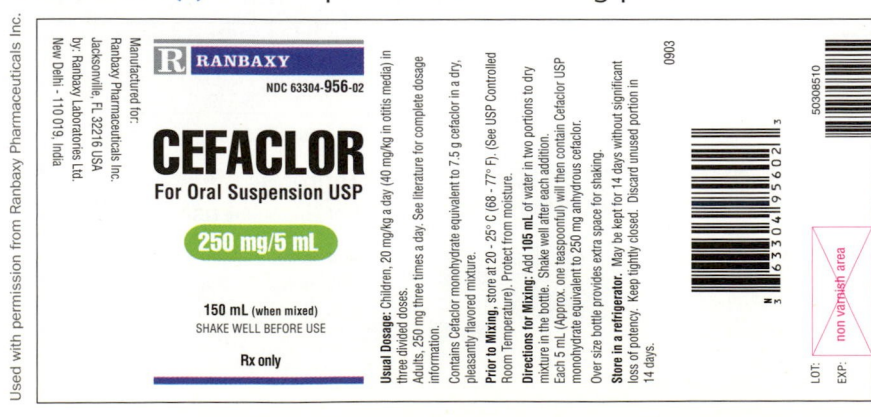

FIGURE 10-3(d)   Oral liquid: Cefaclor 375 mg per 5 mL

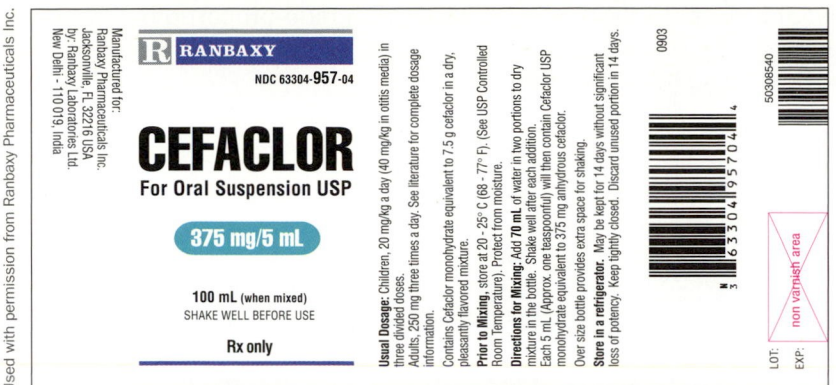

EXAMPLE 1 ■

The doctor orders *cefaclor 100 mg p.o. q.i.d.*

Look at the labels of cefaclor available in Figure 10-3. You choose *cefaclor 125 mg per 5 mL*. Follow the three steps to dosage calculations.

Step 1   **Convert**   No conversion is necessary because the order and supply dosage are both in the same units.

Step 2   **Think**   You want to give less than 125 mg, so you want to give less than 5 mL. Double-check your thinking with ratio-proportion.

Step 3   **Calculate** $\dfrac{\text{Dosage on hand}}{\text{Amount on hand}} = \dfrac{\text{Dosage desired}}{\text{X Amount desired}}$

$\dfrac{125 \text{ mg}}{5 \text{ mL}} \times \dfrac{100 \text{ mg}}{\text{X mL}}$ Cross-multiply

$125\text{X} = 100 \times 5$

$125\text{X} = 500$

$\dfrac{125\text{X}}{125} = \dfrac{500}{125}$ Simplify: Divide both sides of the equation by the number before the unknown X

$\text{X} = 4 \text{ mL}$ Label the units to match the unknown X

Give 4 mL of the cefaclor (concentration 125 mg per 5 mL) orally four times daily.

Notice that the label says the dosage strength (or concentration) is 125 mg per 5 mL. The order is for only 100 mg so you know you will give less than 5 mL. You will give 4 mL of the cefaclor with the dosage strength of 125 mg per 5 mL. Double-check to be sure your calculated dosage is consistent with your reasonable dosage from Step 2. If, for instance, you calculate to give more than 5 mL, then you should suspect a calculation error.

EXAMPLE 2 ■

Suppose, using the same drug order in Example 1, *cefaclor 100 mg p.o. q.i.d.*, you choose a stronger solution, *cefaclor 250 mg per 5 mL*. Follow the three steps to dosage calculations.

Step 1   **Convert**   No conversion is necessary because the order and supply dosage are both in the same units and system.

Step 2   **Think**   You want to give 100 mg, and you have 250 mg per 5 mL so you will give less than half of 5 mL. Double-check your thinking with ratio-proportion.

Step 3   **Calculate**

$$\frac{\text{Dosage on hand}}{\text{Amount on hand}} = \frac{\text{Dosage desired}}{\text{X Amount desired}}$$

$$\frac{250 \text{ mg}}{5 \text{ mL}} \underset{\times}{\times} \frac{100 \text{ mg}}{\text{X mL}} \quad \text{Cross-multiply}$$

$$250\text{X} = 100 \times 5$$

$$250\text{X} = 500$$

$$\frac{250\text{X}}{250} = \frac{500}{250} \quad \begin{array}{l}\text{Simplify: Divide both sides of the equation}\\\text{by the number before the unknown X}\end{array}$$

$$\text{X} = 2 \text{ mL} \quad \text{Label the units to match the unknown X}$$

Give 2 mL of the cefaclor (concentration 250 mg per 5 mL) orally four times daily.

Notice that in both Example 1 and Example 2, the supply quantity is the same (5 mL), but the dosage strength (weight) of medication is different (125 mg per 5 mL versus 250 mg per 5 mL). This results in the calculated dose volume (amount to give) being different (4 mL versus 2 mL). This difference is the result of each liquid's concentration. *Cefaclor 125 mg per 5 mL is half as concentrated as cefaclor 250 mg per 5 mL.* In other words, there is half as much drug in 5 mL of the *125 mg per 5 mL* supply as there is in 5 mL of the *250 mg per 5 mL* supply. Likewise, *cefaclor 250 mg per 5 mL is twice as concentrated as cefaclor 125 mg per 5 mL.* The more concentrated solution allows you to give the patient less volume per dose for the same dosage. This is significant when administering medication to infants and small children when a smaller quantity is needed. Think about this carefully until it is clear.

CAUTION

Think before you calculate. It is important to estimate before you apply any formula. In this way, if you make an error in math or if you set up the problem incorrectly, your thinking will alert you to try again.

EXAMPLE 3 ▪

The doctor orders **potassium chloride 40 mEq p.o. daily.**

The label on the package reads *potassium chloride 20 mEq per 15 mL.* How many mL should you administer?

Step 1   **Convert**   No conversion is necessary.

Step 2   **Think**   You want to give more than 15 mL. In fact, you want to give exactly twice as much as 15 mL. You know this is true because 40 mEq is twice as much as 20 mEq. Therefore, it will take 2 × 15 mL or 30 mL to give 40 mEq. Continue to Step 3 to double-check your thinking.

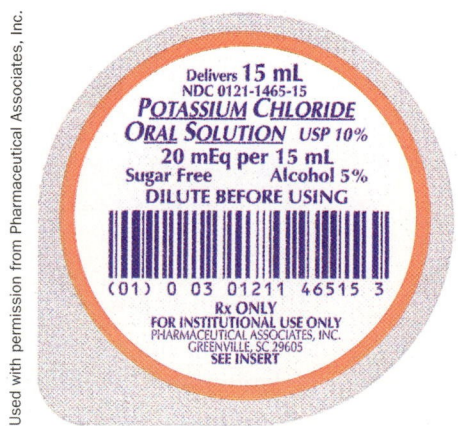

Delivers **15 mL**
NDC 0121-1465-15
POTASSIUM CHLORIDE
ORAL SOLUTION USP 10%
20 mEq per 15 mL
Sugar Free   Alcohol 5%
DILUTE BEFORE USING

(01) 0 03 01211 46515 3

Rx ONLY
FOR INSTITUTIONAL USE ONLY
PHARMACEUTICAL ASSOCIATES, INC.
GREENVILLE, SC 29605
SEE INSERT

Step 3 **Calculate** $\dfrac{\text{Dosage on hand}}{\text{Amount on hand}} = \dfrac{\text{Dosage desired}}{\text{X Amount desired}}$

$$\dfrac{20 \text{ mEq}}{15 \text{ mL}} \times \dfrac{40 \text{ mEq}}{\text{X mL}} \qquad \text{Cross-multiply}$$

$$20\text{X} = 40 \times 15$$

$$20\text{X} = 600$$

$$\dfrac{20\text{X}}{20} = \dfrac{600}{20} \qquad \text{Simplify: Divide both sides of the equation by the number before the unknown X}$$

$$\text{X} = 30 \text{ mL} \qquad \text{Label the units to match the unknown X}$$

Give 30 mL of potassium chloride (concentration 20 mEq per 15 mL) orally daily.

QUICK REVIEW

Look again at Steps 1 through 3 as a valuable dosage calculation checklist.

Step 1 **Convert** Be sure that all measurements are in the same system and all units are in the same size.

Step 2 **Think** Carefully estimate the reasonable amount of the drug that you should administer.

Step 3 **Calculate** $\dfrac{\text{Dosage on hand}}{\text{Amount on hand}} = \dfrac{\text{Dosage desired}}{\text{X Amount desired}}$

Review Set 23

Calculate 1 dose of the drugs ordered.

1. Order: Roxanol Oral Solution 30 mg p.o. q.4h p.r.n. pain

   Supply: Roxanol Oral Solution 20 mg per 5 mL

   Give: _____ mL

2. Order: promethazine c̄ codeine gr $\frac{1}{6}$ p.o. q.6h p.r.n. cough

   Supply: promethazine c̄ codeine solution 10 mg per 5 mL

   Give: _____ mL

3. Order: Penicillin-VK 1 g p.o. 1 h pre-op dental surgery

   Supply: Penicillin-VK oral suspension 250 mg (400,000 units) per 5 mL

   Give: _____ mL

4. Order: amoxicillin 100 mg p.o. q.i.d.

   Supply: 80 mL bottle of Amoxil (amoxicillin) oral pediatric suspension 200 mg per 5 mL

   Give: _____ mL

5. Order: Tylenol 0.325 g p.o. q.4h p.r.n., pain

   Supply: Tylenol 325 mg per 5 mL

   Give: _____ t

6. Order: promethazine HCl 25 mg p.o. at bedtime pre-op

   Supply: promethazine HCl 6.25 mg/t

   Give: _____ mL

7. Order: dicloxacillin 125 mg p.o. q.6h

   Supply: dicloxacillin suspension 62.5 mg per 5 mL

   Give: _____ t

8. Order: Pediazole 300 mg p.o. q.6h

   Supply: Pediazole 200 mg per 5 mL

   Give: _____ mL

9. Order: cefaclor suspension 225 mg p.o. b.i.d.

   Supply: cefaclor suspension 375 mg per 5 mL

   Give: _____ mL

10. Order: **Septra suspension 400 mg p.o. b.i.d.**

    Supply: Septra suspension 200 mg per 5 mL

    Give: _____ mL

11. Order: **Elixophyllin liquid 0.24 g p.o. stat**

    Supply: Elixophyllin liquid 80 mg per 15 mL

    Give: _____ mL

12. Order: **Trilisate liquid 750 mg p.o. t.i.d.**

    Supply: Trilisate liquid 500 mg per 5 mL

    Give: _____ mL

13. Order: **hydrochlorothiazide solution 100 mg p.o. b.i.d.**

    Supply: hydrochlorothiazide solution 50 mg per 5 mL

    Give: _____ t

14. Order: **Pepcid 20 mg p.o. q.i.d.**

    Supply: Pepcid 40 mg per 5 mL

    Give: _____ mL

15. Order: **digoxin elixir 0.25 mg p.o. daily**

    Supply: digoxin elixir 50 mcg/mL

    Give: _____ mL

16. Order: **Zyvox 0.6 g p.o. q.12h**

    Supply: Zyvox 100 mg per 5 mL

    Give: _____ fl oz

17. Order: **cephalexin 375 mg p.o. t.i.d.**

    Supply: cephalexin 250 mg per 5 mL

    Give: _____ t

18. Order: **lactulose 20 g via gastric tube b.i.d. today**

    Supply: lactulose 10 g per 15 mL

    Give: _____ fl oz

19. Order: **erythromycin 1.2 g p.o. q.8h**

    Supply: erythromycin 600 mg per 5 mL

    Give: _____ mL

20. Order: **oxacillin sodium 0.25 g p.o. q.8h**

    Supply: oxacillin sodium 125 mg per 2.5 mL

    Give: _____ t

21. Order: **amoxicillin suspension 100 mg p.o. q.6h**

    Supply: amoxicillin suspension 250 mg per 5 mL

    Give: _____ mL

Use the labels A, B, and C below to calculate 1 dose of the following orders (22, 23, and 24). Indicate the letter corresponding to the label you select.

22. Order: **amoxicillin 500 mg p.o. q.8h**

    Select: _____

    Give: _____

23. Order: **cefpodoxime 200 mg p.o. q.12h**

    Select: _____

    Give: _____

24. Order: **Vistaril 10 mg p.o. q.i.d.**

    Select: _____

    Give: _____

NDC 0069-5440-97

Vistaril®
hydroxyzine pamoate   *Dye Free Formula*
equivalent to
25 mg /5 ml*
hydroxyzine HCl
ORAL SUSPENSION
120 ml
CAUTION: Federal law prohibits dispensing without prescription.

MADE IN U.S.A. 4
FOR ORAL USE ONLY
SHAKE WELL BEFORE USING
STORE BELOW 77°F (25°C)
RECOMMENDED STORAGE

READ ACCOMPANYING PROFESSIONAL INFORMATION

*Each teaspoonful (5 ml) contains hydroxyzine pamoate equivalent to 25 mg hydroxyzine hydrochloride

USUAL DAILY DOSAGE
Adults: 1 to 4 teaspoonfuls 3-4 times daily.
Children: 6 years and over—2 to 4 teaspoonfuls daily in divided doses.
Under 6 years—2 teaspoonfuls daily in divided doses.

Pfizer **LABORATORIES DIVISION**
PFIZER INC., NEW YORK, N.Y. 10017

A

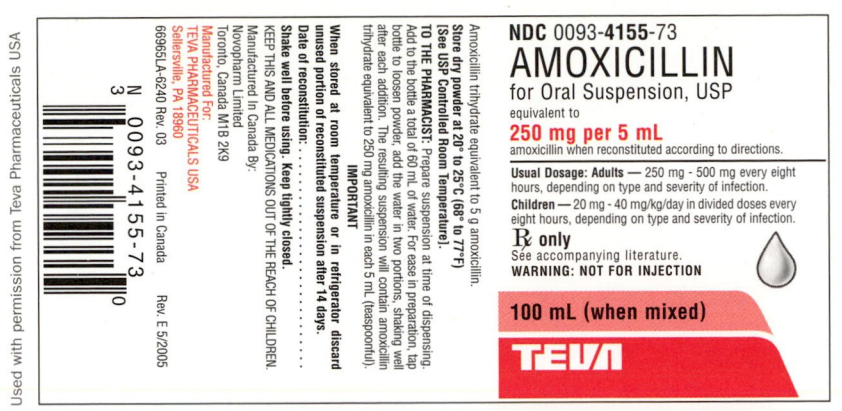

B

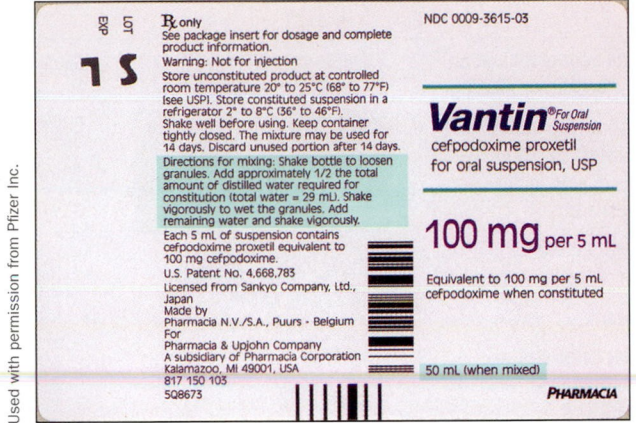

C

Calculate the information requested based on the drugs ordered. The labels provided are the drugs available.

25. Order: *cefaclor 187 mg p.o. t.i.d.*

Give: _____ mL

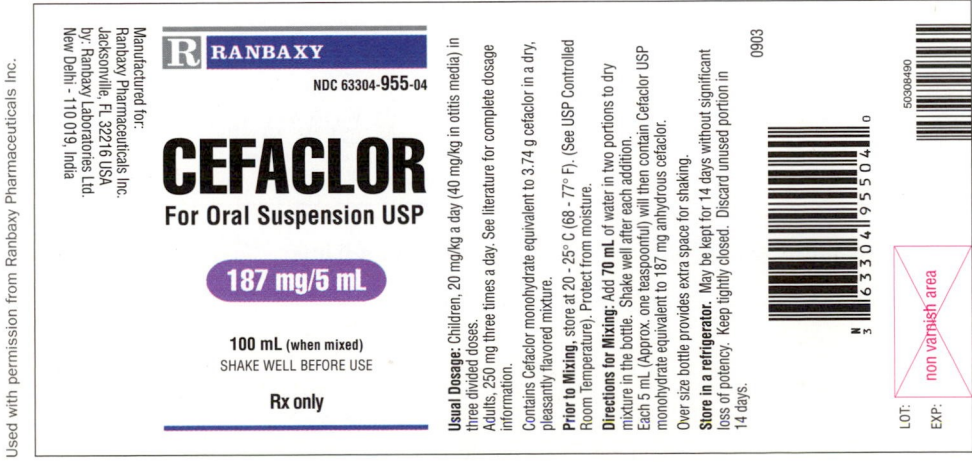

26. Order: *oxycodone hydrochloride*
    (oral solution concentrate) 15 mg p.o.
    q.6h p.r.n., pain

    Give: _____ mL

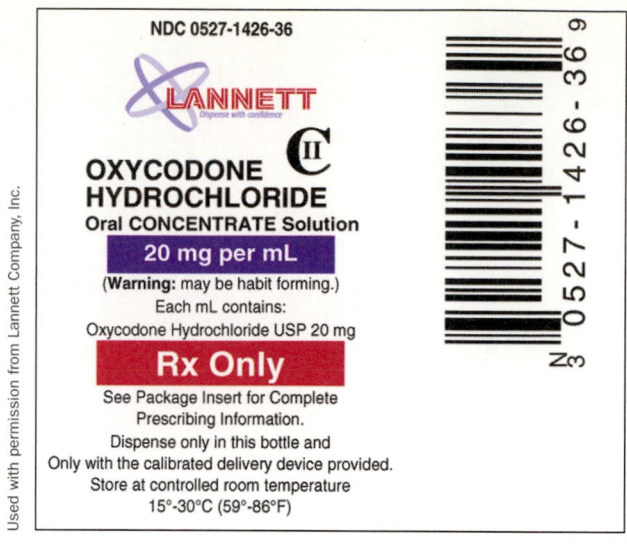

27. Order: *valproic acid*
    0.5 g p.o. t.i.d.

    Give: _____ mL

    How many full doses
    are available in this
    bottle? _____

28. Order: *Biaxin 75 mg p.o.*
    q.12h

    Give: _____ mL

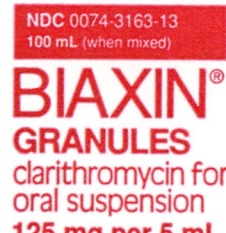

29. Order: *Antacid Plus 30 mL p.o. 30 min. p.c. and bedtime*

    How many containers will be needed for a 24-hour
    period? _____

30. Meals are served at 8 AM, noon, and 6 PM. Using international
    time, what are the administration times for the 30 min p.c.
    dosages for the order in question 29? (Allow 30 minutes
    for each meal to be eaten.) _____

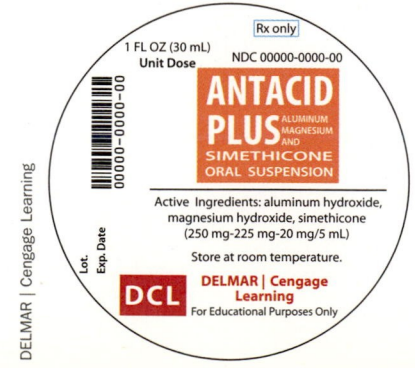

After completing these problems, see pages 520–521 to check
your answers.

SUMMARY

Let's examine where you are in mastering the skill of dosage calculations. You have learned to convert equivalent units within systems of measurements and from one system to another. You have also applied this conversion skill to the calculation of oral dosages—both solid and liquid forms. By now, you know that solving dosage problems requires that all units of measurement first be expressed in the same system and same size.

Next, you learned to think through the dosage ordered and dosage supplied to estimate the amount to be given. *To minimize medication errors, it is essential that you consider the reasonableness of the amount before applying a calculation method or formula.*

Finally, you have learned to set up and solve a drug dosage proportion of two equivalent ratios with one unknown, X. This method is so simple and easy to recall that it will stick with you throughout your career:

$$\frac{\text{Dosage on hand}}{\text{Amount on hand}} = \frac{\text{Dosage desired}}{\text{X Amount desired}}$$

Review the Critical Thinking Skills and work the practice problems for Chapter 10. If you are having difficulty, get help from an instructor before proceeding to Chapter 11. Continue to concentrate on accuracy. Keep in mind that one error can be a serious mistake when you are calculating the dosages of medicines. Medication administration is a legal responsibility. Remember, when you give a medication, you are legally responsible for your actions.

CRITICAL THINKING SKILLS

Inaccuracy in dosage calculation is often attributed to errors in calculating the dosage. Many medication errors can be avoided by first asking the question, "What is the reasonable amount to give?"

ERROR

Incorrect calculation and not assessing the reasonableness of the calculation before administering the medication.

Possible Scenario

The physician ordered **phenobarbital 60 mg p.o. b.i.d.** for a patient with seizures. The pharmacy supplied *phenobarbital 30 mg per tablet.* The nurse did not use Step 2 to think about the reasonable dosage and calculated the dosage this way:

$$\frac{\text{Dosage on hand}}{\text{Amount on hand}} = \frac{\text{Dosage desired}}{\text{X Amount desired}}$$

$$\frac{30 \text{ mg}}{1 \text{ tablet}} \diagdown\diagup \frac{60 \text{ mg}}{\text{X tablets}}$$

$$30 \text{ X} = 60$$

$$\frac{30 \text{X}}{30} = \frac{60}{30}$$

$$\text{X} = 20 \text{ tablets}$$

(Answer is incorrect! But what if the nurse did not realize this?)

Suppose the nurse then gave the patient 20 tablets of the 30 mg per tablet of phenobarbital. The patient would have received 600 mg of phenobarbital, or 10 times the correct dosage. This is a serious error.

Potential Outcome

The patient would likely develop signs of phenobarbital toxicity, such as nystagmus (rapid eye movement), ataxia (lack of coordination), central nervous system depression, respiratory depression, hypothermia, and hypotension. When the error was caught and the physician notified, the patient would likely be given doses of charcoal to hasten elimination of the drug. Depending on the severity of the symptoms, the patient would likely be moved to the intensive care unit for monitoring of respiratory and neurological status.

(Continued)

Prevention

This medication error could have been prevented if the nurse had used the three-step method and esti-mated for the reasonable dosage of the drug to give. The order is for 60 mg of phenobarbital, and the available drug has 30 mg per tablet, so the nurse should give 2 tablets. The incorrect calculation that in-dicated such a large number of tablets to give per dose should have alerted the nurse to a possible error.

Ratio-proportion $\frac{\text{Dosage on hand}}{\text{Amount on hand}} = \frac{\text{Dosage desired}}{\text{X Amount desired}}$ should be used to verify thinking about the *reasonable* dosage. Further, the nurse should double-check the math to find the error.

$$\frac{\text{Dosage on hand}}{\text{Amount on hand}} \diagup\!\!\!\!\diagdown \frac{\text{Dosage desired}}{\text{X Amount desired}}$$

$$\frac{30 \text{ mg}}{1 \text{ tablet}} = \frac{60 \text{ mg}}{\text{X tablets}}$$

$$30 \text{ X} = 60$$

$$\frac{30\text{X}}{30} = \frac{60}{30}$$

$$\text{X} = 2 \text{ tablets} \qquad \text{(Not 20 tablets)}$$

CRITICAL THINKING SKILLS

Oral suspensions used for medications prescribed for children frequently are supplied in various dosage strengths per teaspoon or 5 mL. This allows for dosage adjustments according to the weight of the child. Nurses should exercise caution when identi-fying the dosage strength ordered and administered.

ERROR

Not recognizing that oral suspensions frequently are supplied in different concentrations and docu-menting the wrong dosage strength in the medical record.

Possible Scenario

After being treated for a few days for a respiratory infection, a child's condition worsens and his parents take him to an urgent care clinic that evening. While taking an admission history the nurse learned that the child had been taking 1 teaspoon of amoxicillin three times a day. Unfamiliar with the various con-centrations of this suspension drug, the nurse wrote in the medical record that the child had been receiving 250 mg of amoxicillin with each dose. In fact, amoxicillin is supplied in three dosage strengths: 200 mg per mL, 250 mg per mL, and 400 mg per 5 mL. The child was actually taking 1 teaspoon of the 400 mg per 5 mL concentration. The nurse documented an incorrect medication history.

Potential Outcome

The health care provider who examines the child would need an accurate medical history to evalu-ate the prescribed treatment and determine the best course of action for the child's current condi-tion. The incorrect dosage documented by the nurse was almost half the dosage the child was receiving. Based on this erroneous information the provider might come to the wrong conclusion that the child was not provided a therapeutic dosage to treat the infection.

Prevention

The nurse should have questioned the parents further to determine what concentration of amoxi-cillin was prescribed. If they were unsure of the dosage, then the nurse should document this in the record. When the amount of a medication is provided by the number of tablets, capsules, milliliters, or ounces, always verify the dosage strength. Many oral medications are supplied in more than one strength or concentration. Do not make assumptions; refer to a reputable drug reference to verify the available dosage strengths.

Medication errors can be caused by setting up ratio-proportion problems incorrectly. Let's look at an example to identify the nurse's error.

ERROR

Incorrectly using the ratio-proportion method of dosage calculation.

Possible Scenario

Suppose the physician ordered *Keflex 80 mg p.o. q.i.d.* for a child with an upper respiratory infection, and the Keflex is supplied in an oral suspension with 250 mg per 5 mL. The nurse decided to calculate the dosage using the ratio-proportion method and set up the problem this way:

$$\frac{80 \text{ mg}}{5 \text{ mL}} = \frac{250 \text{ mg}}{X \text{ mL}} \quad \textbf{INCORRECT}$$

$$80X = 1,250$$

$$\frac{80X}{80} = \frac{1,250}{80}$$

$$X = 15.6 \text{ mL}$$

The nurse gave the child 15 mL of Keflex for 2 doses. The next day as the nurse prepared the medication in the medication room, another nurse observed the nurse pour 15 mL in a medicine cup and asked about the dosage. At that point, the nurse realized the error.

Potential Outcome

The child would likely have developed complications from overdosage of Keflex, such as renal impairment and liver damage. When the physician was notified of the errors, he would likely have ordered the medication discontinued and the child's blood urea nitrogen (BUN) and liver enzymes monitored. An incident report would be filed and the family would be notified of the error.

Prevention

This type of calculation error occurred because the nurse set up the ratio-proportion problem incorrectly. The dosage on hand and amount on hand were not both set up on the left (or same) side of the proportion. The problem should have been calculated this way:

$$\frac{250 \text{ mg}}{5 \text{ mL}} = \frac{80 \text{ mg}}{X \text{ mL}} \quad \textbf{CORRECT}$$

$$250X = 400$$

$$\frac{250X}{250} = \frac{400}{250}$$

$$X = 1.6 \text{ mL}$$

In addition, had the nurse used Step 2 in the calculation process, the nurse would have realized the dose required was less than 5 mL, not more. In calculating ratio-proportion problems, remember to keep the weight of medication and the amount of the *known* together on the left side of the proportion, and the weight and the amount of the *unknown* together on the right side. In this scenario the patient would have received almost 10 times the amount of medication ordered by the physician each time the nurse committed the error. You know this because there are 250 mg in 5 mL, and the nurse gave 15 mL. You can use ratio-proportion to determine how many mg of Keflex the child received in the scenario.

$$\frac{250 \text{ mg}}{5 \text{ mL}} = \frac{X \text{ mg}}{15 \text{ mL}}$$

$$5X = 3,750$$

$$X = 750 \text{ mg, not 80 mg as ordered}$$

Obviously the nurse did not think through for the logical amount and either miscalculated the dosage three times or did not bother to calculate the dosage again, preventing identification of the error.

PRACTICE PROBLEMS—CHAPTER 10

Calculate 1 dose of the following drug orders. The tablets are scored in half.

1. Order: **tolbutamide 250 mg p.o. b.i.d.**

   Supply: tolbutamide 0.5 g tablets

   Give: _____ tablet(s)

2. Order: **codeine gr $\frac{1}{2}$ p.o. q.4h p.r.n., pain**

   Supply: codeine 15 mg tablets

   Give: _____ tablet(s)

3. Order: **Synthroid 0.075 mg p.o. daily**

   Supply: Synthroid 150 mcg tablets

   Give: _____ tablet(s)

4. Order: **phenobarbital gr $\frac{1}{6}$ p.o. t.i.d.**

   Supply: phenobarbital elixir 20 mg per 5 mL

   Give: _____ mL

5. Order: **Keflex 500 mg p.o. q.i.d.**

   Supply: Keflex 250 mg per 5 mL

   Give: _____ mL

6. Order: **Inderal 20 mg p.o. q.i.d.**

   Supply: Inderal 10 mg tablets

   Give: _____ tablet(s)

7. Order: **Amoxil 400 mg p.o. q.6h**

   Supply: Amoxil 250 mg per 5 mL

   Give: _____ mL

8. Order: **Diabenese 150 mg p.o. b.i.d.**

   Supply: Diabenese 100 mg tablets

   Give: _____ tablet(s)

9. Order: **Aspirin gr v p.o. daily**

   Supply: Aspirin 325 mg tablets

   Give: _____ tablet(s)

10. Order: **codeine gr $\frac{1}{4}$ p.o. daily**

    Supply: codeine 30 mg tablets

    Give: _____ tablet(s)

11. Order: **Inderal 30 mg p.o. q.i.d.**

    Supply: Inderal 20 mg tablets

    Give: _____ tablet(s)

12. Order: **Synthroid 300 mcg p.o. daily**

    Supply: Synthroid 0.3 mg tablets

    Give: _____ tablet(s)

13. Order: **Lasix 60 mg p.o. daily**

    Supply: Lasix 40 mg tablets

    Give: _____ tablet(s)

14. Order: **Tylenol $\bar{c}$ codeine gr $\frac{1}{8}$ p.o. daily**

    Supply: Tylenol with 7.5 mg codeine tablets

    Give: _____ tablet(s)

15. Order: **penicillin G 400,000 units p.o. q.i.d.**

    Supply: penicillin G 200,000 unit tablets

    Give: _____ tablet(s)

16. Order: **Vasotec 7.5 mg p.o. daily**

    Supply: Vasotec 5 mg and 10 mg tablets

    Select: _____ mg tablets

    and give _____ tablet(s)

17. Order: **Penicillin VK 375 mg p.o. q.i.d.**

    Supply: Penicillin VK 250 mg per 5 mL

    Give: _____ mL

18. Order: **Neomycin 1 g p.o. q6h**

    Supply: Neomycin 500 mg tablets

    Give: _____ tablet(s)

19. Order: **Halcion 0.25 mg p.o. bedtime**

    Supply: Halcion 0.125 mg tablets

    Give: _____ tablet(s)

20. Order: **Roxanol 30 mg p.o. q.4h p.r.n., pain**

    Supply: Roxanol 20 mg/mL

    Give: _____ mL

21. Order: **dexamethasone 750 mcg p.o. b.i.d.**

    Supply: dexamethasone 0.75 mg and 1.5 mg tablets

    Select: _____ mg tablets

    Give: _____ tablet(s)

22. Order: **Edecrin 12.5 mg p.o. b.i.d.**

    Supply: Edecrin 25 mg tablets

    Give: _____ tablet(s)

23. Order: **Urecholine 50 mg p.o. t.i.d.**

    Supply: Urecholine 25 mg tablets

    Give: _____ tablet(s)

24. Order: **Erythrocin 0.5 g p.o. q.12h**

    Supply: Erythrocin 250 mg tablets

    Give: _____ tablet(s)

25. Order: **glyburide 2.5 mg p.o. daily**

    Supply: glyburide 1.25 mg tablets

    Give: _____ tablet(s)

26. Order: **Tranxene 7.5 mg p.o. q.AM**

    Supply: Tranxene 3.75 mg capsules

    Give: _____ capsules

27. Order: **phenobarbital gr $\frac{3}{4}$ p.o. daily**

    Supply: phenobarbital 15 mg, 30 mg, and 60 mg scored tablets

    Select: _____ mg tablets

    Give: _____ tablet(s)

28. Order: **acetaminophen 240 mg p.o. q.4h p.r.n., pain or T greater than 102°F**

    Supply: acetaminophen drops 80 mg per 0.8 mL

    Give: _____ mL

29. Order: **acetaminophen 160 mg p.o. q.4h p.r.n., pain or T greater than 102°F**

    Supply: acetaminophen liquid 160 mg/t

    Give: _____ mL

30. Order: **Coumadin 7.5 mg p.o. daily**

    Supply: Coumadin 2.5 mg tablets

    Give: _____ tablet(s)

See the four medication administration records (MARs) and accompanying labels on the following pages for questions 31 through 49.

Calculate 1 dose of each of the drugs prescribed. Labels A–R provided on pages 202–204 are the drugs you have available. Indicate the letter corresponding to the label you select.

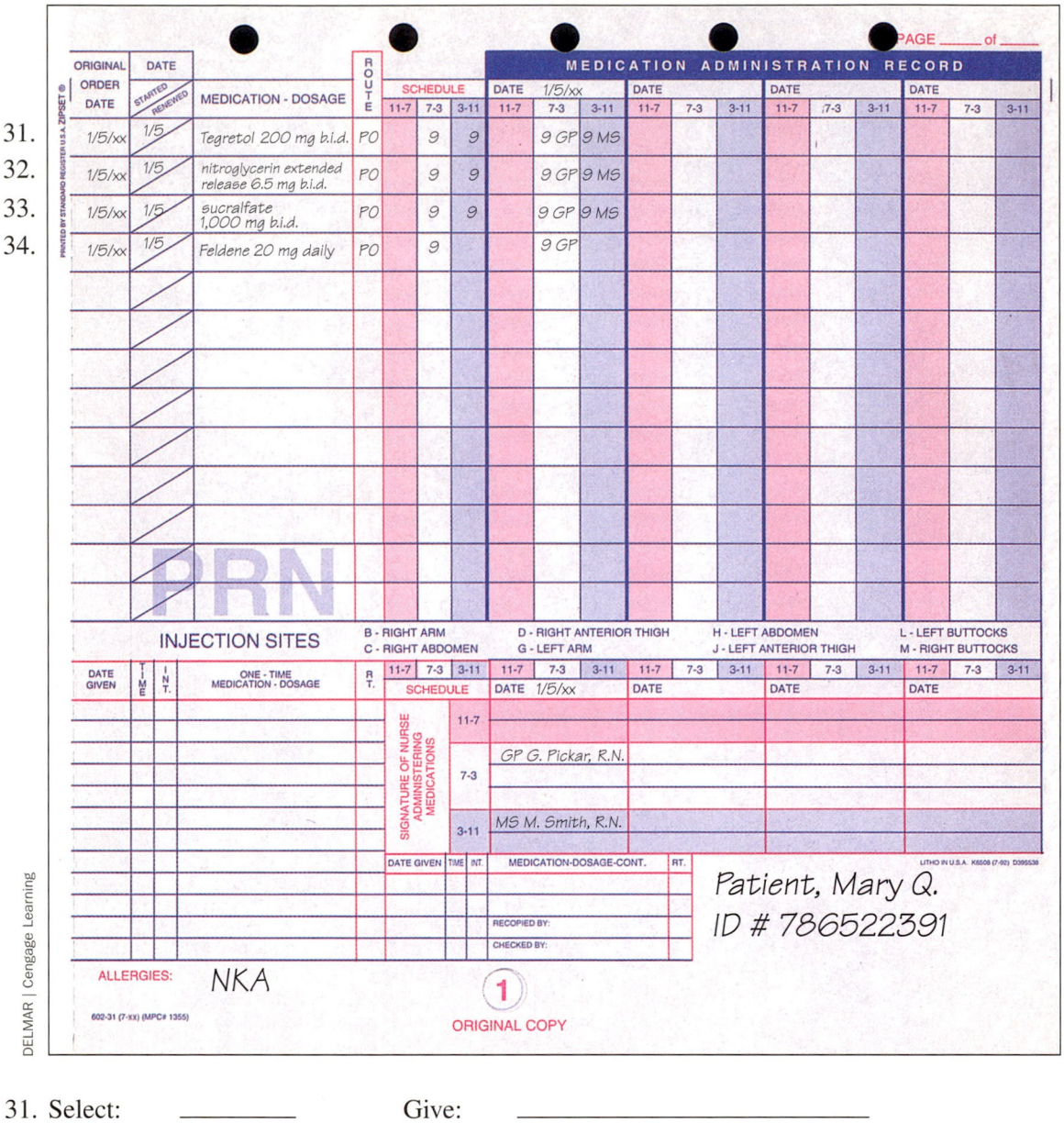

#	ORIGINAL ORDER DATE	DATE STARTED / RENEWED	MEDICATION - DOSAGE	ROUTE	SCHEDULE 11-7	SCHEDULE 7-3	SCHEDULE 3-11	1/5/xx 11-7	1/5/xx 7-3	1/5/xx 3-11
31.	1/5/xx	1/5	Tegretol 200 mg b.i.d.	PO		9	9		9 GP	9 MS
32.	1/5/xx	1/5	nitroglycerin extended release 6.5 mg b.i.d.	PO		9	9		9 GP	9 MS
33.	1/5/xx	1/5	sucralfate 1,000 mg b.i.d.	PO		9	9		9 GP	9 MS
34.	1/5/xx	1/5	Feldene 20 mg daily	PO		9			9 GP	

MEDICATION ADMINISTRATION RECORD

PRN

INJECTION SITES
B - RIGHT ARM   D - RIGHT ANTERIOR THIGH   H - LEFT ABDOMEN   L - LEFT BUTTOCKS
C - RIGHT ABDOMEN   G - LEFT ARM   J - LEFT ANTERIOR THIGH   M - RIGHT BUTTOCKS

SIGNATURE OF NURSE ADMINISTERING MEDICATIONS
11-7
7-3   GP G. Pickar, R.N.
3-11   MS M. Smith, R.N.

Patient, Mary Q.
ID # 786522391

ALLERGIES: NKA

⓵ ORIGINAL COPY

DELMAR | Cengage Learning

31. Select: _____   Give: _____
32. Select: _____   Give: _____
33. Select: _____   Give: _____
34. Select: _____   Give: _____

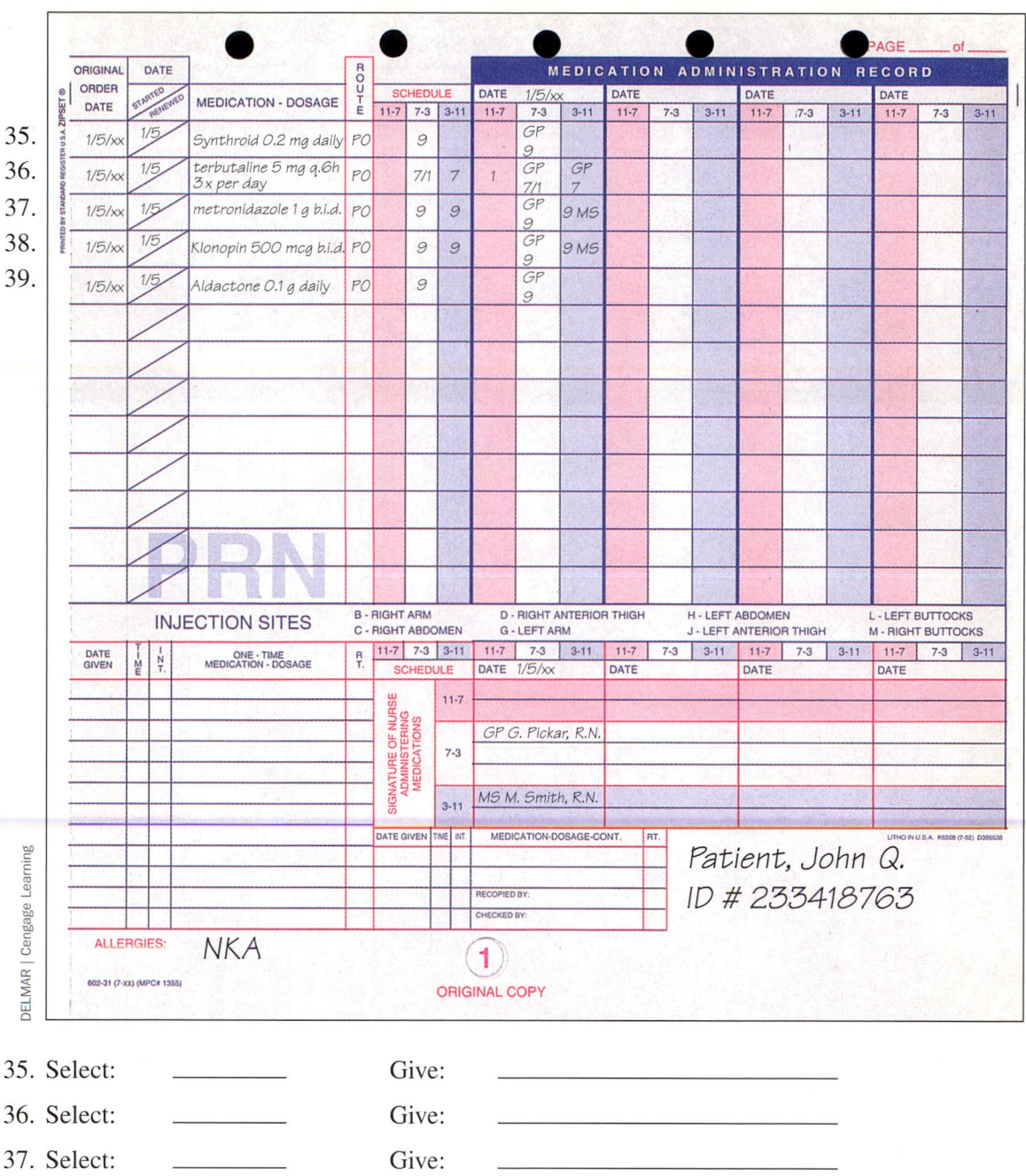

	ORIGINAL ORDER DATE	DATE STARTED RENEWED	MEDICATION - DOSAGE	ROUTE	SCHEDULE 11-7	7-3	3-11	DATE 1/5/xx 11-7	7-3	3-11	DATE 11-7	7-3	3-11	DATE 11-7	7-3	3-11	DATE 11-7	7-3	3-11
35.	1/5/xx	1/5	Synthroid 0.2 mg daily	PO		9		GP 9											
36.	1/5/xx	1/5	terbutaline 5 mg q.6h 3 x per day	PO	7/1	7	1	GP 7/1	GP 7										
37.	1/5/xx	1/5	metronidazole 1 g b.i.d.	PO		9	9	GP 9	9 MS										
38.	1/5/xx	1/5	Klonopin 500 mcg b.i.d.	PO		9	9	GP 9	9 MS										
39.	1/5/xx	1/5	Aldactone 0.1 g daily	PO		9		GP 9											

PRN

MEDICATION ADMINISTRATION RECORD

INJECTION SITES

B - RIGHT ARM	D - RIGHT ANTERIOR THIGH	H - LEFT ABDOMEN	L - LEFT BUTTOCKS
C - RIGHT ABDOMEN	G - LEFT ARM	J - LEFT ANTERIOR THIGH	M - RIGHT BUTTOCKS

SIGNATURE OF NURSE ADMINISTERING MEDICATIONS

11-7	
7-3	GP G. Pickar, R.N.
3-11	MS M. Smith, R.N.

RECOPIED BY:
CHECKED BY:

Patient, John Q.
ID # 233418763

ALLERGIES: NKA

(1) ORIGINAL COPY

602-31 (7-XX) (MPC# 1355)

LITHO IN U.S.A. K6508 (7-92) D395538

DELMAR | Cengage Learning

35. Select: _____   Give: _____

36. Select: _____   Give: _____

37. Select: _____   Give: _____

38. Select: _____   Give: _____

39. Select: _____   Give: _____

PHARMACY MAR

	START	STOP	MEDICATION				SCHEDULED TIMES	OK'D BY	0701 TO 1500	1501 TO 2300	2301 TO 0700
40.	01/05/xx 0800		DIGOXIN 0.5 MG 250 MCG TABS DAILY 2 TABS			TAB PO	1700				
41.	01/05/xx 0800		POTASSIUM CHLORIDE 40 MEQ 20 MEQ PER BID 15 ML-30 ML			PO	0900 2100				
42.	01/05/xx 0800		LOPID 0.6 G 600 MG TABS BID - AC 1 TAB			TAB PO	0730 1630				
43.	01/05/xx 0800		LEVOTHYROXINE 200 MCG 100 MCG TABS DAILY 2 TABS			TAB PO	0900				
44.	01/05/xx 0800		LOPRESSOR 100 MG 50 MG TABS BID 2 TABS			TAB PO	0900 2100				
			▢		▢						
			▢		▢						
			▢		▢						
45.	01/05/xx 0800 PRN		PERCOCET 5 MG 5MG/325MG Q4H TABS - 1 TAB PRN HEADACHE			TAB PO					

Gluteus **Thigh** A. Right H. Right B. Left I. Left **Ventro Gluteal** C. Right J. Right D. Left K. Left E. Abdomen 1 | 2 3 | 4 Page 1 of 2 DAILY	**STANDARD TIMES** DAILY = 0900 BID = Q12H = 0900 & 2100 TID = 0800, 1400, 2200 Q8H = 0800, 1600, 2400 QID = 0800, 1200, 1800, 2200 Q6H = 0600, 1200, 1800, 2400 Q4H = 0400, 0800, 1200... DAILY DIGOXIN = 1700 DAILY WARFARIN = 1600

NURSE'S SIGNATURE INITIAL	
0701- 1500 _____	
1501- 2300 _____	
2301- 0700 _____	
OK'd by _____	

ALLERGIES:
NO KNOWN DRUG ALLERGIES

FROM: 01/05/xx 0701

Patient: DOE, JANE Q.
Patient #   244317789

Physician: J. PHYSICIAN, MD
Room: 407-2 SOUTH
TO: 01/06/xx 0700

40. Select: _____   Give: _____

41. Select: _____   Give: _____

42. Select: _____   Give: _____

43. Select: _____   Give: _____

44. Select: _____   Give: _____

45. Select: _____   Give: _____

PHARMACY MAR

	START	STOP	MEDICATION	SCHEDULED TIMES	OK'D BY	0701 TO 1500	1501 TO 2300	2301 TO 0700
46.	01/05/xx 0800		RANITIDINE 300 MG TAB / 150 MG TABS BEDTIME PO / 2 TABS	2200				
47.	01/05/xx 0800		INDERAL 60 MG CAP / 60 MG CAPS BID PO / 1 CAP	0900 2100				
48.	01/05/xx 0800		LASIX 20 MG TAB / 20 MG TABS BID PO / 1 TAB	0900 2100				
49.	01/05/xx 0800		POTASSIUM CHLORIDE 20 MEQ TAB / 10 MEQ TABS DAILY PO / 2 TABS	0900				

Gluteus	Thigh	STANDARD TIMES	NURSE'S SIGNATURE INITIAL		
A. Right	H. Right	DAILY = 0900	0701-1500 _____	ALLERGIES: NO KNOWN DRUG ALLERGIES	Patient: S., SARAH
B. Left	I. Left	BID = Q12H = 0900 & 2100	1501-2300 _____		Patient # 266734964
Ventro Gluteal		TID = 0800, 1400, 2200			
C. Right	J. Right	Q8H = 0800, 1600, 2400	2301-0700 _____		Physician: J. PHYSICIAN, MD
D. Left	K. Left	QID = 0800, 1200, 1800, 2200			Room: 407-3 SOUTH
E. Abdomen	1 / 2 — 3 / 4	Q6H = 0600, 1200, 1800, 2400 Q4H = 0400, 0800, 1200... DAILY DIGOXIN = 1700	OK'd by _____		
Page 1 of 2	DAILY	DAILY WARFARIN = 1600		FROM: 01/05/xx 0701	TO: 01/06/xx 0700

DELMAR | Cengage Learning

46. Select: _____ Give: _____

47. Select: _____ Give: _____

48. Select: _____ Give: _____

49. Select: _____ Give: _____

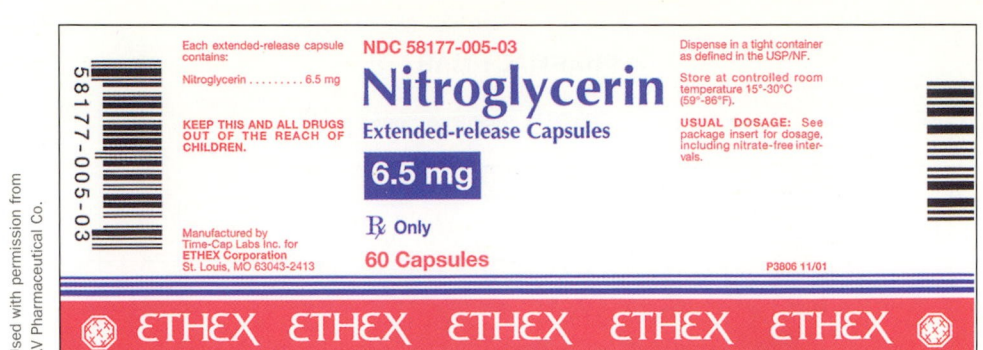

Used with permission from KV Pharmaceutical Co.

Each extended-release capsule contains:

Nitroglycerin . . . . 6.5 mg

KEEP THIS AND ALL DRUGS OUT OF THE REACH OF CHILDREN.

Manufactured by Time-Cap Labs Inc. for ETHEX Corporation St. Louis, MO 63043-2413

NDC 58177-005-03

Nitroglycerin

Extended-release Capsules

6.5 mg

℞ Only

60 Capsules

Dispense in a tight container as defined in the USP/NF.

Store at controlled room temperature 15°-30°C (59°-86°F).

USUAL DOSAGE: See package insert for dosage, including nitrate-free intervals.

P3806 11/01

ETHEX ETHEX ETHEX ETHEX ETHEX

A

Used with permission from Pfizer Inc.

Store below 86°F (30°C)

Dispense in tight, light-resistant containers (USP).

DOSAGE AND USE
See accompanying prescribing information. One capsule per day.

Each capsule contains 20 mg piroxicam.

IMPORTANT: This closure is not child-resistant.

CAUTION: Federal law prohibits dispensing without prescription.

100 Capsules NDC 0069-3230-66

Feldene®
(piroxicam) 20

20 mg

Pfizer Pfizer Labs
Division of Pfizer Inc, NY, NY 10017

6505-01-137-4628

3 0069-3230-66 2

05-4300-00-5
MADE IN USA

1292

B

Used with permission from Aventis Pharmaceuticals.

NDC 0088-1712-53

Carafate®
Tablets
sucralfate

1 gram

120 Tablets

❦ *Aventis*

℞ ONLY

Each CARAFATE® Tablet contains 1g sucralfate.

Dosage and Administration: See package insert for dosage information.

WARNING: Keep out of reach of children.

Pharmacist: Dispense in light-resistant, tight container with child-resistant closure.

Important: This package is not child-resistant.

Store at controlled room temperature 59–86°F (15–30°C).

Aventis Pharmaceuticals Inc. Kansas City, MO 64137 USA ©2000 www.aventispharma-us.com

3 0088-1712-53 6

Exp 50059224

C

© Novartis. Used by permission.

NDC 0083-0052-30

Tegretol® 100 mg
carbamazepine USP

Chewable Tablets

100 tablets

Rx only

Ⓝ NOVARTIS

EXP.
LOT

0083-0052-30 0

©Novartis

5000098
Dosage: See package insert. **Do not store above 30°C (86°F). Protect from light and moisture. Dispense in tight, light-resistant container (USP).**

Keep this and all drugs out of the reach of children.

Novartis Pharmaceuticals Corporation East Hanover, New Jersey 07936

D

Used with permission from Pharmaceutical Associates, Inc.

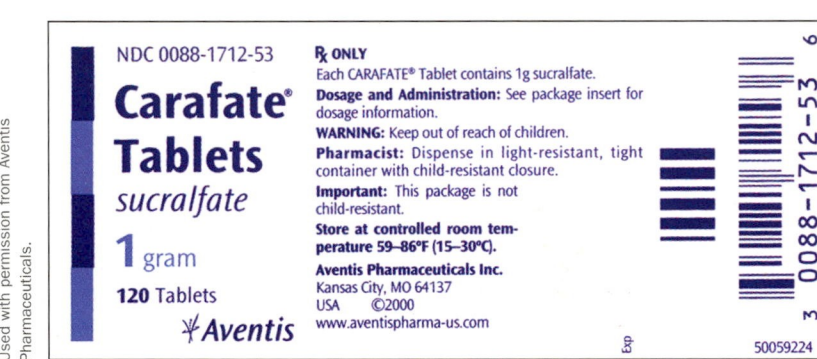

Delivers **15 mL**
NDC 0121-1465-15
POTASSIUM CHLORIDE ORAL SOLUTION USP 10%
20 mEq per 15 mL
Sugar Free   Alcohol 5%
DILUTE BEFORE USING

(01) 0 03 01211 46515 3

Rx ONLY
FOR INSTITUTIONAL USE ONLY
PHARMACEUTICAL ASSOCIATES, INC.
GREENVILLE, SC 29605
SEE INSERT

E

Used with permission from Pfizer Inc.

Store below 25°C (77°F).

Protect from light.

Dispense in tight, light-resistant, child-resistant containers (USP).

DOSAGE AND USE:
See accompanying prescribing information.

Each tablet contains 500 mg metronidazole.

NDC 0025-1821-50

50 Tablets   **Rx only**

Flagyl®
metronidazole tablets USP (500)

500 mg

Distributed by
Pfizer G.D. Searle LLC
Division of Pfizer Inc, NY, NY 10017

FPO (80% x 11.5mm)

0025-1821-50 9

2281

LOT
EXP

05-6605-32-0

F

USUAL DOSAGE:
See package insert for prescribing information.

Dispense in a tight, light-resistant container as defined in the USP with a child-resistant closure.

Store at 20°-25°C (68°-77°F) [See USP Controlled Room Temperature]. Excursion permitted 15°-30°C (59°-86°F)

Rev. 03/05

NDC 0527-1318-01

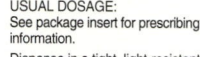

TERBUTALINE SULFATE TABLETS, USP

2.5 mg

Rx Only

100 TABLETS

Each tablet contains:
Terbutaline, USP ...... 2.5 mg

Inactive Ingredients:
Anhydrous lactose, magnesium stearate, microcrystalline cellulose, povidone, and pregelatinized starch.

Manufactured by:
Lannett Company, Inc.
Philadelphia, PA 19136

Exp. Date:

Lot No.:

G

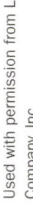

N 3 0527-1318-01 5

NDC 0004-0068-01   27899225

Klonopin®
(clonazepam)

0.5 mg

Each tablet contains 0.5 mg clonazepam.

100 tablets

Bulk Package - Not intended for dispensing.
Dispense in tight, light-resistant containers as defined in USP/NF.
Store at 59°-86°F (15°-30°C).

0004-0068-01

C IV

R only

Roche

Usual dosage: See package insert.
Made in Switzerland
Distributed by:
Roche Laboratories Inc.
Nutley, New Jersey 07110

EXP.   LOT

H

NDC 0048-1070-03
NSN 6505-01-340-0152
Code 3P1073

SYNTHROID®
(Levothyroxine Sodium Tablets, USP)

100 mcg   (0.1 mg)

100 TABLETS

Rx only

BASF Pharma   knoll

See full prescribing information for dosage and administration.

Dispense in a tight, light-resistant container as described in USP.

Store at 25°C (77°F); excursions permitted to 15°-30°C (59°-86°F). [See USP Controlled Room Temperature].

Knoll Pharmaceutical Company
Mount Olive, NJ 07828 USA

7885-04

3 0048-1070-03 6

I

NDC 0039-0067-50

Lasix®   20 mg
furosemide

500 Tablets   ✦ **Aventis**

R ONLY
Each LASIX® Tablet contains 20mg furosemide. **Dosage and Administration:** See package insert for dosage information. **WARNING:** Keep out of reach of children. Do not use if bottle closure seal is broken. **Pharmacist:** Dispense in well-closed, light-resistant container with child-resistant closure. **Store at room temperature.**
Hoechst-Roussel Pharmaceuticals
Division of **Aventis Pharmaceuticals Inc.**
Kansas City, MO 64137 USA   ©2000
www.aventispharma-us.com

3 0039-0067-50 9

50058803   50058803   50058803

J

Each tablet contains 600 mg gemfibrozil.
Usual Adult Dosage–
See package insert for full prescribing information.
Keep this and all drugs out of the reach of children.
Dispense in tight container as defined in the USP.
Store at controlled room temperature 20°- 25°C (68°- 77°F) [see USP]. Protect from light and humidity.
Important–This package for pharmacy stock use.
Manufactured by:
Parke Davis Pharmaceuticals, Ltd.
Vega Baja, PR 00694
Distributed by:
PARKE-DAVIS
Div of Warner-Lambert Co
Morris Plains, NJ 07950 USA
© 1997-'99, PDPL

N 0071-0737-30

Lopid®
(Gemfibrozil Tablets, USP)

600 mg
R only

500 TABLETS

℗ **PARKE-DAVIS**

6505-01-300-7956

3 0071-0737-30 3

05-5894-32-0

Exp date and lot

K

NDC 00000-0000-00

1000 TABLETS

DIGOXIN Tablets

Each scored tablet contains
250 mcg (0.25 mg)
of digoxin

Store at 25°C (77°F) in a dry place (see insert)

Rx only

0000-0000-00

DCL   **DELMAR | Cengage Learning**
For Educational Purposes Only

Lot.
Exp. Date

L

Store below 25°C (77°F).
Protect from light.

Dispense in tight, light-resistant, child-resistant containers (USP).

DOSAGE AND USE:
See accompanying prescribing information.

Each tablet contains 50 mg spironolactone.

100 Tablets   NDC 0025-1041-31
                     Rx only

Aldactone®
spironolactone tablets, USP   50

50 mg

Distributed by
Pfizer   **G.D. Searle LLC**
Division of Pfizer Inc, NY, NY 10017

2139

FPO: UPC @ 80%

3 0025-1041-31 0

05-6587-32-1

M

© Novartis. Used by permission.

NDC 0028-0051-10
6505-01-071-6557

Lopressor® 50 mg

metoprolol tartrate USP

1000 tablets

Rx only

Dosage: See package insert.
Store between 15°C - 30°C (59°F - 86°F).
Protect from moisture.
Dispense in tight, light-resistant container (USP).

Novartis Pharmaceuticals Corporation
East Hanover, New Jersey 07936

PHARMACIST: Container closure is not child-resistant.
Keep this and all drugs out of the reach of children.

EXP
LOT

645122

Ⓝ 3 0028-0051-10 6

N

Used with permission from Endo Pharmaceuticals Inc.

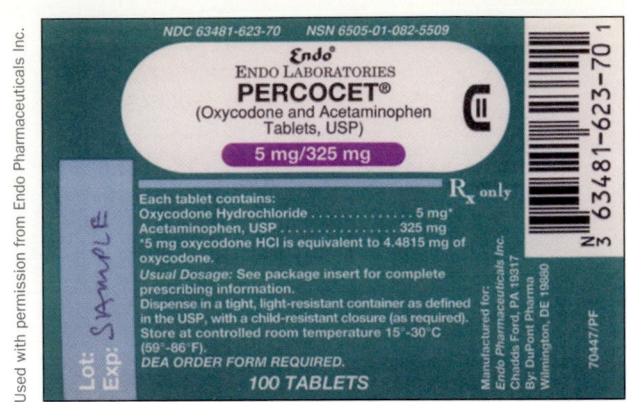

O

Used with permission from Akrimax Pharmaceuticals, LLC

NDC 24090-470-88   100 Capsules

Inderal® LA
(propranolol hydrochloride)
Long-Acting Capsules

60 mg

SEALED FOR YOUR PROTECTION

℞ only

AKRIMAX PHARMACEUTICALS

Store at 20° to 25°C (68° to 77°F); excursions permitted to 15° to 30°C (59° to 86°F). [See USP Controlled Room Temperature.] Protect from light, moisture, freezing, and excessive heat. Dispense in a tight, light-resistant container as defined in the USP.

Ⓝ 3 24090-470-88 9

P

Used with permission from Teva Pharmaceuticals USA

NDC 0172-4357-49

RANITIDINE
Tablets USP

150 mg*

★Each tablet contains:
ranitidine hydrochloride, USP
equivalent to 150 mg ranitidine

60 TABLETS

TEVA

℞ only Usual Adult Dosage: See package insert for full prescribing information.
Store at 20° to 25°C (68° to 77°F) [See USP Controlled Room Temperature], in a dry place.
PROTECT FROM LIGHT
Replace cap securely after each opening.
Dispense in a tight, light-resistant container as defined in the USP, with a child-resistant closure (as required).
KEEP THIS AND ALL MEDICATIONS OUT OF THE REACH OF CHILDREN.

Manufactured By:
IVAX PHARMACEUTICALS, INC.
Miami, FL 33137
Manufactured For:
TEVA PHARMACEUTICALS USA
Sellersville, PA 18960

Iss. 10/2006

LOT: EXP:

Ⓝ 3 0172-4357-49 5

Q

DELMAR | Cengage Learning

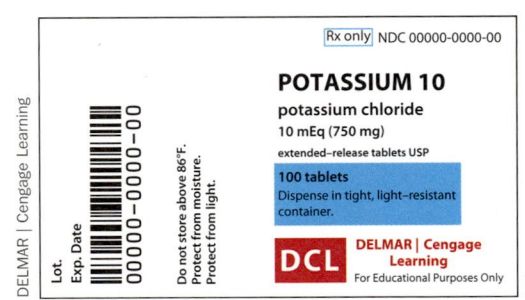

R

50. Describe the strategy to prevent this medication error.

Possible Scenario

Suppose the physician ordered **Penicillin VK 5 mL (250 mg) p.o. q.i.d.** for a patient with an upper respiratory tract infection. The pharmacy supplied Penicillin VK 125 mg per 5 mL. In a rush to administer the medication on time, the nurse read the order as *Penicillin VK 5 mL,* checked the label for Penicillin VK and poured that amount and administered the drug. In a hurry, the nurse failed to recognize that 5 mL of the supply dosage of 125 mg per 5 mL did not provide the ordered dosage of 250 mg and underdosed the patient.

Potential Outcome

The patient received one-half of the ordered dosage of antibiotic needed to treat the respiratory infection. If this error was not caught, the patient's infection would not be halted. This would add to the patient's illness time and might lead to a more severe infection. Additional tests might be required to determine why the patient was not responding to the medication.

Prevention

_____

_____

After completing these problems, see pages 521–522 to check your answers.

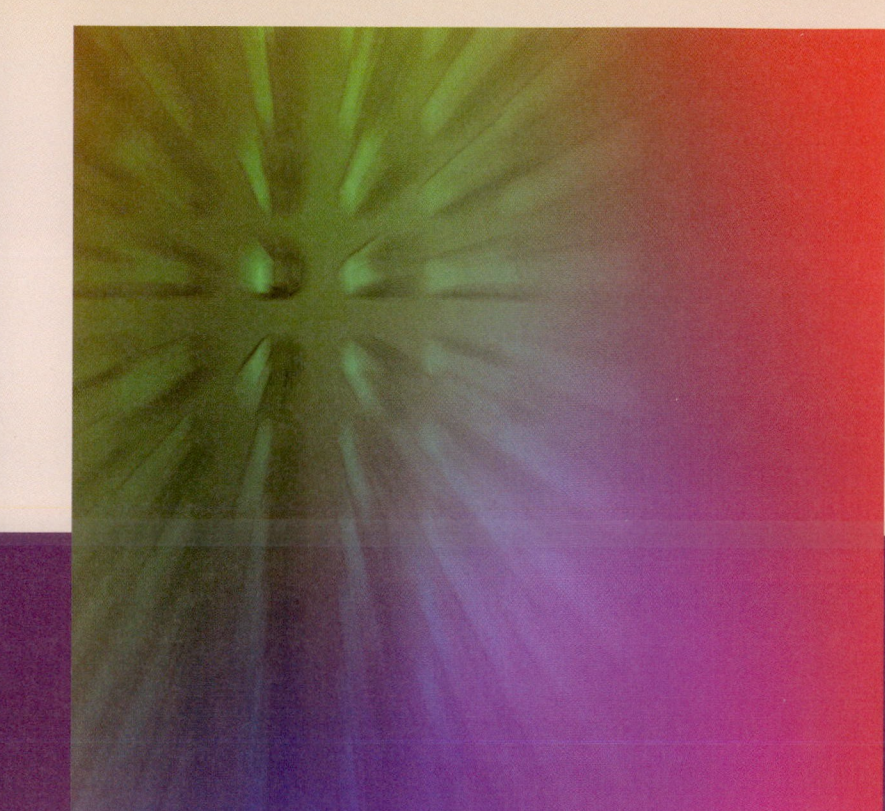

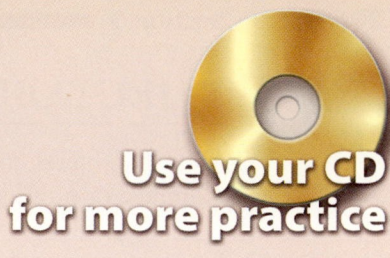
Use your CD
for more practice

11

Parenteral Dosage of Drugs

OBJECTIVES

Upon mastery of Chapter 11, you will be able to calculate the parenteral dosages of drugs. To accomplish this you will also be able to:

- Apply the three steps for dosage calculations: convert, think, and calculate.
- Use ratio-proportion to calculate the amount to give.
- Measure insulin in a matching insulin syringe.
- Compare the calibration of U-100 insulin syringe units to milliliters (100 units/mL).

The term *parenteral* is used to designate routes of administration other than gastrointestinal, such as the injection routes of IM, subcut, ID, and IV. In this chapter, intramuscular (IM), subcutaneous (subcut), and intravenous (IV) injections will be emphasized. Intravenous flow-rate calculations are discussed in Chapters 15–17.

Intramuscular indicates an injection given into a muscle, such as promethazine given IM for nausea and vomiting. *Subcutaneous* means an injection given into the subcutaneous tissue, such as an insulin injection for the management of diabetes given subcut. *Intravenous* refers to an injection given directly into a vein, either by direct injection (IV push) or diluted in a larger volume of intravenous fluid and administered as part of an intravenous infusion. When a patient has an IV site or IV infusing, the IV injection route is frequently used to administer parenteral drugs rather than the IM route. *Intradermal* (ID) means an injection given under the skin, such as an allergy test or tuberculin skin test.

INJECTABLE SOLUTIONS

Most parenteral medications are prepared in liquid or solution form and packaged in dosage vials, ampules, or prefilled syringes (Figure 11-1). Injectable drugs are measured in syringes.

FIGURE 11-1   Parenteral solutions

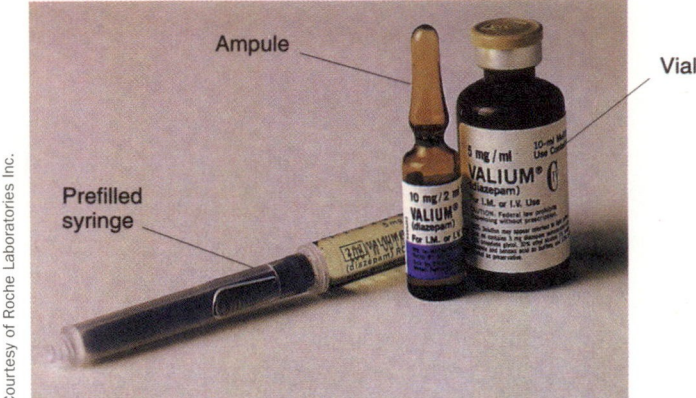

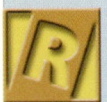

RULE

The maximum dosage volume to be administered per intramuscular injection site for:

1. An average 150 lb adult = 3 mL (maximum for deltoid site is 2 mL)

2. Children age 6 to 12 years = 2 mL

3. Children birth to age 5 years = 1 mL

For example, if you must give an adult patient 4 mL of a drug, divide the dose into two injections of 2 mL each. The condition of the patient must be considered when applying this rule. Adults or children who have decreased muscle or subcutaneous tissue mass or poor circulation may not be able to tolerate the maximum dosage volumes.

To solve parenteral dosage problems, apply the same steps used for the calculation of oral dosages.

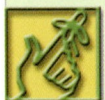

REMEMBER

Step 1	**Convert**	Ensure that all units of measurement are in the same system and all units are the same size.
Step 2	**Think**	Estimate the logical amount.
Step 3	**Calculate**	$\dfrac{\text{Dosage on hand}}{\text{Amount on hand}} = \dfrac{\text{Dosage desired}}{\text{X Amount desired}}$

Use the following rules to help you decide which size syringe to select to administer parenteral dosages.

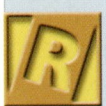

RULE

As you calculate parenteral dosages:

1. Round the amount to be administered (X) to tenths if the amount is greater than 1 mL, and measure it in a 3 mL syringe.

2. Measure amounts of less than 1 mL rounded to hundredths and all amounts less than 0.5 mL in a 1 mL syringe.

3. Amounts of 0.5 to 1 mL, calculated in tenths, can be accurately measured in either a 1 mL or 3 mL syringe.

Let's look at some examples of appropriate syringe selections for the dosages to be measured and review how to read the calibrations. Refer to Chapter 6, *Equipment Used in Dosage Measurement,* regarding how to measure medication in a syringe. To review, the top black ring should align with the desired calibration, not the raised midsection and not the bottom ring. Look carefully at the illustrations that follow.

EXAMPLE 1 ■

Measure 0.33 mL in a 1 mL syringe.

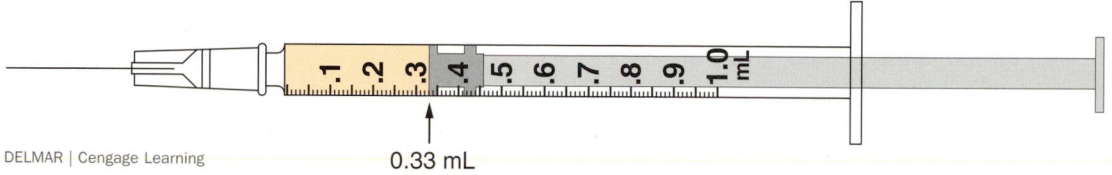

DELMAR | Cengage Learning   0.33 mL

EXAMPLE 2 ■

Round 1.33 mL to 1.3 mL, and measure in a 3 mL syringe.

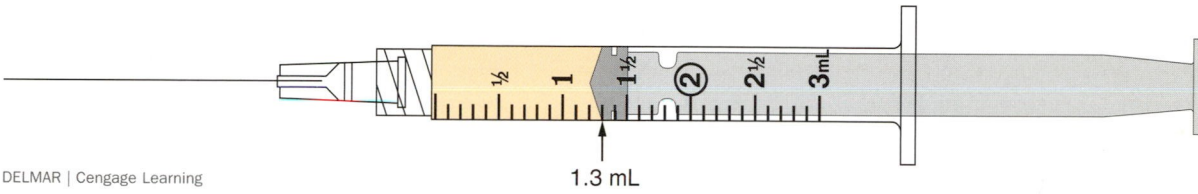

DELMAR | Cengage Learning   1.3 mL

EXAMPLE 3 ■

Measure 0.6 mL in either a 1 mL or 3 mL syringe. (Notice that the amount is measured in tenths and is greater than 0.5 mL, so the 3 mL syringe would be acceptable.)

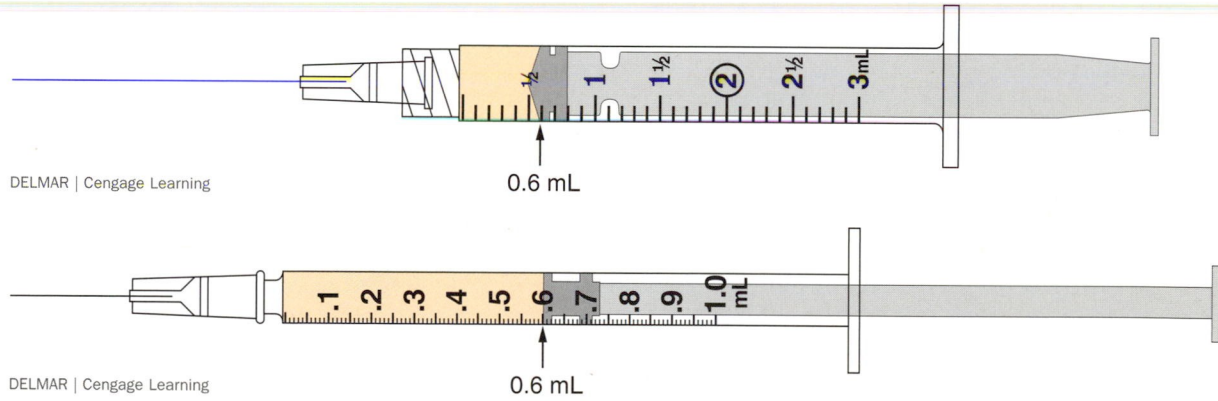

DELMAR | Cengage Learning   0.6 mL

DELMAR | Cengage Learning   0.6 mL

EXAMPLE 4 ■

Measure 0.65 mL in a 1 mL syringe. (Notice that the amount is measured in hundredths and is less than 1 mL.)

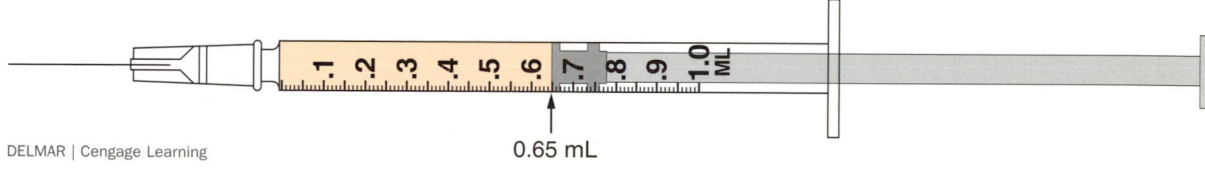

DELMAR | Cengage Learning   0.65 mL

An amber color has been added to selected syringe drawings throughout the text to *simulate a specific amount of medication,* as indicated in the example or problem. Because the color used may not correspond to the actual color of the medications named, **it must not be used as a reference for identifying medications.**

Let's look at some examples of parenteral dosage calculations.

EXAMPLE 1 ■

The drug order reads Vistaril 100 mg IM stat.

Available is Vistaril intramuscular solution 50 mg/mL in a 10 mL multiple-dose vial. How many milliliters should be administered to the patient?

FOR INTRAMUSCULAR USE ONLY.
USUAL ADULT DOSE: Intramuscularly: 25 - 100 mg stat; repeat every 4 to 6 hours, as needed.
See accompanying prescribing information.
Each mL contains 50 mg of hydroxyzine hydrochloride, 0.9% benzyl alcohol and sodium hydroxide to adjust to optimum pH.
To avoid discoloration, protect from prolonged exposure to light.
Rx only

10 mL NDC 0049-5460-74
Vistaril®
(hydroxyzine hydrochloride)
Intramuscular Solution
50 mg/mL
Pfizer **Roerig**
Division of Pfizer Inc, NY, NY 10017
05-1111-32-4
MADE IN USA

Store below 86°F (30°C).
PROTECT FROM FREEZING.
PATIENT: _____
ROOM NO.: _____
9249

Used with permission from Pfizer Inc.

Step 1	**Convert**	No conversion is necessary.
Step 2	**Think**	You want to give more than 1 mL. In fact, you want to give twice as much because 100 mg is twice as much as 50 mg.

Step 3   **Calculate**

$$\frac{\text{Dosage on hand}}{\text{Amount on hand}} = \frac{\text{Dosage desired}}{\text{X Amount desired}}$$

$$\frac{50 \text{ mg}}{1 \text{ mL}} \times \frac{100 \text{ mg}}{\text{X mL}} \qquad \text{Cross-multiply}$$

$$50\text{X} = 100$$

$$\frac{50\text{X}}{50} = \frac{100}{50} \qquad \text{Simplify: Divide both sides of the equation by the number before the unknown X}$$

$$\text{X} = 2 \text{ mL} \qquad \text{Label the units to match the unknown X}$$

2 mL given intramuscularly immediately

Select a 3 mL syringe and measure 2 mL of Vistaril 50 mg/mL. Look carefully at the illustration to clearly identify the part of the black rubber stopper that measures the exact dosage.

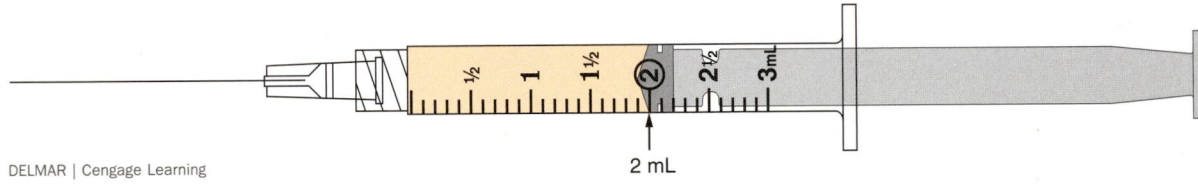

DELMAR | Cengage Learning

2 mL

EXAMPLE 2 ■

The drug order reads Nubain 5 mg subcut q.4h p.r.n., pain.

The 10 mL multiple dose vial is labeled Nubain 20 mg/mL injection.

NDC 63481-509-05
NUBAIN®
(Nalbuphine HCl) Rx only
20 mg/mL injection
10 mL Multiple Dose Vial
Each mL contains: 20 mg nalbuphine HCl, 0.94% sodium citrate hydrous, 1.26% citric acid anhydrous, and 0.2% of a 9:1 mixture of methyl and propylparaben, as preservatives. pH is adjusted, if necessary, to 3.5 to 3.7 with hydrochloric acid.
FOR IM, SC OR IV USE
Usual Dosage: See package insert for complete prescribing information.
Store at 25°C (77°F); excursions permitted to 15°-30°C (59°-86°F).
PROTECT FROM EXCESSIVE LIGHT.
Manufactured for:
Endo Pharmaceuticals Inc.
Chadds Ford, PA 19317
70361/OK
Lot: _____
Exp: _____

Used with permission from Endo Pharmaceuticals Inc.

Step 1	**Convert**	No conversion necessary.
Step 2	**Think**	You want to give less than 1 mL. Actually you want to give $\frac{1}{4}$ or 0.25 of a mL.

Step 3   **Calculate**

$$\frac{\text{Dosage on hand}}{\text{Amount on hand}} = \frac{\text{Dosage desired}}{\text{X Amount desired}}$$

$$\frac{20 \text{ mg}}{1 \text{ mL}} \times \frac{5 \text{ mg}}{\text{X mL}} \qquad \text{Cross-multiply}$$

$$20\text{X} = 5$$

$$\frac{20\text{X}}{20} = \frac{5}{20} \qquad \text{Simplify: Divide both sides of the equation by the number before the unknown X}$$

$$\text{X} = 0.25 \text{ mL} \qquad \text{Label the units to match the unknown X}$$

0.25 mL given subcutaneously as needed for pain every 4 hours

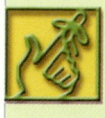

REMEMBER

Dosages measured in hundredths (such as 0.25 mL) and all amounts less than 0.5 mL should be prepared in a 1 mL syringe, which is calibrated in hundredths. However, if the route is IM, you may need to change needles to a more appropriate length.

Select a 1 mL syringe and measure 0.25 mL of Nubain 20 mg/mL. Look carefully at the illustration to clearly identify the part of the black rubber stopper that measures the exact dosage.

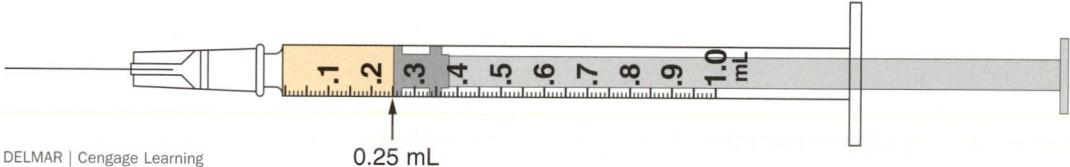

DELMAR | Cengage Learning

0.25 mL

EXAMPLE 3 ■

Drug order: ketorolac tromethamine
    12 mg IV q.6h p.r.n., pain

Supply: ketorolac tromethamine injection
    15 mg/mL

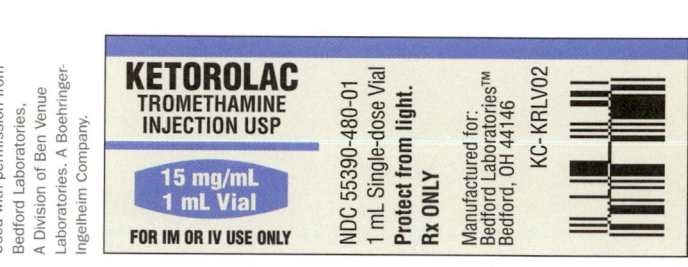

Used with permission from Bedford Laboratories, A Division of Ben Venue Laboratories. A Boehringer Ingelheim Company.

KETOROLAC
TROMETHAMINE
INJECTION USP

15 mg/mL
1 mL Vial

FOR IM OR IV USE ONLY

NDC 55390-480-01
1 mL Single-dose Vial
Protect from light.
Rx ONLY

Manufactured for:
Bedford Laboratories™
Bedford, OH 44146

KC-KRLV02

Step 1	Convert	No conversion is necessary.
Step 2	Think	You want to give less than 1 mL but more than 0.5 mL.
Step 3	Calculate	$\dfrac{\text{Dosage on hand}}{\text{Amount on hand}} = \dfrac{\text{Dosage desired}}{\text{X Amount desired}}$

$$\frac{15\ mg}{1\ mL} \diagtimes \frac{12\ mg}{X\ mL} \qquad \text{Cross-multiply}$$

$$15X = 12$$

$$\frac{15X}{15} = \frac{12}{15} \qquad \text{Simplify: Divide both sides of the equation by the number before the unknown X}$$

$$X = 0.8\ mL \qquad \text{Label the units to match the unknown X}$$

0.8 mL given intramuscularly every 6 hours as needed for pain

Select a 1 mL or 3 mL syringe and draw up all of the contents of the 1 mL single-dose vial. Then discard 0.2 mL to administer 0.8 mL of ketorolac 15 mg/mL.

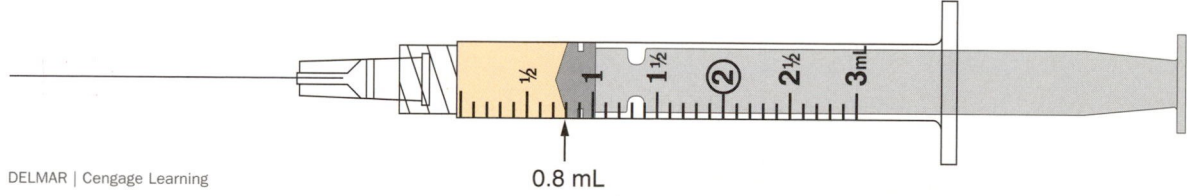

DELMAR | Cengage Learning

0.8 mL

EXAMPLE 4 ■

Order: heparin 8,000 units subcut b.i.d.

Supply: A vial of heparin sodium injection
    10,000 units/mL

| Step 1 | Convert | No conversion is necessary. |
| Step 2 | Think | You want to give less than 1 mL but more than 0.5 mL. |

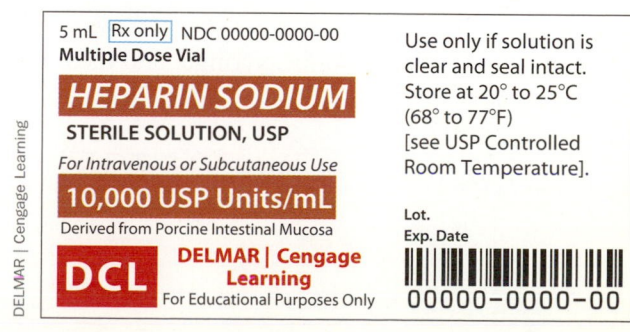

5 mL Rx only NDC 00000-0000-00
Multiple Dose Vial

HEPARIN SODIUM
STERILE SOLUTION, USP
For Intravenous or Subcutaneous Use

10,000 USP Units/mL
Derived from Porcine Intestinal Mucosa

DCL **DELMAR | Cengage Learning**
For Educational Purposes Only

Use only if solution is clear and seal intact.
Store at 20° to 25°C (68° to 77°F)
[see USP Controlled Room Temperature].

Lot.
Exp. Date

00000-0000-00

DELMAR | Cengage Learning

Step 3 **Calculate**

$$\frac{\text{Dosage on hand}}{\text{Amount on hand}} = \frac{\text{Dosage desired}}{\text{X Amount desired}}$$

$$\frac{10{,}000 \text{ units}}{1 \text{ mL}} \diagdown\diagup \frac{8{,}000 \text{ units}}{\text{X mL}} \qquad \text{Cross-multiply}$$

$$10{,}000\text{X} = 8{,}000$$

$$\frac{10{,}000\text{X}}{10{,}000} = \frac{8{,}000}{10{,}000} \qquad \text{Simplify: Divide both sides of the equation by the number before the unknown X}$$

$$\text{X} = 0.8 \text{ mL} \qquad \text{Label the units to match the unknown X}$$

0.8 mL given subcutaneously twice daily

Select a 1 mL or a 3 mL syringe and measure 0.8 mL of heparin 10,000 units/mL. Heparin is a potent anticoagulant drug. It is safest to measure it in a 1 mL syringe.

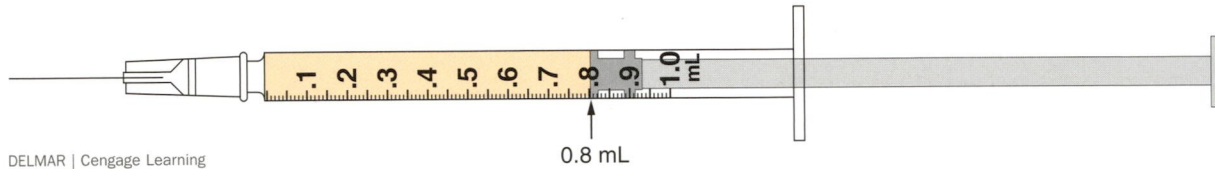

0.8 mL

EXAMPLE 5 ■

Order: **clindamycin**
300 mg
IV q.12h

Supply: clindamycin
injection
150 mg/mL

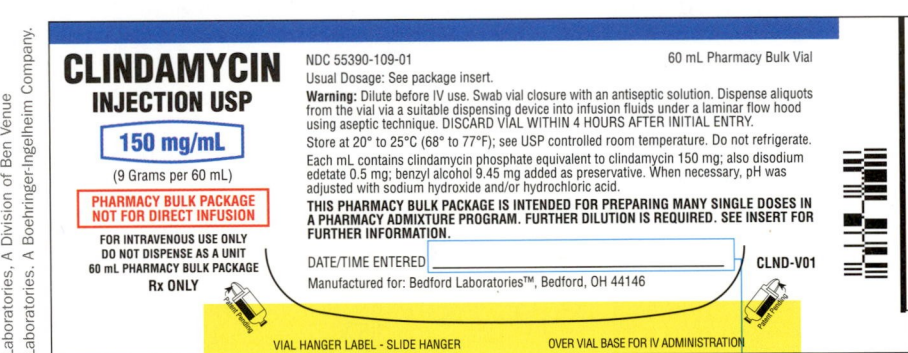

Step 1 **Convert** No conversion is necessary.

Step 2 **Think** You want to give more than 1 mL. Actually, you want to give 300 mg, which is 2 times 150 mg and 2 times 1 mL, or 2 mL. Calculate to double-check your estimate.

Step 3 **Calculate**

$$\frac{\text{Dosage on hand}}{\text{Amount on hand}} = \frac{\text{Dosage desired}}{\text{X Amount desired}}$$

$$\frac{150 \text{ mg}}{1 \text{ mL}} \diagdown\diagup \frac{300 \text{ mg}}{\text{X mL}} \qquad \text{Cross-multiply}$$

$$150\text{X} = 300$$

$$\frac{150\text{X}}{150} = \frac{300}{150} \qquad \text{Simplify: Divide both sides of the equation by the number before the unknown X}$$

$$\text{X} = 2 \text{ mL} \qquad \text{Label the units to match the unknown X}$$

2 mL given intramuscularly every 12 hours

Select a 3 mL syringe, and measure 2 mL of clindamycin 150 mg/mL.

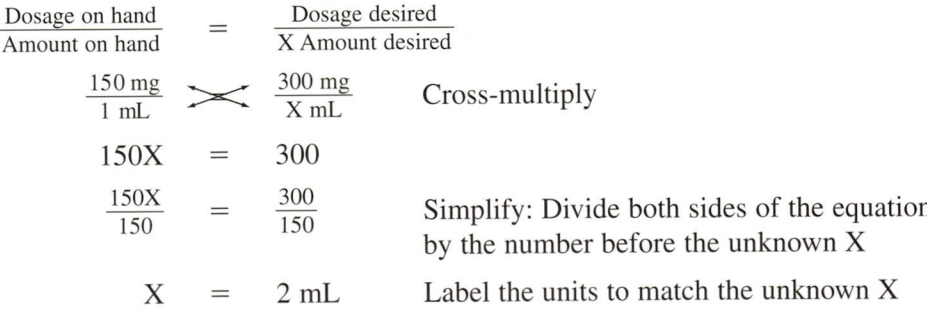

2 mL

EXAMPLE 6 ■

Order: Robinul 150 mcg IM stat

Supply: Robinul 0.2 mg/mL

Step 1 **Convert** Order: Robinul 150 mcg

Convert 0.2 mg to mcg to eliminate decimal fraction.

Equivalent: 1 mg = 1,000 mcg

$$\frac{1 \text{ mg}}{1{,}000 \text{ mcg}} \bowtie \frac{0.2 \text{ mg}}{X \text{ mcg}} \qquad \text{Cross-multiply}$$

$$X \quad = \quad 1{,}000 \times 0.2 \qquad 0.200. \text{ Move the decimal three places to the right. Add zeros to complete the operation.}$$

$$X \quad = \quad 200 \text{ mcg} \qquad \text{Label the units to match the unknown X}$$

Step 2 **Think** You want to give less than 1 mL but more than 0.5 mL. Be careful with the units and decimals. Don't be fooled into thinking 0.2 mg is less than 150 mcg. After conversion you can clearly see that 0.2 mg is more than 150 mcg because 0.2 mg = 200 mcg, which is more than 150 mcg.

Step 3 **Calculate** $$\frac{\text{Dosage on hand}}{\text{Amount on hand}} = \frac{\text{Dosage desired}}{X \text{ Amount desired}}$$

$$\frac{200 \text{ mcg}}{1 \text{ mL}} \bowtie \frac{150 \text{ mcg}}{X \text{ mL}} \qquad \text{Cross-multiply}$$

$$200X \quad = \quad 150$$

$$\frac{200X}{200} = \frac{150}{200} \qquad \text{Simplify: Divide both sides of the equation by the number before the unknown X}$$

$$X \quad = \quad 0.75 \text{ mL} \qquad \text{Label the units to match the unknown X}$$

0.75 mL given intramuscularly immediately

Select a 1 mL syringe, and measure 0.75 mL of Robinul 0.2 mg/mL. You may have to change needles because this is an IM injection.

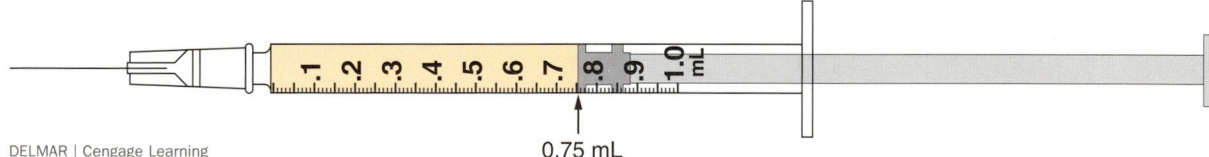

0.75 mL

EXAMPLE 7 ■

The drug order reads morphine sulfate gr $\frac{1}{6}$ IV q.4h p.r.n., pain.

The label on the single-dose vial states morphine sulfate 10 mg/mL.

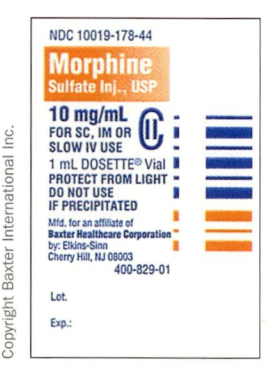

Step 1 **Convert** Order: morphine sulfate gr $\frac{1}{6}$

Convert gr to mg to eliminate the fraction.

Equivalent: gr i = 60 mg

$$\frac{\text{gr } 1}{60 \text{ mg}} \bowtie \frac{\text{gr } \frac{1}{6}}{X \text{ mg}} \qquad \text{Cross-multiply}$$

$$X = 60 \times \frac{1}{6} \qquad X = \frac{60}{1} \times \frac{1}{6}$$

$$X = \frac{\overset{10}{\cancel{60}}}{\underset{1}{\cancel{6}}} 10 \text{ mg} \qquad\qquad \text{Label the units to match the unknown X}$$

Order: **morphine sulfate gr** $\dfrac{1}{6}$ = 10 mg

Supply: morphine sulfate 10 mg/mL

Step 2 Think Now it is obvious that you want to give 1 mL.

Step 3 Calculate $\dfrac{\text{Dosage on hand}}{\text{Amount on hand}} = \dfrac{\text{Dosage desired}}{\text{X Amount desired}}$

$$\dfrac{10 \text{ mg}}{1 \text{ mL}} \times\!\!\!\!\times \dfrac{10 \text{ mg}}{\text{X mL}} \qquad \text{Cross-multiply}$$

$$10X = 10$$

$$\dfrac{10X}{10} = \dfrac{10}{10} \qquad\qquad \begin{array}{l}\text{Simplify: Divide both sides of the equation}\\ \text{by the number before the unknown X}\end{array}$$

$$X = 1 \text{ mL} \qquad\qquad \text{Label the units to match the unknown X}$$

1 mL given intramuscularly every 4 hours as needed for pain

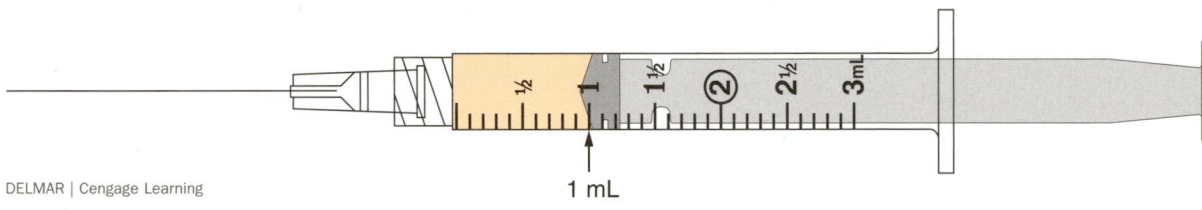

1 mL

QUICK REVIEW

- To solve parenteral dosage problems, apply the three steps to dosage calculations:

  STEP 1 Convert

  STEP 2 Think

  STEP 3 Calculate $\dfrac{\text{Dosage on hand}}{\text{Amount on hand}} = \dfrac{\text{Dosage desired}}{\text{X Amount desired}}$

- Prepare a maximum of 3 mL per IM injection site for an average-size adult, 2 mL per site for adult deltoid site and children ages 6 through 12, and 0.5 to 1 mL for children under age 6.

- Calculate dose volumes and prepare injectable fractional doses in a syringe using these guidelines:

  - Standard doses more than 1 mL: Round to tenths and measure in a 3 mL syringe. The 3 mL syringe is calibrated to 0.1 mL increments. Example: 1.53 mL is rounded to 1.5 mL and drawn up in a 3 mL syringe.

  - Small (less than 0.5 mL) doses: Round to hundredths and measure in a 1 mL syringe. Critical care and children's doses less than 1 mL calculated in hundredths should also be measured in a 1 mL syringe. The 1 mL syringe is calibrated in 0.01 mL increments. Example: 0.257 mL is rounded to 0.26 mL and drawn up in a 1 mL syringe.

  - Amounts of 0.5 to 1 mL calculated in tenths can be accurately measured in either a 1 mL or 3 mL syringe.

Review Set 24

Calculate the amount you will prepare for each dose. The labels provided represent the drugs available. Draw an arrow to the syringe calibration that corresponds to the amount you will administer. Indicate doses that have to be divided.

1. Order: *Depo-Provera 1 g IM stat*

   Give: _____ mL

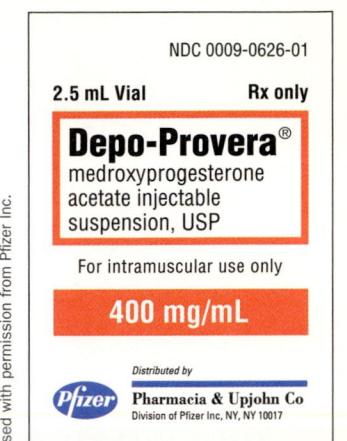

Used with permission from Pfizer Inc.

NDC 0009-0626-01

2.5 mL Vial   Rx only

Depo-Provera®
medroxyprogesterone
acetate injectable
suspension, USP

For intramuscular use only

400 mg/mL

Distributed by
Pfizer **Pharmacia & Upjohn Co**
Division of Pfizer Inc, NY, NY 10017

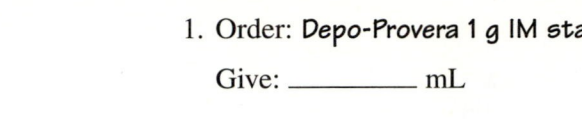

2. Order: *Bicillin C-R 900/300 2,400,000 units IM stat*

   Give: _____ mL

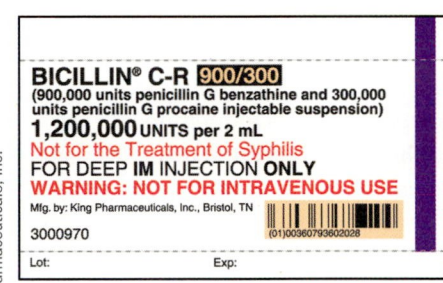

Used with permission from King Pharmaceuticals, Inc.

BICILLIN® C-R 900/300
(900,000 units penicillin G benzathine and 300,000
units penicillin G procaine injectable suspension)
1,200,000 UNITS per 2 mL
Not for the Treatment of Syphilis
FOR DEEP **IM** INJECTION **ONLY**
WARNING: NOT FOR INTRAVENOUS USE
Mfg. by: King Pharmaceuticals, Inc., Bristol, TN
3000970
(01)00360793602028
Lot: Exp:

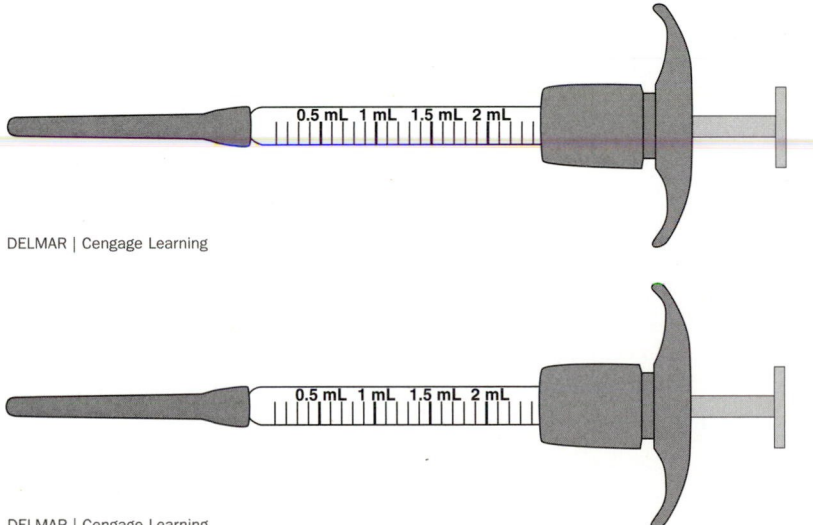

3. Order: *digoxin 600 mcg IV stat*

   Give: _____ mL

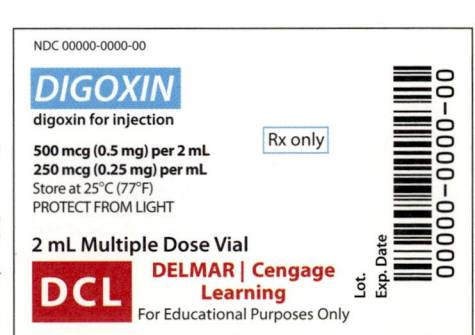

NDC 00000-0000-00

DIGOXIN
digoxin for injection

500 mcg (0.5 mg) per 2 mL
250 mcg (0.25 mg) per mL
Store at 25°C (77°F)
PROTECT FROM LIGHT

2 mL Multiple Dose Vial

DCL **DELMAR | Cengage Learning**
For Educational Purposes Only

Rx only

Exp. Date   Lot.

00000-0000-00

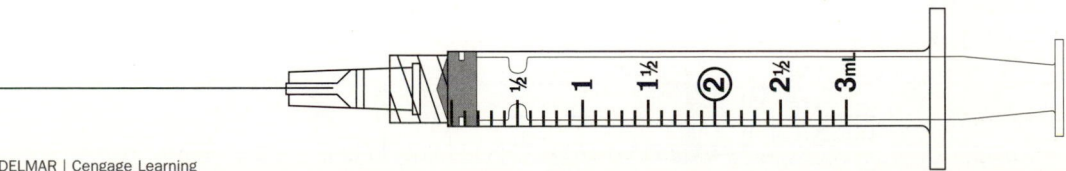

4. Order: **dexamethasone sodium phosphate 1.5 mg IV q.12h**

Give: _____ mL

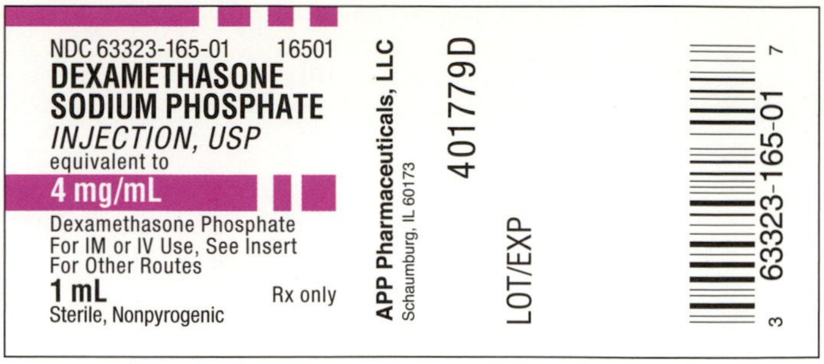

NDC 63323-165-01   16501

DEXAMETHASONE SODIUM PHOSPHATE
INJECTION, USP
equivalent to

4 mg/mL

Dexamethasone Phosphate
For IM or IV Use, See Insert
For Other Routes
1 mL   Rx only
Sterile, Nonpyrogenic

APP Pharmaceuticals, LLC
Schaumburg, IL 60173

401779D

LOT/EXP

3 63323-165-01 7

Reprinted with permission of APP Pharmaceuticals, LLC.

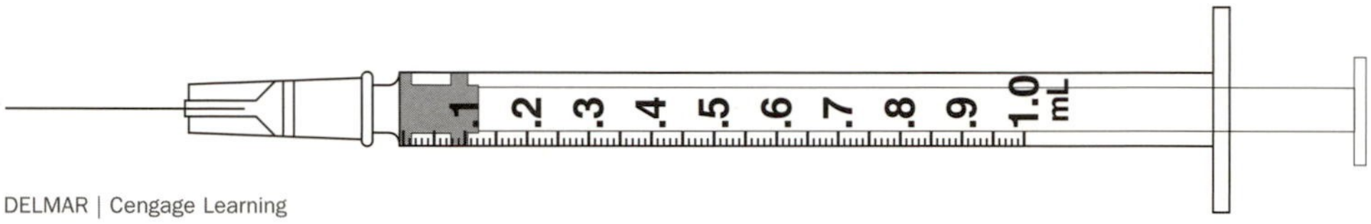

DELMAR | Cengage Learning

5. Order: **terbutaline 250 mcg subcut stat and repeat q.15–30 min if no significant improvement in status asthmaticus**

Give: _____ mL

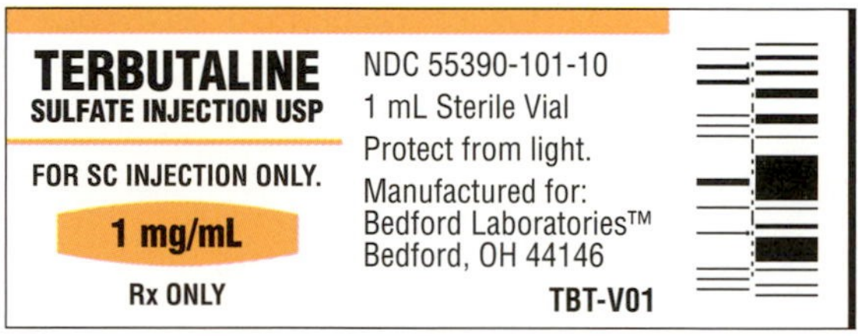

TERBUTALINE
SULFATE INJECTION USP

FOR SC INJECTION ONLY.

1 mg/mL

Rx ONLY

NDC 55390-101-10
1 mL Sterile Vial
Protect from light.
Manufactured for:
Bedford Laboratories™
Bedford, OH 44146

TBT-V01

Used with permission from Bedford Laboratories, A Division of Ben Venue Laboratories, A Boehringer-Ingelheim Company.

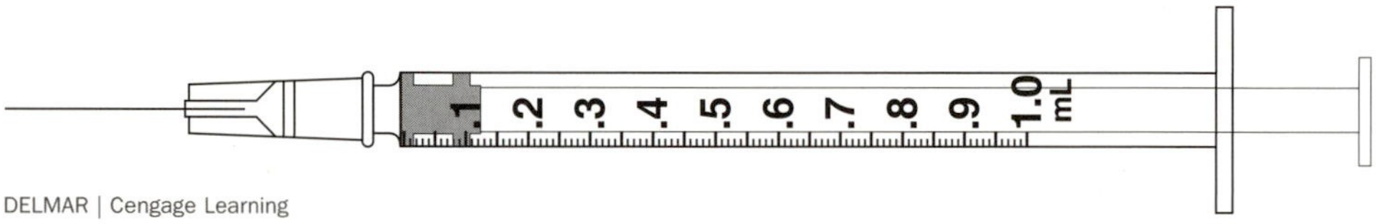

DELMAR | Cengage Learning

6. Order: **heparin 4,000 units subcut q.8h**

Give: _____ mL

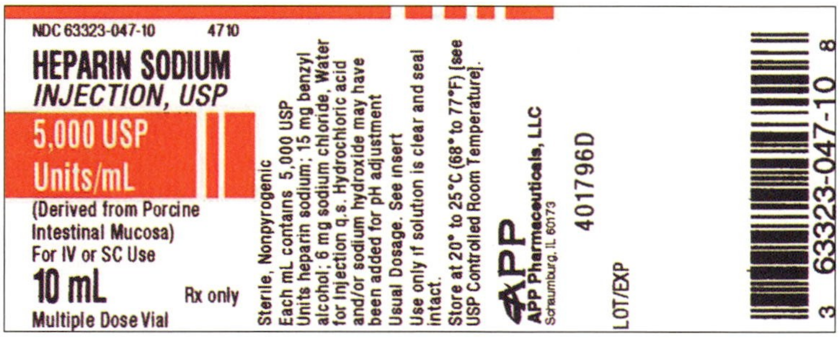

NDC 63323-047-10   4710

HEPARIN SODIUM
INJECTION, USP

5,000 USP Units/mL

(Derived from Porcine
Intestinal Mucosa)
For IV or SC Use
10 mL   Rx only
Multiple Dose Vial

Sterile, Nonpyrogenic
Each mL contains 5,000 USP
Units heparin sodium; 15 mg benzyl
alcohol; 6 mg sodium chloride. Water
for injection q.s. Hydrochloric acid
and/or sodium hydroxide may have
been added for pH adjustment
Usual Dosage. See insert
Use only if solution is clear and seal
intact.
Store at 20° to 25°C (68° to 77°F) [see
USP Controlled Room Temperature].

APP
APP Pharmaceuticals, LLC
Schaumburg, IL 60173

401796D

LOT/EXP

3 63323-047-10 8

Reprinted with permission of APP Pharmaceuticals, LLC.

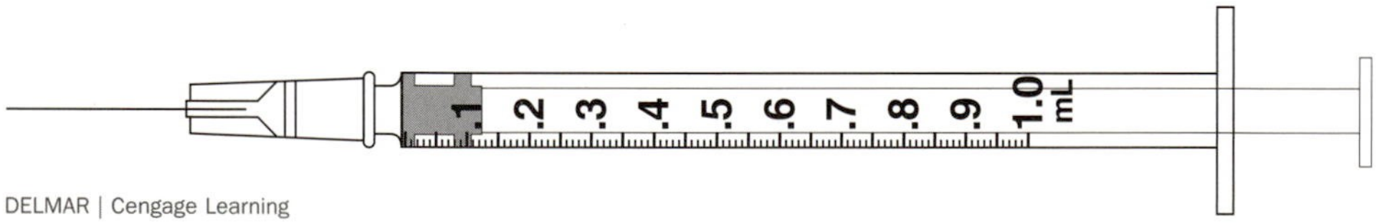

DELMAR | Cengage Learning

7. Order: **ondansetron 3 mg IV stat**

Give: _____ mL

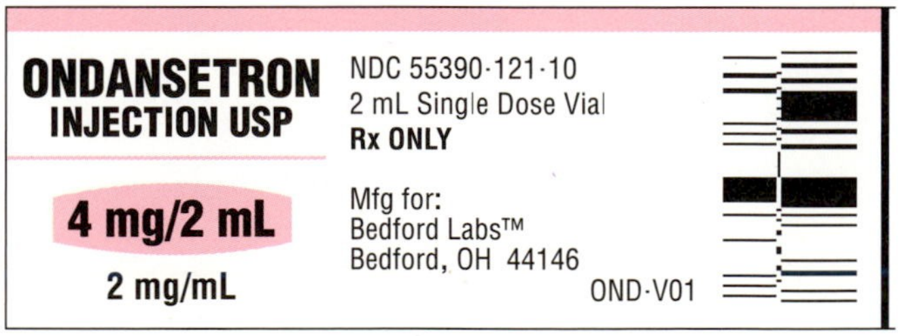

ONDANSETRON
INJECTION USP

Rx ONLY

4 mg/2 mL

2 mg/mL

NDC 55390-121-10
2 mL Single Dose Vial

Mfg for:
Bedford Labs™
Bedford, OH 44146

OND-V01

Used with permission from Bedford Laboratories, A Division of Ben Venue Laboratories, A Boehringer-Ingelheim Company.

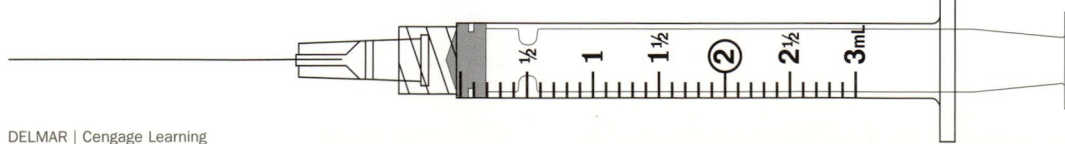

DELMAR | Cengage Learning

8. Order: ketorolac 18 mg IV
   q.6h p.r.n., pain

   Give: _____ mL

KETOROLAC
TROMETHAMINE
INJECTION USP

30 mg/mL
1 mL Vial
FOR IM OR IV USE ONLY

NDC 55390-481-01
1 mL Single-dose Vial
Protect from light.
Rx ONLY

Manufactured for:
Bedford Laboratories™
Bedford, OH 44146
KC-KRLVA03

9. Order: bumetanide
   500 mcg IV bolus stat

   Give: _____ mL

BUMETANIDE
INJECTION, USP

For IV or IM Use

1 mg/4 mL

0.25 mg/mL

Rx ONLY

NDC 55390-500-05   4 mL VIAL

Each mL contains: 0.25 mg bumetanide, 0.85% sodium chloride, 0.4% ammonium acetate as buffers, 0.01% edetate disodium, 1% benzyl alcohol as preservative and pH adjusted to approximately 7 with sodium hydroxide.

Usual Dosage: See package insert.

Store at controlled room temperature 15° to 30° C (59° to 86°F).

Manufactured for:
Bedford Laboratories™
Bedford, OH 44146   **BMVA04**

10. Order: morphine sulfate gr $\frac{1}{4}$ IV q.4h p.r.n., pain

    Give: _____ mL

NDC 10019-179-44
Morphine
Sulfate Inj., USP
15 mg/mL
FOR SC, IM OR
SLOW IV USE
1 mL
DOSETTE® Vial
PROTECT FROM LIGHT
DO NOT USE
IF PRECIPITATED
Mfd. for an affiliate of
Baxter Healthcare Corporation
by: Elkins-Sinn
Cherry Hill, NJ 08003
400-833-00

Lot:

Exp.:

11. Order: methotrexate 30 mg IV
    daily × 5 days

    Give: _____ mL

Exp. Date:

NDC 10019-940-17
Methotrexate
Injection, USP
PRESERVATIVE FREE R only
50 mg (25 mg/mL)
Sterile Isotonic Liquid
2 mL Single Dose Vial
Mfd. for **Baxter Healthcare Corp.** affiliate
by: Bigmar Pharmaceuticals SA
Barbengo, Switzerland

See package insert for routes of administration.
Usual Dosage: Consult package insert for dosage and full prescribing information.
Each mL contains methotrexate sodium equivalent to 25 mg methotrexate.
Inactive ingredients: Sodium Chloride 0.490% w/v and Water for Injection. Sodium hydroxide and/or hydrochloric acid may be added to adjust pH to 8.5-8.7 during manufacture.
Store at controlled room temperature 15°-30°C (59°-86°F).
PROTECT FROM LIGHT. Retain in carton until time of use. Discard any unused portion.   10-1038A   460-222-00

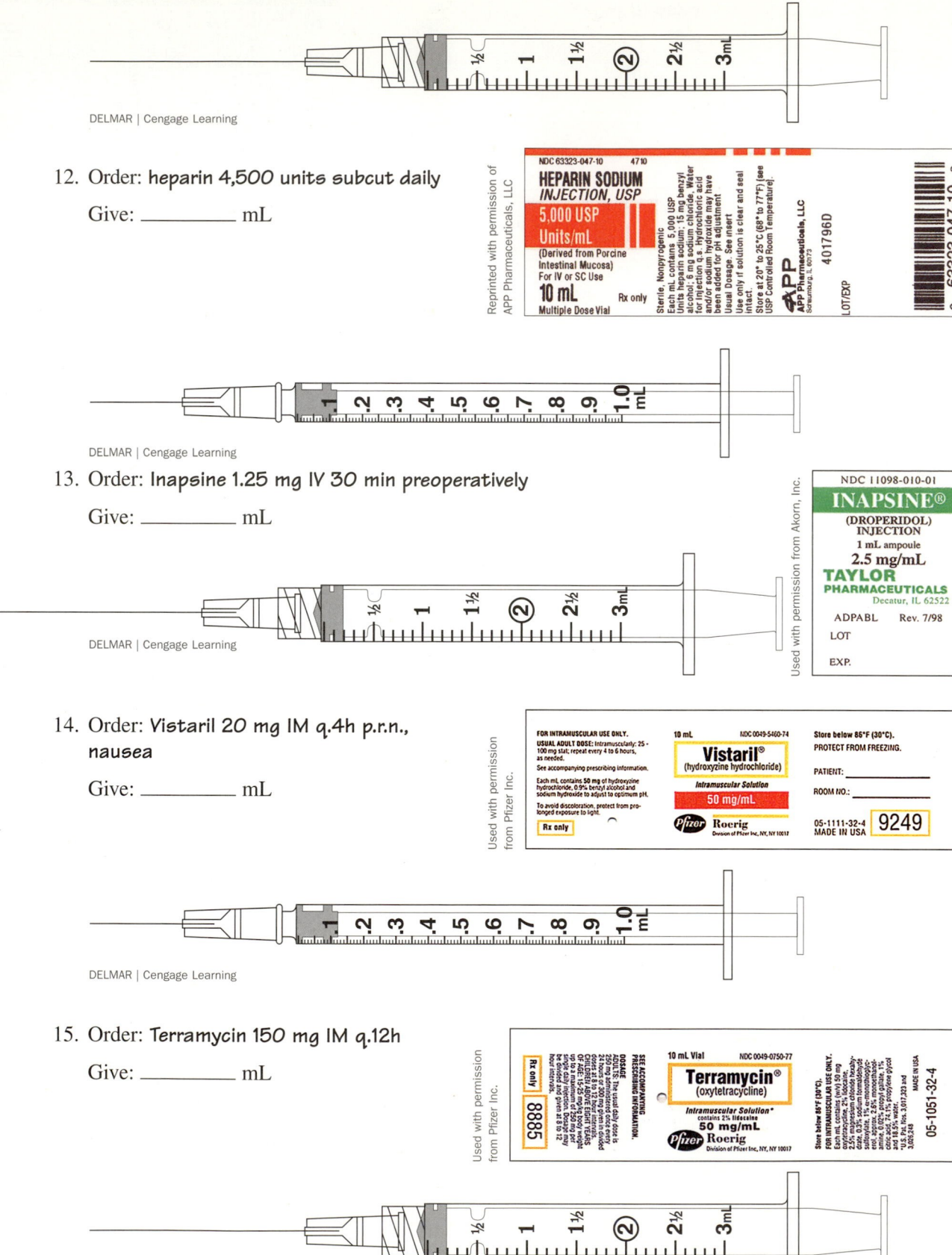

DELMAR | Cengage Learning

12. Order: **heparin 4,500 units subcut daily**

Give: _____ mL

NDC 63323-047-10   4710

HEPARIN SODIUM
INJECTION, USP

**5,000 USP
Units/mL**

(Derived from Porcine
Intestinal Mucosa)
For IV or SC Use
10 mL   Rx only
Multiple Dose Vial

Reprinted with permission of APP Pharmaceuticals, LLC

APP
APP Pharmaceuticals, LLC
Schaumburg, IL 60173

401796D

LOT/EXP

3 63323-047-10 8

DELMAR | Cengage Learning

13. Order: **Inapsine 1.25 mg IV 30 min preoperatively**

Give: _____ mL

NDC 11098-010-01

INAPSINE®
(DROPERIDOL)
INJECTION
1 mL ampoule
2.5 mg/mL

TAYLOR
PHARMACEUTICALS
Decatur, IL 62522

ADPABL   Rev. 7/98

LOT

EXP.

Used with permission from Akorn, Inc.

DELMAR | Cengage Learning

14. Order: **Vistaril 20 mg IM q.4h p.r.n.,
nausea**

Give: _____ mL

FOR INTRAMUSCULAR USE ONLY.
USUAL ADULT DOSE: Intramuscularly: 25 -
100 mg stat; repeat every 4 to 6 hours,
as needed.
See accompanying prescribing information.

Each mL contains 50 mg of hydroxyzine
hydrochloride, 0.9% benzyl alcohol and
sodium hydroxide to adjust to optimum pH.

To avoid discoloration, protect from prolonged exposure to light.

Rx only

10 mL   NDC 0049-5460-74

Vistaril®
(hydroxyzine hydrochloride)

Intramuscular Solution
50 mg/mL

Pfizer Roerig
Division of Pfizer Inc, NY, NY 10017

Store below 86°F (30°C).
PROTECT FROM FREEZING.

PATIENT: _____

ROOM NO.: _____

05-1111-32-4   **9249**
MADE IN USA

Used with permission from Pfizer Inc.

DELMAR | Cengage Learning

15. Order: **Terramycin 150 mg IM q.12h**

Give: _____ mL

Rx only   **8885**

10 mL Vial   NDC 0049-0750-77

Terramycin®
(oxytetracycline)

*Intramuscular Solution**
contains 2% lidocaine
50 mg/mL

Pfizer Roerig
Division of Pfizer Inc, NY, NY 10017

05-1051-32-4

Used with permission from Pfizer Inc.

DELMAR | Cengage Learning

16. Order: **cyancobalamin 100 mcg IM daily x 7 days**

    Give: _____ mL

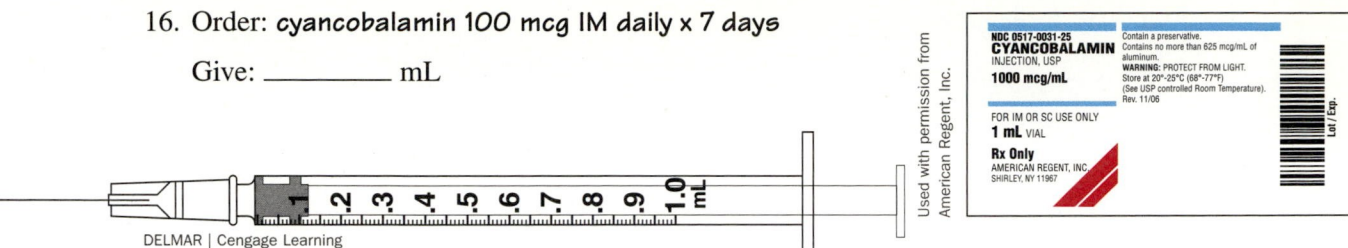

DELMAR | Cengage Learning

17. Order: **clindamycin 0.6 g IV q.12h**

    Give: _____ mL

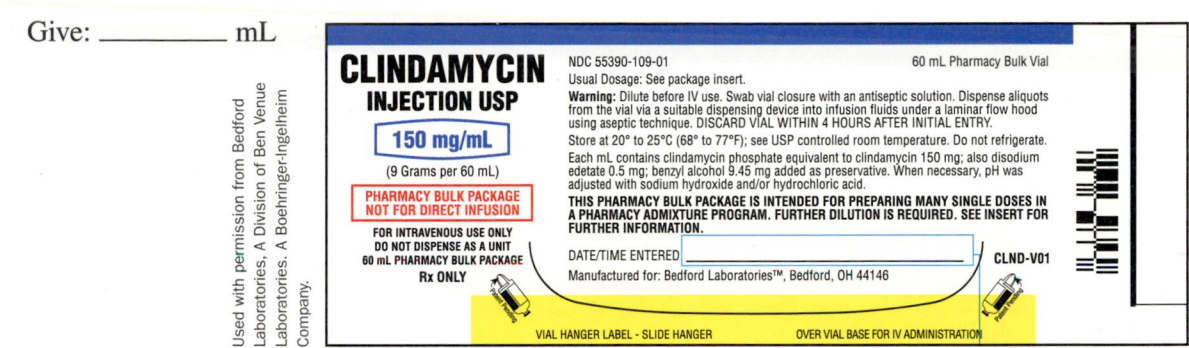

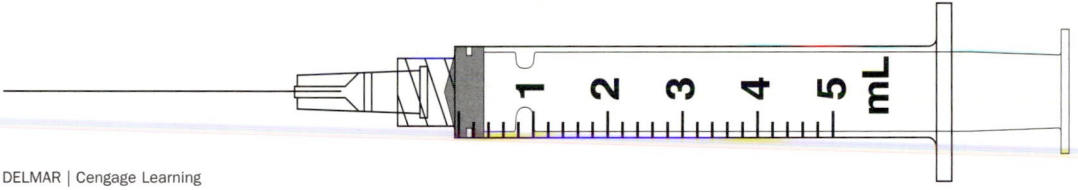

DELMAR | Cengage Learning

18. Order: **ranitidine 20 mg IV q.6h**

    Give: _____ mL

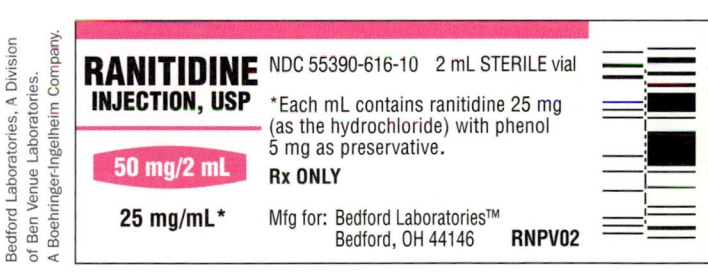

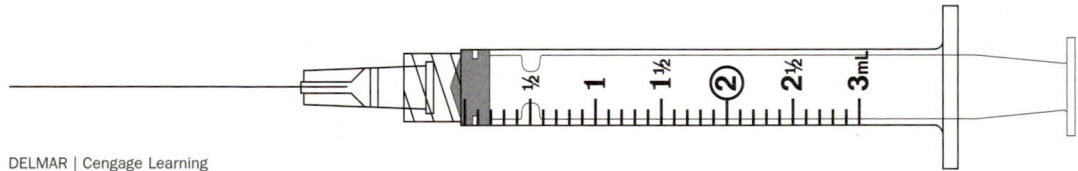

DELMAR | Cengage Learning

19. Order: **promethazine 12.5 mg IM stat**

    Give: _____ mL

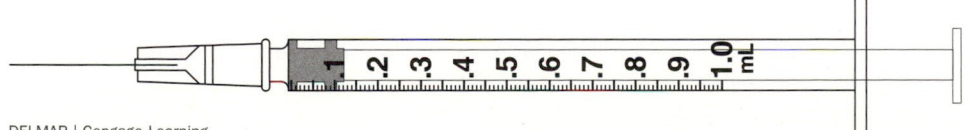

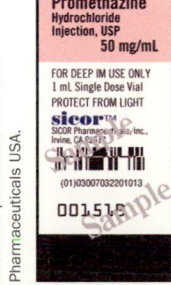

DELMAR | Cengage Learning

20. Order: furosemide 15 mg IV daily

Give: _____ mL

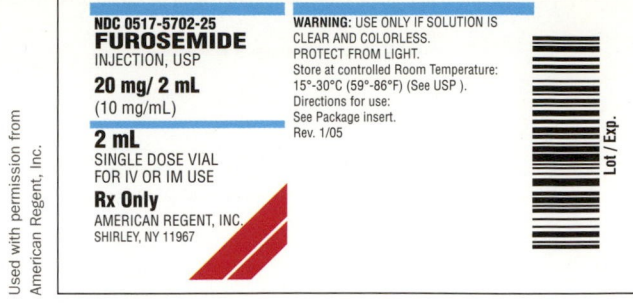

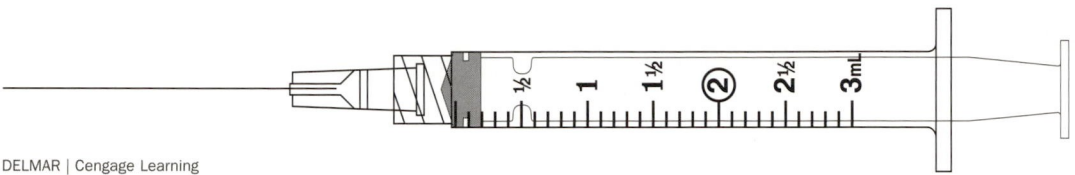

DELMAR | Cengage Learning

After completing these problems, see pages 523–526 to check your answers.

INSULIN

Insulin, a hormone made in the pancreas, is necessary for the metabolism of glucose, proteins, and fats. Patients who are deficient in insulin (insulin-dependent diabetics) are required to take insulin by injection daily. Insulin is a ready-to-use solution that is measured in units.

MATH TIP

The common supply dosage of insulin is **100 units per mL**, which is abbreviated on the label as **U-100**.

Think: U-100 = 100 units per mL

Insulin is also available as **500 units per mL (U-500)**. This supply dosage is used in special circumstances for diabetic patients with marked insulin resistance (such as daily requirements of more than 200 units).

Think: U-500 = 500 units per mL

CAUTION

Accuracy in insulin preparation and administration is critical. Inaccuracy is potentially life-threatening. It is essential for nurses to understand the information on the insulin label, to correctly interpret the insulin order, and to select the correct syringe to accurately measure insulin for administration. It is critical to understand that U-500 insulin (500 units/mL) is five times as concentrated as U-100 insulin (100 units/mL). **Extreme caution must be exercised in the administration of U-500 insulin because inadvertent overdose may result in irreversible insulin shock and death.**

Insulin Labels

Figure 11-2 identifies the essential components of insulin labels. Notice the difference in U-100 and U-500 insulin. The insulin label includes important information. For example, the *brand* and *generic names,* the *supply dosage* or *concentration,* and the *storage* instructions are details routinely found on most parenteral drug labels. Chapter 8 explains these and other typical drug label components. Compare the U-100 and U-500 insulin labels to find important identifiers.

FIGURE 11-2 (a) U-100 insulin label and (b) U-500 insulin label

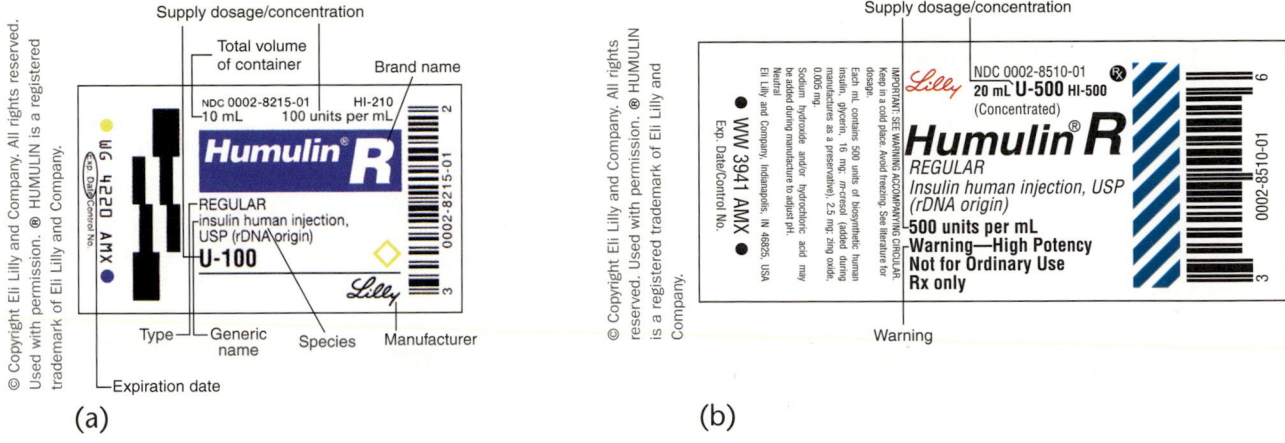

(a)

(b)

Insulin Action Times

Figure 11-3 (a–j) shows a sampling of insulin labels arranged by action times as described by McCulloch (2008).

- Rapid acting—5-15 min, peak in 45-75 min, 2-4 hr duration: *lispro, aspart, and glulisine*

- Short acting—30 min, peak in 2-4 hr, 5-8 hr duration: *regular*

- Intermediate acting—2 hr, peak in 6-10 hr, 18-28 hr duration: *NPH*

- Long acting—2 hr, no peak, 6-24 hr duration: *detemir and glargine*

Regular and NPH insulin are the two types used most frequently and they are often mixed. Notice the uppercase, bold letters on these two insulin types: ***R** for regular insulin and **N** for NPH insulin.* These letters are important visual identifiers when selecting the insulin type. Further, note the different concentrations of regular insulin: *regular U-100 (100 units/mL) and regular U-500 (500 units/mL).*

CAUTION

Insulin repeatedly is at the top of the list of high risk medications that can lead to errors and patient harm (Cohen, 2007; ISMP, 2008; Onufer, 2002). Avoid a potentially life-threatening medication error. Carefully read the label, and compare it to the drug order to ensure that you select the correct action time and type of insulin. Then accurately measure the correct dose amount.

FIGURE 11-3 Labels for insulin types grouped by action times

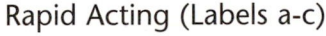

Rapid Acting (Labels a-c)

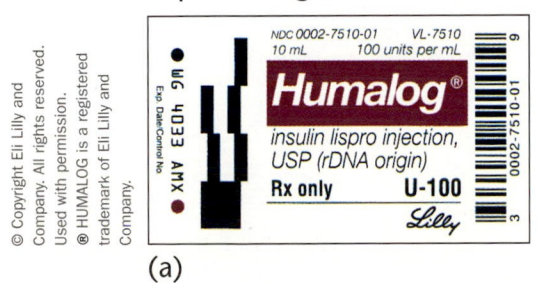

(a)

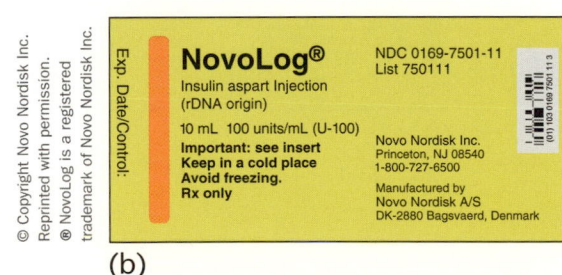

(b)

Continued

FIGURE 11-3 continued

Rapid Acting

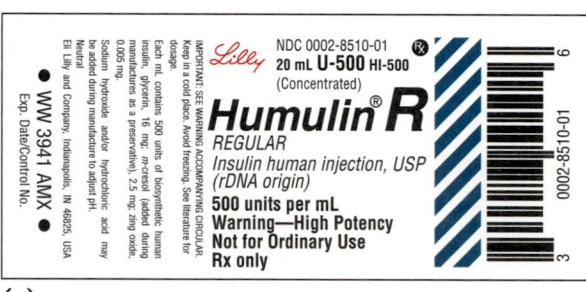

(c)

Short Acting (Labels d-f)

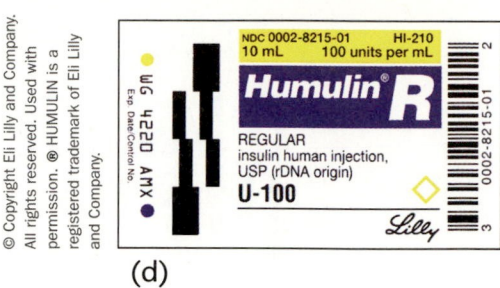

(d)

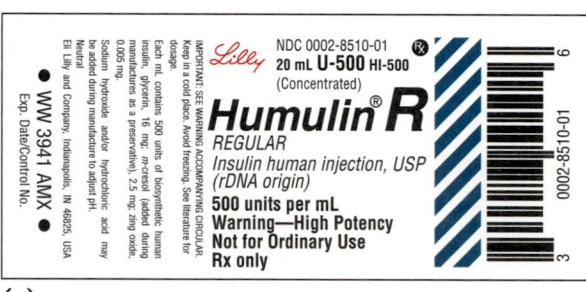

(e)

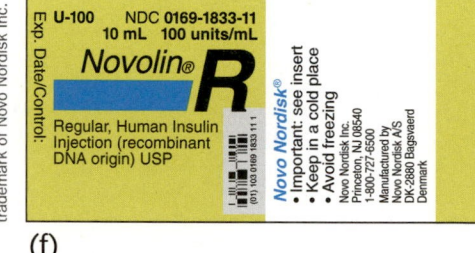

(f)

Intermediate Acting (Labels g and h)

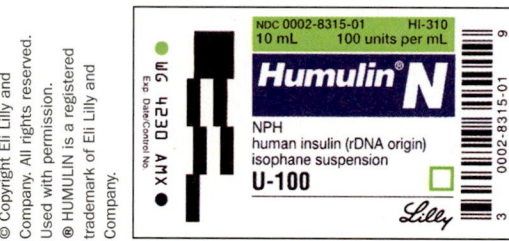

(g)

(h)

Long Acting (Labels i and j)

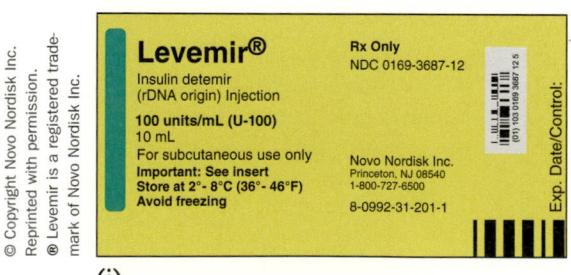

(i)

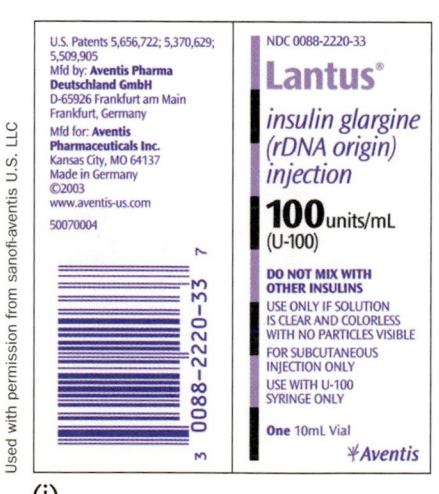

(j)

Premixed, Combination Insulin

There are several premixed insulin combinations that are commercially available. Figure 11-4 (a–e) depicts five of these preparations. It is important to carefully read the labels to understand what types of insulin are included in each combination. Notice that Novolin 70/30 (Figure 11-4a) includes 70% NPH U-100 insulin and 30% regular U-100 insulin in each unit. Therefore, if the physician orders 10 units of 70/30 U-100 insulin, the patient would receive 7 units of NPH insulin (70% or 0.7 × 10 units = 7 units) and 3 units of regular insulin (30% or 0.3 × 10 units = 3 units) in the 70/30 concentration. If the physician orders 20 units of 70/30 insulin, the patient would receive 14 units (0.7 × 20 = 14) of NPH and 6 units (0.3 × 20 = 6) of regular insulin.

The Humulin 50/50 U-100 insulin concentration means there is 50% NPH U-100 insulin and 50% regular U-100 insulin in each unit. Therefore, if the physician orders 12 units of 50/50 U-100 insulin, the patient would receive 6 units of NPH U-100 insulin (50% or 0.5 × 12 units = 6 units) and 6 units of regular U-100 insulin (50% or 0.5 × 12 units = 6 units).

It is easy to mistake one 70/30 or 50/50 preparation for another. For example, check out the differences on the label for Novolin 70/30 (Figure 11-4a) and Novolog 70/30 (Figure 11-4e). The Novolin is a combination of NPH and regular U-100 insulin; but the Novolog is a combination of aspart protamine and aspart. These are all different action times and selecting the wrong combination could be a serious and life-threatening error.

FIGURE 11-4 Premixed, combination insulins

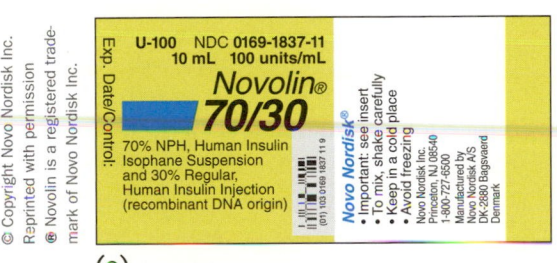

(a)

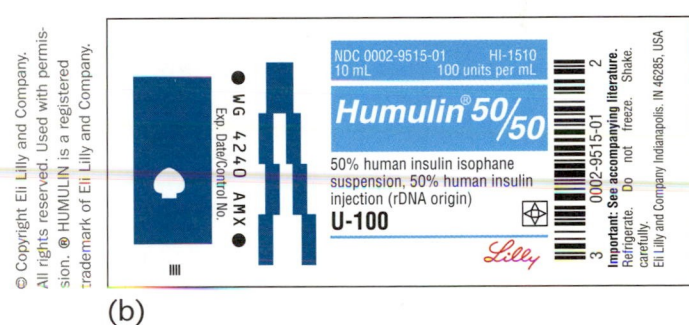

(b)

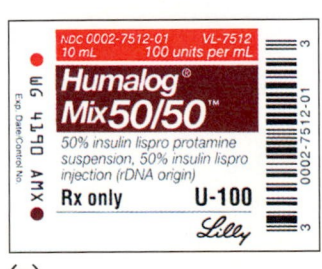

(c)

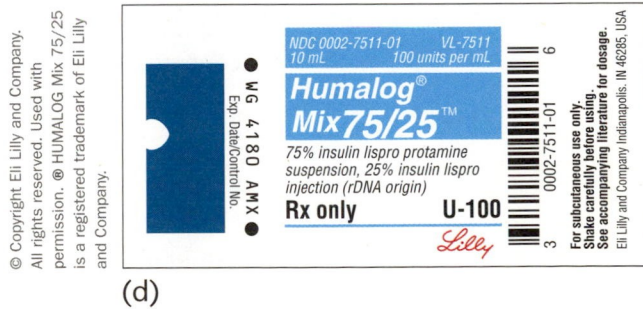

(d)

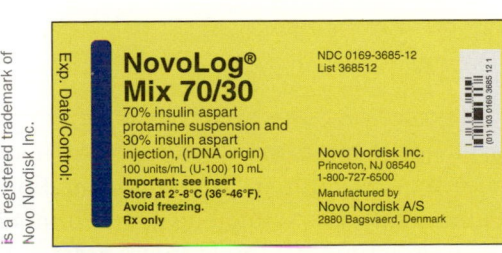

(e)

Interpreting the Insulin Order

Insulin orders must be written clearly and contain specific information to ensure correct administration and prevent errors. An insulin order should contain:

1. The *brand and generic names, and action time.* Patients are instructed to stay with the same manufacturer's brand name insulin. Slight variations between brands can affect an individual's response. Verify both the usual brand name used and the actual insulin supplied with the patient before administration. Look for one of the four action times: rapid-acting (e.g., lispro), short-acting (e.g., regular), intermediate-acting (e.g., NPH), and long-acting (e.g., detemir).

2. The *supply dosage (concentration)* and *number of units* to be given—for example, U-100 regular insulin 40 units.

3. The *route* of administration and *time* or *frequency.* All insulin may be administered subcutaneously (subcut), and regular U-100 insulin may additionally be administered intravenously (IV).

EXAMPLES ■

Humulin R regular U-100 insulin 14 units subcut stat

Novolin N NPH U-100 insulin 24 units subcut $\frac{1}{2}$ hour $\overline{a}$ breakfast

Insulin Coverage—The "Sliding Scale"

A special insulin order is sometimes needed to "cover" a patient's increasing blood sugar (glucose) level that is not yet regulated. Because of the rapid action, lispro or regular insulin will be used. The physician will specify the amount of insulin in units, which "slide" up or down based on a specific blood sugar level range. Sliding scales are individualized for each patient. Here's an example of a sliding-scale order:

EXAMPLE ■

Order: Humulin R regular U-100 insulin subcut a.c. based on glucose reading at 1600

INSULIN SLIDING SCALE	
Insulin Dose	**Glucose Reading***
No coverage	Glucose less than 160
2 units	160–220
4 units	221–280
6 units	281–340
8 units	341–400

*Glucose greater than 400: Hold insulin; call MD stat.

For example, if the patient's blood glucose is 290, you would administer 6 units of Humulin R regular U-100 insulin.

Insulin Administration

The primary route of insulin administration is by subcutaneous injection. Regular U-100 insulin can also be administered intravenously. The schedule and frequency for insulin administration varies based on the needs of the individual patient. The insulin pump is one method for insulin administration (Figure 11-5). Insulin pumps deliver rapid- or short-acting insulin 24 hours a day through a catheter placed under the skin. Pumps can be programmed to deliver a basal rate and/or bolus doses. Basal insulin is delivered continuously over 24 hours to keeps blood glucose levels in range between meals and overnight. The basal rate can be programmed to deliver different rates at different times of the day and night. Bolus doses can be delivered at mealtimes to provide control for additional food intake.

FIGURE 11-5 Insulin pump

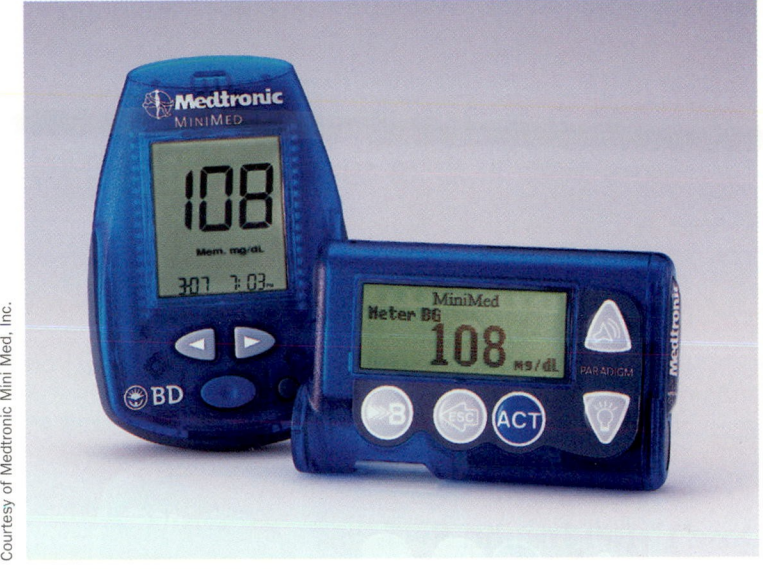

Courtesy of Medtronic Mini Med, Inc.

Measuring Insulin in an Insulin Syringe

The insulin syringe and measurement of insulin were introduced in Chapter 6. This critical skill warrants your attention again. Once you understand (a) how insulin is packaged, (b) about different concentrations (i.e., U-100 or U-500), and (c) how to use the insulin syringe, you will find insulin dosage simple.

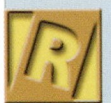

RULE

- Measure U-100 insulin in a U-100 insulin syringe only. Do not use a 3 mL or 1 mL syringe to measure U-100 insulin.

- Use U-100 insulin syringes to measure U-100 insulin only. Do not measure other drugs supplied in units or U-500 insulin in a U-100 insulin syringe.

- Measure U-500 insulin in a 1 mL syringe. Take extra precautions when measuring and administering U-500 insulin to note that the concentration is 500 units/mL. Correct dosage requires a calculation.

- Two nurses must check insulin dosage before administration to the patient.

Measuring U-100 insulin with the insulin syringe is simple. The insulin syringe makes it possible to obtain a correct dosage without mathematical calculation. Let's look at three different U-100 insulin syringes. They are the *standard* (100 unit) capacity and the *lo-dose* (50 unit and 30 unit) capacity.

Standard U-100 Insulin Syringe

EXAMPLE ■

The Standard U-100 insulin syringe in Figure 11-6 is a dual-scale syringe with 100 units/mL capacity. It is calibrated on one side in even-numbered, 2 unit increments (2, 4, 6, . . .) with every 10 units labeled (10, 20, 30, . . .). It is calibrated on the reverse side in odd-numbered, 2 unit increments (1, 3, 5, . . .) with every 10 units labeled (5, 15, 25, . . .). The measurement of 73 units of U-100 insulin is illustrated in Figure 11-6.

FIGURE 11-6   Standard U-100 insulin syringe measuring 73 units

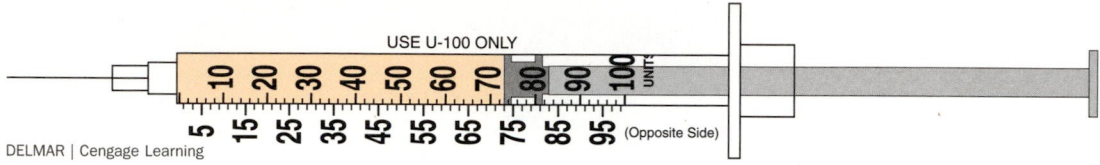

DELMAR | Cengage Learning

CAUTION

Look carefully at the increments on the dual scale. The volume from one mark to the next (on either side) is 2 units. You are probably comfortable counting by twos for even numbers. Pay close attention when counting by twos with odd numbers.

Lo-Dose U-100 Insulin Syringes

EXAMPLE 1 ■

The Lo-Dose U-100 insulin syringe in Figure 11-7 is a single-scale syringe with 50 units per 0.5 mL capacity. It is calibrated in 1 unit increments with every 5 units (5, 10, 15, . . .) labeled up to 50 units. The enlarged 50 unit calibration of this syringe makes it easy to read and use to measure low dosages of insulin. To measure 32 units, withdraw U-100 insulin to the 32 unit mark (Figure 11-7).

FIGURE 11-7   50-U Lo-Dose U-100 insulin syringe measuring 32 units

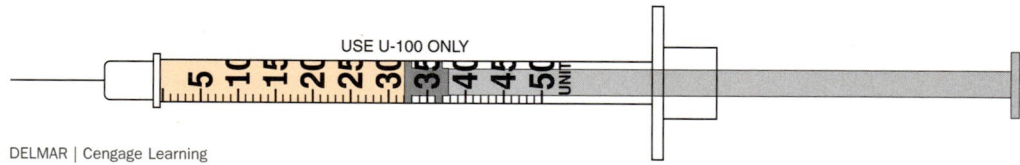

DELMAR | Cengage Learning

EXAMPLE 2 ■

The Lo-Dose U-100 insulin syringe in Figure 11-8 is a single-scale syringe with 30 units per 0.3 mL capacity. It is calibrated in 1 unit increments with every 5 units (5, 10, 15, . . .) labeled up to 30 units. The enlarged 30 unit calibration accurately measures small amounts of insulin, such as for children. To measure 12 units, withdraw U-100 insulin to the 12 unit mark (Figure 11-8).

FIGURE 11-8   30-U Lo-Dose U-100 insulin syringe measuring 12 units

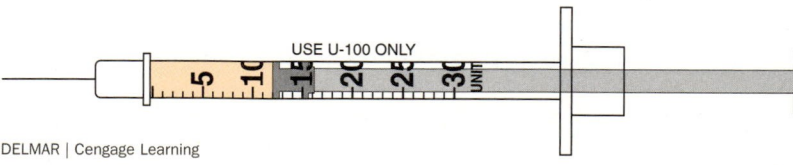

DELMAR | Cengage Learning

CAUTION

Always choose the smallest capacity U-100 insulin syringe available for accurate U-100 insulin measurement. Use Standard and Lo-Dose U-100 syringes to measure U-100 insulin only. Although the Lo-Dose U-100 insulin syringes only measure a maximum of 30 or 50 units, they are still intended for the measurement of U-100 insulin only.

Be cautious when measuring. The Lo-Dose U-100 syringe is calibrated in 1 unit increments; the Standard U-100 insulin syringe is calibrated in 2 unit increments on the even and odd scales.

Prefilled U-100 Insulin Pens

The re-usable U-100 insulin pen is equipped with a disposable 3 mL U-100 insulin cartridge to deliver multiple doses of U-100 insulin Figures 11-9 and 11-10 show samples of the insulin pen and a cartridge label.

FIGURE 11-9   Sample Reusable U-100 insulin pen with memory feature

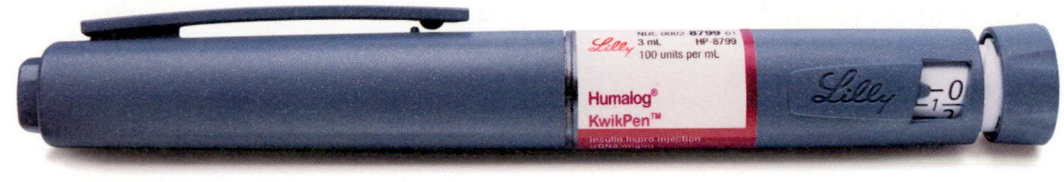

Eli Lilly and Company.

FIGURE 11-10   Sample U-100 insulin pen cartridge label

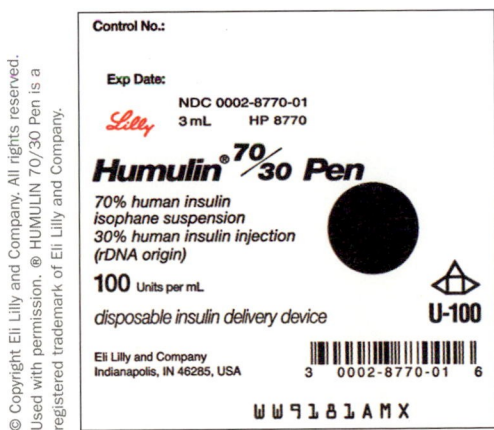

Measuring U-500 Insulin in a 1 mL Syringe

There is no special insulin syringe for the measurement of U-500 insulin. It is recommended that a 1 mL syringe be used. To be safe, physicians should prescribe the exact dosage and dose amount with the order. If you are unsure of the order, be sure to ask for clarification. Do not guess! Because U-500 insulin is concentrated, it is five times as potent as U-100 insulin. **Dosage errors can be life-threatening**. Always double check calculations and preparation with two nurses.

EXAMPLE ■

Order: Humulin R U-500 regular insulin 240 units (0.48 mL) subcut stat
Supply: Humulin R U-500 regular insulin

Is the dose amount correct as ordered? Do a calculation check.

Step 1	**Convert**	Recall that U-500 = 500 units/mL
Step 2	**Think**	There are 500 units in 1 mL; 240 units is slightly less than half of 500 units and 0.48 mL is a little less than ½ or 0.5 mL. Calculate to confirm your thinking.

Step 3 Calculate

$$\frac{\text{Dosage on hand}}{\text{Amount on hand}} \quad \diagup\!\!\!\!\diagdown \quad \frac{\text{Dosage desired}}{\text{X Amount desired}}$$

$$\frac{500 \text{ units}}{1 \text{ mL}} = \frac{240 \text{ units}}{\text{X mL}}$$

$$500X = 240$$

$$\frac{500X}{500} = \frac{240}{500}$$

$$X = 0.48 \text{ mL}$$

The dose amount of 0.48 mL is correct.

Combination Insulin Dosage

The patient may have two types of insulin prescribed to be administered at the same time. When possible, a pre-mixed U-100 insulin preparation is prescribed (Figure 11-4). However, if the preparation desired is not available, then the nurse must mix the U-100 insulins. To avoid injecting the patient twice, it is common practice to draw up both insulins into the same syringe.

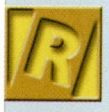

RULE
Draw up clear insulin first, then draw up cloudy insulin.
Regular insulin is clear. NPH insulin is cloudy.
THINK: *First clear, then cloudy.* **THINK:** *First regular, then NPH.*

EXAMPLE 1 ■

Order: Novolin R regular U-100 insulin 12 units with Novolin N NPH U-100 insulin 40 units subcut ā breakfast.

To accurately draw up both insulins into the same syringe, you will need to know the total units of both insulins: 12 + 40 = 52 units. Withdraw 12 units of the regular U-100 insulin (clear) and then withdraw 40 more units of the NPH U-100 insulin (cloudy) up to the 52 unit mark (Figure 11-11). In this case, the smallest capacity syringe you can use is the Standard U-100 insulin syringe. Notice that the NPH insulin is drawn up last and is closest to the needle in the diagram. In reality, the drugs mix right away.

FIGURE 11-11 (a) Combination insulin dosage (b) regular U-100 insulin label, and (c) NPH U-100 insulin label

(a)

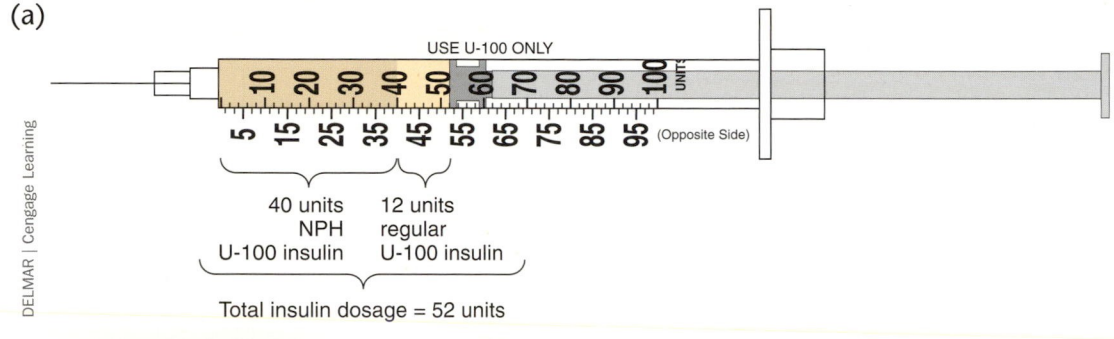

(b)

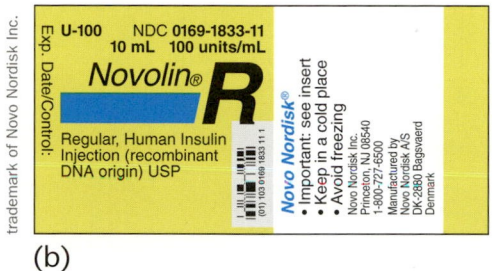

(c)

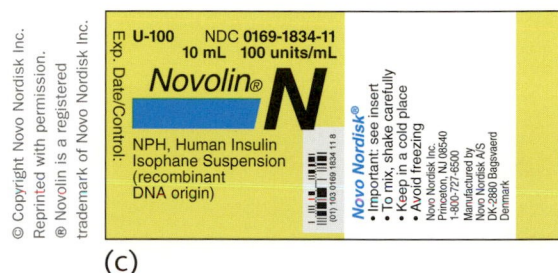

The second example gives step-by-step directions for this procedure. Look closely at Figures 11-12 and 11-13, which demonstrate the procedure, as you study Example 2. Notice that to withdraw regular insulin (clear) first and then NPH insulin (cloudy), you must inject the dose amount of air into the NPH insulin *before* you inject the dose amount of air into the regular insulin.

EXAMPLE 2 ■

The physician orders Novolin R regular U-100 insulin 10 units with Novolin N NPH U-100 insulin 30 units subcut $\frac{1}{2}$ hour ā dinner.

1. Draw back and inject 30 units of air into the NPH insulin vial (cloudy liquid). Remove needle.

2. Draw back and inject 10 units of air into the regular insulin vial (clear liquid) and leave the needle in the vial.

3. Turn the vial of regular U-100 insulin upside down, and draw out the insulin to the 10-unit mark on the U-100 syringe. Make sure all air bubbles are removed.

4. Roll the vial of the NPH U-100 insulin in your hands to mix; do not shake it. Insert the needle into the NPH insulin vial, turn the vial upside down, and slowly draw back to the 40 unit mark, being careful not to exceed the 40 unit calibration. In Figure 11-13, 10 units of regular U-100 + 30 units of NPH U-100 = 40 units of insulin total.

CAUTION

If you withdraw too much of the second insulin (NPH), you must discard the entire medication and start over.

CAUTION

Long-acting types of insulin should not be mixed or diluted with any other insulin preparations. Mixing long-acting insulin with other insulin solutions may interfere with blood sugar control, which could be serious and life-threatening.

FIGURE 11-12   Procedure for drawing up combination insulin dosage: 10 units Novolin R regular U-100 insulin with 30 units Novolin N NPH U-100 insulin

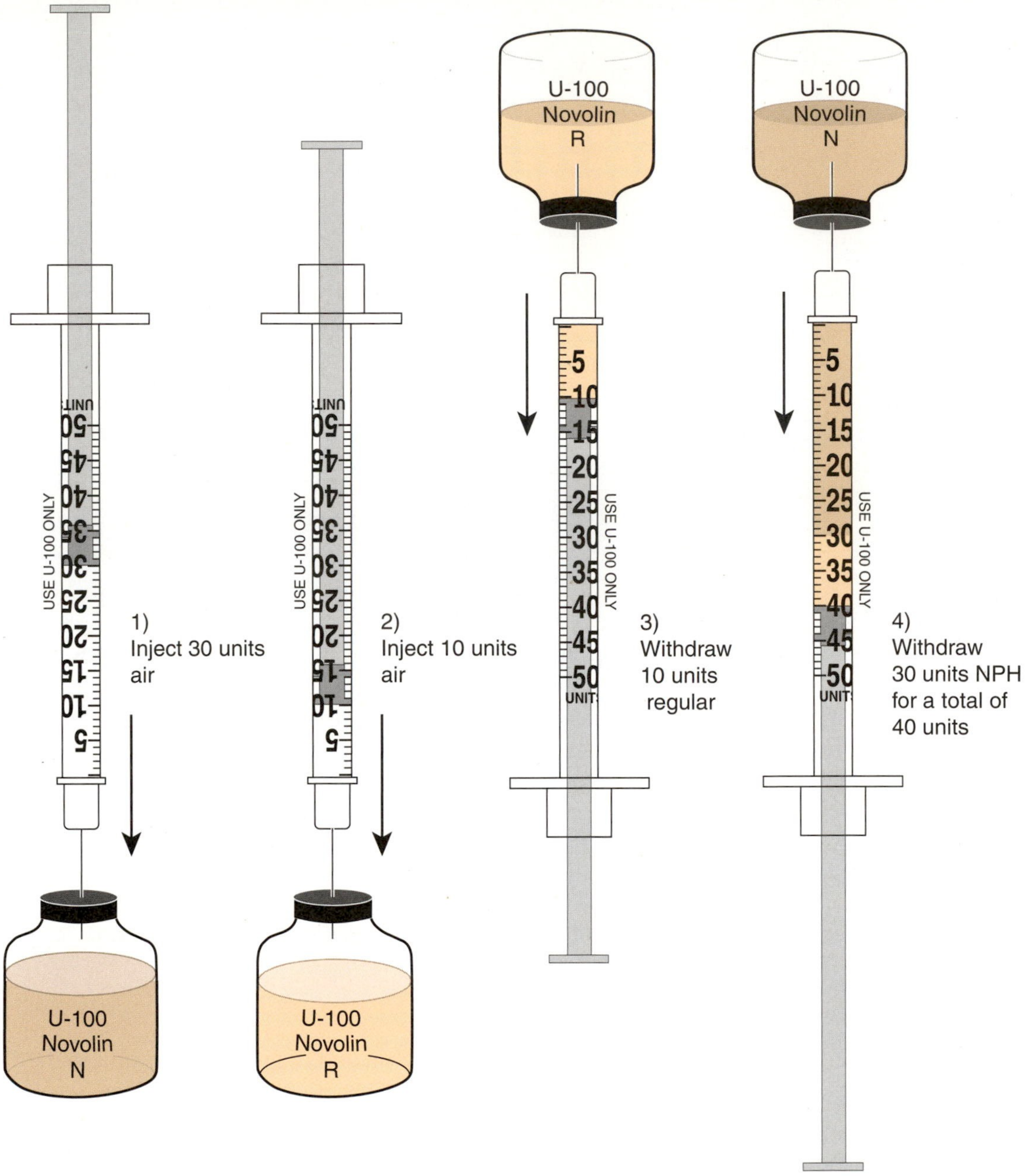

1) Inject 30 units air

2) Inject 10 units air

3) Withdraw 10 units regular

4) Withdraw 30 units NPH for a total of 40 units

DELMAR | Cengage Learning

FIGURE 11-13   Combination insulin dosage

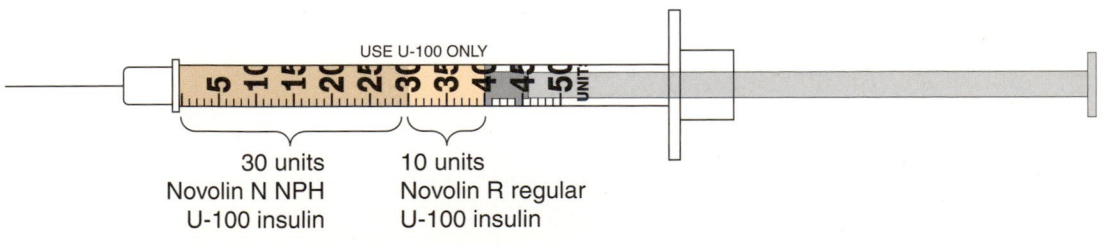

30 units Novolin N NPH U-100 insulin

10 units Novolin R regular U-100 insulin

Total insulin dosage = 40 units

DELMAR | Cengage Learning

Avoiding Insulin Dosage Errors

Insulin dosage errors are costly and, unfortunately, too common. They can be avoided by following two important rules.

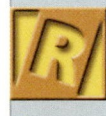

RULE

1. Insulin dosages must be checked by two nurses.

2. When combination dosages are prepared, two nurses must verify each step of the process.

QUICK REVIEW

- Carefully read the physician's order, and match the supply dosage for type, brand, and concentration of insulin.

- Always measure U-100 insulin in a U-100 insulin syringe.

- An insulin syringe is used to *only* measure U-100 insulin. Insulin syringes must not be used to measure other medications measured in units or U-500 insulin preparations.

- Use the smallest capacity U-100 insulin syringe possible to most accurately measure U-100 insulin doses.

- When drawing up combination insulin doses, think *clear first, then cloudy*.

- Do not mix long-acting insulin with any other insulin or solution.

- Avoid insulin dosage errors. The insulin dosage should be checked by two nurses.

- There are 100 units per mL for U-100 insulin.

- There are 500 units per mL for U-500 insulin.

- Measure U-500 insulin in a 1 mL syringe after careful dosage calculation.

Review Set 25

For each of the following insulin labels, identify:

- Brand name

- Generic name

- Action time (rapid-acting, short-acting, intermediate-acting, or long-acting)

- Concentration in units per mL

- Syringe you would select to measure a prescribed dosage

1. Brand name　　　　————————

　Generic name　　　————————

　Action time　　　　————————

　Concentration　　　————————

　Syringe　　　　　　————————

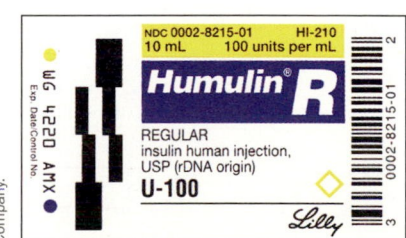

2. Brand name   _____

     Generic name   _____

     Action time   _____

     Concentration   _____

     Syringe   _____

3. Brand name   _____

     Generic name   _____

     Action time   _____

     Concentration   _____

     Syringe   _____

4. Brand name   _____

     Generic name   _____

     Action time   _____

     Concentration   _____

     Syringe   _____

5. Brand name   _____

     Generic name   _____

     Action time   _____

     Concentration   _____

     Syringe   _____

6. Brand name   _____

     Generic name   _____

     Action time   _____

     Concentration   _____

     Syringe   _____

U-100   NDC 0169-1834-11
10 mL   100 units/mL
Novolin® N
NPH, Human Insulin Isophane Suspension (recombinant DNA origin)
Novo Nordisk®
• Important: see insert
• To mix, shake carefully
• Keep in a cold place
• Avoid freezing
Novo Nordisk Inc. Princeton, NJ 08540 1-800-727-6500
Manufactured by Novo Nordisk A/S DK-2880 Bagsvaerd Denmark
© Copyright Novo Nordisk Inc. Reprinted with permission. ® Novolin is a registered trademark of Novo Nordisk Inc.

NovoLog®
Insulin aspart Injection (rDNA origin)
NDC 0169-7501-11
List 750111
10 mL 100 units/mL (U-100)
Important: see insert Keep in a cold place Avoid freezing. Rx only
Novo Nordisk Inc. Princeton, NJ 08540 1-800-727-6500
Manufactured by Novo Nordisk A/S DK-2880 Bagsvaerd, Denmark
© Copyright Novo Nordisk Inc. Reprinted with permission. ® NovoLog is a registered trademark of Novo Nordisk Inc.

NDC 0002-7510-01   VL-7510
10 mL   100 units per mL
Humalog®
insulin lispro injection, USP (rDNA origin)
Rx only   U-100
Lilly
© Copyright Eli Lilly and Company. All rights reserved. Used with permission. ® HUMALOG is a registered trademark of Eli Lilly and Company.

Lilly   NDC 0002-8510-01
20 mL U-500 HI-500 (Concentrated)
Humulin® R
REGULAR
Insulin human injection, USP (rDNA origin)
500 units per mL
Warning—High Potency
Not for Ordinary Use
Rx only
WW 3941 AMX
© Copyright Eli Lilly and Company. All rights reserved. Used with permission. ® HUMULIN is a registered trademark of Eli Lilly and Company.

U.S. Patents 5,656,722; 5,370,629; 5,509,905
Mfd by: **Aventis Pharma Deutschland GmbH** D-65926 Frankfurt am Main Frankfurt, Germany
Mfd for: **Aventis Pharmaceuticals Inc.** Kansas City, MO 64137 Made in Germany ©2003 www.aventis-us.com
50070004
NDC 0088-2220-33
Lantus®
insulin glargine (rDNA origin) injection
100units/mL (U-100)
DO NOT MIX WITH OTHER INSULINS
USE ONLY IF SOLUTION IS CLEAR AND COLORLESS WITH NO PARTICLES VISIBLE
FOR SUBCUTANEOUS INJECTION ONLY
USE WITH U-100 SYRINGE ONLY
One 10mL Vial
Aventis
Used with permission from sanofi-aventis U.S. LLC

---

7. Describe the three syringes available to measure U-100 insulin. _____

_____

8. What would be your preferred syringe choice to measure 35 units of U-100 insulin?

_____

9. There are 60 units of U-100 insulin per _____ mL.

10. There are 125 units of U-500 insulin per _____ mL.

11. Sixty-five (65) units of U-100 insulin should be measured in a(n) _____ syringe.

12. True or False? The 50 unit Lo-Dose U-100 insulin syringe is intended to measure U-50 insulin only. _____

Identify the U-100 insulin dosage indicated by the colored area of the syringe.

13. _____ units

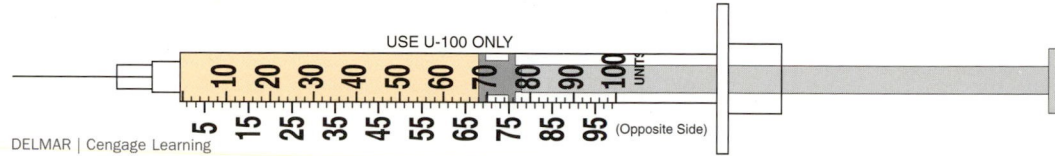

14. _____ units

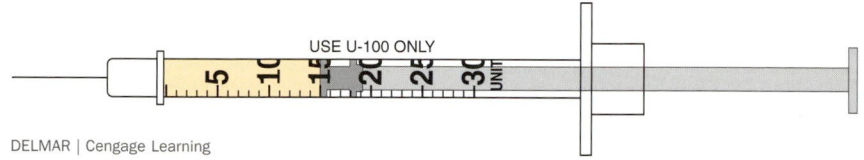

15. _____ units

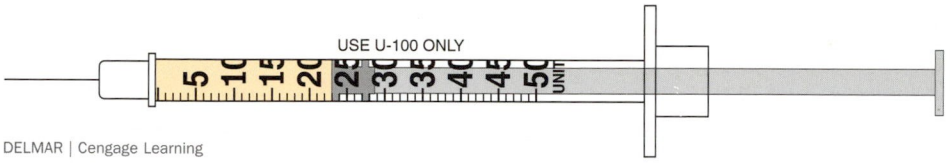

16. _____ units

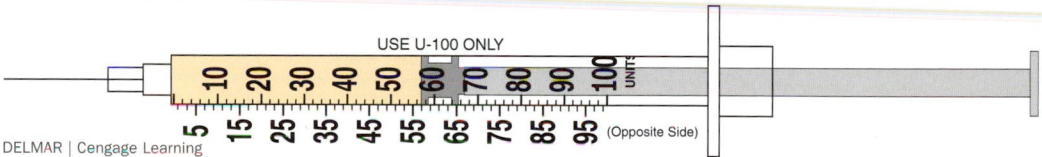

Draw an arrow on the syringe to identify the given dosages.

17. 80 units U-100 insulin

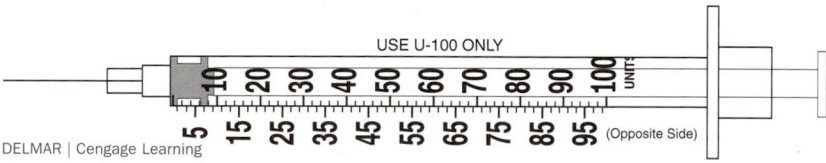

18. 15 units U-100 insulin

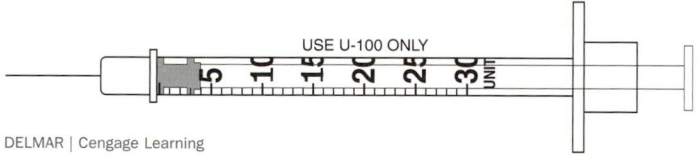

19. 66 units U-100 insulin

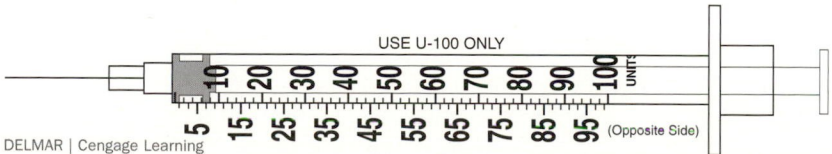

20. 16 units U-100 insulin

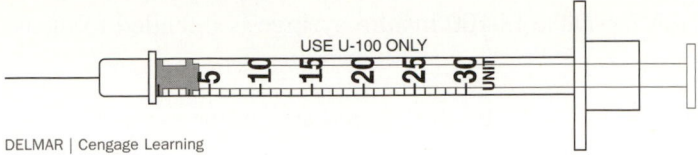

DELMAR | Cengage Learning

21. 200 units of U-500 insulin

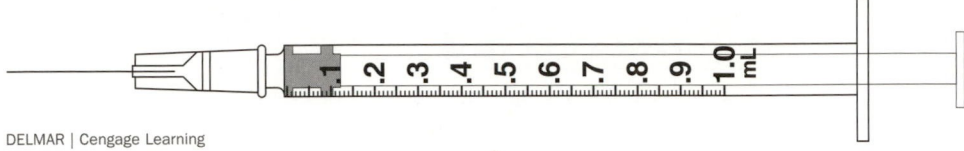

DELMAR | Cengage Learning

Draw arrows, and label the dosage for each of the combination insulin orders to be measured in the same syringe. Label and measure the insulins in the correct order, indicating which insulin will be drawn up first.

22. Novolin R regular U-100 insulin 21 units with Novolin N NPH U-100 insulin 15 units subcut stat

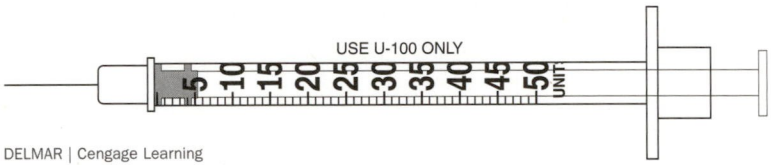

DELMAR | Cengage Learning

23. Humulin R regular U-100 insulin 16 units with Humulin N NPH U-100 insulin 42 units subcut stat

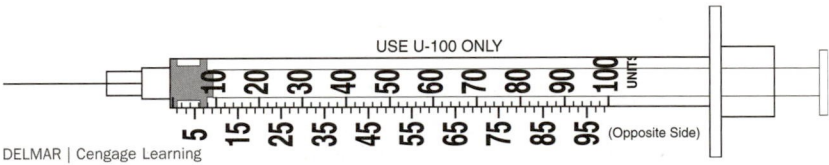

DELMAR | Cengage Learning

24. Humulin R regular U-100 insulin 32 units with Humulin N NPH U-100 insulin 40 units subcut $\bar{a}$ dinner

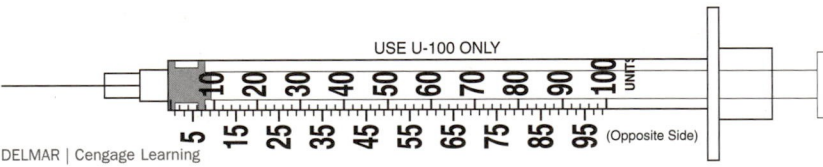

DELMAR | Cengage Learning

25. Humulin R regular U-100 insulin 8 units with Humulin N NPH U-100 insulin 12 units subcut stat

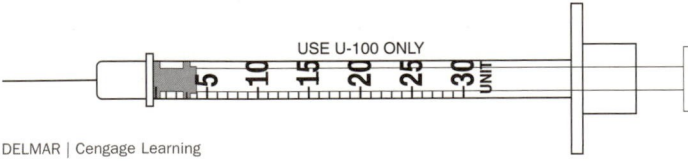

DELMAR | Cengage Learning

Use the following medication order and insulin sliding scale to answer questions 26 through 30.

Order: Humulin R regular U-100 insulin subcut a.c. per sliding scale.

INSULIN SLIDING SCALE	
Insulin Dose	**Glucose Reading***
No coverage	Glucose less than 160
2 units	160–220
4 units	221–280
6 units	281–340
8 units	341–400

*Glucose greater than 400: Hold insulin; call MD stat.

26. When will you check the patient's blood glucose level to determine the amount of insulin to give?

   _____

27. At what range of blood glucose levels will you administer insulin? _____

28. The patient's blood glucose level before breakfast is 250. What should you do? _____

   _____

29. The patient's blood glucose level before lunch is 150. How much insulin should you give now?

   _____

30. The patient's blood glucose level before dinner is 410. What should you do now?

   _____

After completing these problems, see pages 526–528 to check your answers.

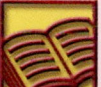

SUMMARY

You are now prepared to solve many of the dosage calculations you will encounter in your health care career. Oral and parenteral drug orders, written in the forms presented thus far, account for a large percentage of prescriptions. You have learned to think through the process from order to supply to amount administered and to apply the dosage calculation ratio-proportion method.

$$\frac{\text{Dosage on hand}}{\text{Amount on hand}} = \frac{\text{Dosage desired}}{\text{X Amount desired}}$$

Work the practice problems for Chapter 11. After completing the practice problems, you should feel comfortable and confident working dosage calculations. If not, seek additional instruction. Concentrate on accuracy. Remember, one error in dosage calculation can be a serious mistake for your patient.

CRITICAL THINKING SKILLS

Although the majority of concentrations of parenteral medication solutions are based on the dosage per 1 mL, some medications have 2 mL, 10 mL, or another volume as the quantity. Failing to identify the quantity of the supplied medication will result in an incorrect dose.

ERROR

Making the assumption that the dosage of the supplied medication was provided in a supply of 1 mL and failing to identify the correct volume to use as the *quantity* in the dosage calculation ratio-proportion.

Possible Scenario

A patient experienced nausea and vomiting following abdominal surgery. The doctor ordered *droperidol 0.5 mg IV slow push q.4h p.r.n., nausea and vomiting.* The nurse selected the correct medication from the stock supply and set up and calculated the dosage calculation as follows.

$$\frac{5 \text{ mg}}{1 \text{ mL}} \quad \bowtie \quad \frac{0.5 \text{ mg}}{X \text{ mL}}$$

$$5X = 0.5 \qquad \textbf{INCORRECT}$$

$$\frac{5X}{5} = \frac{0.5}{5}$$

$$X = 0.1 \text{ mL}$$

Assuming the supplied concentration was 5 mg per mL, the nurse incorrectly set up the first ratio as $\frac{5 \text{ mg}}{1 \text{ mL}}$. The 2 mL single-dose ampule was actually labeled in large letters as 5 mg/2 mL and in smaller letters (2.5 mg/mL). The dose the nurse administered was 0.1 mL. The **correct** calculation should have been either of the following.

$$\frac{5 \text{ mg}}{2 \text{ mL}} \quad \bowtie \quad \frac{0.5 \text{ mg}}{X \text{ mL}} \qquad \textbf{or} \qquad \frac{2.5 \text{ mg}}{1 \text{ mL}} \quad \bowtie \quad \frac{0.5 \text{ mg}}{X \text{ mL}}$$

$$5X = 1 \qquad\qquad 2.5X = 0.5$$

$$\frac{5X}{5} = \frac{1}{5} \qquad\qquad \frac{2.5X}{2.5} = \frac{0.5}{2.5}$$

$$X = 0.2 \text{ mL} \qquad\qquad X = 0.2 \text{ mL}$$

The correct amount to be administered was 0.2 mL. The patient received half the ordered dose. The patient stopped vomiting but continued with a significant amount of nausea. The nurse medicated the patient again as soon as the p.r.n. medication was due, but the patient experienced unnecessary discomfort in the meantime.

Potential Outcome

The nurse may have picked up the error the next time the medication was administered, but chances are that the same mistake would be repeated. The patient might again not have adequate relief of nausea and remain in significant discomfort. Not realizing that the patient received an incorrect dose, the nurse might contact the physician to increase the ordered dose for this patient. When the next nurse assigned to this patient calculated the correct volume of the increased dose, the patient could then be given a dose that was considerably higher than administered previously. With the higher dose, possibly ordered unnecessarily, the patient would be at greater risk for side effects and adverse reactions, such as increased sedation, hypotension, or tachycardia.

Prevention

The supply concentration always involves two values used in the first ratio—the dosage strength expressed as the weight of the drug per a certain volume or capacity amount, in this case 5 mg per 2 mL or 2.5 mg/mL. Carefully read the label to be sure you understand and copy down the correct supply dosage when setting up the proportion. Although drug labels often express the dosage strength of the drug as per 1 mL, do not assume that this is the case. Always read the label for the exact supply dosage strength or concentration.

CRITICAL THINKING SKILLS

Many insulin errors occur when the nurse fails to clarify an incomplete order. Let's look at an example of an insulin error when the order did not include the type of insulin to be given.

ERROR

Failing to clarify an insulin order when the type of insulin is not specified.

Possible Scenario

Suppose the physician who intended for a patient to receive NPH U-100 insulin, wrote an insulin order this way:

| Humulin U-100 insulin 50 units subcut a.c. breakfast | **INCORRECT** |

Because the physician did not specify the type of insulin, the nurse assumed it was regular insulin and noted that on the medication administration record. Suppose the patient was given the regular U-100 insulin instead of the insulin intended by the physician. Several hours later the patient developed signs of hypoglycemia (low blood glucose), including shakiness, tremors, confusion, and sweating.

Potential Outcome

A stat blood glucose would likely reveal a dangerously low glucose level. The patient would be given a glucose infusion to increase the blood sugar. The nurse may not realize the error until she and the doctor check the original order and find that the incomplete order was filled in by the nurse. When the doctor did not specify the type of insulin, the nurse assumed the physician meant regular, which is short-acting, when in fact intermediate-acting NPH insulin was desired.

Prevention

This error could have been avoided by remembering all the essential components of an insulin order: brand or generic name, type of insulin (such as regular or NPH), supply dosage, the amount to give in units, and the frequency. When you fill in an incomplete order, you are essentially practicing medicine without a license. This would be a clear malpractice incident. It does not make sense to put you and your patient in such jeopardy. A simple phone call would clarify the situation for everyone involved. Further, the nurse should have double-checked the dosage with another licensed practitioner. Had the nurse done so, the error could have been discovered prior to administration.

PRACTICE PROBLEMS—CHAPTER 11

Calculate the amount you will prepare for 1 dose. Indicate the syringe you will select to measure the medication.

1. Order: **Dilaudid 4 mg IV q.4h p.r.n., pain**

   Supply: Dilaudid 10 mg/mL

   Give: _____ mL   Select _____ syringe

2. Order: **morphine sulfate gr $\frac{1}{4}$ IV stat**

   Supply: morphine sulfate 10 mg/mL

   Give: _____ mL   Select _____ syringe

3. Order: Lanoxin 0.6 mg IV stat

   Supply: Lanoxin 500 mcg per 2 mL

   Give: _____ mL   Select _____ syringe

4. Order: hydroxyzine 15 mg IM stat

   Supply: hydroxyzine 25 mg/mL

   Give: _____ mL   Select _____ syringe

5. Order: Cleocin 300 mg IV q.i.d.

   Supply: Cleocin 0.6 g per 4 mL

   Give: _____ mL   Select _____ syringe

6. Order: Reglan 50 mg added to 50 mL IV PB bag as one time order to infuse over 30 min.

   Supply: 30 mL single-dose vial Reglan 5 mg/mL

   Give: _____ mL   Select _____ syringe

7. Order: hydroxyzine 40 mg IM q.4h p.r.n., agitation

   Supply: hydroxyzine 50 mg/mL

   Give: _____ mL   Select _____ syringe

8. Order: Valium 5 mg IV q.4h p.r.n., agitation

   Supply: Valium 10 mg per 2 mL

   Give: _____ mL   Select _____ syringe

9. Order: glycopyrrolate 200 mcg IM stat

   Supply: glycopyrolate 0.2 mg/mL

   Give: _____ mL   Select _____ syringe

10. Order: Dilantin 100 mg IV q.8h

    Supply: Dilantin 100 mg per 2 mL ampule

    Give: _____ mL   Select _____ syringe

11. Order: atropine gr $\frac{1}{100}$ IM on call to O.R.

    Supply: atropine 0.4 mg/mL

    Give: _____ mL   Select _____ syringe

12. Order: Valium 3 mg IV stat

    Supply: Valium 10 mg per 2 mL

    Give: _____ mL   Select _____ syringe

13. Order: heparin 6,000 units subcut q.12h

    Supply: heparin 10,000 units/mL vial

    Give: _____ mL   Select _____ syringe

14. Order: **tobramycin sulfate 75 mg IV q.8h**

    Supply: tobramycin sulfate 40 mg/mL

    Give: _____ mL   Select _____ syringe

15. Order: **morphine sulfate gr $\frac{1}{10}$ IV q.3h p.r.n., pain**

    Supply: morphine sulfate 10 mg/mL ampule

    Give: _____ mL   Select _____ syringe

16. Order: **atropine gr $\frac{1}{150}$ IM on call to O.R.**

    Supply: atropine 0.4 mg/mL

    Give: _____ mL   Select _____ syringe

17. Order: **ketorolac 20 mg IV q.6h p.r.n., severe pain**

    Supply: ketorolac 30 mg/mL

    Give: _____ mL   Select _____ syringe

18. Order: **gentamicin 40 mg IV q.8h**

    Supply: gentamicin 80 mg per 2 mL

    Give: _____ mL   Select _____ syringe

19. Order: **hydromorphone 3 mg IV q.4h p.r.n., pain**

    Supply: hydromorphone 10 mg/mL

    Give: _____ mL   Select _____ syringe

20. Order: **morphine sulfate 8 mg IV q.4h p.r.n., pain**

    Supply: morphine sulfate 5 mg/mL

    Give: _____ mL   Select: _____ syringe

21. Order: **vitamin B$_{12}$ 0.75 mg IM daily**

    Supply: vitamin B$_{12}$ 1,000 mcg/mL

    Give: _____ mL   Select _____ syringe

22. Order: **phytonadione 15 mg IM stat**

    Supply: phytonadione 10 mg/mL

    Give: _____ mL   Select _____ syringe

23. Order: **promethazine 35 mg IM q.4h p.r.n., nausea and vomiting**

    Supply: promethazine 50 mg/mL

    Give: _____ mL   Select _____ syringe

24. Order: **heparin 8,000 units subcut stat**

    Supply: heparin 10,000 units/mL

    Give: _____ mL   Select _____ syringe

25. Order: **morphine sulfate gr $\frac{1}{6}$ subcut q.4h p.r.n., pain**

    Supply: morphine sulfate 8 mg/mL

    Give: _____ mL   Select _____ syringe

26. Order: **Lanoxin 0.4 mg IV stat**

    Supply: Lanoxin 500 mcg per 2 mL

    Give: _____ mL   Select _____ syringe

27. Order: **Lasix 60 mg IV stat**

    Supply: Lasix 20 mg per 2 mL ampule

    Give: _____ mL   Select _____ syringe

28. Order: **heparin 4,000 units subcut q.6h**

    Supply: heparin 5,000 units/mL

    Give: _____ mL   Select _____ syringe

29. Order: **hydralazine 30 mg IV q.6h**

    Supply: hydralazine 20 mg/mL

    Give: _____ mL   Select _____ syringe

30. Order: **lidocaine 50 mg IV stat**

    Supply: lidocaine 2%

    Give: _____ mL   Select _____ syringe

31. Order: **verapamil 4 mg IV push stat**

    Supply: verapamil 2.5 mg/mL

    Give: _____ mL   Select _____ syringe

32. Order: **heparin 3,500 units subcut q.12h**

    Supply: heparin 5,000 units/mL

    Give: _____ mL   Select _____ syringe

33. Order: **neostigmine 0.5 mg IM stat**

    Supply: neostigmine 1:2,000

    Give: _____ mL   Select _____ syringe

34. Order: **Cipro 100 mg added to 100 mL IV PB q.12h**

    Supply: Cipro 400 mg per 40 mL

    Give: _____ mL   Select _____ syringe

35. Order: **Novolin R regular U-100 insulin 16 units subcut a.c.**

    Supply: Novolin R regular U-100 insulin, with Standard 100 units and Lo-Dose 30 units U-100 insulin syringes

    Give: _____ units   Select _____ syringe

36. Order: Novolin N NPH U-100 insulin 25 units subcut ā breakfast

    Supply: Novolin N NPH U-100 insulin with Standard 100 units and Lo-Dose 50 units U-100 insulin syringes

    Give: _____ units   Select _____ syringe

Calculate 1 dose of each of the drug orders numbered 37 through 48. Draw an arrow on the syringe indicating the calibration line that corresponds to the dose to be administered. The labels provided on pages 241–242 are the medications you have available. Indicate dosages that must be divided.

37. haloperidol decanoate 150 mg IM monthly

    Give: _____ mL

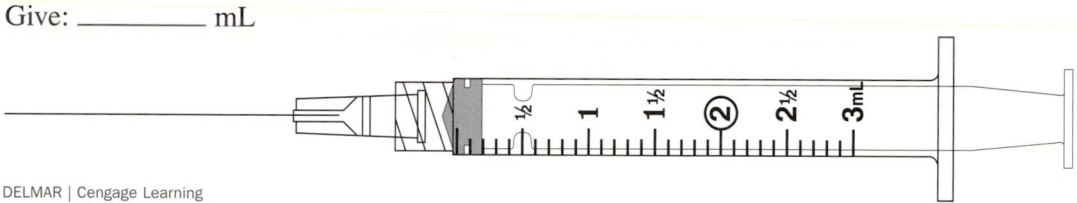

DELMAR | Cengage Learning

38. gentamicin 50 mg IV q.8h

    Give: _____ mL

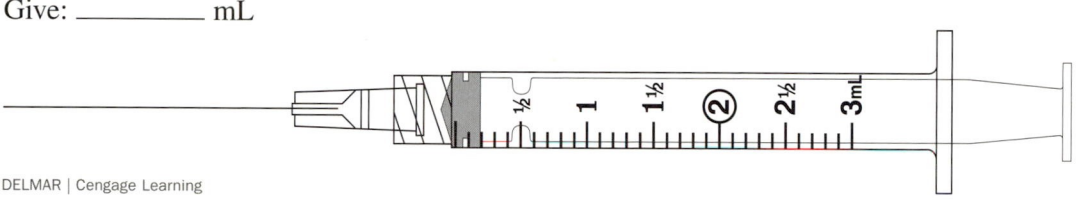

DELMAR | Cengage Learning

39. Inapsine 1 mg IV stat

    Give: _____ mL

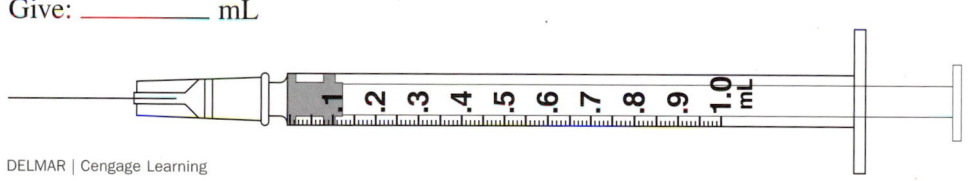

DELMAR | Cengage Learning

40. furosemide 15 mg IV stat

    Give: _____ mL

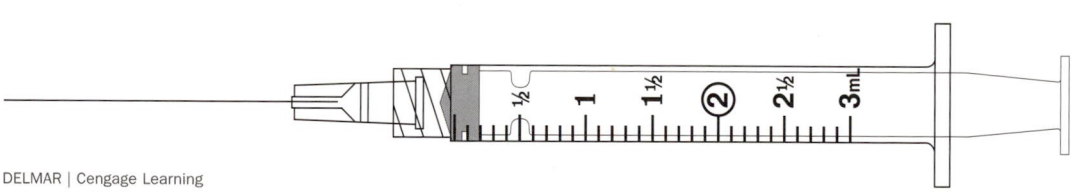

DELMAR | Cengage Learning

41. naloxone 0.2 mg IV stat

    Give: _____ mL

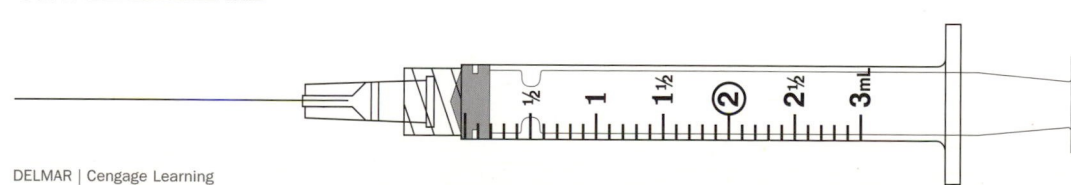

DELMAR | Cengage Learning

42. Humulin R regular U-100 insulin 22 units subcut stat

    Give: _____ units

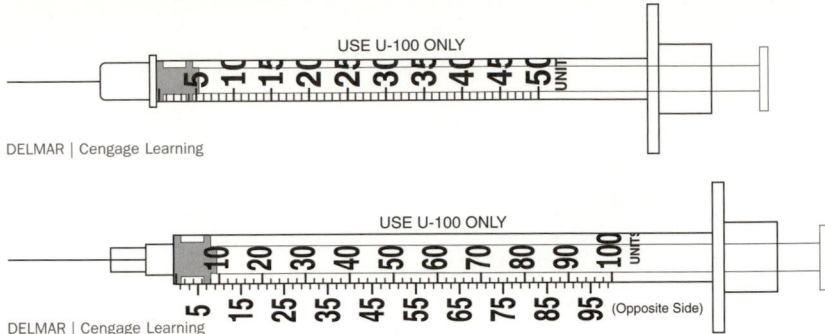

DELMAR | Cengage Learning

43. ketoralac 24 mg IV q.6h p.r.n., pain

    Give: _____ mL

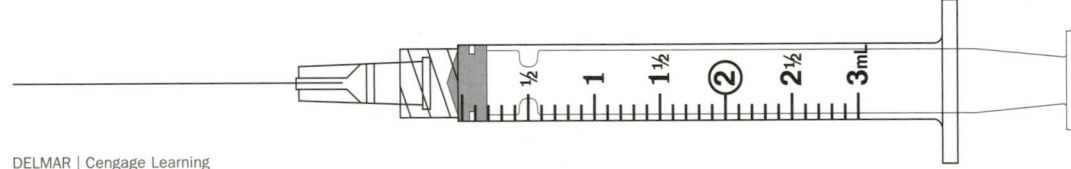

DELMAR | Cengage Learning

44. promethazine 15 mg IM q.4h p.r.n., nausea and vomiting

    Give: _____ mL

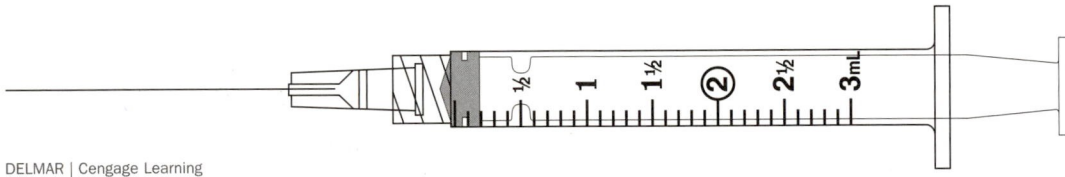

DELMAR | Cengage Learning

45. nitroglycerin 25 mg added to 100 mL IV piggyback, titrate according to standard protocol

    Give: _____ mL

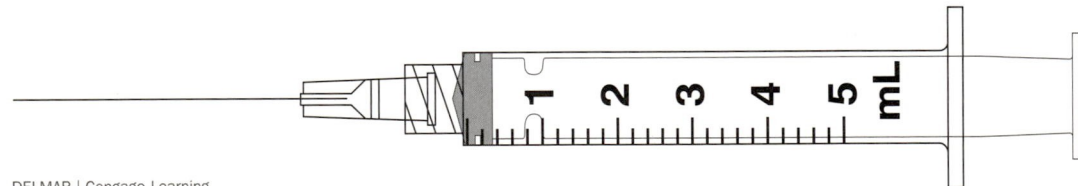

DELMAR | Cengage Learning

46. cyanocobalamin 250 mcg IM daily × 7 days

    Give: _____ mL

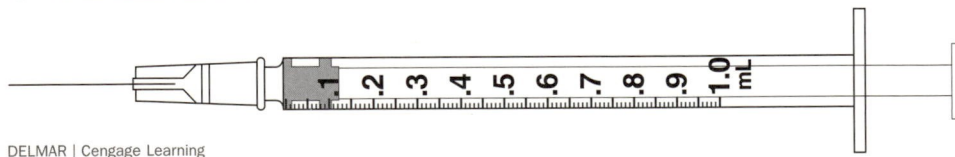

DELMAR | Cengage Learning

47. Novolin R regular U-100 insulin 32 units with Novolin N NPH U-100 insulin 54 units subcut ā breakfast

    Give: _____ total units

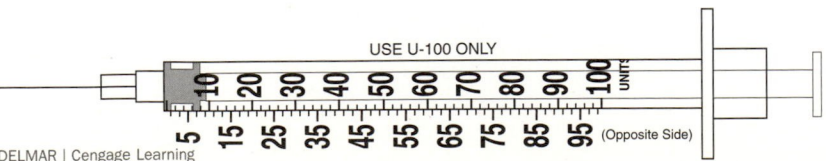

DELMAR | Cengage Learning

48. Novolin 70/30 U-100 insulin 46 units subcut c̄ dinner

Give: _____ units

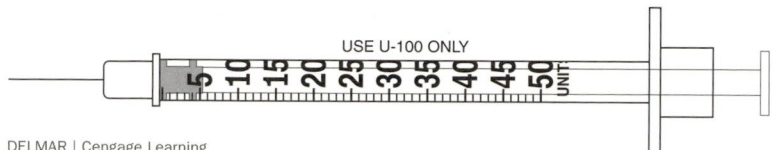

USE U-100 ONLY

DELMAR | Cengage Learning

Used with permission from American Regent, Inc.

NDC 0517-5702-25
FUROSEMIDE
INJECTION, USP

20 mg/ 2 mL
(10 mg/mL)

2 mL
SINGLE DOSE VIAL
FOR IV OR IM USE

Rx Only
AMERICAN REGENT, INC.
SHIRLEY, NY 11967

WARNING: USE ONLY IF SOLUTION IS CLEAR AND COLORLESS. PROTECT FROM LIGHT.
Store at controlled Room Temperature: 15°-30°C (59°-86°F) (See USP).
Directions for use:
See Package insert.
Rev. 1/05

Lot / Exp.

Reprinted with permission of APP Pharmaceuticals, LLC

NDC 63323-010-20   1020

GENTAMICIN

INJECTION, USP
equivalent to

40 mg/mL

Gentamicin   Rx only
For IM or IV Use.
Must be diluted for IV use.

20 mL Multiple Dose Vial

Sterile

Each mL contains: Gentamicin sulfate equivalent to 40 mg gentamicin; 1.8 mg methylparaben and 0.2 mg propylparaben as preservatives; 3.2 mg sodium metabisulfite; 0.1 mg disodium edetate; Water for Injection q.s. Sodium hydroxide and/or sulfuric acid may have been added for pH adjustment. Usual Dosage: See insert.
Warning: Patients treated with gentamicin sulfate and other aminoglycosides should be under close observation because of the potential toxicity. See Warnings and Precautions in the insert.
Store at 20° to 25°C (68° to 77°F) [see USP Controlled Room Temperature].

APP
APP Pharmaceuticals, LLC
Schaumburg, IL 60173

401897D

LOT/EXP

3 63323-010-20 1

Used with permission from Bedford Laboratories. A Division of Ben Venue Laboratories. A Boehringer-Ingelheim Company.

KETOROLAC
TROMETHAMINE
INJECTION USP

30 mg/mL
1 mL Vial

FOR IM OR IV USE ONLY

NDC 55390-481-01
1 mL Single-dose Vial
Protect from light.
Rx ONLY

Manufactured for:
Bedford Laboratories™
Bedford, OH 44146

KC- KRLVA03

© Novo Nordisk Inc. Reprinted with permission. ® Novolin is a registered trademark of Novo Nordisk Inc.

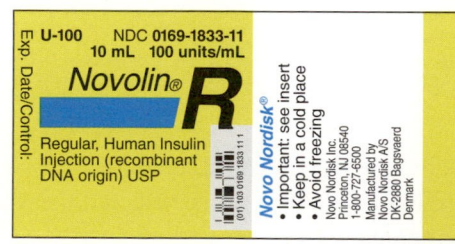

Exp. Date/Control:

U-100   NDC 0169-1833-11
10 mL   100 units/mL

Novolin **R**

Novo Nordisk®
• **Important: see insert**
• Keep in a cold place
• Avoid freezing

Regular, Human Insulin Injection (recombinant DNA origin) USP

Novo Nordisk Inc.
Princeton, NJ 08540
1-800-727-6500
Manufactured by
Novo Nordisk A/S
DK-2880 Bagsvaerd
Denmark

(01) 103 0169 1833 11 1

© Novo Nordisk Inc. Reprinted with permission. ® Novolin is a registered trademark of Novo Nordisk Inc.

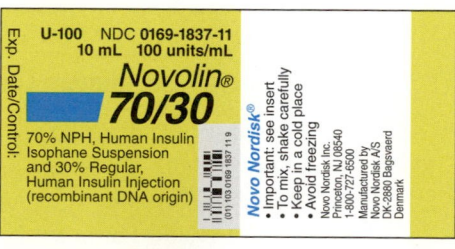

Exp. Date/Control:

U-100   NDC 0169-1837-11
10 mL   100 units/mL

Novolin **70/30**

Novo Nordisk®
• **Important: see insert**
• To mix, shake carefully
• Keep in a cold place
• Avoid freezing

70% NPH, Human Insulin Isophane Suspension and 30% Regular, Human Insulin Injection (recombinant DNA origin)

Novo Nordisk Inc.
Princeton, NJ 08540
1-800-727-6500
Manufactured by
Novo Nordisk A/S
DK-2880 Bagsvaerd
Denmark

(01) 103 0169 1837 11 9

Used with permission from Teva Pharmaceuticals USA

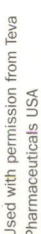

Do not refrigerate or freeze.
PROTECT FROM LIGHT.
Retain in carton until contents are used.

NDC 0703-7023-01   ℞only

Haloperidol
Decanoate Injection
100 mg*/mL
* as haloperidol

IM Use Only
5 mL Multiple Dose Vial
Sterile

sicor™ SICOR Pharmaceuticals, Inc., Irvine, CA 92618

Usual Dosage: See Package Insert.
The dose of haloperidol decanoate should be expressed in terms of its haloperidol content.
Store at controlled room temperature 15°–30°C (59° to 86°F).

702304

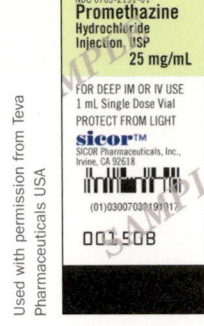

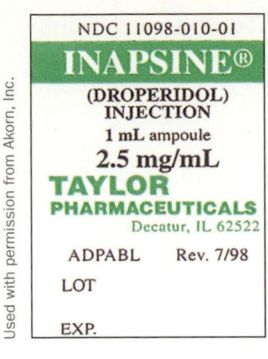

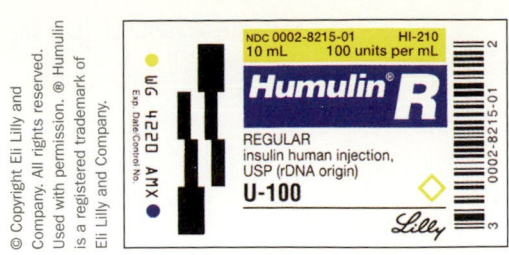

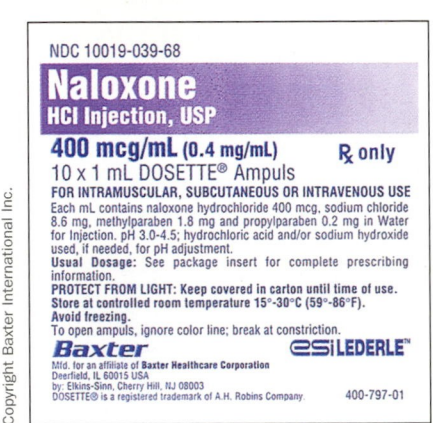

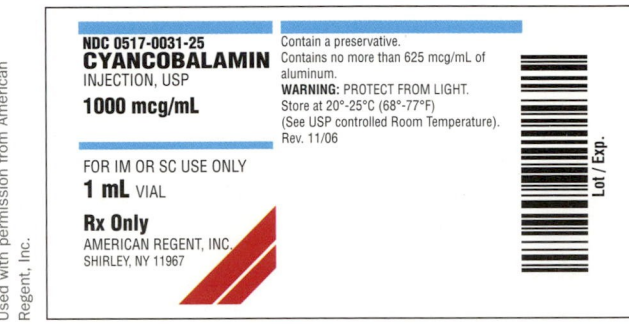

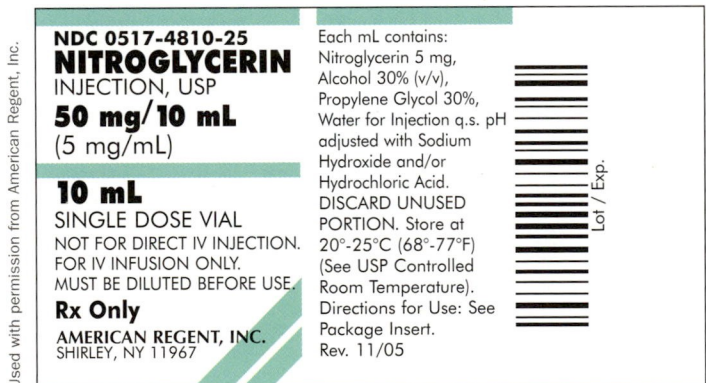

49. Describe the strategy you would implement to prevent this medication error.

Possible Scenario

Suppose the physician ordered Humulin R U-100 insulin 40 units mixed with Humulin N U-100 insulin 20 units to be administered subcut before breakfast. The nurse selected the vials of Humulin R and Humulin N U-100 insulin from the medication drawer and injected 40 units of air in the Humulin N vial and 20 units of air in the Humulin R vial, drew up 20 units of Humulin R, and then drew up 40 units of Humulin N.

Potential Outcome

The patient received the incorrect dosage of insulin because the nurse drew up 20 units of Humulin R and 40 units of Humulin N instead of the dosage that was ordered: 40 units of Humulin R and 20 units of Humulin N. Because the patient received too little short-acting insulin (one-half the amount ordered), the patient would likely show signs of hyperglycemia, such as urinary frequency, thirst, and potential visual changes. Not only would this patient feel uncomfortable at the time of the hyperglycemia, it would also be more difficult for the physician to get control of the patient's blood sugars in the future. Also, the increased dose of NPH insulin may put the patient at risk for hypoglycemia later in the day, and high blood sugars may increase the risk of infection.

Prevention

_____

_____

50. Describe the strategy you would implement to prevent this medication error.

Possible Scenario

Suppose the physician ordered **Novolin R U-100 insulin 10 units subcut stat** for a patient with a blood glucose of 300. The nurse selected the Novolin R U-100 insulin from the patient's medication drawer and selected a 1 mL syringe to administer the dose. The nurse looked at the syringe for the 10 unit mark and was confused as to how much should have been drawn up. The nurse finally decided to draw up 1 mL of insulin into the syringe, administered the dose, and then began to question whether the correct dosage was administered. The nurse called the supervisor for advice.

Potential Outcome

The patient would have received 10 times the correct dosage of insulin. Because this was a short-acting insulin, the patient would likely show signs of severe hypoglycemia, such as loss of consciousness, seizures, myocardial infarction, and potential death. There is substantial risk of harm for this patient.

Prevention

_____

_____

After completing these problems, see pages 528–531 to check your answers.

REFERENCES

Cohen, H. (2007). Protecting patients from harm: Reduce the risk of high alert drugs. _Nursing2007_, September 2007, p. 49-55.

Institute for Safe Medication Practices. (2008). ISMP's list of high alert medications. Retrieved October 4, 2009 from http://www.ismp.org/Tools/highalertmedications.pdf

McCulloch, D. (2008). General principles of insulin therapy in diabetes mellitus. _Up to Date_. www.uptodate.com. Section Editor: Nathan, D. Deputy Editor: Mulder, J. Last updated Oct 26, 2007; last literature review Oct 1, 2008. Retrieved February 28, 2009.

Onufer, C. (2002). Could you be in danger?: Insulin. The #1 drug error in hospitals. _Diabetes Health_. Retrieved October 4, 2009 from http://www.diabeteshealth.com/read/2002/11/01/3039/could-u-be-in-danger-insulin--the-1-drug-error-in-hospitals/

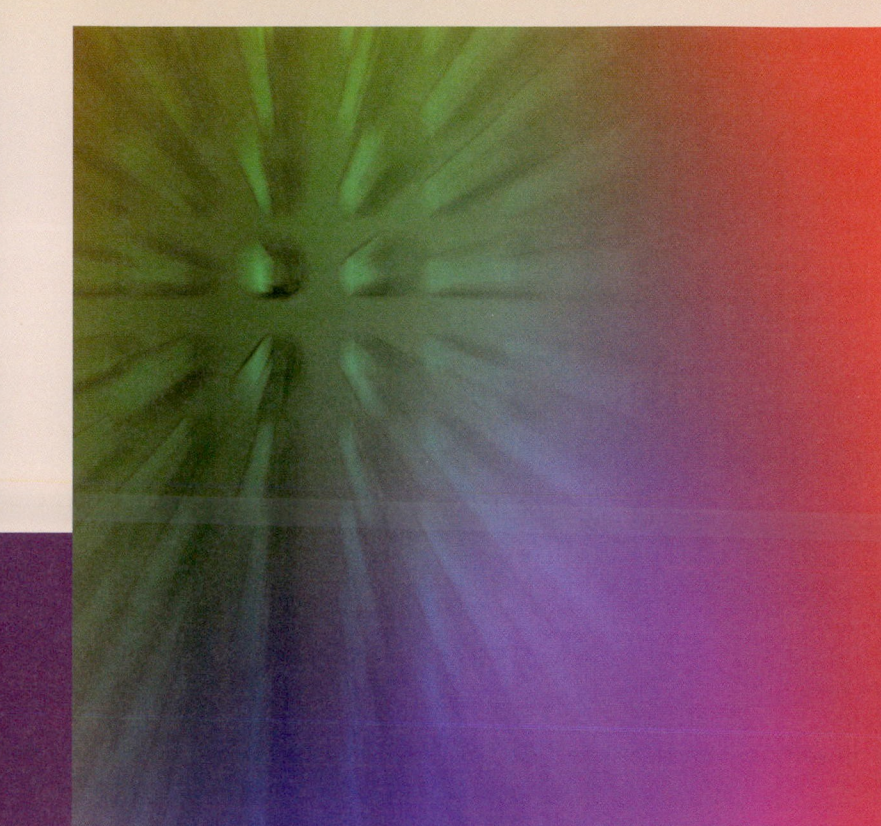

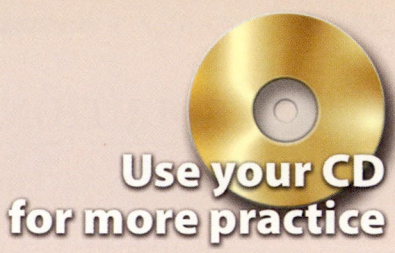
Use your CD
for more practice

12

Reconstitution of Solutions

OBJECTIVES

Upon mastery of Chapter 12, you will be prepared to reconstitute injectable and noninjectable solutions. To accomplish this you will also be able to:

- Define and apply the terms *solvent (diluent), solute,* and *solution.*
- Reconstitute and label medications supplied in powder or dry form.
- Differentiate between varying directions for reconstitution and select the correct set to prepare the dosage ordered.
- Calculate the amount of solute and solvent needed to prepare a desired strength and quantity of an irrigating solution or enteral feeding.

Some parenteral medications are supplied in powder form and must be mixed with water or some other liquid before administration. As more health care is provided in the home setting, nurses and other health care workers must dilute topical irrigants, soaks, and nutritional feedings. This process of mixing and diluting solutions is referred to as *reconstitution.*

The process of reconstitution is comparable to the preparation of hot chocolate from a powdered mix. By adding the correct amount of hot water (referred to as the *solvent* or *diluent*) to the package of powdered hot chocolate drink mix (referred to as the *solute*), you prepare a tasty, hot beverage (the resulting *solution*).

The properties of solutions are important concepts to understand. Learn them well now because we will apply them again when we examine intravenous solutions.

SOLUTION PROPERTIES

As you look at Figures 12-1 and 12-2, let's define the terms of reconstitution.

FIGURE 12-1   Concentrated liquid solute: 50 milliliters of concentrated solute diluted with 50 milliliters of solvent make 100 milliliters of diluted solution

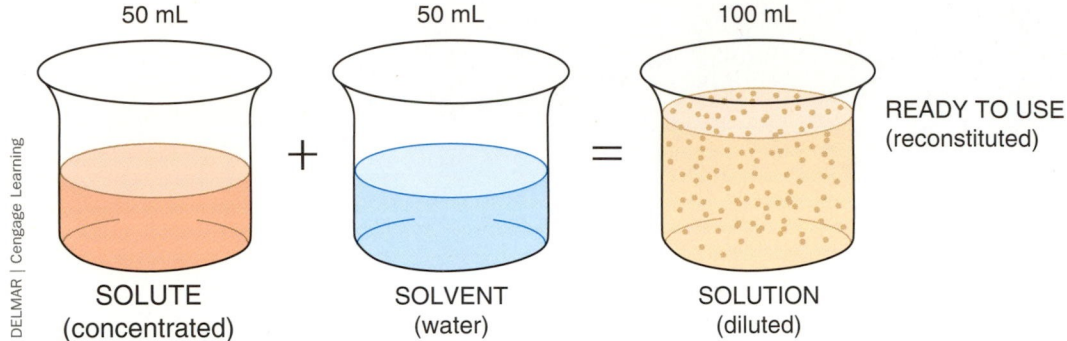

50 mL   50 mL   100 mL

SOLUTE
(concentrated)
+
SOLVENT
(water)
=
SOLUTION
(diluted)

READY TO USE
(reconstituted)

DELMAR | Cengage Learning

FIGURE 12-2(a)   Solid solute: The solid powder form of 500 mg of Zithromax is reconstituted with 4.8 mL of sterile water as the diluent to make 5 mL of Zithromax IV solution with the supply dosage of 100 mg/mL

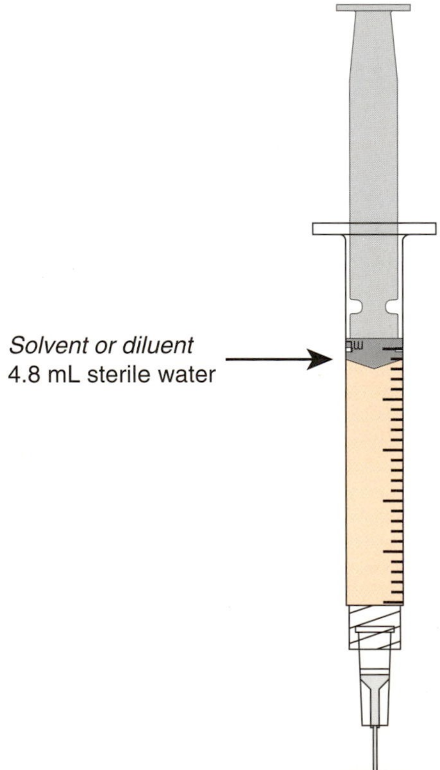

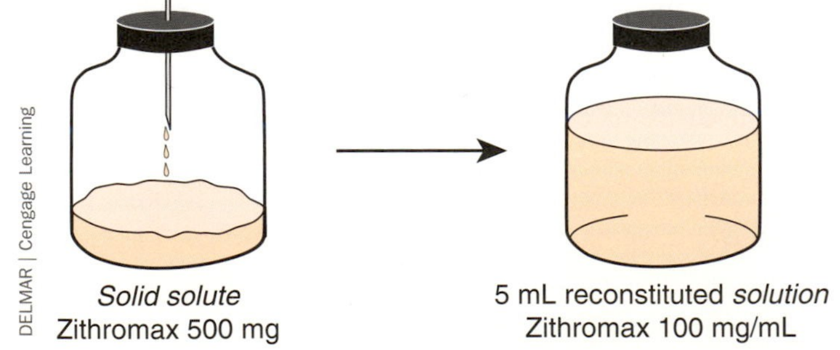

FIGURE 12-2(b)   Zithromax 500 mg label

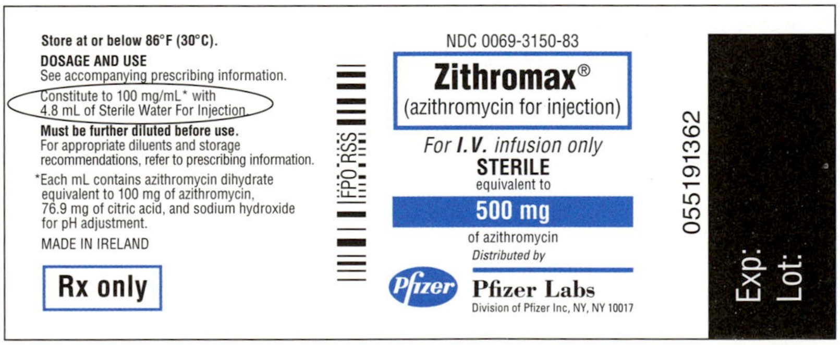

Solvent or diluent
4.8 mL sterile water

Used with permission from Pfizer Inc.

Store at or below 86°F (30°C).
DOSAGE AND USE
See accompanying prescribing information.
Constitute to 100 mg/mL* with
4.8 mL of Sterile Water For Injection.
Must be further diluted before use.
For appropriate diluents and storage
recommendations, refer to prescribing information.
*Each mL contains azithromycin dihydrate
equivalent to 100 mg of azithromycin,
76.9 mg of citric acid, and sodium hydroxide
for pH adjustment.
MADE IN IRELAND

Rx only

NDC 0069-3150-83

Zithromax®
(azithromycin for injection)

For I.V. infusion only
STERILE
equivalent to
500 mg
of azithromycin
Distributed by
Pfizer **Pfizer Labs**
Division of Pfizer Inc, NY, NY 10017

055191362

Exp:
Lot:

Solid solute
Zithromax 500 mg

5 mL reconstituted *solution*
Zithromax 100 mg/mL

DELMAR | Cengage Learning

- *Solute*—a substance to be dissolved or diluted. It can be in solid or liquid form.

- *Solvent*—a substance (liquid) that dissolves another substance to prepare a solution. *Diluent* is a synonymous term.

- *Solution*—the resulting mixture of a solute plus a solvent.

To prepare a therapeutic solution, you will add a solvent or diluent (usually normal saline or water) to a solute (solid substance or concentrated stock solution) to obtain the required strength of a stated volume of a solution. This means that the solid substance or concentrate, called a solute, is diluted with a solvent to obtain a reconstituted solution of a weaker strength. However, the amount of the drug that was in the pure solute or concentrated stock solution still equals the amount of pure drug in the diluted solution. Only the solvent has been added to the solute, expanding the total volume.

Figure 12-1 shows that the amount of pure drug (solute) remains the same in the concentrated form and in the resulting solution. However, in solution, notice the solute particles are dispersed or suspended throughout the resulting weaker solution. The particles evident in Figure 12-1 are for illustration purposes only. In a solution, the solute would be dissolved.

The *strength* of a solution or *concentration* was briefly discussed in Chapters 8 and 10. Solution strength indicates the ratio of solute to solvent. Consider how each of these substances—solute and solvent—contributes a certain number of parts to the total solution.

Look at the Zithromax 500 mg label (Figure 12-2b). The label directions indicate that 4.8 mL of sterile water (solvent) should be added to the powder (solid solute) to prepare the reconstituted solution. As the label indicates, the resulting supply dosage would be 100 mg of Zithromax per 1 mL of solution.

Let's thoroughly examine the reconstitution of powdered injectable medications.

RECONSTITUTION OF INJECTABLE MEDICATIONS IN POWDER FORM

Some medications are unstable when stored in solution or liquid form. Thus they are packaged in powdered form and must be dissolved or reconstituted by a liquid solvent or diluent and mixed thoroughly. Reconstitution is a necessary step in medication preparation to create a measurable and usable dosage form. The pharmacist often does this before dispensing liquid medications, for oral as well as parenteral routes. However, nurses need to understand reconstitution and know how to accomplish it. Some medications must be prepared by the nurse just prior to administration because they become unstable when stored in solution form.

CAUTION

Before reconstituting injectable drugs, read and follow the label or package insert directions carefully, including checking the drug and diluent expiration dates. Consult a pharmacist with any questions.

Let's look at the rules for reconstituting injectable medications from powder to liquid form. Follow these rules carefully to ensure that the patient receives the correct dosage of the intended solution.

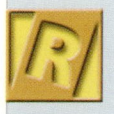

RULE

When reconstituting injectable medications, you must determine both the type and amount of diluent to be used.

Some powdered medications are packaged by the manufacturer with special diluents for reconstitution. Sterile water and 0.9% sodium chloride (normal saline) are most commonly used as diluents in

FIGURE 12-3 Reconstitution diluent for parenteral powdered drugs

ⓐ **20 mL** Single-dose
Sterile Water
for Inj., USP
FOR DRUG DILUENT USE
◀◀◀ *ABBOTT LABORATORIES, NORTH CHICAGO, IL60064, USA*

NDC 0074-4887-20
Contains no antimicrobial or other added substance. Sterile, nonpyrogenic. Do not give intravenously unless rendered nearly isotonic. Caution: Federal (USA) law prohibits dispensing without prescription.   06-6360-2/R6-3/89

parenteral medications. Both sterile water (Figure 12-3) and normal saline are available *preservative-free* when intended for a single use only, as well as in *bacteriostatic* form with preservative when intended for more than one use. Carefully check the instructions, expiration date, and vial label for the appropriate diluent.

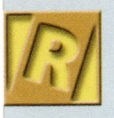

RULE
When reconstituting injectable medications, you must determine the volume in mL of diluent to be used for the route as ordered, then reconstitute the drug and note the resulting supply dosage on the vial.

Because many reconstituted parenteral medications can be administered either intramuscularly (IM) or intravenously (IV), it is essential to verify the route of administration before reconstituting the medication. Remember that the intramuscular volume of 3 mL or less per adult injection site (or 2 mL if deltoid site) is determined by the patient's age and condition and the intramuscular site selected. The directions take this into account by stating the minimum volume or quantity of diluent that should be added to the powdered drug for IM use. Often the powdered drug itself adds volume to the solution. The powder displaces the liquid as it dissolves and increases the total resulting volume. The resulting volume of the reconstituted drug is usually given on the label. This resulting volume determines the liquid's concentration or supply dosage.

Look at the directions on the cefazolin label (Figure 12-4a). It states, "To prepare solution add 2 mL Sterile Water for Injection or 0.9% Sodium Chloride Injection. Provides an approximate volume of 2.2 mL (225 mg per mL)." Notice that when 2 mL of diluent are added and the powder is dissolved, the bulk of the powder adds an additional 0.2 mL for a total solution volume of 2.2 mL. (The amount of diluent added will vary with each medication.) Thus, the supply dosage available after reconstitution is *225 mg of cefazolin per mL of solution*. Figure 12-4 demonstrates the reconstitution procedure for cefazolin 500 mg, to fill the order of **cefazolin 225 mg IV q.6h.**

Single-dose vials contain only enough medication for 1 dose, and the resulting contents are administered after the powder is diluted. But in some cases the nurse also may dilute a powdered medication in a multiple-dose vial that will yield more than 1 dose. When this is the case, it is important to clearly label the vial after reconstitution. Labeling is discussed in the next section.

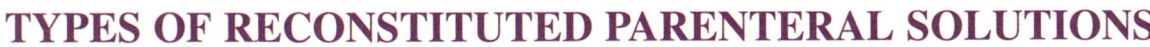

TYPES OF RECONSTITUTED PARENTERAL SOLUTIONS

There are two types of reconstituted parenteral solutions: single strength and multiple strength. The simplest type to dilute is a *single-strength* solution. This type usually has the recommended dilution directions and resulting supply dosage printed on the label, such as the cefazolin 500 mg label in Figure 12-4 and the Zithromax label in Figure 12-5a.

Some medications have several directions for dilution that allow the nurse to select the best supply dosage. This is called a *multiple-strength* solution and requires even more careful reading of the instructions, such as the Pfizerpen label shown in Figure 12-5b. Sometimes these directions for reconstitution will not fit on the vial label. You must consult the package insert or other printed instructions to ensure accurate dilution of the parenteral medication.

Let's look at some examples to clarify what the health care professional needs to do to correctly reconstitute and calculate dosages of parenteral medications supplied in powder form.

FIGURE 12-4(a) Cefazolin 500 mg powder

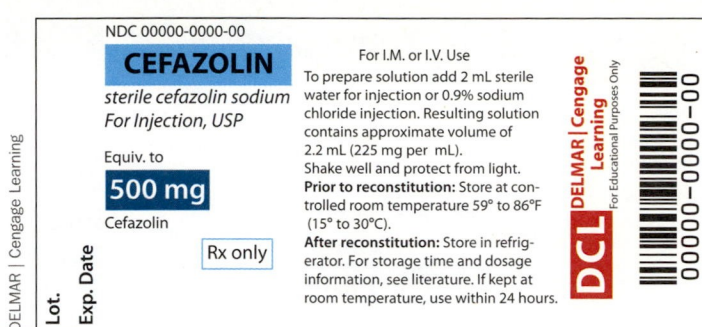

FIGURE 12-4(b) Cefazolin reconstitution procedure to fill the order
cefazolin 225 mg IV q.6h

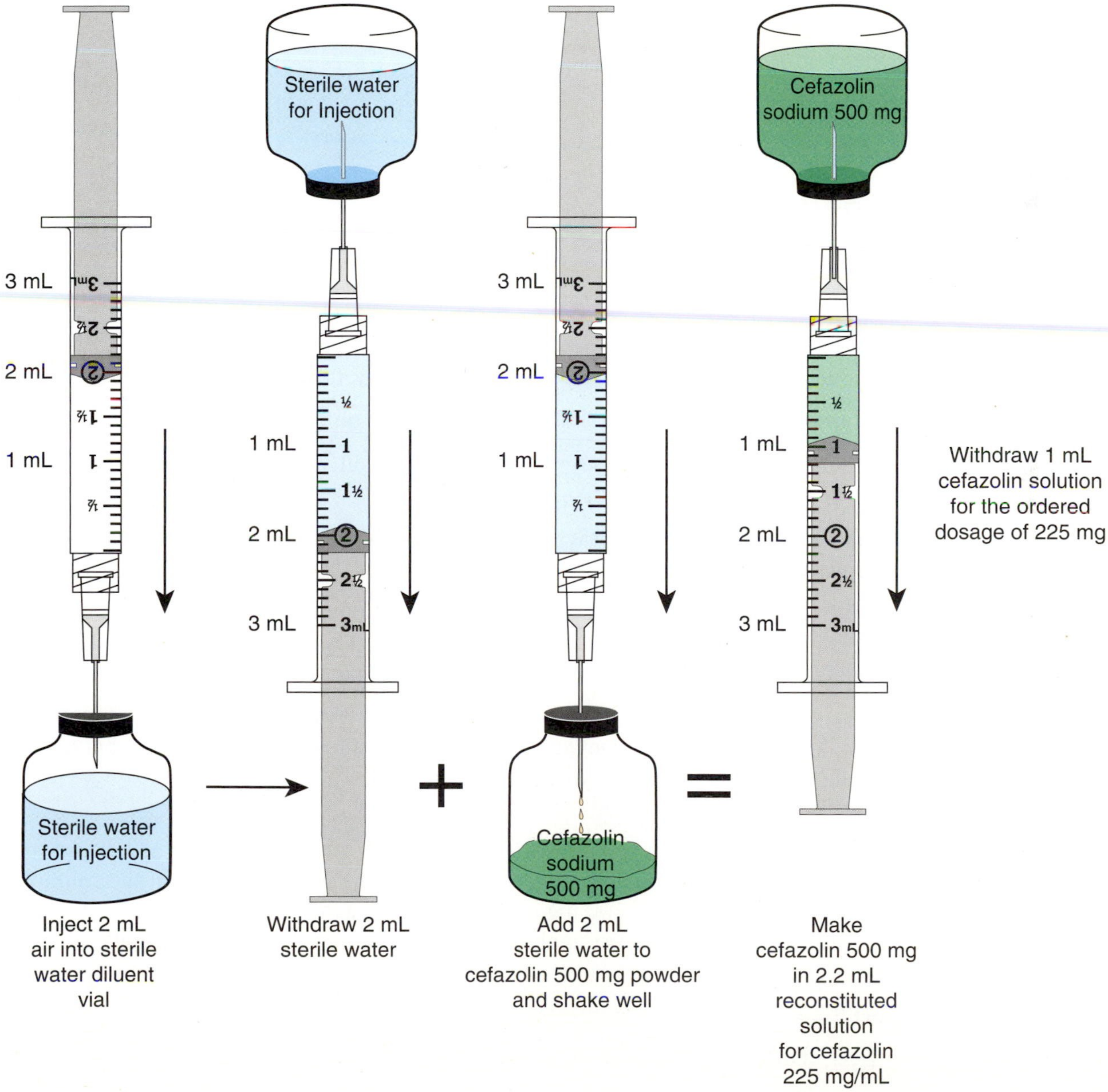

Sterile water
for Injection

Cefazolin
sodium 500 mg

Withdraw 1 mL
cefazolin solution
for the ordered
dosage of 225 mg

Sterile water
for Injection

Cefazolin
sodium
500 mg

Inject 2 mL
air into sterile
water diluent
vial

Withdraw 2 mL
sterile water

Add 2 mL
sterile water to
cefazolin 500 mg powder
and shake well

Make
cefazolin 500 mg
in 2.2 mL
reconstituted
solution
for cefazolin
225 mg/mL

FIGURE 12-5(a) Zithromax label: single-strength solution

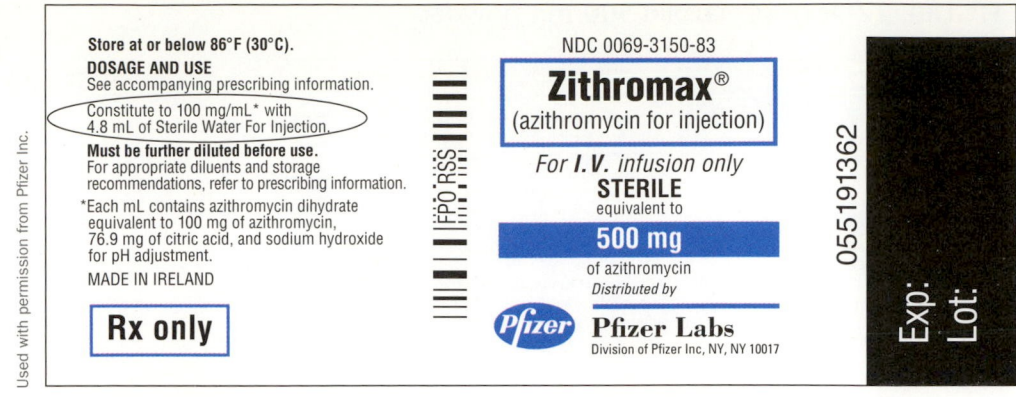

FIGURE 12-5(b) Pfizerpen label: multiple-strength solution

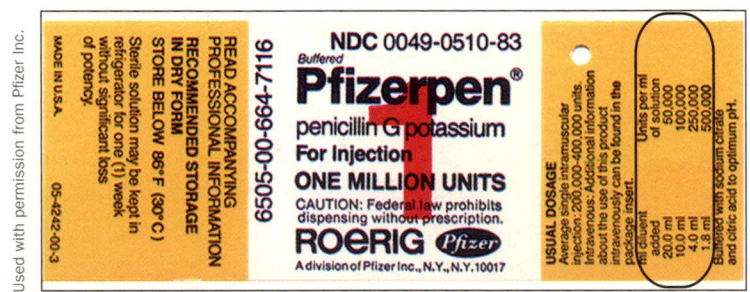

Single-Strength Solution

EXAMPLE 1 ■

Order: **Zithromax 400 mg IV daily × 2 days**

Supply: 500 mg vial of powdered Zithromax with directions on the left side of the label that state, "Constitute to 100 mg/mL with 4.8 mL of Sterile Water for injection;" See Figure 12-5(a).

Carefully sort through and analyze the information provided on the label.

■ First, how much and what type of diluent must you add? The directions state to *add 4.8 mL of Sterile Water.*

■ Second, what is the resulting supply dosage or concentration? When reconstituted, the *supply dosage is Zithromax 100 mg/mL.*

■ Third, what is the resulting total volume of the reconstituted solution? The *total volume is 5 mL.* The powder added 0.2 mL to the solution. You know this because the supply dosage is 100 mg/mL, and you added 4.8 mL of diluent. Therefore, it is only logical that the total volume is 5 mL.

■ Finally, to fill the order as prescribed, how many full doses are available in this vial? The order is for 400 mg, and the single-dose vial contains 500 mg. This is enough for 1 full dose, but not enough for 2 full doses. Two doses would require 800 mg.

Now, let's put it all together.

This means you have available a vial of 500 mg of Zithromax to which you will add 4.8 mL of sterile water as the diluent. The powdered drug displaces 0.2 mL. The resulting 5 mL of the solution contains 500 mg of the drug, and there are 100 mg of Zithromax in each 1 mL of solution.

After reconstitution, you are ready to apply the same three steps of dosage calculation that you learned in Chapters 10 and 11.

Step 1	**Convert**	No conversion is necessary.
		Order: **Zithromax 400 mg IV daily × 2 days**
		Supply: 100 mg/mL
Step 2	**Think**	You want to give more than 1 mL. In fact, you want to give 4 times 1 mL.

Step 3 **Calculate** $\dfrac{\text{Dosage on hand}}{\text{Amount on hand}} = \dfrac{\text{Dosage desired}}{\text{X Amount desired}}$

$\dfrac{100 \text{ mg}}{1 \text{ mL}} \quad\diagdown\!\!\!\!\!\diagup\quad \dfrac{400 \text{ mg}}{\text{X mL}}$ Cross-multiply

$100X = 400$

$\dfrac{100X}{100} = \dfrac{400}{100}$ Simplify: Divide both sides of the equation by the number before the unknown X

$X = 4 \text{ mL}$ Label the units to match the unknown X

Give 4 mL Zithromax reconstituted to 100 mg/mL, intravenously each day for 2 days. The dose would be further diluted in an IV solution.

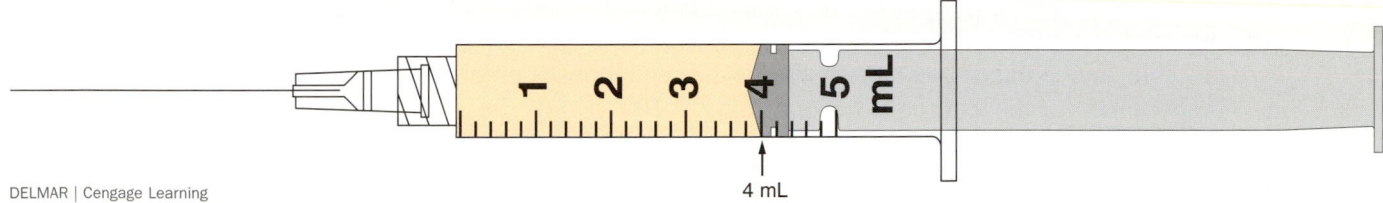

4 mL

This vial of Zithromax 500 mg contains only 1 full ordered dose of reconstituted drug. Any remaining medication is usually discarded. Because this vial provides only 1 dose, you will not have to label and store any of the reconstituted drug.

EXAMPLE 2 ■

Suppose the drug order reads **Zithromax 250 mg IV daily.**

Using the same size vial of Zithromax and the same dilution instructions as in the previous example, you would now have 2 full doses of Zithromax, making this a *multiple-dose vial*. The supply is the same, 100 mg/mL.

$\dfrac{\text{Dosage on hand}}{\text{Amount on hand}} = \dfrac{\text{Dosage desired}}{\text{X Amount desired}}$

$\dfrac{100 \text{ mg}}{1 \text{ mL}} \quad\diagdown\!\!\!\!\!\diagup\quad \dfrac{250 \text{ mg}}{\text{X mL}}$ Cross-multiply

$100X = 250$

$\dfrac{100X}{100} = \dfrac{250}{100}$ Simplify: Divide both sides of the equation by the number before the unknown X

$X = 2.5 \text{ mL}$ Label the units to match the unknown X

Select a 3 mL syringe and measure 2.5 mL of Zithromax reconstituted to 100 mg/mL.

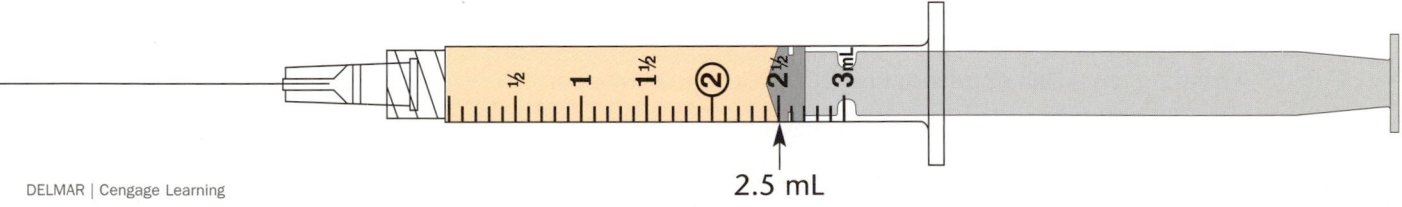

2.5 mL

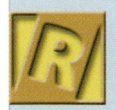

RULE

When reconstituting multiple-dose injectable medications, verify the length of drug potency. Store the reconstituted drug appropriately with a reconstitution label attached.

If multiple doses result from the reconstitution of a powdered drug, the solution must be used in a timely manner. Because the drug potency (or stability) may be several hours to several days, check the drug label, package information sheet, or *Hospital Formulary* for how long the drug may be used after reconstitution. Store the drug appropriately at room temperature or refrigerate per the manufacturer's instructions. The package insert for Zithromax states, "Reconstituted solution is stable for 24 hours at or below room temperature (86° F) and 7 days when refrigerated."

CAUTION

The length of potency is different from the expiration date. The expiration date is provided by the manufacturer on the label. It indicates the last date the drug may be reconstituted and used.

When you reconstitute or mix a multiple-dose vial of medication in powdered form, it is important that the vial be clearly labeled with the *date and time* of preparation, the strength or *supply dosage* you prepared, *length of potency, storage directions,* and your *initials.* Because the medication becomes unstable after storage for long periods, the date and time are especially important. Figure 12-6 shows the proper label for the Zithromax reconstituted to 100 mg/mL. Because there are 2 doses of reconstituted drug in this vial, and 2 doses will be administered 24 hours apart (now at 0800, then again the next day at 0800), this drug should be refrigerated. Refrigeration will protect the potency of the drug in case the second dose is administered slightly later than 0800. Indicate the need for refrigeration on the label.

FIGURE 12-6   Reconstitution label for Zithromax

1/10/xx, 0800, reconstituted
as 100 mg/mL. Expires 1/17/xx,
0800. Keep refrigerated. G.D.P.

DELMAR | Cengage Learning

Multiple-Strength Solution

Some parenteral powdered medications have directions for preparing several different solution strengths to allow you to select a particular dosage strength (Figure 12-7). This results in a reasonable amount to be given to a particular patient.

FIGURE 12-7   Pfizerpen label

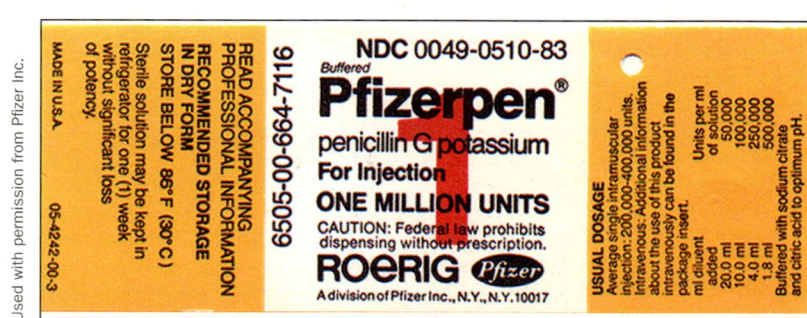

Used with permission from Pfizer Inc.

EXAMPLE ■

Order: **penicillin G potassium 300,000 units IM q.6h**

Supply: Pfizerpen (penicillin G potassium) 1,000,000 units vial

This vial contains a total of 1,000,000 units of penicillin. The reconstitution instructions are shown on the right side of the label. The instructions detail four different parenteral solution supply dosages or concentrations that are determined by the added diluent volume. The left column provides a choice of suggested volumes of diluent. The right column indicates the final solution strength in units per mL. Let's look at each of the four instructions. Notice how these reconstituted concentrations differ and when each might be selected.

Add 20 mL Diluent

Refer to the first set of directions, which indicates to add 20 mL diluent to prepare 50,000 units per milliliter of solution. Is this a good choice for preparing the medication to fill the order? What do we know?

- First, to follow the first set of directions, how much and what type of diluent must you add? The directions state to *add 20 mL of diluent.* (You must check the package insert to determine the type of diluent because this information is not stated on the label. The package insert recommends Water for Injection or Sterile Isotonic Sodium Chloride Solution for Parenteral Use.)

- Second, what is the concentration of the reconstituted penicillin? When adding 20 mL of diluent, the *supply dosage or concentration is 50,000 units/mL.*

- Third, what is the resulting total volume of this reconstituted solution? The *total volume is 20 mL.* You know this because the supply dosage is 50,000 units/mL or 1,000,000 units per 20 mL. The volume of diluent is large enough that the powder dissolves without adding any significant additional volume.

- Finally, how many full doses of penicillin as ordered are available in this vial? The vial contains 1,000,000 units, and the order is for 300,000 units. There are *3 full doses* (plus some extra) in this vial. If you choose this concentration, a reconstitution label would be required.

This means that when you add 20 mL of sterile diluent to this vial of powdered penicillin, the result is 1,000,000 units of penicillin in 20 mL of solution, with a concentration of 50,000 units per mL.

Apply the three steps of dosage calculation.

Step 1 **Convert**   No conversion is necessary.

Order: penicillin G potassium 300,000 units IM q.6h

Supply: 50,000 units/mL

Step 2 **Think**   You want to give more than 1 mL. In fact, you want to give 6 times 1 mL.

Step 3 **Calculate** $\dfrac{\text{Dosage on hand}}{\text{Amount on hand}} = \dfrac{\text{Dosage desired}}{\text{X Amount desired}}$

$$\dfrac{50,000 \text{ units}}{1 \text{ mL}} \quad \underset{\times}{} \quad \dfrac{300,000 \text{ units}}{\text{X mL}} \quad \text{Cross-multiply}$$

$$50,000\text{X} \;=\; 300,000$$

$$\dfrac{50,000\text{X}}{50,000} = \dfrac{300,000}{50,000} \quad \text{Simplify: Divide both sides of the equation by the number before the unknown X}$$

$$\text{X} \;=\; 6 \text{ mL} \quad \text{Label the units to match the unknown X}$$

Because each dose is 6 mL and the total volume is 20 mL, you would have enough for 2 additional full doses. However, this is an IM dose, and 3 mL is the maximum volume for a large, adult muscle. To administer this order using this concentration, you would need to inject the patient with two 3 mL syringes filled with 3 mL of penicillin each. Therefore, this is a poor choice of reconstitution instructions to prepare this order.

Add 10 mL Diluent

Refer to the second set of directions on the penicillin label, which indicates to add 10 mL of diluent for 100,000 units per mL of solution. Would this prepare an appropriate concentration to fill the order? What do we know?

- First, to correctly follow the second set of directions, how much and what type of diluent must you add? The directions state to add *10 mL of diluent.* (You must check the package insert to determine the type of diluent because this information is not stated on the label. The package insert recommends Water for Injection or Sterile Isotonic Sodium Chloride Solution for Parenteral Use.)

- Second, what is the concentration of the reconstituted penicillin? When adding 10 mL of diluent, the *supply dosage or concentration is 100,000 units/mL.*

- Third, what is the resulting total volume of this reconstituted solution? The *total volume is 10 mL.* You know this because the supply dosage is 100,000 units/mL or 1,000,000 units per 10 mL. The solution volume is large enough that the powder does not add significant volume to the solution.

- Finally, how many full doses of penicillin as ordered are available in this vial? The vial contains 1,000,000 units, and the order is for 300,000 units. There are *3 full doses* (plus some extra) in this vial. If you select this set of instructions, you will need to add a reconstitution label to the vial after mixing.

This means when you add 10 mL of sterile diluent to this vial of powdered penicillin, the result is 1,000,000 units of penicillin in 10 mL of solution with a concentration of 100,000 units per mL.

Apply the three steps of dosage calculation.

Step 1 Convert   No conversion is necessary.

Order: **penicillin G potassium 300,000 units IM q.6h**

Supply: 100,000 units/mL

Step 2 Think   You want to give more than 1 mL. In fact, you want to give 3 times 1 mL.

Step 3 Calculate

$$\frac{\text{Dosage on hand}}{\text{Amount on hand}} = \frac{\text{Dosage desired}}{\text{X Amount desired}}$$

$$\frac{100{,}000 \text{ units}}{1 \text{ mL}} \quad\times\quad \frac{300{,}000 \text{ units}}{\text{X mL}} \qquad \text{Cross-multiply}$$

$$100{,}000\text{X} = 300{,}000$$

$$\frac{100{,}000\text{X}}{100{,}000} = \frac{300{,}000}{100{,}000} \qquad \text{Simplify: Divide both sides of the equation by the number before the unknown X}$$

$$\text{X} = 3 \text{ mL} \qquad \text{Label the units to match the unknown X}$$

Because each dose is 3 mL and the total volume is 10 mL, you would have enough for 2 additional full doses. As an IM dose, 3 mL is the maximum volume for a large, adult muscle. Although this is a safe volume and would require only one injection, perhaps another concentration would result in a lesser volume that would be more readily absorbed.

Add 4 mL Diluent

Refer to the third set of directions on the penicillin label, which indicates to add 4 mL of diluent for 250,000 units per mL of solution. Would this prepare an appropriate concentration to fill the order?

What is different about this set of directions? Let's analyze the information provided on the label.

- First, to follow the third set of directions, how much and what type of diluent must you add? The directions state to *add 4 mL of diluent.* (Remember, you must check the package insert to determine the type of diluent because this information is not stated on the label. The package insert recommends Water for Injection or Sterile Isotonic Sodium Chloride Solution for Parenteral Use.)

- Second, what is the supply dosage of the reconstituted penicillin? When adding 4 mL of diluent, the supply dosage is *250,000 units/mL.*

- Third, what is the resulting total volume of this reconstituted solution? The *total volume is 4 mL.* You know this because the supply dosage is 250,000 units/mL or 1,000,000 units per 4 mL. The powder does not add significant volume to the solution.

- Finally, how many full doses of penicillin are available in this vial? The vial contains 1,000,000 units, and the order is for 300,000 units. Regardless of the concentration, there are still *3 full doses* (plus some extra) in this vial. A reconstitution label would be needed.

This means that when you add 4 mL of sterile diluent to the vial of powdered penicillin, the result is 4 mL of solution with 250,000 units of penicillin per mL.

Calculate 1 dose.

Step 1   Convert   No conversion is necessary.

Order: *penicillin G potassium 300,000 units IM q.6h*

Supply: 250,000 units/mL

Step 2   Think   You want to give more than 1 mL but less than 2 mL.

Step 3   Calculate $\dfrac{\text{Dosage on hand}}{\text{Amount on hand}} = \dfrac{\text{Dosage desired}}{\text{X Amount desired}}$

$$\dfrac{250{,}000 \text{ units}}{1 \text{ mL}} \quad\diagdown\!\!\!\!\diagup\quad \dfrac{300{,}000 \text{ units}}{\text{X mL}} \qquad \text{Cross-multiply}$$

$$250{,}000\text{X} = 300{,}000$$

$$\dfrac{250{,}000\text{X}}{250{,}000} = \dfrac{300{,}000}{250{,}000} \qquad \text{Simplify: Divide both sides of the equation by the number before the unknown X}$$

$$\text{X} = 1.2 \text{ mL} \qquad \text{Label the units to match the unknown X}$$

Because each dose is 1.2 mL and the total volume is 4 mL, you would have enough for 2 additional full doses. As an IM dose, 3 mL is the maximum volume for a large, adult muscle. This concentration would result in a reasonable volume that would be readily absorbed. This is a good choice of concentration instructions to use to prepare this order.

Select a 3 mL syringe, and measure 1.2 mL of Pfizerpen reconstituted to 250,000 units/mL.

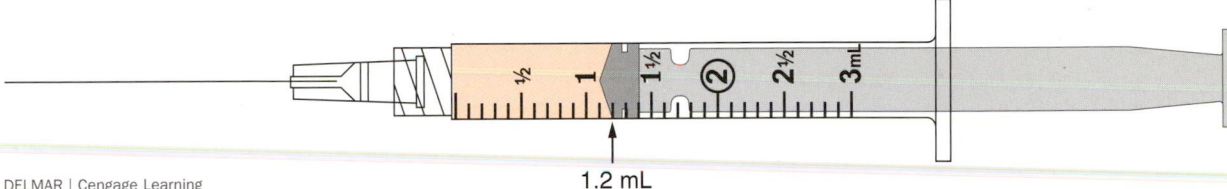

DELMAR | Cengage Learning

1.2 mL

CAUTION

The supply dosage of a reconstituted drug is an essential detail that the preparer must write on the multiple-dose vial label. Once a powdered drug is reconstituted, there is no way to verify how much diluent was actually added unless it is properly labeled.

Be sure to add a label to the reconstituted Pfizerpen 250,000 units/mL vial (Figure 12-8).

FIGURE 12-8 Reconstitution label for Pfizerpen 1,000,000 units with 4 mL diluent

DELMAR | Cengage Learning

1/30/xx, 0800, reconstituted as 250,000 units/mL. Expires 2/06/xx, 0800. Keep refrigerated. G.D.P.

Add 1.8 mL Diluent

The fourth set of directions instructs you to add 1.8 mL diluent for a solution concentration of 500,000 units/mL. Let's examine this information.

■ First, to fulfill the fourth set of directions, how much and what type of diluent must you add? The directions state to *add 1.8 mL of diluent.* (You must check the package insert to determine the type of diluent because this information is not stated on the label. Use Water for Injection or Sterile Isotonic Sodium Chloride Solution for Parenteral Use.)

■ Second, what is the supply dosage of the reconstituted penicillin? When adding 1.8 mL of diluent, the supply dosage is *500,000 units/mL.*

- Third, what is the resulting total volume of this reconstituted solution? The *total volume is 2 mL.* You know this because the supply dosage is 500,000 units/mL or 1,000,000 units per 2 mL. The powder displaces 0.2 mL of the solution, causing the resulting total volume to be larger than the volume of diluent used. (Notice that this is the most concentrated, or the strongest, of the four concentrations.)

- Finally, how many full doses of penicillin are available in this vial? The vial contains 1,000,000 units, and the order is for 300,000 units. Notice that regardless of the concentration, there are *3 full doses* (plus some extra) in this vial. You must prepare a different reconstitution label because this is a different concentration.

Following the fourth set of directions, you add 1.8 mL of diluent to prepare 2 mL of solution with a resulting concentration of 500,000 units of penicillin in each 1 mL.

Calculate 1 dose.

Step 1   Convert   No conversion is necessary.

Order: **penicillin G potassium 300,000 units IM q.6h**

Supply: 500,000 units/mL

Step 2   Think   You want to give less than 1 mL.

Step 3   Calculate

$$\frac{\text{Dosage on hand}}{\text{Amount on hand}} = \frac{\text{Dosage desired}}{\text{X Amount desired}}$$

$$\frac{500{,}000 \text{ units}}{1 \text{ mL}} \diagdown\!\!\!\!\diagup \frac{300{,}000 \text{ units}}{\text{X mL}} \qquad \text{Cross-multiply}$$

$$500{,}000\text{X} = 300{,}000$$

$$\frac{500{,}000\text{X}}{500{,}000} = \frac{300{,}000}{500{,}000} \qquad \text{Simplify: Divide both sides of the equation by the number before the unknown X}$$

$$\text{X} = 0.6 \text{ mL} \qquad \text{Label the units to match the unknown X}$$

Because each dose is 0.6 mL and the total volume is 2 mL, you would have enough for 2 additional full doses. This supply dosage would result in a reasonable volume for an IM injection for an infant, small child, or anyone with wasted muscle mass.

Select a 3 mL syringe, and measure 0.6 mL of penicillin reconstituted to 500,000 units/mL.

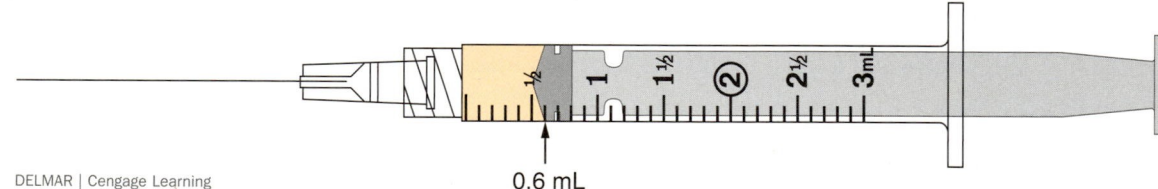

DELMAR | Cengage Learning

0.6 mL

Finally, add the label to the reconstituted penicillin G 500,000 units/mL vial (Figure 12-9).

FIGURE 12-9   Reconstitution label for Pfizerpen 1,000,000 units with 1.8 mL diluent

DELMAR | Cengage Learning

1/30/xx, 0800, reconstituted as 500,000 units/mL. Expires 2/06/xx, 0800. Keep refrigerated. G.D.P.

As you can see from these four possible reconstituted strengths, 3 full doses are available from this multiple-dose vial in each case. The added diluent volume is the vital factor that determines the resulting concentration. The *supply dosage* ultimately determines the *injectable volume per dose.*

MATH TIP

When multiple directions for diluting are given, the smaller the amount of diluent added, the greater or stronger the resulting solution concentration will be.

RECONSTITUTED PARENTERAL SOLUTIONS WITH VARIOUS ROUTES

A variety of drugs are labeled and packaged with reconstitution instructions. Some drugs are for IM use only and some are for IV use only, whereas others may be used for either. Some are even suitable for subcut, IM, or IV administration. Carefully check the route and related reconstitution directions. The following material gives examples of several types of directions you will encounter.

Drugs with Injection Reconstitution Instructions—Either IM or IV

EXAMPLE ■

Order: Solu-Medrol 200 mg IV q.6h

Supply: 500 mg vial of powdered Solu-Medrol for IM or IV injection (Figure 12-10) with directions on the left side of the label that state, "Reconstitute with 8 mL Bacteriostatic Water for Injection with Benzyl Alcohol . . . Each 8 mL (when mixed with 8 mL diluent) contains methylprednisolone sodium succinate equivalent to methylprednisolone 500 mg." These instructions will apply to orders for either the intramuscular or intravenous route.

FIGURE 12-10   Solu-Medrol 500 mg label

> Store at controlled room temperature 20° to 25°C (68° to 77°F) [see USP]. Protect from light.
>
> Reconstitute with 8 mL Bacteriostatic Water for Injection with Benzyl Alcohol.
>
> Store solution at controlled room temperature 20° to 25°C (68° to 77°F) and use within 48 hours after mixing. **Protect from light.**
>
> **DOSAGE AND USE:**
> See accompanying prescribing information.
>
> *Each 8 mL (when mixed with 8 mL of diluent) contains methylprednisolone sodium succinate equivalent to methylprednisolone, 500 mg. Also contains monobasic sodium phosphate anhydrous, 6.4 mg; dibasic sodium phosphate dried, 69.6 mg.
>
> When necessary, pH was adjusted with sodium hydroxide.
> Lyophilized in container.
>
> Used with permission from Pfizer Inc.
>
> NDC 0009-0758-01
>
> 1 Vial
> 4–125 mg Doses   Rx only
>
> **Solu-Medrol®**
> methylprednisolone sodium succinate for injection, USP
>
> For intramuscular or intravenous use
>
> **500 mg***
>
> Recommended Diluent Contains Benzyl Alcohol as a Preservative (This Package Does Not Contain Diluent)
>
> Distributed by
> **Pfizer** Pharmacia & Upjohn Co
> Division of Pfizer Inc, NY, NY 10017
>
> 3 N 0009-0758-01 1
>
> 1681

What do we know?

- First, to fill the order, how much and what type of diluent must you add? The directions state to *Reconstitute with 8 mL of bacteriostatic water for injection with Benzyl Alcohol.*

- Second, what is the supply dosage of the reconstituted Solu-Medrol? When adding 8 mL of diluent, the *supply dosage is 500 mg per 8 mL.*

- Third, what is the resulting total volume of this reconstituted solution? The *total volume is 8 mL.* Any amount that the powdered drug displaces in solution is insignificant and does not add volume. You know this because the instructions state, " . . . each 8 mL contains methylprednisolone, 500 mg."

- Finally, how many full doses of Solu-Medrol are available in this vial? The vial contains 500 mg, and the order is for 200 mg. There are *2 full doses* in the vial (plus some extra). A reconstitution label is needed. The label indicates that the reconstituted drug can be stored for 48 hours.

This means that you have available a vial of 500 mg of Solu-Medrol to which you will add 8 mL of diluent. The final yield of the solution is 500 mg per 8 mL, which is your supply dosage.

Calculate 1 dose.

Step 1 **Convert**   No conversion is necessary.

Order: Solu-Medrol 200 mg IV q.6h

Supply: 500 mg per 8 mL

Step 2 **Think**   You want to give more than 1 mL and less than 4 mL.

Step 3 **Calculate**

$$\frac{\text{Dosage on hand}}{\text{Amount on hand}} = \frac{\text{Dosage desired}}{\text{X Amount desired}}$$

$$\frac{500 \text{ mg}}{8 \text{ mL}} \ \times \ \frac{200 \text{ mg}}{\text{X mL}} \qquad \text{Cross-multiply}$$

$$500\text{X} = 1{,}600$$

$$\frac{500\text{X}}{500} = \frac{1{,}600}{500} \qquad \text{Simplify: Divide both sides of the equation by the number before the unknown X}$$

$$\text{X} = 3.2 \text{ mL} \qquad \text{Label the units to match the unknown X}$$

1/30/xx, 0800, reconstituted as 500 mg/8 mL. Expires 2/01/xx, 0800, store at room temperature 68°–77°F. G.D.P.

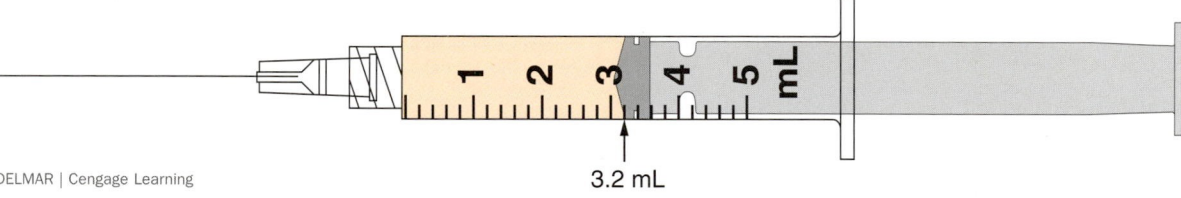

3.2 mL

Drugs with Different IM and IV Reconstitution Instructions

Notice that the ceftriaxone has one set of instructions for IM use (Figure 12-11) and another set for IV administration (Figure 12-12). The nurse must carefully check the route ordered and then follow the directions that correspond to that route. In such cases, it is important not to interchange the dilution instructions for IM and IV administrations.

FIGURE 12-11(a)   Ceftriaxone 1 g label

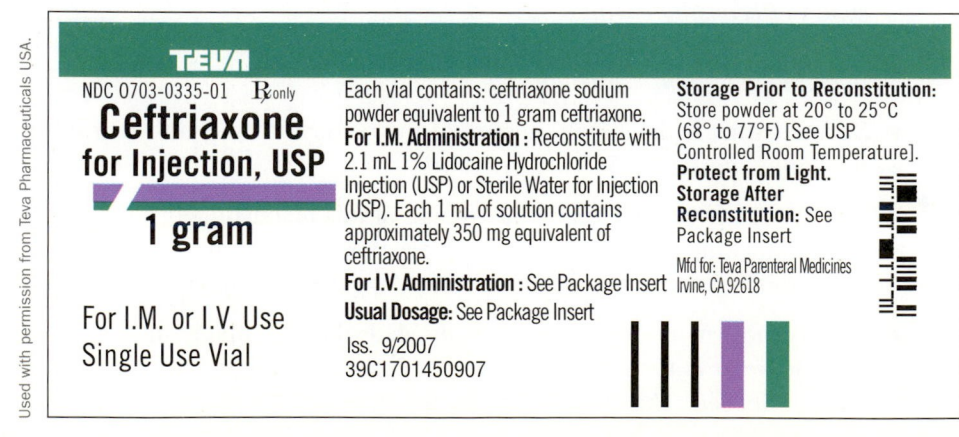

TEVA

NDC 0703-0335-01 ℞only

Ceftriaxone for Injection, USP

1 gram

For I.M. or I.V. Use
Single Use Vial

Each vial contains: ceftriaxone sodium powder equivalent to 1 gram ceftriaxone. **For I.M. Administration :** Reconstitute with 2.1 mL 1% Lidocaine Hydrochloride Injection (USP) or Sterile Water for Injection (USP). Each 1 mL of solution contains approximately 350 mg equivalent of ceftriaxone.
For I.V. Administration : See Package Insert
Usual Dosage: See Package Insert

Iss. 9/2007
39C1701450907

Storage Prior to Reconstitution: Store powder at 20° to 25°C (68° to 77°F) [See USP Controlled Room Temperature].
Protect from Light.
Storage After Reconstitution: See Package Insert

Mfd for: Teva Parenteral Medicines Irvine, CA 92618

FIGURE 12-11(b)   Package insert storage information for intramuscular administration

Ceftriaxone for injection, USP *intramuscular* solutions remain stable (loss of potency less than 10%) for the following time periods:

Diluent	Concentration mg/mL	Storage	
		Room Temp. (25°C)	Refrigerated (4°C)
Sterile Water for Injection	100 250, 350	2 days 24 hours	10 days 3 days
0.9% Sodium Chloride Solution	100 250, 350	2 days 24 hours	10 days 3 days
5% Dextrose Solution	100 250, 350	2 days 24 hours	10 days 3 days
Bacteriostatic Water + 0.9% Benzyl Alcohol	100 250, 350	24 hours 24 hours	10 days 3 days
1% Lidocaine Solution (without epinephrine)	100 250, 350	24 hours 24 hours	10 days 3 days

EXAMPLE 1 ■

Order: *ceftriaxone 250 mg IM q.12h*

Supply: 1 g vial of powdered ceftriaxone (Figure 12-11a) with IM reconstitution directions on the label that state, "For IM Administration: Reconstitute with 2.1 mL 1% Lidocaine Hydrochloride Injection (USP) or Sterile Water for Injection (USP). Each 1 mL of solution contains approximately 350 mg equivalent of ceftriaxone."

■ First, to fill the order, how much and what type of diluent must you add? The directions state to *add 2.1 mL of diluent.* Two diluents are recommended on the label: *1% Lidocaine Hydrochloride Injection (USP) or Sterile Water for Injection (USP).* Use sterile water for injection.

■ Second, what is the supply dosage of the reconstituted ceftriaxone? The resulting *supply dosage is 350 mg/mL.*

■ Third, what is the resulting total volume of this reconstituted solution? The total volume is larger than the volume of the diluent. We know this because the resulting supply dosage is 350 mg/mL or 1,050 mg per 3 mL. While 1,050 mg is approximately equal to the supplied dose of 1 g, 3 mL is considerably larger than 2.1 mL, the volume of the diluent. The solution volume is not sufficient to dilute the powder without adding additional volume. Therefore, you cannot use 2.1 mL in your calculation.

■ Finally, how many full doses of ceftriaxone are available in this vial? The vial contains 1 g or 1,000 mg. The order is for 250 mg. There are 4 full doses in the vial. The package insert states that the *solution reconstituted with sterile water for injection is stable at room temperature for 24 hours and refrigerated for 3 days.* A reconstitution label is needed.

   This means that you have available a vial of 1 g of ceftriaxone to which you will add 2.1 mL of sterile water for injection as the diluent. The final yield of the solution has a volume greater than the diluent with a supply dosage of 350 mg/mL.

Step 1   **Convert**   No conversion is necessary.

                    Order: *ceftriaxone 250 mg IM q.12h*

                    Supply: 350 mg/mL

Step 2   **Think**   You want to give less than 1 mL.

Step 3 **Calculate** $\dfrac{\text{Dosage on hand}}{\text{Amount on hand}} = \dfrac{\text{Dosage desired}}{X \text{ Amount desired}}$

$$\dfrac{350 \text{ mg}}{1 \text{ mL}} \times \dfrac{250 \text{ mg}}{X \text{ mL}} \qquad \text{Cross-multiply}$$

$$350X = 250$$

$$\dfrac{350X}{350} = \dfrac{250}{350} \qquad \text{Simplify: Divide both sides of the equation by the number before the unknown X}$$

$$X = 0.71 \text{ mL} \qquad \text{Label the units to match the unknown X}$$

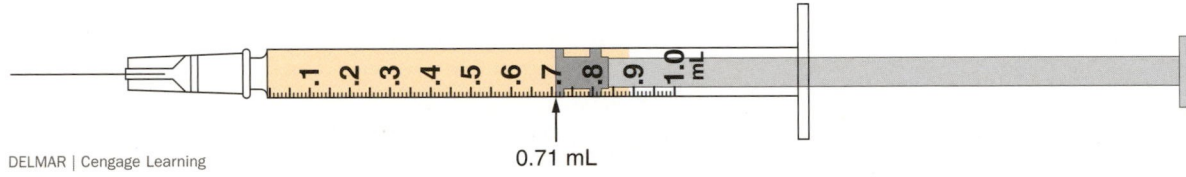

> 1/30/xx, 0800, reconstituted as 350 mg/mL for IM use. Expires 2/2/xx, refrigerate. G.D.P.

DELMAR | Cengage Learning

0.71 mL

CAUTION

Because this is an IM dose, you may need to change needles. Change needles prior to drawing up medication. Changing needles after the medication is measured may alter the actual dose of medication injected.

EXAMPLE 2 ■

Order: *ceftriaxone 400 mg IV q.12h*

Supply: 1 g vial of powdered ceftriaxone (Figure 12-11a) with IV reconstitution directions that state, "See Package Insert." The package insert provides instructions to "Reconstitute vials with an appropriate IV diluent (see COMPATIBILITY AND STABILITY). Add 9.6 mL to 1 g vial. After reconstitution, each 1 mL of solution contains approximately 100 mg equivalent of ceftriaxone" (Figure 12-12).

FIGURE 12-12 Ceftriaxone for injection package insert information for IV administration

Intravenous Administration

Ceftriaxone for injection, USP should be administered intravenously by infusion over a period of 30 minutes. Concentrations between 10 mg/mL and 40 mg/mL are recommended; however, lower concentrations may be used if desired. Reconstitute vials with an appropriate IV diluent (see **COMPATIBILITY AND STABILITY**).

Vial Dosage Size	Amount of Diluent to be Added
250 mg	2.4 mL
500 mg	4.8 mL
1 g	9.6 mL
2 g	19.2 mL

After reconstitution, each 1 mL of solution contains approximately 100 mg equivalent of ceftriaxone. Withdraw entire contents and dilute to the desired concentration with the appropriate IV diluent.

- First, to fill the order, how much and what type of diluent must you add? The directions state to *add 9.6 mL of appropriate IV diluent* to 1 g vial. The package insert lists Sterile Water for Injection as one of five appropriate IV diluents.

- Second, what is the supply dosage of the reconstituted ceftriaxone? The resulting *supply dosage is 100 mg/mL.*

- Third, what is the resulting total volume of this reconstituted solution? The *total volume is larger than the volume of the diluent.* We know this because the resulting supply dosage is 100 mg/mL or 1,000 mg per 10 mL. The solution volume is not sufficient to dilute the powder without adding additional volume. Therefore you cannot use 9.6 mL, the volume of the diluent, in your calculation.

- Finally, how many full doses of ceftriaxone are available in this vial? The vial contains 1 g or 1,000 mg. The order is for 400 mg. There are *2 full doses in the vial.* The package insert states that the *reconstituted solution is stable at room temperature for 24 hours and refrigerated for 3 days.* A reconstitution label is needed.

This means that you have available a vial of 1 g of ceftriaxone to which you will add 9.6 mL of diluent for IV administration. The final yield of the solution has a volume greater than the diluent with a supply dosage of 100 mg/mL. Most IV antibiotics are then further diluted in an approved IV solution and infused over a specified time period. You will learn more about this in Section 4.

Calculate 1 dose.

Step 1 Convert No conversion is necessary.

Order: *ceftriaxone 400 mg IV q.12h*

Supply: 100 mg/mL

Step 2 Think You want to give more than 1 mL. In fact, you want to give 4 times this amount, or 4 mL.

Step 3 Calculate

$$\frac{\text{Dosage on hand}}{\text{Amount on hand}} = \frac{\text{Dosage desired}}{\text{X Amount desired}}$$

$$\frac{100 \text{ mg}}{1 \text{ mL}} \quad \times \quad \frac{400 \text{ mg}}{\text{X mL}} \qquad \text{Cross-multiply}$$

$$100\text{X} = 400$$

$$\frac{100\text{X}}{100} = \frac{400}{100} \qquad \text{Simplify: Divide both sides of the equation by the number before the unknown X}$$

$$\text{X} = 4 \text{ mL} \qquad \text{Label the units to match the unknown X}$$

> 1/30/xx 0800, reconstituted as
> 100 mg/mL for IV use. Expires 1/31/xx,
> 0800, store at room temperature. G.D.P.

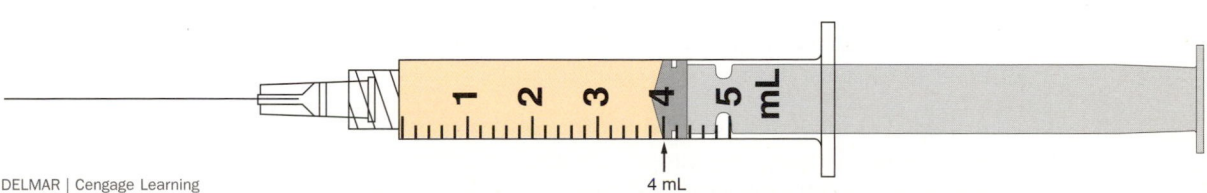

4 mL

Drugs with Instructions to "See Package Insert" for Dilution and Administration

Some labels only give the dosage strength contained in the vial and other minimal information that is insufficient to properly reconstitute or safely store the drug. To prepare the powdered medication, you must see the package insert. Look at the amphotericin B label (Figure 12-13a) and the accompanying package insert information (Figure 12-13b). The label instructs you to "See insert for reconstitution and dosage information." The following example demonstrates the use of the package insert for calculating the dosage.

EXAMPLE ■

Order: *amphotericin B 37.5 mg IV daily*

Supply: amphotericin B 50 mg

Look at the preparation instructions given in the package insert (Figure 12-13b).

FIGURE 12-13(a)   Amphotericin B 50 mg label

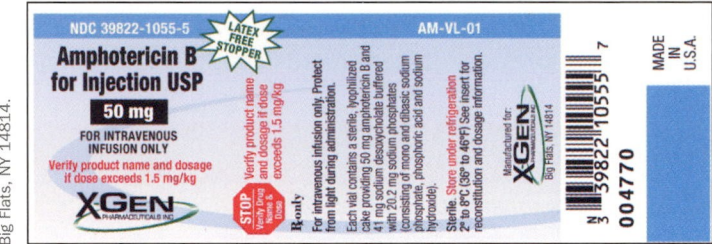

Used with permission from X-GEN Pharmaceuticals, Inc., Big Flats, NY 14814.

FIGURE 12-13(b)   Amphotericin B package insert reconstitution information

Used with permission from X-GEN Pharmaceuticals, Inc., Big Flats, NY 14814.

> **Preparation of Solutions**
> Reconstitute as follows: An initial concentrate of 5 mg amphotericin B per mL is first prepared by rapidly expressing 10 mL Sterile Water for Injection USP *without a bacteriostatic agent* directly into the lyophilized cake, using a sterile needle (minimum diameter: 20 gauge) and syringe. Shake the vial immediately until the colloidal solution is clear. The infusion solution, providing 0.1 mg amphotericin B per mL, is then obtained by further dilution (1:50) with 5% Dextrose Injection USP *of pH above 4.2.* The pH of each container of Dextrose Injection should be ascertained before use. Commercial Dextrose Injection usually has a pH above 4.2; however, if it is below 4.2, then 1 or 2 mL of buffer should be added to the Dextrose Injection before it is used to dilute the concentrated solution of amphotericin B. The recommended buffer has the following composition:
>
> | | |
> |---|---|
> | Dibasic sodium phosphate (anhydrous) | 1.59 g |
> | Monobasic sodium phosphate (anhydrous) | 0.96 g |
> | Water for Injection USP | qs 100.0 mL |

■ First, to fill the order, how much and what type of diluent must you add? The directions advise the preparer, for initial concentration, to *add 10 mL of Sterile Water for Injection USP without a bacteriostatic agent.* Further the directions state, "The infusion solution, providing 0.1 mg amphotericin B per mL, is then obtained by further dilution (1:50) with 5% Dextrose Injection USP of pH above 4.2." This means that before administration to the patient, the initial concentration of 5 mg/mL must be further diluted for infusion to 0.1 mg/mL or 1:50 concentration. (We will use the latter information after we calculate the dosage.)

■ Second, what is the supply dosage of the reconstituted amphotericin B? When adding 10 mL of diluent, the *supply dosage is 5 mg/mL.*

■ Third, what is the resulting total volume of this reconstituted solution? The *total volume is 10 mL.* You know this because the supply dosage is 5 mg/mL or 50 mg per 10 mL. The powder does not add significant volume to this solution.

■ Finally, how many full doses of amphotericin B are available in this vial? The vial contains 50 mg, and the order is for 37.5 mg. There is enough for *1 full dose* (plus some extra) in the vial but not enough for 2 full doses. No reconstitution label is needed.

This means that you have available a vial of 50 mg of amphotericin B to which you will add 10 mL of diluent. The final yield of the solution is 5 mg/mL, which is your supply dosage. Each 1 mL (5 mg) must be further diluted with 49 mL of IV solution for administration.

Calculate 1 dose of the initial concentration (before further dilution).

Step 1	**Convert**	No conversion is necessary.

Order: **amphotericin B 37.5 mg IV daily**

Supply: amphotericin B 5 mg/mL

Step 2	**Think**	You want to give more than 1 mL but less than 10 mL.

Step 3 **Calculate**

$$\frac{\text{Dosage on hand}}{\text{Amount on hand}} = \frac{\text{Dosage desired}}{\text{X Amount desired}}$$

$$\frac{5\text{ mg}}{1\text{ mL}} \;\;\Large\times\normalsize\;\; \frac{37.5\text{ mg}}{\text{X mL}}\qquad \text{Cross-multiply}$$

$$5X = 37.5$$

$$\frac{5X}{5} = \frac{37.5}{5}\qquad \text{Simplify: Divide both sides of the equation by the number before the unknown X}$$

$$X = 7.5\text{ mL}\qquad \text{Label the units to match the unknown X}$$

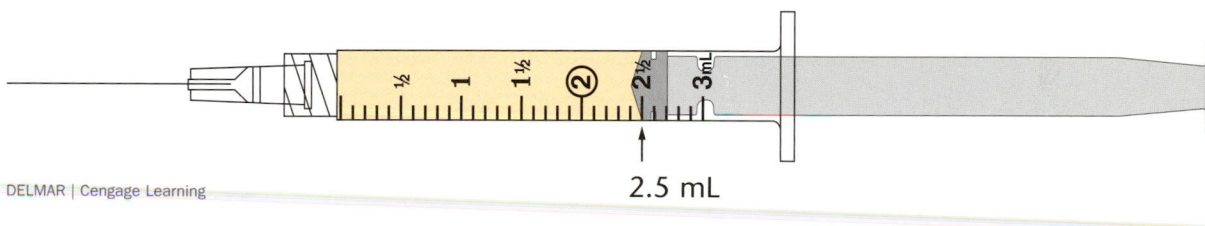

2.5 mL

DELMAR | Cengage Learning

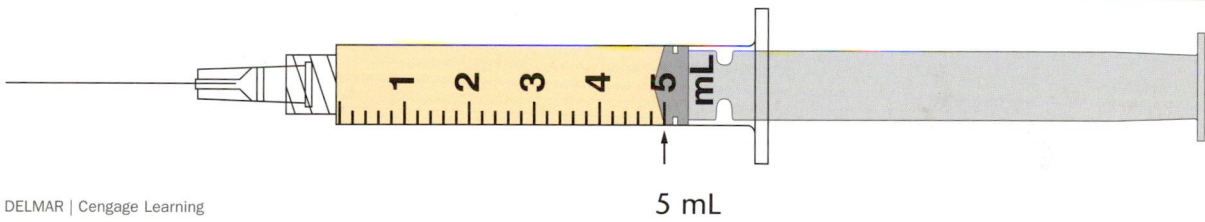

5 mL

DELMAR | Cengage Learning

Recall that the instructions indicate that further dilution of the initial concentration is required before administration: *The infusion solution, providing 0.1 mg amphotericin B per mL, is then obtained by further dilution (1:50) with 5% Dextrose injection.* This may be accomplished by adding 49 mL of 5% Dextrose and Water Injection to each 1 mL (5 mg) of amphotericin B solution. We have 7.5 mL of concentrated amphotericin solution to dilute; therefore, we need to add it to *7.5 × 49 = 367.5 or 368 mL* of IV solution before administering this drug intravenously.

QUICK REVIEW

- Check expiration dates of the drug and diluent before beginning reconstitution.

It is important that you remember the following points when reconstituting drugs.

- If any medicine remains for future use after reconstitution, clearly label:
  1. Date and time of preparation.
  2. Strength or concentration per volume.

(Continued)

3. Potency expiration.

4. Recommended storage.

5. Your initials.

■ Read all instructions carefully. If no instructions accompany the vial, confer with the pharmacist before proceeding.

■ When reconstituting multiple-strength parenteral powders, select the dosage strength that is appropriate for the patient's age, size, and condition.

■ Carefully select the correct reconstitution directions for IM or IV administration.

Review Set 26

Calculate the amount you will prepare for each dose. The labels provided are the drugs available. Draw an arrow to the syringe calibration that corresponds with the amount you will draw up and prepare a reconstitution label, if needed.

1. Order: ceftriaxone 400 mg IV q.6h

Package Insert States: "Reconstituted solution is stable at room temperature for 24 hours and refrigerated for 3 days."

Reconstitute with _____ mL diluent for a concentration of _____ mg/mL

Give: _____ mL

How many full doses are available in this vial? _____ dose(s)

Prepare a reconstitution label for the remaining solution.

<table>
<tr><td></td></tr>
</table>

Reconstitution label

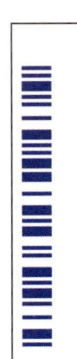

Rocephin®
(Ceftriaxone for Injection USP)
500 mg

EXP

Single-Use Vial

Batch

R only   ◇Roche◇

For I.M. or I.V. Use
Equivalent to 500 mg ceftriaxone

For I.M. Administration:
Reconstitute with 1 mL
1% Lidocaine Hydrochloride
Injection (USP) or Sterile Water
for Injection (USP). Each 1 mL of
solution contains approximately
350 mg equivalent of ceftriaxone
as ceftriaxone sodium.

For I.V. Administration:
Reconstitute with 4.8 mL of an
I.V. diluent specified in the
accompanying package insert.
Each 1 mL of solution contains
approximately 100 mg equivalent
of ceftriaxone as ceftriaxone
sodium. **Withdraw entire**
contents and dilute to the desired
concentration with the appropriate
I.V. diluent. USUAL DOSAGE: See
package insert.

Storage Prior to Reconstitution:
Store at 20°–25°C (68°–77°F) [see
USP Controlled Room Temperature].

Protect From Light.

Storage After Reconstitution:
See package insert.

Made in Switzerland
Distributed by:
Roche Laboratories Inc.
Nutley, New Jersey 07110

10075457 USA 111

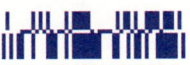

(01) 103 0004 1963 02 7

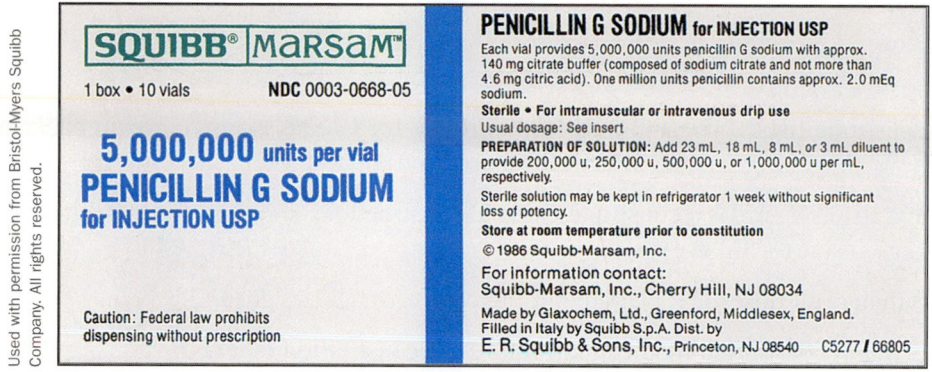

2. Order: penicillin G 150,000 units IV q.12h

SQUIBB® MARSAM™

1 box • 10 vials   NDC 0003-0668-05

5,000,000 units per vial
PENICILLIN G SODIUM
for INJECTION USP

Caution: Federal law prohibits
dispensing without prescription

PENICILLIN G SODIUM for INJECTION USP
Each vial provides 5,000,000 units penicillin G sodium with approx.
140 mg citrate buffer (composed of sodium citrate and not more than
4.6 mg citric acid). One million units penicillin contains approx. 2.0 mEq
sodium.
Sterile • For intramuscular or intravenous drip use
Usual dosage: See insert
PREPARATION OF SOLUTION: Add 23 mL, 18 mL, 8 mL, or 3 mL diluent to
provide 200,000 u, 250,000 u, 500,000 u, or 1,000,000 u per mL,
respectively.
Sterile solution may be kept in refrigerator 1 week without significant
loss of potency.
Store at room temperature prior to constitution
© 1986 Squibb-Marsam, Inc.
For information contact:
Squibb-Marsam, Inc., Cherry Hill, NJ 08034
Made by Glaxochem, Ltd., Greenford, Middlesex, England.
Filled in Italy by Squibb S.p.A. Dist. by
E. R. Squibb & Sons, Inc., Princeton, NJ 08540   C5277 / 66805

Describe the four concentrations and calculate the amount to give for each of the supply dosage concentrations.

Reconstitute with _____ mL diluent for a concentration of _____ units/mL

Give _____ mL

Reconstitute with _____ mL diluent for a concentration of _____ units/mL

Give _____ mL

Reconstitute with _____ mL diluent for a concentration of _____ units/mL

Give _____ mL

Reconstitute with _____ mL diluent for a concentration of _____ units/mL

Give _____ mL

Indicate the concentration you would choose and explain the rationale for your selection

Select _____ units/mL and give _____ mL. Rationale: _____

_____

How many full doses are available in this vial? _____ dose(s)

Prepare a reconstitution label for the remaining solution.

Reconstitution label

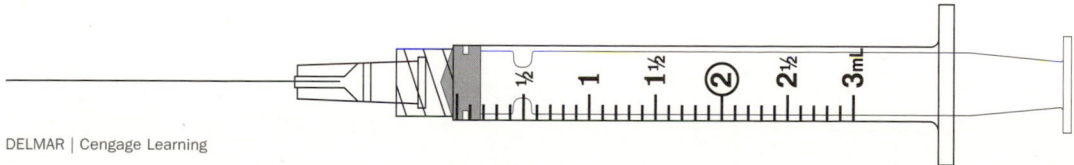

3. Order: **ampicillin 375 mg IV q.6h**

NDC 00000-0000-00		

AMPICILLIN

For Injection, USP

ampicillin sodium
equivalent to

500 mg ampicillin

For IM or IV Use

Lot.
Exp. Date

Rx only

For IM Use: add 1.7 mL diluent. The resulting solution provides 250 mg ampicillin per mL. IM or IV Injection: USE SOLUTION WITHIN 1 HOUR. IV Infusion: See package insert. Usual dosage: Children: 25 to 50 mg/kg/day in equally divided doses at 6 hour intervals. Adults: 250 to 500 mg every 6 hours. Package insert includes detailed precautions and indications. Store at controlled room temperature 15°–30°C (59°–86°F).

DELMAR | Cengage Learning
For Educational Purposes Only

DCL

00000-0000-00

(Reconstitute for IM use and then further dilute for IV use as instructed in package insert.) Reconstitute with _____ mL diluent for a concentration of _____ mg/mL

Give: _____ mL (reconstitute using IM instructions and then further dilute as instructed in package insert for IV use)

How many full doses are available in this vial? _____ dose(s)

Does this reconstituted medication require a reconstitution label? _____

Explain: _____

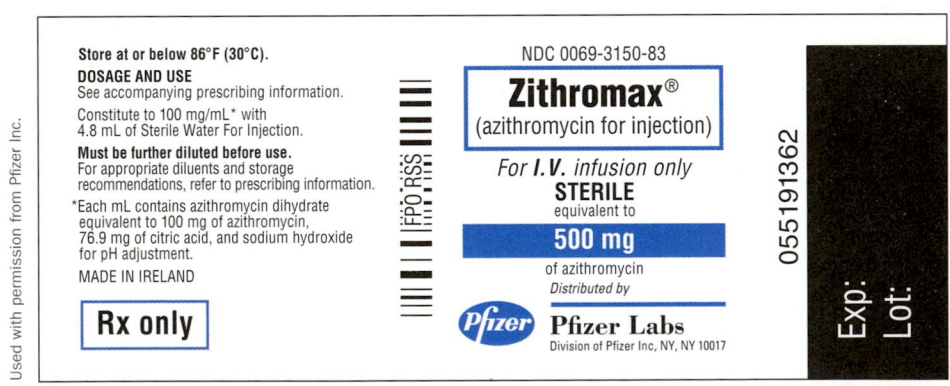

DELMAR | Cengage Learning

4. Order: **Zithromax 0.5 g IV daily**

Store at or below 86°F (30°C).

DOSAGE AND USE
See accompanying prescribing information.
Constitute to 100 mg/mL* with
4.8 mL of Sterile Water For Injection.
Must be further diluted before use.
For appropriate diluents and storage
recommendations, refer to prescribing information.

*Each mL contains azithromycin dihydrate
equivalent to 100 mg of azithromycin,
76.9 mg of citric acid, and sodium hydroxide
for pH adjustment.

MADE IN IRELAND

Rx only

Used with permission from Pfizer Inc.

NDC 0069-3150-83

Zithromax®
(azithromycin for injection)

For I.V. infusion only
STERILE
equivalent to

500 mg
of azithromycin
Distributed by

Pfizer **Pfizer Labs**
Division of Pfizer Inc, NY, NY 10017

055191362

Exp:
Lot:

Reconstitute with _____ mL diluent for a concentration of _____ mg/mL

Give: _____ mL

How many full doses are available in this vial? _____ dose(s)

Does this reconstituted medication require a reconstitution label? _____

Explain: _____

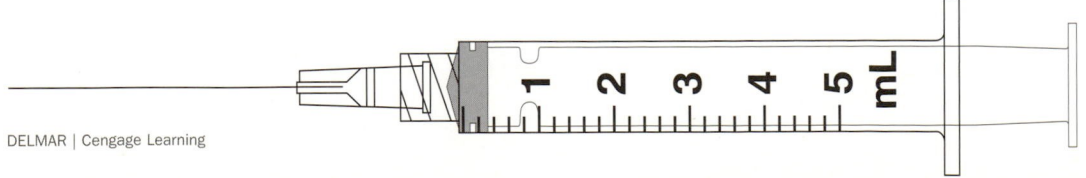

DELMAR | Cengage Learning

5. Order: **Rocephin 750 mg IM daily**

   Reconstitute with _____ mL diluent for an initial concentration
   of _____ mg/mL

   Give: _____ mL

   How many full doses are available in this vial? _____ dose(s)

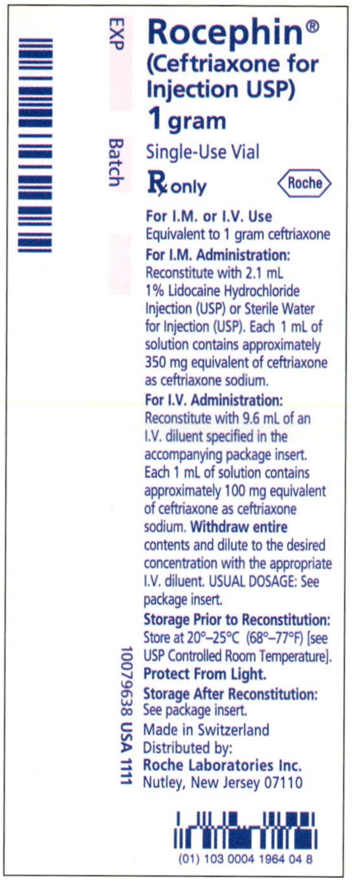

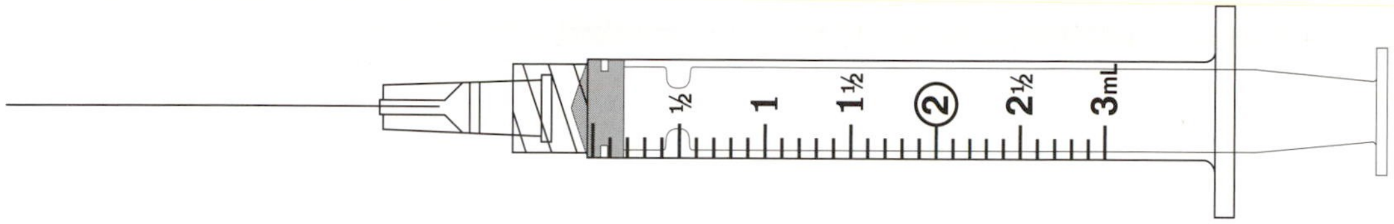

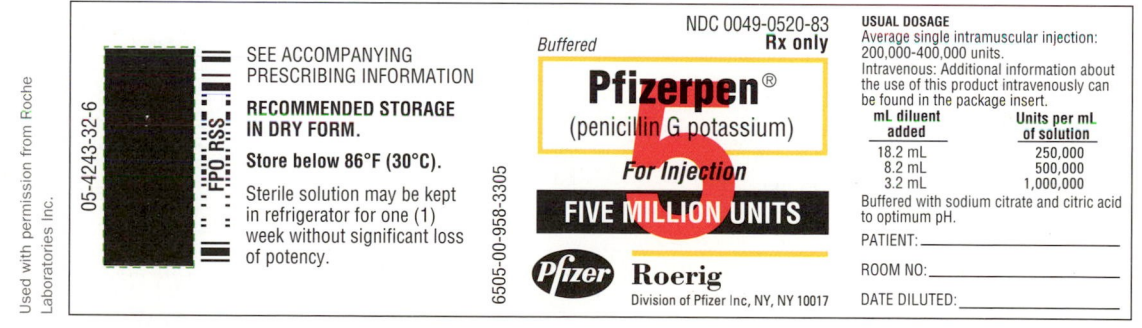

DELMAR | Cengage Learning

Used with permission from Pfizer Inc.

Rocephin®
(Ceftriaxone for Injection USP)
1 gram
Single-Use Vial
Rx only   (Roche)

EXP

Batch

For I.M. or I.V. Use
Equivalent to 1 gram ceftriaxone
For I.M. Administration:
Reconstitute with 2.1 mL
1% Lidocaine Hydrochloride
Injection (USP) or Sterile Water
for Injection (USP). Each 1 mL of
solution contains approximately
350 mg equivalent of ceftriaxone
as ceftriaxone sodium.
For I.V. Administration:
Reconstitute with 9.6 mL of an
I.V. diluent specified in the
accompanying package insert.
Each 1 mL of solution contains
approximately 100 mg equivalent
of ceftriaxone as ceftriaxone
sodium. **Withdraw entire**
contents and dilute to the desired
concentration with the appropriate
I.V. diluent. USUAL DOSAGE: See
package insert.
Storage Prior to Reconstitution:
Store at 20°–25°C (68°–77°F) [see
USP Controlled Room Temperature].
Protect From Light.
Storage After Reconstitution:
See package insert.
Made in Switzerland
Distributed by:
Roche Laboratories Inc.
Nutley, New Jersey 07110

10079638 USA 1111

(01) 103 0004 1964 04 8

6. Order: **penicillin G potassium 1,000,000 units IV q.6h**

Used with permission from Roche Laboratories Inc.

05-4243-32-6

FPO RSS

SEE ACCOMPANYING
PRESCRIBING INFORMATION
**RECOMMENDED STORAGE
IN DRY FORM.**
Store below 86°F (30°C).
Sterile solution may be kept
in refrigerator for one (1)
week without significant loss
of potency.

6505-00-958-3305

NDC 0049-0520-83
Rx only

Buffered

Pfizerpen®
(penicillin G potassium)
5
For Injection
FIVE MILLION UNITS

Pfizer **Roerig**
Division of Pfizer Inc, NY, NY 10017

USUAL DOSAGE
Average single intramuscular injection:
200,000-400,000 units.
Intravenous: Additional information about
the use of this product intravenously can
be found in the package insert.

mL diluent added	Units per mL of solution
18.2 mL	250,000
8.2 mL	500,000
3.2 mL	1,000,000

Buffered with sodium citrate and citric acid
to optimum pH.

PATIENT: _____

ROOM NO: _____

DATE DILUTED: _____

   Describe the three concentrations and calculate the amount to give for each of the supply dosage
   concentrations.

   Reconstitute with _____ mL diluent for a concentration of _____ units/mL

   Give _____ mL

   Reconstitute with _____ mL diluent for a concentration of _____ units/mL

   Give _____ mL

   Reconstitute with _____ mL diluent for a concentration of _____ units/mL

   Give _____ mL

Indicate the concentration you would choose and explain the rationale for your selection.

Select _____ units/mL and give _____ mL. Rationale: _____

_____

How many full doses are available in this vial? _____ dose(s)

Prepare a reconstitution label for the remaining solution.

[box]

Reconstitution label

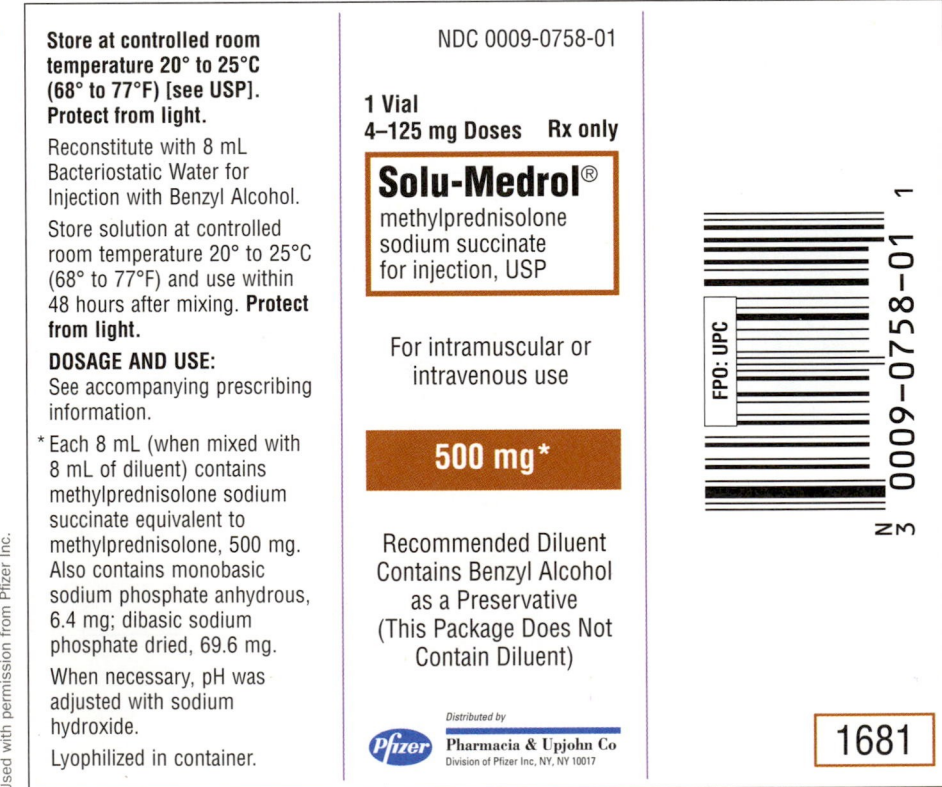

DELMAR | Cengage Learning

7. Order: **Methylprednisolone 175 mg IV daily**

Store at controlled room temperature 20° to 25°C (68° to 77°F) [see USP]. Protect from light.	NDC 0009-0758-01	

Store at controlled room temperature 20° to 25°C (68° to 77°F) [see USP]. Protect from light.

Reconstitute with 8 mL Bacteriostatic Water for Injection with Benzyl Alcohol.

Store solution at controlled room temperature 20° to 25°C (68° to 77°F) and use within 48 hours after mixing. **Protect from light.**

DOSAGE AND USE:
See accompanying prescribing information.

*Each 8 mL (when mixed with 8 mL of diluent) contains methylprednisolone sodium succinate equivalent to methylprednisolone, 500 mg. Also contains monobasic sodium phosphate anhydrous, 6.4 mg; dibasic sodium phosphate dried, 69.6 mg.

When necessary, pH was adjusted with sodium hydroxide.

Lyophilized in container.

Used with permission from Pfizer Inc.

NDC 0009-0758-01

1 Vial
4–125 mg Doses   **Rx only**

Solu-Medrol®
methylprednisolone
sodium succinate
for injection, USP

For intramuscular or
intravenous use

500 mg*

Recommended Diluent
Contains Benzyl Alcohol
as a Preservative
(This Package Does Not
Contain Diluent)

Distributed by
Pfizer **Pharmacia & Upjohn Co**
Division of Pfizer Inc, NY, NY 10017

FPO: UPC

3 0009-0758-01 1

1681

Reconstitute with _____ mL diluent for a concentration of _____ mg per _____ mL
or _____ mg/mL.

Give: _____ mL

How many full doses are available in this vial? _____ dose(s)

Prepare a reconstitution label for the remaining solution.

```
┌─────────────────────────────────────────────┐
│                                             │
│                                             │
│                                             │
│                                             │
│                                             │
└─────────────────────────────────────────────┘
```

Reconstitution label

DELMAR | Cengage Learning

8. Order: **cytarabine 200 mg IV daily × 7 days**

CYTARABINE
FOR INJECTION USP

NDC 55390-132-10   LYOPHILIZED

See package insert for complete prescribing information.
Each vial contains 500 mg and, if necessary, hydrochloric
acid and/or sodium hydroxide for pH adjustment.

FOR INTRAVENOUS,
SUBCUTANEOUS, OR
INTRATHECAL USE

When reconstituted with 10 mL Bacteriostatic Water for
Injection USP with benzyl alcohol, each mL contains 50 mg
cytarabine. **Do not use a diluent containing benzyl alcohol
for intrathecal and high dose investigational use.**

500 mg

Store both powder and reconstituted solution at 20° to 25°C
(68° to 77°F). [See USP Controlled Room Temperature.]
Use reconstituted solution within 48 hours. Discard
solution if a slight haze develops.

Rx ONLY

Manufactured for:
Bedford Laboratories™
Bedford, OH 44146   CYB-VB06

Used with permission from Bedford Laboratories. A Division of Ben Venue Laboratories. A Boehringer-Ingelheim Company.

Reconstitute with _____ mL diluent for a concentration of _____ mg/mL

Give: _____ mL

How many full doses are available in this vial? _____ dose(s)

Prepare a reconstitution label for the remaining solution.

```
┌─────────────────────────────────────────────┐
│                                             │
│                                             │
│                                             │
│                                             │
│                                             │
└─────────────────────────────────────────────┘
```

Reconstitution label

DELMAR | Cengage Learning

9. Order: penicillin G potassium 500,000 units IV q.6h

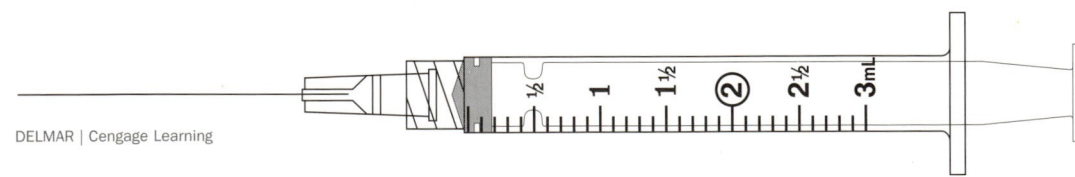

Used with permission from Pfizer Inc.

MADE IN U.S.A.

05-42-42-00-3

READ ACCOMPANYING
PROFESSIONAL INFORMATION
RECOMMENDED STORAGE
IN DRY FORM
STORE BELOW 86°F (30°C)

Sterile solution may be kept in
refrigerator for one (1) week
without significant loss
of potency.

6505-00-664-7116

NDC 0049-0510-83
Buffered
Pfizerpen®
penicillin G potassium
For Injection
ONE MILLION UNITS
CAUTION: Federal law prohibits
dispensing without prescription.
ROERIG *Pfizer*
A division of Pfizer Inc., N.Y., N.Y. 10017

USUAL DOSAGE
Average single intramuscular
injection 200,000-400,000 units.
Intravenous: Additional information
about the use of this product
intravenously can be found in the
package insert.

ml diluent added	Units per ml of solution
20.0 ml	50,000
10.0 ml	100,000
4.0 ml	250,000
1.8 ml	500,000

Buffered with sodium citrate
and citric acid to optimum pH.

PATIENT:

ROOM NO.:

DATE DILUTED:

Describe the four concentrations and calculate the amount to give for each of the supply dosage concentrations.

Reconstitute with _____ mL diluent for a concentration of _____ units/mL

Give _____ mL

Reconstitute with _____ mL diluent for a concentration of _____ units/mL

Give _____ mL

Reconstitute with _____ mL diluent for a concentration of _____ units/mL

Give _____ mL

Reconstitute with _____ mL diluent for a concentration of _____ units/mL

Give _____ mL

Indicate the concentration you would choose and explain the rationale for your selection.

Select _____ units/mL and give _____ mL. Rationale: _____

_____

How many full doses are available in this vial? _____ dose(s)

Prepare a reconstitution label for the remaining solution.

Reconstitution label

DELMAR | Cengage Learning

10. Order: Unasyn 1,500 mg IV q.6h

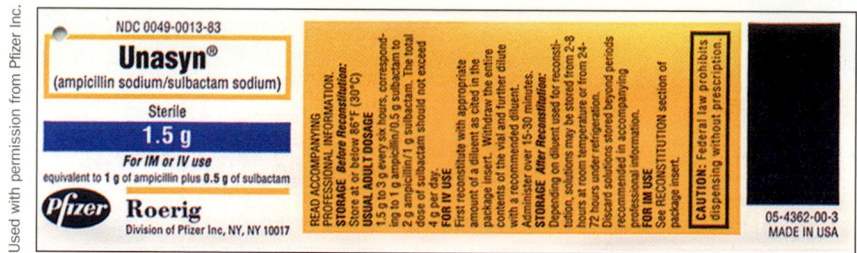

Package insert directions state:

Unasyn Vial Size	Volume Diluent to Be Added	Withdrawal Volume
1.5 g	3.2 mL	4.0 mL
3.0 g	6.4 mL	8.0 mL

Reconstitute with _____ mL diluent for a concentration of _____ g per _____ mL
or _____ mg/mL.

Give: _____ mL

How many full doses are in this vial? _____ dose(s)

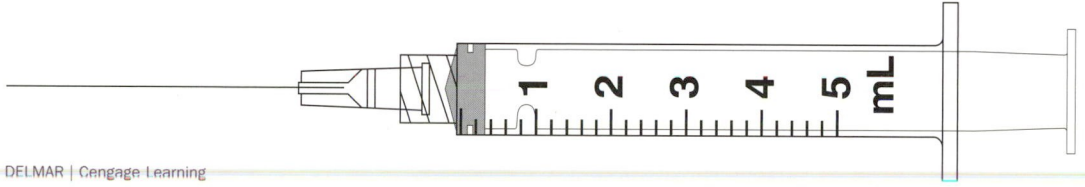

DELMAR | Cengage Learning

11. Order: methylprednisolone succinate 24 mg IV daily

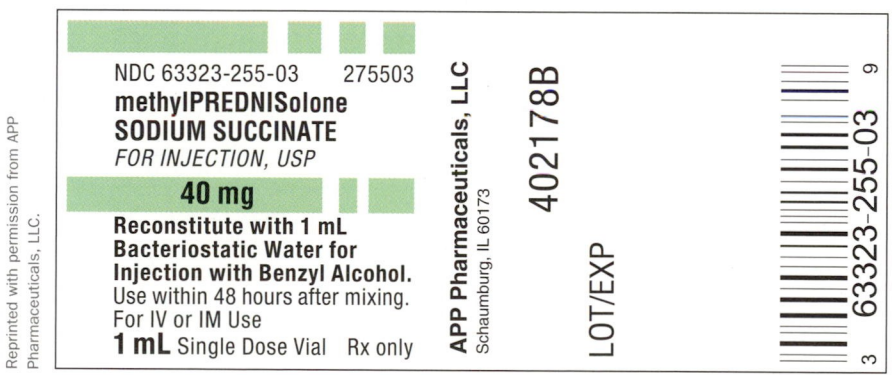

Reconstitute with _____ mL diluent for a concentration of _____ mg/mL

Give _____ mL

How many full doses are available in this vial? _____ dose(s)

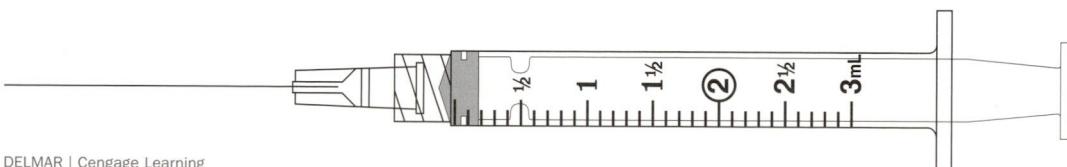

DELMAR | Cengage Learning

12. Order: *Ceftriaxone 750 mg IV q.12h*

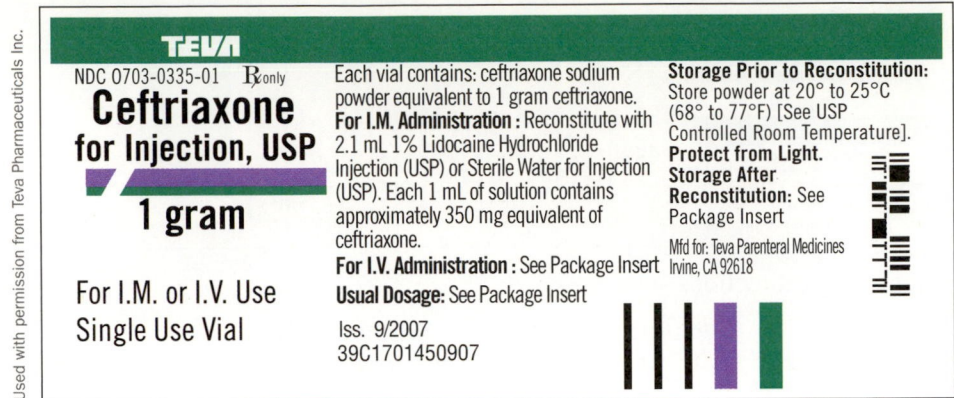

Package insert for ceftriaxone states, "Reconstituted solution is stable at room temperature for 24 hours and refrigerated for 3 days." Administration instructions:

Intravenous Administration

Ceftriaxone for injection, USP should be administered intravenously by infusion over a period of 30 minutes. Concentrations between 10 mg/mL and 40 mg/mL are recommended; however, lower concentrations may be used if desired. Reconstitute vials with an appropriate IV diluent (see **COMPATIBILITY AND STABILITY**).

Vial Dosage Size	Amount of Diluent to be Added
250 mg	2.4 mL
500 mg	4.8 mL
1 g	9.6 mL
2 g	19.2 mL

After reconstitution, each 1 mL of solution contains approximately 100 mg equivalent of ceftriaxone. Withdraw entire contents and dilute to the desired concentration with the appropriate IV diluent.

Reconstitute with _____ mL diluent for a concentration of _____ g per _____ mL or _____ mg/mL.

Give: _____ mL

How many full doses are available in this vial? _____ dose(s)

Will the drug remain potent to use all available doses? _____

Explain: _____

Prepare a reconstitution label for the remaining solution.

Reconstitution label

13. Order: **cefepime 1,500 mg IV q.12h in 100 mL D₅W (5% Dextrose and Water IV solution) IVPB**

   Supply: Maxipime (cefepime) 2 g powder for injection in vial

   Directions: See package insert below.

Administration

For Intravenous Infusion, constitute the 500 mg, 1 g, or 2 g vial, and add an appropriate quantity of the resulting solution to an IV container with one of the compatible IV fluids listed in the **Compatibility and Stability** subsection. **THE RESULTING SOLUTION SHOULD BE ADMINISTERED OVER APPROXIMATELY 30 MINUTES.**

Table 14: Preparation of Solutions of MAXIPIME

Single-Dose Vials for Intravenous/Intramuscular Administration	Amount of Diluent to be added (mL)	Approximate Available Volume (mL)	Approximate Cefepime Concentration (mg/mL)
cefepime vial content			
500 mg (IV)	5.0	5.6	100
500 mg (IM)	1.3	1.8	280
1 g (IV)	10.0	11.3	100
1 g (IM)	2.4	3.6	280
2 g (IV)	10.0	12.5	160
ADD-Vantage®			
1 g vial	50	50	20
1 g vial	100	100	10
2 g vial	50	50	40
2 g vial	100	100	20

Compatibility and Stability

Intravenous: MAXIPIME is compatible at concentrations between 1 mg/mL and 40 mg/mL with the following IV infusion fluids: 0.9% Sodium Chloride Injection, 5% and 10% Dextrose Injection, M/6 Sodium Lactate Injection, 5% Dextrose and 0.9% Sodium Chloride Injection, Lactated Ringers and 5% Dextrose Injection, Normosol-R™ and Normosol-M™ in 5% Dextrose Injection. These solutions may be stored up to 24 hours at controlled room temperature 20°–25° C (68°–77° F) or 7 days in a refrigerator 2°–8° C (36°–46°F). MAXIPIME in ADD-Vantage® vials is stable at concentrations of 10–40 mg/mL in 5% Dextrose Injection or 0.9% Sodium Chloride Injection for 24 hours at controlled room temperature 20°–25° C or 7 days in a refrigerator 2°–8° C.

Reconstitute vial with _____ mL diluent for an initial concentration of _____ g per _____ mL or _____ mg/mL

Give: _____ mL

How many full doses are available in this vial? _____ dose(s)

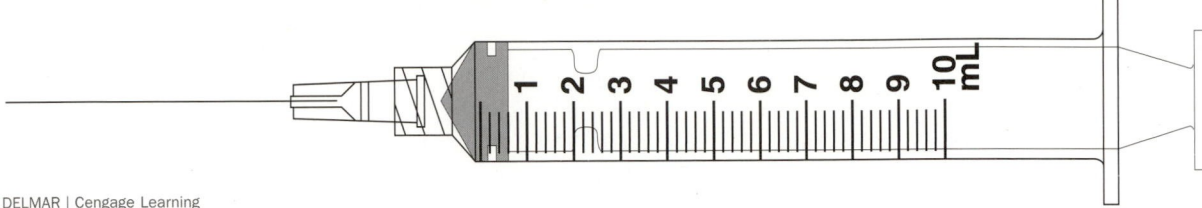

Reconstitution label

14. Order: *cephradine 250 mg IV q.6h*

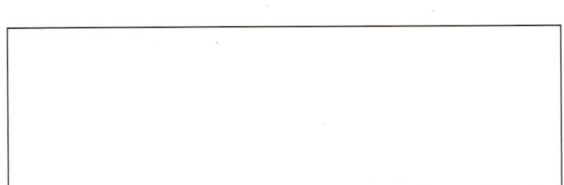

SQUIBB

1 box • 10 vials   NDC 0003-1476-10

250 mg per vial
VELOSEF®
Cephradine for Injection USP

E. R. Squibb & Sons, Inc.
Princeton, NJ 08540
Made in USA

VELOSEF®
Cephradine for Injection USP

Each vial contains 250 mg cephradine with 79 mg anhydrous sodium carbonate; total sodium content is approximately 34 mg (1.5 mEq)
For Intramuscular or Intravenous use
To prepare IM solution add 1.2 mL sterile diluent. To prepare IV solution add 5 mL sterile diluent. Use solution within 2 hours if stored at room temperature. Solution retains full potency for 24 hours when stored at 5° C.
See insert for detailed information
Usual adult dosage: 500 mg to 1 gram qid—See insert
Caution: Federal law prohibits dispensing without prescription
Store at room temperature; avoid excessive heat
Protect from light   US Patent 3,940,483   M5366F / D7610

Reconstitute with _____ mL diluent for a concentration of _____ mg/mL

Give: _____ mL

How many full doses are available in this vial? _____ dose(s)

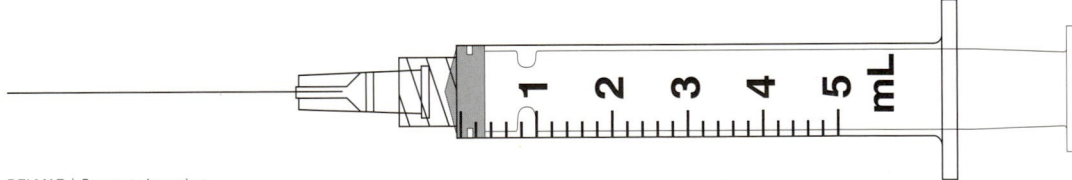

15. Order: *cefazolin 250 mg IV q.6h*

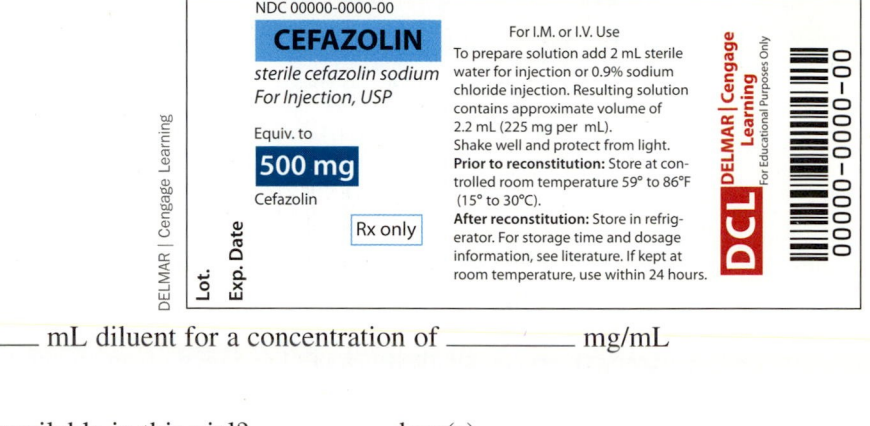

Reconstitute with _____ mL diluent for a concentration of _____ mg/mL

Give: _____ mL

How many full doses are available in this vial? _____ dose(s)

Prepare a reconstitution label for the remaining solution.

Reconstitution label

After completing these problems, see pages 531–537 to check your answers.

RECONSTITUTION OF NONINJECTABLE SOLUTIONS

Now let's look at reconstitution of noninjectable solutions, such as nutritional formulas and irrigating solutions. In most cases, the nurse or health care professional must dilute a liquid concentrate (solute) with water or saline (solvent) to make a weaker solution.

Solution Concentration

An important concept for understanding solution concentration or strength is that the amount of solvent used to decrease the total concentration is determined by the desired final strength of the solution. The *less* solvent added, the *more concentrated* the final solution strength; the *more* solvent added, the *less concentrated* the final solution strength. Think of orange juice concentrate as a way to illustrate this concept. The directions call for three cans of water to be added to one can of orange juice concentrate. The result is "reconstituted juice," a ready-to-drink beverage. If you like a stronger orange taste, you might add only two cans of water, making it a *more* concentrated juice, but you get *less total volume* to drink. If you have several people wanting to drink orange juice, you might choose to add four cans of water to the final total volume. You get *more* volume, but the orange juice is *less* concentrated; therefore, it is more dilute because you have increased the water (solvent) content. Note that in either case, the amount of orange juice concentrate in the final solution is the same.

Medical notation to express the strength of a solution uses either a ratio, percent, or fraction. The fraction is the preferred form because it is easily applied in calculations and helps explain the ratio of solute to total solution. Recall that a ratio or percent can also be expressed as a fraction.

RULE

When a fraction expresses the strength of a solution, made from a liquid concentrate:

■ The numerator of the fraction is the number of parts of solute.

■ The denominator of the fraction is the total number of parts of total solution.

■ The difference between the denominator (final solution) and the numerator (parts of solute) is the number of parts of solvent.

Let's describe some solutions made from liquid concentrates.

EXAMPLE 1 ■

$\frac{1}{4}$ **strength reconstituted orange juice** made from canned frozen concentrate

$$\frac{1}{4} \text{ strength} = \frac{1 \text{ part (can) of frozen orange juice concentrate}}{4 \text{ parts (cans) of total reconstituted orange juice}}$$

■ 1 part (can) frozen orange juice concentrate (*solute,* numerator)

■ 4 parts (cans) of total reconstituted orange juice (*solution,* denominator)

■ $4 - 1 = 3$ parts (cans) of water (*solvent*)

Three cans of water added to 1 can frozen orange juice concentrate makes 4 cans of a final reconstituted orange juice solution. The resulting $\frac{1}{4}$ strength reconstituted orange juice is comparable to the strength of fresh juice.

EXAMPLE 2 ■

$\frac{1}{3}$ **strength nutritional formula**

■ 1 part concentrate formula as the solute

■ 3 parts of total solution

■ $3 - 1 = 2$ parts solvent (water)

Therefore, 1 can of nutritional formula concentrate and 2 cans of water make a $\frac{1}{3}$ strength nutritional formula.

Calculating Solutions

To prepare a prescribed solution of a certain strength from a solute, you can apply ratio-proportion similar to what you learned for calculating dosages.

RULE

To prepare solutions,

1. Apply ratio-proportion to find the amount of solute (X)

   $$\text{Ratio for desired solution strength} = \frac{X \text{ Amount of solute}}{\text{Quantity of desired solution}}$$

2. Quantity of desired solution − Amount of solute = Amount of solvent

The unknown X you are solving for is the quantity or amount of solute you will need to add to the solvent to prepare the desired solution. Let's look at how this rule is applied in health care.

TOPICAL SOLUTIONS / IRRIGANTS

Topical or irrigating solutions may be mixed from powders, salts, or liquid concentrates. Asepsis in mixing, storage, and use is essential. Liquids can quickly harbor microorganisms. Our focus here is to review the essentials of reconstitution, but nurses and other health care professionals need to be alert at all times to the chain of infection.

Most often nurses and other health care professionals will further dilute ready-to-use solutions, which are called *full-strength* or stock solutions, to create a less concentrated liquid. Consider the desired solution strength as well as the final volume needed for the task.

EXAMPLE 1 ■

Hydrogen peroxide, which is usually available full strength as a 3% solution, can be drying to the skin and should not be directly applied undiluted. For use as a topical antiseptic, the therapeutic protocol is to reconstitute hydrogen peroxide to $\frac{1}{2}$ strength with normal saline used as the solvent. You decide to make 4 fluid ounces that can be kept in a sterile container at the patient's bedside for traction pin care.

Step 1	**Convert**	No conversion is necessary.
Step 2	**Think**	The fraction represents the desired solution strength: $\frac{1}{2}$ strength means 1 part solute (hydrogen peroxide) to 2 total parts solution. The amount of solvent is $2 - 1 = 1$ part saline. Because you need 4 fl oz of solution, you estimate that you will need $\frac{1}{2}$ of it as solute and $\frac{1}{2}$ of it as solvent, or 2 fl oz hydrogen peroxide and 2 fl oz saline to make a total of 4 fl oz of $\frac{1}{2}$ strength hydrogen peroxide.
Step 3	**Calculate**	Remember that $\frac{1}{2}$ strength $= \frac{1 \text{ part solute}}{2 \text{ parts total solution}}$. Here, the desired solution strength is $\frac{1}{2}$. The quantity of solution desired is 4 fl oz. You want to know how much solute (X fl oz) you will need.

$$\frac{1}{2} \quad \diagdown\!\!\!\!\diagup \quad \frac{X \text{ fl oz} \text{ (solute)}}{4 \text{ fl oz} \text{ (solution)}}$$

$$2X = 4$$

$$\frac{2X}{2} = \frac{4}{2}$$

$$X = 2 \text{ fl oz (solute)}$$

X (2 fl oz) is the quantity of solute (full-strength hydrogen peroxide) you will need to prepare the desired solution (4 fl oz of $\frac{1}{2}$ strength hydrogen peroxide). The amount of solvent is 4 fl oz − 2 fl oz = 2 fl oz. If you add 2 fl oz of full-strength hydrogen peroxide (solute) to 2 fl oz of normal saline (solvent), you will prepare 4 fl oz of a $\frac{1}{2}$ strength hydrogen peroxide topical antiseptic.

EXAMPLE 2 ■

Suppose a physician orders a patient's wound irrigated with $\frac{2}{3}$ **strength hydrogen peroxide and normal saline solution q.4h while awake.** You will need 60 mL per irrigation and will do three irrigations during your 12-hour shift. You will need to prepare 60 mL × 3 irrigations = 180 mL total solution. How much stock hydrogen peroxide and normal saline will you need?

Step 1	**Convert**	No conversion is necessary.
Step 2	**Think**	You want to make $\frac{2}{3}$ strength, which means 2 parts solute (concentrated hydrogen peroxide) to 3 total parts solution. The amount of solvent is $3 - 2 = 1$ part saline. Because you need 180 mL of solution, you estimate that you will need $\frac{2}{3}$ of it as solute ($\frac{2}{3} \times 180$ mL = 120 mL) and $\frac{1}{3}$ of it as solvent ($\frac{1}{3} \times 180$ mL = 60 mL).

Step 3 **Calculate** $\frac{2}{3}$ ✕ $\frac{X\ mL\ \text{(solute)}}{180\ mL\ \text{(solution)}}$

$$3X = 360$$

$$\frac{3X}{3} = \frac{360}{3}$$

$$X = 120\ mL\ \text{(solute)}$$

120 mL is the quantity of solute (hydrogen peroxide) you will need to prepare the desired solution (180 mL of $\frac{2}{3}$ strength). Because you want to make a total of 180 mL of solution for wound irrigation, the amount of solvent you need is 180 mL − 120 mL = 60 mL of normal saline. Therefore, to make 180 mL of $\frac{2}{3}$ strength hydrogen peroxide, mix 120 mL full-strength hydrogen peroxide and 60 mL normal saline.

ORAL AND ENTERAL FEEDINGS

The principles of reconstitution are frequently applied to nutritional liquids for children and adults with special needs. Premature infants require increased calories for growth yet cannot take large volumes of fluid. Children who suffer from intestinal malabsorption require incremental changes as their bodies adjust to more concentrated formulas. Adults, especially the elderly, also experience nutritional problems that can be remedied with liquid nutrition. Prepared solutions that are taken orally or through feeding tubes are usually available and ready to use from manufacturers. Nutritional solutions may also be mixed from powders or liquid concentrates. Figure 12-14 shows examples of the three forms of one nutritional formula. Directions on the label detail how much water should be added to the powdered form or liquid concentrate. Nutritionists provide further expertise in creating complex solutions for special patient needs.

As mentioned previously, health care professionals must be alert at all times to the chain of infection. Asepsis in mixing, storage, and use of nutritional liquids is essential. Because they contain sugars, such liquids have an increased risk for contamination during preparation and spoilage during storage and use. These are important concepts to teach a patient's family members.

FIGURE 12-14 Nutritional formulas

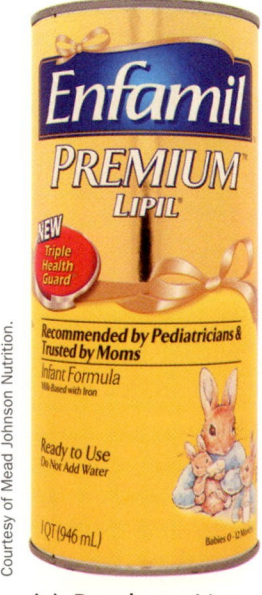 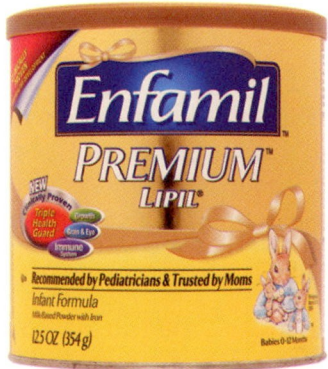 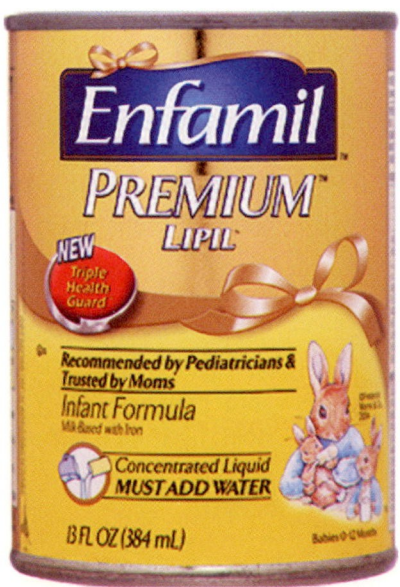

Courtesy of Mead Johnson Nutrition.

(a) Ready to Use

(b) Powder for Reconstitution

(c) Concentrated Liquid for Reconstitution

Diluting Ready-to-Use Nutritional Liquids

Ready-to-use nutritional liquids are those solutions that are normally administered directly from the container without any further dilution. Most ready-to-use formulas contain 20 calories per fluid ounce and are used for children and adults. The manufacturer balances the solute (nutrition) and solvent (water) to create a balanced, full-strength solution. However, some children and adults require less than full-strength formula for a short period to normalize intestinal absorption. Nutritional formulas are diluted with sterile water or tap water for oral use. Consult the facility policy regarding the use of tap water to reconstitute nutritional formulas. Let's look at a few typical examples.

EXAMPLE 1 ■

A physician orders **Ensure $\frac{1}{4}$ strength 120 mL q.2h via NG tube × 3 feedings** for a patient who is recovering from gastric surgery. Available are 4 and 8 fl oz cans of Ensure ready-to-use formula.

Step 1 Convert   Approximate equivalent: 1 fl oz = 30 mL

$$\frac{1\ fl\ oz}{30\ mL} \diagdown\!\!\!\!\diagup \frac{4\ fl\ oz}{X\ mL} \qquad \text{and} \qquad \frac{1\ fl\ oz}{30\ mL} \diagdown\!\!\!\!\diagup \frac{8\ fl\ oz}{X\ mL}$$

$$X = 120\ mL \qquad\qquad\qquad\qquad X = 240\ mL$$

Step 2 Think   You need 120 mL total reconstituted formula for each of 3 feedings. This is a total of 120 mL × 3 = 360 mL. But you must dilute the full-strength formula to $\frac{1}{4}$ strength. You know that $\frac{1}{4}$ strength means 1 part formula to 4 parts solution. The solvent needed is 4 − 1 = 3 parts water. You will need $\frac{1}{4}$ of the solution as solute ($\frac{1}{4}$ × 360 mL = 90 mL) and $\frac{3}{4}$ of the solution as solvent ($\frac{3}{4}$ × 360 mL = 270 mL). Therefore, if you mix 90 mL of full-strength formula with 270 mL of water, you will have 360 mL of $\frac{1}{4}$ strength formula.

Step 3 Calculate $\frac{1}{4} \diagdown\!\!\!\!\diagup \frac{X\ mL}{360\ mL}$

$$4X = 360$$

$$\frac{4X}{4} = \frac{360}{4}$$

$$X = 90\ mL\ \text{(full-strength Ensure)}$$

You need 90 mL of the formula (solute). Use 90 mL from the 4 fl oz can because it contains 120 mL. (You will have 30 mL left over.) The amount of solvent needed is 360 mL − 90 mL = 270 mL water. Add 270 mL water to 90 mL of full-strength Ensure to make a total of 360 mL of $\frac{1}{4}$ strength Ensure. You now have enough for 3 full feedings. Administer 120 mL to the patient for each feeding.

EXAMPLE 2 ■

The physician orders **800 mL of $\frac{3}{4}$ strength Sustacal through a gastrostomy tube over 8 hours** to supplement a patient while he sleeps. Sustacal ready-to-use formula comes in 10 fl oz cans.

Step 1 Convert   Approximate equivalent: 1 fl oz = 30 mL

$$\frac{1\ fl\ oz}{30\ mL} \diagdown\!\!\!\!\diagup \frac{10\ fl\ oz}{30\ mL}$$

$$X = 300\ mL$$

Step 2 Think The ordered solution strength is $\frac{3}{4}$. This means "3 parts solute to 4 total parts in solution." You know that $\frac{3}{4}$ of the 800 mL will be solute or full-strength Sustacal ($\frac{3}{4} \times$ 800 mL = 600 mL) and $\frac{1}{4}$ of the solution will be solvent or water ($\frac{1}{4} \times$ 800 mL = 200 mL). This proportion of solute to solvent will reconstitute the Sustacal to the required $\frac{3}{4}$ strength and total volume of 800 mL.

Step 3 Calculate

$$\frac{3}{4} \bowtie \frac{\text{X mL}}{\text{800 mL}}$$

$$4\text{X} = 2{,}400$$

$$\frac{4\text{X}}{4} = \frac{2{,}400}{4}$$

$$\text{X} = 600 \text{ mL (full-strength Sustacal)}$$

You need 600 mL of the formula (solute). Because the 10 fl oz can contains 300 mL, you will need 2 cans (600 mL) to prepare the $\frac{3}{4}$ strength Sustacal as ordered. The amount of solvent needed is 800 mL − 600 mL = 200 mL water. Add 200 mL water to 600 mL (or 2 cans) of full-strength Sustacal to make a total of 800 mL of $\frac{3}{4}$ strength Sustacal for the full feeding.

QUICK REVIEW

■ *Solute*—a concentrated or solid substance to be dissolved or diluted.

■ *Solvent*—or diluent, a liquid substance that dissolves another substance to prepare a solution.

■ *Solution*—the resulting mixture of a solute plus a solvent.

■ When a fraction expresses the strength of a desired solution to be made from a liquid concentrate:

  ■ The *numerator* of the fraction is the number of parts of *solute*.

  ■ The *denominator* of the fraction is the total number of parts of *solution*.

  ■ The *difference between the denominator and the numerator* is the number of parts of *solvent*.

■ To prepare solutions:

  1. Ratio for desired solution strength $= \dfrac{\text{X Amount of solute}}{\text{Quantity of desired solution}}$

  2. Quantity of desired solution − Amount of solute = Amount of solvent.

Review Set 27

Explain how you would prepare each of the following solutions using liquid stock hydrogen peroxide as the solute and saline as the solvent.

1. 480 mL of $\frac{1}{3}$ strength for wound irrigation _____

2. 4 fl oz of $\frac{1}{4}$ strength for skin cleansing _____

3. 240 mL of $\frac{3}{4}$ strength for skeletal pin care _____

4. 16 fl oz of $\frac{1}{2}$ strength for wound care _____

Explain how you would prepare each of the following from ready-to-use nutritional formulas for the specified time period. Note which supply would require the least discard of unused formula.

5. $\frac{1}{3}$ strength Ensure 900 mL via NG tube over 9 h. Supply: Ensure 4, 8, and 12 fl oz cans

_____

6. $\frac{1}{4}$ strength Isomil 4 fl oz p.o. q.4 h for 24 h. Supply: Isomil 3, 6, and 12 fl oz cans _____

7. $\frac{2}{3}$ strength Sustacal 300 mL p.o. q.i.d. Supply: Sustacal 5 and 10 fl oz cans _____

8. $\frac{1}{2}$ strength Ensure 26 fl oz via gastrostomy tube over 5 h. Supply: 4, 8, and 12 fl oz cans

9. $\frac{1}{2}$ strength Sustacal 250 mL p.o. q.i.d. Supply: Sustacal 5 and 10 fl oz cans _____

10. $\frac{3}{4}$ strength Isomil 8 fl oz p.o. q.4 h for 24 h. Supply: Isomil 3, 6, and 12 fl oz cans _____

11. $\frac{2}{3}$ strength Ensure 6 fl oz via gastrostomy tube over 2 h. Supply: 4, 8, and 12 fl oz cans

12. $\frac{1}{4}$ strength Ensure 16 fl oz via NG tube over 6 h. Supply: Ensure 4, 8, and 12 fl oz cans

After completing these problems, see page 537 to check your answers.

CRITICAL THINKING SKILLS

Often, when reconstituting a medication, the powdered drug itself adds volume to the solution. In this case the resulting volume will be greater than the volume of the diluent used to prepare the solution. Care must be taken to verify the actual volume of the reconstituted solution or the dose administered may be incorrect.

ERROR

Misinterpreting the reconstitution instructions on the label of a powdered drug and incorrectly calculating a dose of medication using the volume of the diluent added as the quantity (Q) in the dosage calculation formula.

Possible Scenario

An adult patient has an order for **penicillin G potassium 1,000,000 units IM q.6h.** The supply of penicillin G potassium was stored in powdered form, and the nurse needed to reconstitute the powder to solution. The nurse first determined what would be an appropriate solution concentration and circled the reconstitution instructions. The drug was labeled as pictured below.

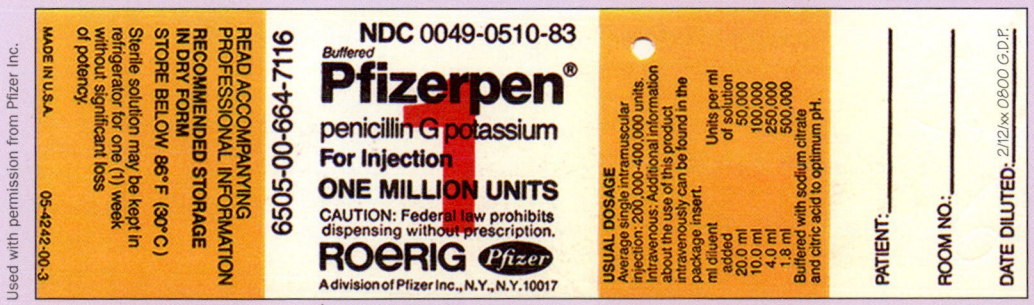

(Continued)

After adding 1.8 mL of the recommended diluent the nurse set up the dosage calculation as:

$$\frac{\text{Dosage on hand}}{\text{Amount on hand}} = \frac{\text{Dosage desired}}{\text{X Amount desired}}$$

$$\frac{500,000 \text{ units}}{1.8 \text{ mL}} \bowtie \frac{1,000,000 \text{ units}}{\text{X mL}}$$

$$500,000\text{X} = 1,800,000 \qquad \textbf{INCORRECT}$$

$$\frac{500,000\text{X}}{500,000} = \frac{1,800,000}{500,000}$$

$$\text{X} = 3.6 \text{ mL}$$

The calculated volume exceeded the maximum amount for an intramuscular injection. Because this was the most concentrated solution recommended, the nurse decided the medication would need to be divided into two syringes, each containing 1.8 mL. There was not enough solution in one vial so the nurse mixed up two vials. Prior to the nurse administering the two intramuscular injections, the patient questioned why he was getting two injections when every other time the nurses only gave him one injection. The nurse returned to the medication room and asked another nurse to verify the calculation. The second nurse pointed out that the solution strengths were provided in units per mL as printed on the top of the right column. There were actually 500,000 units in 1 mL, not in 1.8 mL, which was the volume of the diluent. The **correct** calculation and reconstitution label should have been:

$$\frac{\text{Dosage on hand}}{\text{Amount on hand}} = \frac{\text{Dosage desired}}{\text{X Amount desired}}$$

$$\frac{500,000 \text{ units}}{1 \text{ mL}} \bowtie \frac{1,000,000 \text{ units}}{\text{X mL}}$$

$$500,000\text{X} = 1,000,000 \qquad \textbf{CORRECT}$$

$$\frac{500,000\text{X}}{500,000} = \frac{1,000,000}{500,000}$$

$$\text{X} = 2 \text{ mL}$$

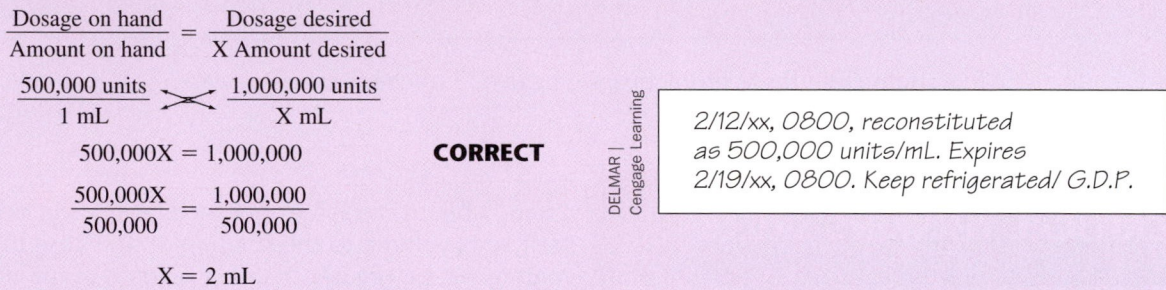

2/12/xx, 0800, reconstituted as 500,000 units/mL. Expires 2/19/xx, 0800. Keep refrigerated/ G.D.P.

DELMAR | Cengage Learning

The nurse now recognized the mistake. There was exactly enough solution left in one vial to add to a syringe containing 1.8 mL to make the required volume of 2 mL. The other medication and syringe were discarded. The nurse then administered the correct dose to the patient in one intramuscular injection.

Potential Outcome

The dose of penicillin the nurse originally prepared was almost twice the ordered dose. If two intramuscular injections were administered, the patient would have experienced unnecessary discomfort. Receiving 1 extra dose of penicillin likely would not have had serious physical consequences, but the patient might have experienced additional side effects of the medication if more additional doses were given. An extra vial of penicillin and syringe were used and discarded, adding unnecessary costs to the patient and hospital. Further, the incident might have lessened the patient's confidence in the nursing care provided, causing increased stress to this hospitalization.

Prevention

Always read the entire label to assure you have all the needed information. The nurse made an error in this case by only reading the last line of the reconstitution instructions. The error could also have been avoided if the nurse stopped to ask, "Does this make sense?" The total dose of the powdered penicillin G potassium in the vial was 1,000,000 units, which was the ordered dose. The nurse should have recognized the calculation error when the incorrect calculated dose required an additional vial to be reconstituted. Ultimately, a mistake was avoided because the nurse listened to the patient. An educated, informed patient is one more way medication errors can be prevented.

CRITICAL THINKING SKILLS

Errors in formula dilution occur when the nurse fails to correctly calculate the amount of solute and solvent needed for the required solution strength.

ERROR

Incorrect calculation of solute and solvent.

Possible Scenario

Suppose the physician ordered $\frac{1}{3}$ strength Isomil 90 mL p.o. q.3h for four feedings for an infant recovering from gastroenteritis. The concentration will be increased after these feedings. The nurse knows she will give all four feedings during her 12 hour shift, so she makes up 360 mL of formula. She takes a 3 fl oz bottle of ready-to-use Isomil and adds three 3 fl oz bottles of water for oral use. She thinks, "One-third means one bottle of formula and three bottles of water. The amount I need even works out!"

Potential Outcome

What the nurse has actually mixed is a $\frac{1}{4}$ strength solution. Because the infant is getting a more dilute solution than intended, the amount of water to solute is increased and the incremental tolerance of more concentrated formula could be jeopardized. Thinking the child is tolerating $\frac{1}{3}$ strength, the physician might increase it to $\frac{2}{3}$ strength, and the infant may have problems digesting this more concentrated formula. His progress could be slowed or even set back.

Prevention

The nurse should have thought through the meaning of the terms of a solution. If so, she would have recognized that $\frac{1}{3}$ strength meant 1 part solute (formula) to 3 total parts of solution with 2 parts water, not 1 part formula to 3 parts water. She should have applied the calculation formula or ratio-proportion to determine the amount of solute (full-strength Isomil) needed and the amount of solvent (water) to add. If she did not know how to prepare the formula, she should have conferred with another nurse or called the pharmacy or dietary services for assistance. Never guess. Think and calculate with accuracy.

PRACTICE PROBLEMS—CHAPTER 12

Calculate the amount you will prepare for 1 dose. Indicate the syringe you will select to measure the medication.

1. Order: **Zosyn 2.5 g IV q.8h**

   Supply: 3.375 g vial of powdered Zosyn

   Directions: Reconstitute Zosyn with 5 mL of a diluent from the list for a total solution volume of 5 mL

   The concentration is _____ g per _____ mL

   Give: _____ mL

   Select: _____ syringe

2. Order: Ampicillin 500 mg IV q.6h

   Supply: Ampicillin 500 mg

   Directions: Reconstitute with 1.7 mL diluent for a concentration of 250 mg/mL (and then further dilute for IV use as instructed)

   Give: _____ mL

   Select: _____ syringe

3. Order: Ancef 500 mg IV q.6h

   Supply: Ancef 1 g

   Directions: Reconstitute with 2.5 mL diluent to yield 3 mL with concentration of 330 mg/mL

   Give: _____ mL

   Select: _____ syringe

4. Order: ceftriaxone 900 mg IV q.12h in 50 mL 5% Dextrose and Water IV solution

   Supply: *See label*

   Add _____ mL diluent to the vial for a concentration of _____ mg/mL

   Give: _____ mL

   How many full doses are available in this vial? _____

   Select: _____ syringe

5. Order: cefepime 500 mg IV q.12h

   Supply: Maxipime (cefepime) 1 g powder for injection vial

   Directions: Reconstitute with 2.4 mL diluent for an approximate available volume of 3.6 mL and a concentration of 280 mg/mL

   Give: _____ mL

   Select: _____ syringe

How many full doses are available in this vial? _____ dose(s)

Prepare a reconstitution label for the remaining solution. The drug is stable for up to 7 days refrigerated and 24 hours at controlled room temperature.

```
┌─────────────────────────────────────────┐
│                                           │
│                                           │
│                                           │
│                                           │
│                                           │
└─────────────────────────────────────────┘
```

Reconstitution label

Label text:

EXP

Batch

Rocephin®
(Ceftriaxone for Injection USP)
1 gram

Single-Use Vial

R only   ◇Roche◇

For I.M. or I.V. Use
Equivalent to 1 gram ceftriaxone

For I.M. Administration:
Reconstitute with 2.1 mL
1% Lidocaine Hydrochloride
Injection (USP) or Sterile Water
for Injection (USP). Each 1 mL of
solution contains approximately
350 mg equivalent of ceftriaxone
as ceftriaxone sodium.

For I.V. Administration:
Reconstitute with 9.6 mL of an
I.V. diluent specified in the
accompanying package insert.
Each 1 mL of solution contains
approximately 100 mg equivalent
of ceftriaxone as ceftriaxone
sodium. **Withdraw entire**
contents and dilute to the desired
concentration with the appropriate
I.V. diluent. USUAL DOSAGE: See
package insert.

Storage Prior to Reconstitution:
Store at 20°–25°C (68°–77°F) [see
USP Controlled Room Temperature].
Protect From Light.
Storage After Reconstitution:
See package insert.
Made in Switzerland
Distributed by:
Roche Laboratories Inc.
Nutley, New Jersey 07110

10079638 USA 111

(01) 103 0004 1964 04 8

6. Order: **Synercid 375 mg IV q.8h**

   Supply: Synercid 500 mg

   Directions: Reconstitute with 5 mL sterile water for a concentration of 100 mg/mL

   Give: _____ mL

   Select: _____ syringe

   How many full doses are available in this vial? _____ dose(s)

Calculate 1 dose of each of the drug orders numbered 7 through 15. The labels shown on pages 286–288 are the medications you have available. Indicate which syringe you would select to measure the dose to be administered. Specify if a reconstitution label is required for multiple-dose vials.

7. Order: **cefazolin 300 mg IV q.8h**

   Reconstitute with _____ mL diluent for a concentration of _____ mg/mL and give _____ mL

   Select: _____ syringe

   How many full doses are available in this vial? _____ dose(s)

   Is a reconstitution label required? _____

8. Order: **methylprednisolone sodium succinate 200 mg IV q.6h**

   Reconstitute with _____ mL diluent for a concentration of _____ mg per _____ mL or _____ mg/mL and give _____ mL

   Select: _____ syringe

   How many full doses are available in this vial? _____ dose(s)

   Is a reconstitution label required? _____

9. Order: **ceftriaxone 1.25 g IV q.12h**

   Reconstitute with _____ mL diluent for a concentration of _____ mg/mL and give _____ mL

   Select: _____ syringe

   How many full doses are available in this vial? _____ dose(s)

   Is a reconstitution label required? _____

10. Order: **penicillin G sodium 500,000 units IM q.12h**

    If smallest volume for injection is desired, reconstitute with _____ mL diluent for a concentration of _____ units/mL and give _____ mL

    Select: _____ syringe

    How many full doses are available in this vial? _____ dose(s)

    Is a reconstitution label required? _____

11. Order: ceftriaxone 200 mg IM q.12h

    Reconstitute with _____ mL diluent for a concentration of _____ mg/mL and give _____ mL

    Select: _____ syringe

    How many full doses are available in this vial? _____ dose(s)

    Is a reconstitution label required? _____

12. Order: Vantin 200 mg p.o. q.12h

    Reconstitute with _____ mL diluent for a concentration of _____ mg/mL and give _____ mL

    How many full doses are available in this bottle? _____ dose(s)

    Is a reconstitution label required? _____

13. Order: cefazolin 400 mg IV q.6h

    Reconstitute with _____ mL diluent for a concentration of _____ mg/mL and give _____ mL

    Select: _____ syringe

    How many full doses are available in this vial? _____ dose(s)

    Is a reconstitution label required? _____

14. Order: penicillin G potassium 2,000,000 units IM q.8h

    Reconstitute with ___ mL diluent for a concentration of ___ units/mL and give ___ mL

    Select: _____ syringe

    How many full doses are available in this vial? ___ dose(s)

    Is a reconstitution label required? ____

15. penicillin G potassium 1,000,000 units IM q.8h

    Reconstitute with ___ mL diluent for a concentration of ___ units/mL and give ___ mL

    Select: _____ syringe

    How many full doses are available in this vial? ___ dose(s)

    Is a reconstitution label required? ____

SQUIBB® MARSAM™

1 box • 10 vials   NDC 0003-0668-05

**5,000,000 units per vial
PENICILLIN G SODIUM
for INJECTION USP**

Caution: Federal law prohibits dispensing without prescription

PENICILLIN G SODIUM for INJECTION USP

Each vial provides 5,000,000 units penicillin G sodium with approx. 140 mg citrate buffer (composed of sodium citrate and not more than 4.6 mg citric acid). One million units penicillin contains approx. 2.0 mEq sodium.

Sterile • For intramuscular or intravenous drip use
Usual dosage: See insert

PREPARATION OF SOLUTION: Add 23 mL, 18 mL, 8 mL, or 3 mL diluent to provide 200,000 u, 250,000 u, 500,000 u, or 1,000,000 u per mL, respectively.

Sterile solution may be kept in refrigerator 1 week without significant loss of potency.

Store at room temperature prior to constitution
© 1986 Squibb-Marsam, Inc.

For information contact:
Squibb-Marsam, Inc., Cherry Hill, NJ 08034

Made by Glaxochem, Ltd., Greenford, Middlesex, England.
Filled in Italy by Squibb S.p.A. Dist. by
E. R. Squibb & Sons, Inc., Princeton, NJ 08540   C5277 / 66805

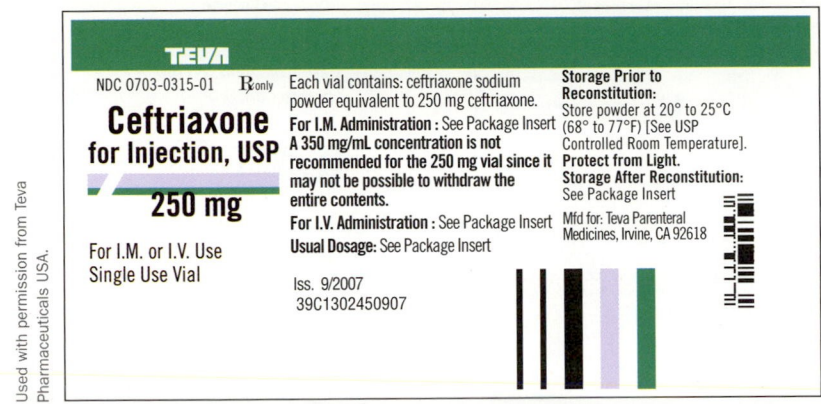

Intramuscular Administration: Reconstitute ceftriaxone for injection powder with the appropriate diluent (see **COMPATIBILITY AND STABILITY**). Inject diluent into vial, shake vial thoroughly to form solution. Withdraw entire contents of vial into syringe to equal total labeled dose.

After reconstitution, each 1 mL of solution contains approximately 250 mg or 350 mg equivalent of ceftriaxone according to the amount of diluent indicated below. If required, more dilute solutions could be utilized. **A 350 mg/mL concentration is not recommended for the 250 mg vial since it may not be possible to withdraw the entire contents.**

As with all intramuscular preparations, ceftriaxone for injection, USP should be injected well within the body of a relatively large muscle; aspiration helps to avoid unintentional injection into a blood vessel.

Vial Dosage Size	Amount of Diluent to be Added	
	250 mg/mL	350 mg/mL
250 mg	0.9 mL	—
500 mg	1.8 mL	1.0 mL
1 g	3.6 mL	2.1 mL
2 g	7.2 mL	4.2 mL

Intravenous Administration

Ceftriaxone for injection, USP should be administered intravenously by infusion over a period of 30 minutes. Concentrations between 10 mg/mL and 40 mg/mL are recommended; however, lower concentrations may be used if desired. Reconstitute vials with an appropriate IV diluent (see **COMPATIBILITY AND STABILITY**).

Vial Dosage Size	Amount of Diluent to be Added
250 mg	2.4 mL
500 mg	4.8 mL
1 g	9.6 mL
2 g	19.2 mL

After reconstitution, each 1 mL of solution contains approximately 100 mg equivalent of ceftriaxone. Withdraw entire contents and dilute to the desired concentration with the appropriate IV diluent.

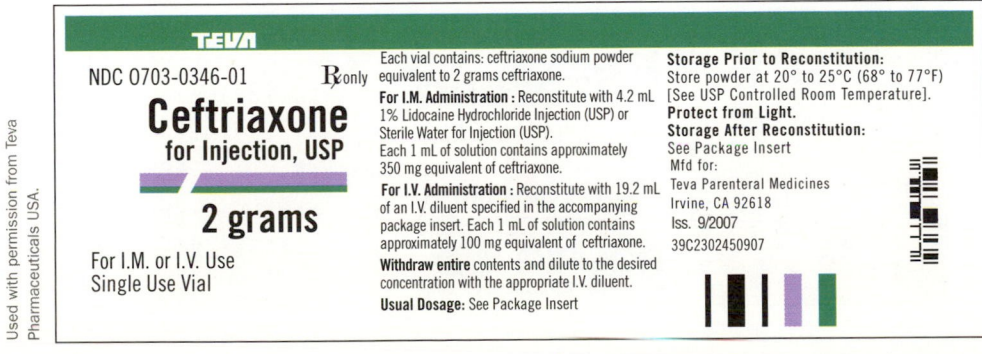

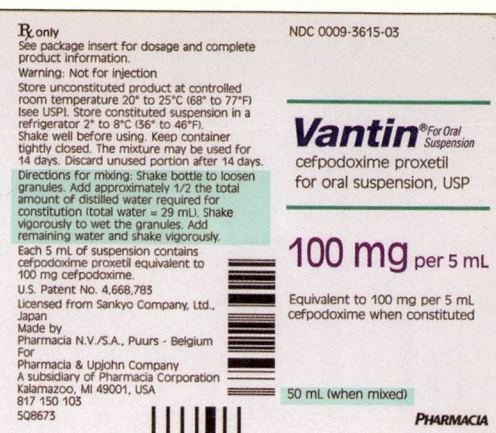

Used with permission from Pfizer Inc.

Rx only
See package insert for dosage and complete product information.

Warning: Not for injection

Store unconstituted product at controlled room temperature 20° to 25°C (68° to 77°F) [see USP]. Store constituted suspension in a refrigerator 2° to 8°C (36° to 46°F). Shake well before using. Keep container tightly closed. The mixture may be used for 14 days. Discard unused portion after 14 days.

Directions for mixing: Shake bottle to loosen granules. Add approximately 1/2 the total amount of distilled water required for constitution (total water = 29 mL). Shake vigorously to wet the granules. Add remaining water and shake vigorously.

Each 5 mL of suspension contains cefpodoxime proxetil equivalent to 100 mg cefpodoxime.

U.S. Patent No. 4,668,783
Licensed from Sankyo Company, Ltd., Japan
Made by
Pharmacia N.V./S.A., Puurs - Belgium
For
Pharmacia & Upjohn Company
A subsidiary of Pharmacia Corporation
Kalamazoo, MI 49001, USA
817 150 103
5Q8673

NDC 0009-3615-03

Vantin® For Oral Suspension
cefpodoxime proxetil
for oral suspension, USP

100 mg per 5 mL

Equivalent to 100 mg per 5 mL cefpodoxime when constituted

50 mL (when mixed)

PHARMACIA

NDC 00000-0000-00

CEFAZOLIN

sterile cefazolin sodium
For Injection, USP

Equiv. to

500 mg

Cefazolin

Rx only

Lot.
Exp. Date

For I.M. or I.V. Use
To prepare solution add 2 mL sterile water for injection or 0.9% sodium chloride injection. Resulting solution contains approximate volume of 2.2 mL (225 mg per mL).
Shake well and protect from light.
Prior to reconstitution: Store at controlled room temperature 59° to 86°F (15° to 30°C).
After reconstitution: Store in refrigerator. For storage time and dosage information, see literature. If kept at room temperature, use within 24 hours.

DCL DELMAR | Cengage Learning
For Educational Purposes Only

DELMAR | Cengage Learning

00000-0000-00

Used with permission from Pfizer Inc.

Store at controlled room temperature 20° to 25°C (68° to 77°F) [see USP].
Protect from light.

Reconstitute with 8 mL Bacteriostatic Water for Injection with Benzyl Alcohol.

Store solution at controlled room temperature 20° to 25°C (68° to 77°F) and use within 48 hours after mixing. **Protect from light.**

DOSAGE AND USE:
See accompanying prescribing information.

* Each 8 mL (when mixed with 8 mL of diluent) contains methylprednisolone sodium succinate equivalent to methylprednisolone, 500 mg. Also contains monobasic sodium phosphate anhydrous, 6.4 mg; dibasic sodium phosphate dried, 69.6 mg. When necessary, pH was adjusted with sodium hydroxide.

Lyophilized in container.

NDC 0009-0758-01

1 Vial
4–125 mg Doses   Rx only

Solu-Medrol®
methylprednisolone sodium succinate
for injection, USP

For intramuscular or intravenous use

500 mg*

Recommended Diluent Contains Benzyl Alcohol as a Preservative (This Package Does Not Contain Diluent)

Distributed by
Pfizer **Pharmacia & Upjohn Co**
Division of Pfizer Inc, NY, NY 10017

FPO: UPC

3 0009-0758-01 1

1681

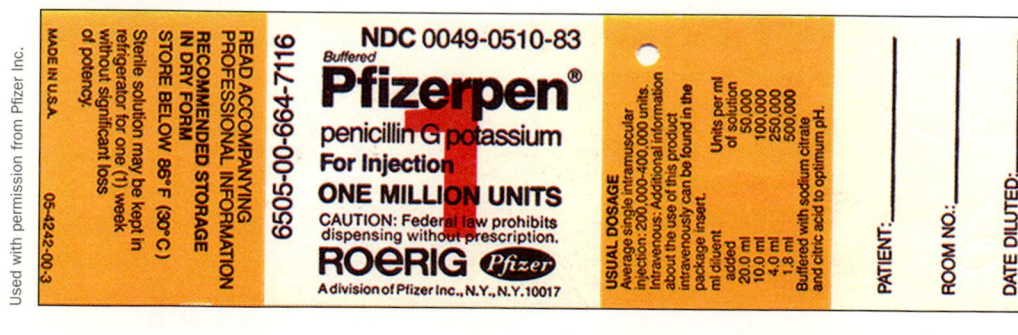

Used with permission from Pfizer Inc.

SEE ACCOMPANYING PRESCRIBING INFORMATION

RECOMMENDED STORAGE IN DRY FORM.

Store below 86°F (30°C).

Sterile solution may be kept in refrigerator for one (1) week without significant loss of potency.

05-4243-32-6   FPO: RSS

6505-00-958-3305

Buffered   NDC 0049-0520-83
   Rx only

Pfizerpen®
(penicillin G potassium)

For Injection

FIVE MILLION UNITS

Pfizer **Roerig**
Division of Pfizer Inc, NY, NY 10017

USUAL DOSAGE
Average single intramuscular injection: 200,000-400,000 units.
Intravenous: Additional information about the use of this product intravenously can be found in the package insert.

mL diluent added	Units per mL of solution
18.2 mL	250,000
8.2 mL	500,000
3.2 mL	1,000,000

Buffered with sodium citrate and citric acid to optimum pH.

PATIENT: _____

ROOM NO: _____

DATE DILUTED: _____

Used with permission from Pfizer Inc.

MADE IN U.S.A.
READ ACCOMPANYING PROFESSIONAL INFORMATION
RECOMMENDED STORAGE IN DRY FORM
STORE BELOW 86° F (30°C)
Sterile solution may be kept in refrigerator for one (1) week without significant loss of potency.

05-4242-00-3

6505-00-664-7116

NDC 0049-0510-83

Buffered
Pfizerpen®
penicillin G potassium
For Injection
ONE MILLION UNITS
CAUTION: Federal law prohibits dispensing without prescription.
ROERIG **Pfizer**
A division of Pfizer Inc., N.Y., N.Y. 10017

USUAL DOSAGE
Average single intramuscular injection: 200,000-400,000 units.
Intravenous: Additional information about the use of this product intravenously can be found in the package insert.

ml diluent added	Units per ml of solution
20.0 ml	50,000
10.0 ml	100,000
4.0 ml	250,000
1.8 ml	500,000

Buffered with sodium citrate and citric acid to optimum pH.

PATIENT: _____

ROOM NO.: _____

DATE DILUTED: _____

Explain how you would prepare each of the following hydrogen peroxide (solute) and normal saline (solvent) irrigation orders:

16. 16 fl oz of $\frac{1}{8}$ strength solution _____

17. 320 mL of $\frac{3}{8}$ strength solution _____

18. 80 mL of $\frac{5}{8}$ strength solution _____

19. 18 fl oz of $\frac{2}{3}$ strength solution _____

20. 1 pt of $\frac{7}{8}$ strength solution _____

21. 1 L of $\frac{1}{4}$ strength solution _____

Explain how you would prepare each of the following from ready-to-use nutritional formulas for the specified time period. Note how many cans or bottles of supply are needed and how much unused formula would remain from the used supply.

22. Order: $\frac{1}{4}$ strength Enfamil 12 mL via NG tube q.h. for 10h

    Supply: Enfamil 3 fl oz bottles

    _____

23. Order: $\frac{3}{4}$ strength Sustacal 360 mL over 4h via gastrostomy tube

    Supply: Sustacal 10 fl oz cans

    _____

24. Order: $\frac{2}{3}$ strength Ensure. Give 90 mL q.h. for 5h via NG tube

    Supply: Ensure 8 fl oz cans

    _____

25. Order: $\frac{3}{8}$ strength Enfamil. Three patients need 32 fl oz of the $\frac{3}{8}$ strength Enfamil for one feeding each.

    Supply: Enfamil 6 fl oz bottles

    _____

26. Order: $\frac{1}{8}$ strength Ensure. Give 160 mL stat via NG tube

    Supply: Ensure 4 fl oz cans

    _____

27. Order: $\frac{1}{2}$ strength Ensure 55 mL hourly for 10h via gastrostomy tube

    Supply: Ensure 12 fl oz cans

    _____

The nurse is making up $\frac{1}{4}$ strength Enfamil formula for several infants in the nursery.

28. If 8 fl oz cans of ready-to-use Enfamil are available, how many cans of formula will be needed to make 48 fl oz of reconstituted $\frac{1}{4}$ strength Enfamil? _____ can(s)

29. How many fl oz of water will be added to the Enfamil in question 28 to correctly reconstitute the $\frac{1}{4}$ strength Enfamil? _____ fl oz

30. Describe the strategy you would implement to prevent this medication error.

Possible Scenario

Suppose a physician ordered **penicillin G potassium 1,000,000 units** IM **stat** for a patient with a severe staph infection. Look at the label of the medication on hand.

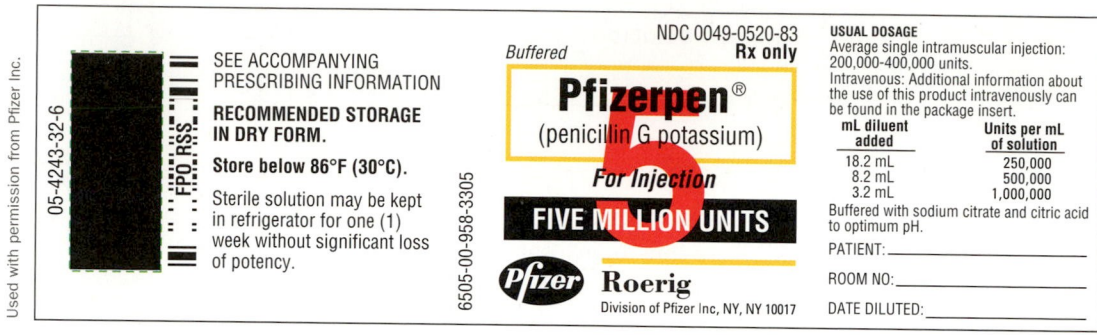

The nurse, in a hurry to give the stat medication, selected the first concentration given on the label: 250,000 units/mL. Next the nurse calculated the dosage using ratio-proportion.

$$\frac{\text{Dosage on hand}}{\text{Amount on hand}} = \frac{\text{Dosage desired}}{\text{X Amount desired}}$$

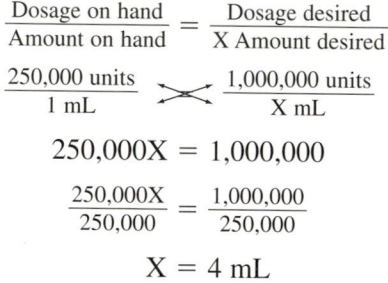

$$\frac{250,000 \text{ units}}{1 \text{ mL}} \diagdown \frac{1,000,000 \text{ units}}{\text{X mL}}$$

$$250,000\text{X} = 1,000,000$$

$$\frac{250,000\text{X}}{250,000} = \frac{1,000,000}{250,000}$$

$$\text{X} = 4 \text{ mL}$$

The nurse added 18.2 mL diluent to the vial and drew up 4 mL of medication. It was not until the nurse drew up the 4 mL that the error was recognized. The nurse realized that 4 mL IM should not be administered in one injection site. The nurse called the pharmacy for another vial of penicillin G and prepared the dose again, using 3.2 mL of diluent for a concentration of 1,000,000 units/mL. To give 1,000,000 units the nurse easily calculated to give 1 mL, which was a safe volume of medication for IM injection in adults.

Potential Outcome

If the nurse selected a 5 mL syringe and changed the needle appropriate for an IM injection to give 4 mL in one injection, the patient would likely have developed an abscess at the site. A 4 mL dose is an excessive volume of medication to administer into the muscle. The patient's hospital stay would likely have been lengthened. Further, the nurse and the hospital may have faced a malpractice suit. The alternative would have been to divide the dose into two injections. Although the patient would have safely received the correct dosage, to give two injections when only one was necessary would have been poor nursing judgment.

Prevention

_____

_____

After completing these problems, see pages 538–540 to check your answers.

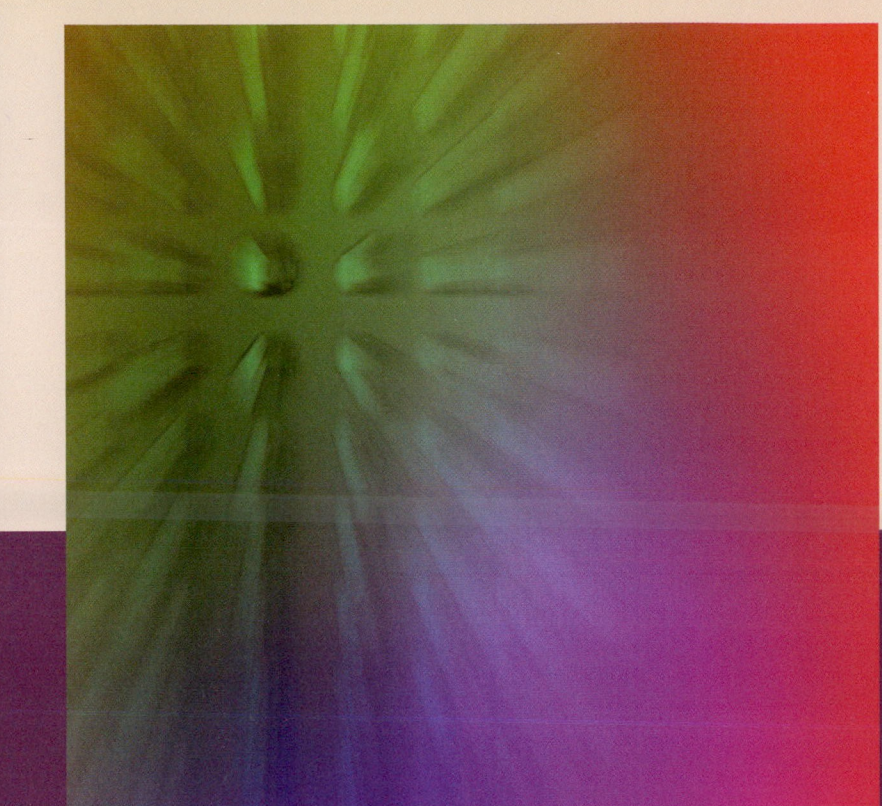
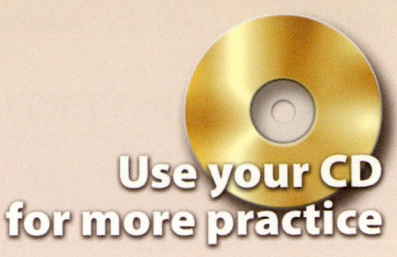

Use your CD for more practice

13

Alternative Dosage Calculation Methods: Formula and Dimensional Analysis

OBJECTIVES

Upon mastery of Chapter 13, you will be able to calculate the dosages of drugs using either the Formula or dimensional analysis methods. To accomplish this, you will also be able to:

- Convert all units of measurement to the same system and same size units using conversion factor method.
- Estimate the reasonable amount of the drug to be administered.
- Use the formula $\frac{D}{H} \times Q = X$ to calculate drug dosage.
- Solve both unit of measurement conversion and dosage calculation using dimensional analysis.

Y ou may prefer to calculate drug dosages by a formula method or dimensional analysis method. They are presented here as an alternative to the ratio-proportion method found in Chapters 10 to 12.

Try all three methods: *ratio-proportion*, $\frac{D}{H} \times Q = X$, and *dimensional analysis*. Choose the one that is easiest and most logical to you.

CONVERTING USING THE CONVERSION FACTOR METHOD

In Chapter 4 you learned to convert units of measurement to the same system and same size units using ratio-proportion. An alternate method of performing conversions is the conversion factor method. To convert using this method:

- Recall the equivalents

- Multiply or divide by the conversion factor

The following information will help you remember when to multiply and when to divide.

The *conversion factor* is a number used with either multiplication or division to change a measurement from one unit of measurement to its equivalent in another unit of measurement.

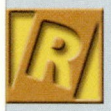

RULE

To convert from a larger to a smaller unit of measurement, multiply by the conversion factor.
THINK: "*Larger* is going down to *smaller*, so you will multiply." Larger ↓ Smaller → Multiply (×)

Stop and think about this. You know this is true because it takes *more* parts of a *smaller* unit to make an equivalent amount of a larger unit. To get *more* parts, *multiply*. Most metric conversions for dosage calculations are simply derived by multiplying or dividing by 1,000. Recall from Chapter 4 that multiplying by 1,000 is the same as moving the decimal point three places to the right.

EXAMPLE 1 ▪

How many grams are equivalent to 4.5 kg?

You know that in metric measurement, 1 kg = 1,000 g. It takes 1,000 of the gram units to equal 1 of the kilogram units. Grams are smaller than kilograms; therefore, more are needed to make an equivalent amount. THINK: Larger ↓ Smaller → Multiply (×). The conversion factor for kilograms to grams is *1,000 g/kg*. Multiply by the conversion factor or move the decimal 3 places to the right.

kilograms (larger unit) × conversion factor (g/kg) = grams (smaller unit)

4.5 k̸g̸ × 1,000 mg/k̸g̸ = 4,500 g; or 4.500. = 4,500 g

Therefore, 4.5 kg = 4,500 g

EXAMPLE 2 ▪

Convert: gr $\frac{3}{4}$ to mg

Known approximate equivalent: gr i = 60 mg

Larger ↓ Smaller → Multiply (×)

Conversion factor: *60 mg/gr*

g̸r̸ $\frac{3}{4}$ × 60 mg/g̸r̸ = 45 mg

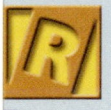

RULE

To convert from a smaller to a larger unit of measurement, divide by the conversion factor.
THINK: "*Smaller* is going up to *larger*, so you will divide." Smaller ↑ Larger → Divide (÷)

You know this is true because it takes *fewer* parts of the *larger* unit to make an equivalent amount of a smaller unit. To get *fewer* parts, *divide*. For most of these metric conversions in dosage calculations, move the decimal point 3 places to the left.

EXAMPLE 3 ▪

Convert: 100 mcg to mg

Known approximate equivalent: 1 mg = 1,000 mcg

Smaller ↑ Larger → Divide (÷)

Conversion factor: *1,000 mcg/mg*

100 mcg ÷ 1,000 mcg/mg = 0.1 mg; or .100. = 0.1 mg

EXAMPLE 4 ▪

Convert: 150 lb to kg

Known approximate equivalent: 1 kg = 2.2 lb

Smaller ↑ Larger → Divide (÷)

Conversion factor: *2.2 lb/kg*

150 lb ÷ 2.2 lb/kg = 68.18 kg

QUICK REVIEW

Use the conversion factor method to convert from one unit of measurement to another.

- Recall the equivalents.

- Identify the conversion factor.

- MULTIPLY by the conversion factor to convert to a smaller unit.
  THINK: Larger ↓ Smaller → Multiply (×)

- DIVIDE by the conversion factor to convert to a larger unit.
  THINK: Smaller ↑ Larger → Divide (÷)

- Most metric conversions in dosage calculations are derived by multiplying or dividing by 1,000.

Review Set 28

Use the conversion factor method to convert each of the following amounts to the unit indicated. Indicate the equivalent used in the conversion.

	Equivalent			Equivalent
1. 50 mL = _____ L _____		11. 2.5 mL = _____ t _____		
2. 300 mg = gr _____ _____		12. gr $\frac{1}{2}$ = _____ mg _____		
3. 84 lb = _____ kg _____		13. 10 mg = gr _____ _____		
4. gr x = _____ mg _____		14. 0.6 mg = gr _____ _____		
5. gr $\frac{1}{8}$ = _____ mg _____		15. 7.5 cm = _____ in _____		
6. 75 mL = _____ fl oz _____		16. 16 g = _____ mg _____		
7. 750 mL = _____ L _____		17. 15 mL = _____ fl oz _____		
8. $1\frac{1}{2}$ fl oz = _____ mL _____		18. 3 oz = _____ lb _____		
9. 15 mg = gr _____ _____		19. 2 qt = _____ L _____		
10. 625 mcg = _____ mg _____		20. 15 kg = _____ lb _____		

21. The medicine order states to administer a potassium chloride supplement added to at least 150 mL of juice. How many fluid ounces of juice should you pour? _____ fl oz

22. A child should have 5 mL of liquid Children's Tylenol (acetaminophen) every 4 hours as needed for fever above 100°F. To relate these instructions to the child's mother, you may advise her to give her child _____ teaspoon(s) of Tylenol per dose.

23. The doctor advises his patient to drink at least 2,000 mL of fluid per day. The patient should have approximately _____ 8-fluid-ounce glasses of water per day.

24. A child needs 15 mL of a drug. How many teaspoonsful should he receive?   _____ t

25. The doctor orders codeine gr $\frac{1}{4}$. This is equivalent to how many milligrams?   _____ mg

After completing these problems, see page 540 to check your answers.
For more practice, rework Review Sets 13 and 14 in Chapter 4 using the conversion factor method.

USING THE FORMULA METHOD TO CALCULATE DOSAGES

You can substitute the formula method for ratio-proportion in Step 3 of the *Three-Step Approach to Dosage Calculations.*

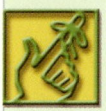

REMEMBER
Three-Step Approach to Dosage Calculations

Step 1 **Convert**   Ensure that all measurements are in the same system of measurement and the same size unit of measurement. If not, convert before proceeding.

Step 2 **Think**   Estimate what is a *reasonable amount* of the drug to administer.

Step 3 **Calculate**   Apply the formula: $\frac{D}{H} \times Q = X$

$$\frac{D \text{ (desired)}}{H \text{ (have)}} \times Q \text{ (quantity)} = X \text{ (amount)}$$

In this formula, *D* represents the *desired* dosage or the dosage ordered. You will find this in the doctor's or the health care practitioner's order. *H* represents the dosage you *have* on hand per a *quantity*, *Q*. Both *H* and *Q* constitute the *supply dosage* found on the label of the drug available. *X* is the unknown and represents the amount of the supply dosage form you want to give, such as *number of tablets* or *mL* of the drug available. Most of the time *Q* is per 1 tablet/capsule or per 1 mL; but this is not always the case. Always identify and insert *Q* in the formula.

EXAMPLE 1 ■

Order: *gentamicin 60 mg IV q.8h*

Supply: gentamicin 40 mg/mL

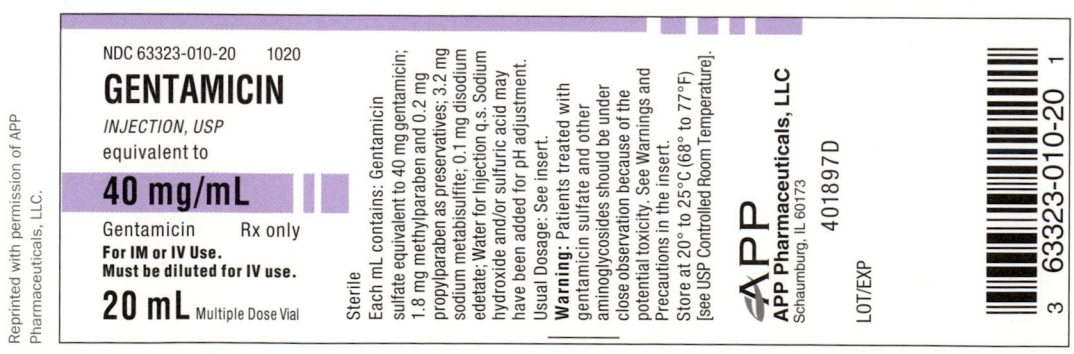

Step 1	Convert	No conversion is necessary.
Step 2	Think	You want to give more than 1 mL; but less than 2 mL.

Step 3 Calculate

$$\frac{D\ (desired)}{H\ (have)} \times Q\ (quantity) = X\ (amount)$$

$$\frac{D}{H} \times Q\ (quantity) = \frac{\overset{3}{\cancel{60}}\ mg}{\underset{2}{\cancel{40}}\ mg} \times 1\ mL = \frac{3}{2}\ mL = 1.5\ mL$$

Give 1.5 mL intravenously every 8 hours.

EXAMPLE 2 ■

Order: Ritalin 10 mg p.o. daily

Supply: Ritalin 5 mg tablets

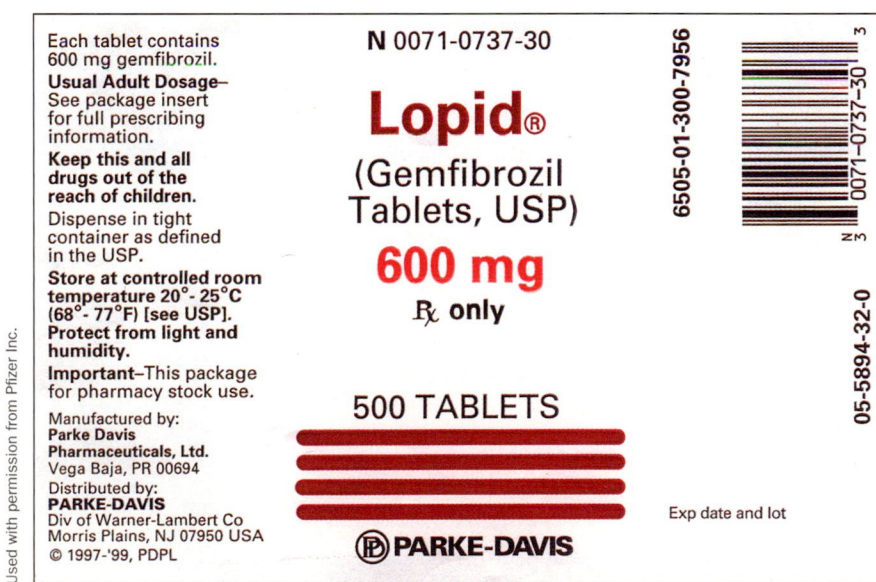

Step 1	Convert	No conversion is necessary.
Step 2	Think	You want to give more than 1 tablet. In fact, you want to give twice as many or 2 tablets.

Step 3 Calculate

$$\frac{D}{H} \times Q = \frac{\overset{2}{\cancel{10}}\ mg}{\underset{1}{\cancel{5}}\ mg} \times 1\ tab = 2\ tab$$

Give 2 tablets orally daily.

EXAMPLE 3 ■

Order: Lopid 0.6 g p.o. b.i.d

Supply: Lopid 600 mg tablets

Step 1 Convert

Equivalent 1 g = 1,000 mg

Larger ↓ Smaller → Multiply (×); or move decimal 3 places to right

Conversion factor: *1,000 mg/g*

0.6 g × 1,000 mg/g = 600 mg; or 0.600. = 600 mg

Step 2	**Think**	You want to give 600 mg and each tablet supplies 600 mg. It is obvious that you want to give 1 tablet.
Step 3	**Calculate**	$\dfrac{D}{H} \times Q = \dfrac{600\ \cancel{mg}}{600\ \cancel{mg}} \times 1\ \text{tab} = 1\ \text{tab}$

Give 1 tablet orally twice daily.

EXAMPLE 4 ■

Order: *codeine gr $\frac{1}{4}$ p.o. q.6h p.r.n., severe cough*

Supply: codeine 30 mg tablets

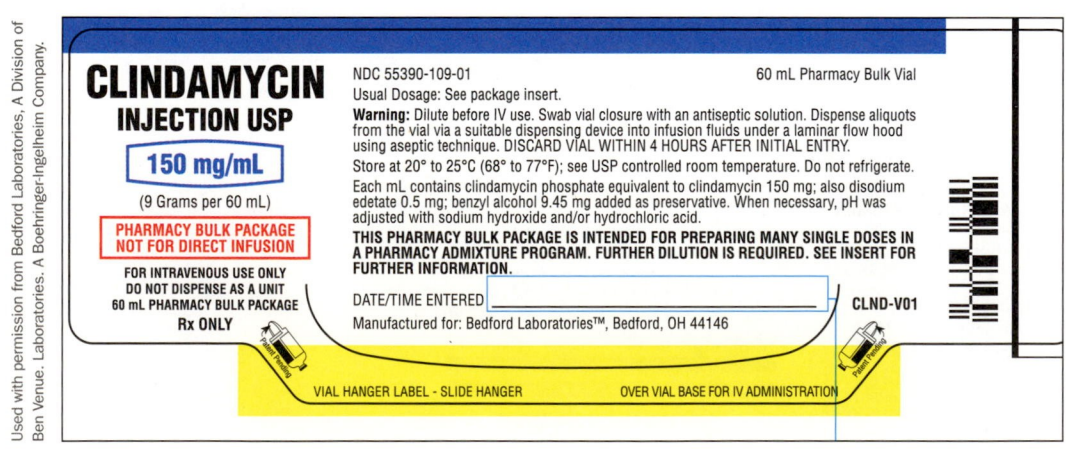

Step 1	**Convert**	Equivalent gr i = 60 mg
		Larger ↓ Smaller → Multiply (×)
		Conversion factor: *60 mg/gr*
		$\cancel{gr}\ \frac{1}{4} \times 60\ \text{mg/}\cancel{gr} = 15\ \text{mg}$
Step 2	**Think**	You want to give less than 1 tablet. Actually, you want to give $\frac{1}{2}$ tablet.
Step 3	**Calculate**	$\dfrac{D}{H} \times Q = \dfrac{\overset{1}{\cancel{15}}\ \cancel{mg}}{\underset{2}{\cancel{30}}\ \cancel{mg}} \times 1\ \text{tab} = \dfrac{1}{2} \times 1\ \text{tab} = \dfrac{1}{2}\ \text{tablet}$

Give $\frac{1}{2}$ tablet orally every 6 hours as needed for cough.

EXAMPLE 5 ■

Order: *clindamycin 0.6 g IV q.12h*

Supply: (clindamycin) 150 mg/mL

Step 1	**Convert**	Equivalent: 1 g = 1,000 mg
		Larger ↓ Smaller → Multiply (×) or move decimal 3 places to right
		The conversion factor is *1,000 mg/g.*
		0.6 $\cancel{g}$ × 1,000 mg/$\cancel{g}$ = 600 mg; or 0.600. = 600 mg

Step 2   **Think**   You want to give more than 2 mL. In fact, you want 2 times 2 mL or 4 mL.

Step 3   **Calculate** $\dfrac{D}{H} \times Q = \dfrac{\overset{4}{\cancel{600}} \text{ mg}}{\underset{1}{\cancel{150}} \text{ mg}} \times 1 \text{ mL} = \dfrac{4}{1} \text{ mL} = 4 \text{ mL}$

Give 4 mL intravenously every 12 hours.

QUICK REVIEW

When calculating dosages using the formula method:

Step 1   **Convert**   To units of the same system and the same size.

Step 2   **Think**   Estimate for a reasonable amount to give.

Step 3   **Calculate** $\dfrac{D}{H} \times Q = X$

$\dfrac{D \text{ (desired)}}{H \text{ (have)}} \times Q \text{ (quantity)} = X \text{ (amount)}$

- Drug dosages cannot be accurately calculated until all units of measurement are in the same system and the same size.

- Always **convert** first, then **think** or reason for the logical answer before you finally **calculate**.

- For most dosage calculation problems:

  - convert to smaller size unit. Example: g → mg

  - convert from the apothecary or household system to the metric system. Example: gr → mg

- Consider the reasonableness of the calculated amount to give. Example: You would question giving more than 3 tablets or capsules per dose for oral administration.

Review Set 29

Use the formula method to calculate the amount you will prepare for each dose.

1. Order: **Premarin 1.25 mg p.o. daily**

   Supply: Premarin 0.625 mg tablets

   Give: _____ tablet(s)

2. Order: **cimetidine 150 mg p.o. q.i.d. c̄ meals & bedtime**

   Supply: cimetidine liquid 300 mg per 5 mL

   Give: _____ mL

3. Order: **Thiamine 80 mg IM stat**

   Supply: Thiamine 100 mg/mL

   Give: _____ mL

4. Order: **ketorlac 20 mg IV q.6h p.r.n., pain**

   Supply: ketorlac 15 mg/mL

   Give: _____ mL

5. Order: **lithium 450 mg p.o. t.i.d.**

   Supply: lithium 300 mg per 5 mL

   Give: _____ mL

6. Order: **Ativan 2.4 mg IM bedtime p.r.n., anxiety**

   Supply: Ativan 4 mg/mL

   Give: _____ mL

7. Order: **Prednisone 7.5 mg p.o. daily**

   Supply: Prednisone 5 mg (scored) tablets

   Give: _____ tablet(s)

8. Order: **hydrochlorothiazide 30 mg p.o. b.i.d.**

   Supply: hydrochlorothiazide 50 mg per 5 mL

   Give: _____ mL

9. Order: **Theophylline 160 mg p.o. q.6h**

   Supply: Theophylline 80 mg per 15 mL

   Give: _____ mL

10. Order: **Tofranil 20 mg IM bedtime**

    Supply: Tofranil 25 mg per 2 mL

    Give: _____ mL

11. Order: **Indocin 15 mg p.o. t.i.d.**

    Supply: Indocin Suspension 25 mg per 5 mL

    Give: _____ mL

12. Order: **Ativan 2 mg IM 2 h pre-op**

    Supply: Ativan 4 mg/mL

    Give: _____ mL

13. Order: **phenobarbital gr $\frac{1}{2}$ p.o. t.i.d.**

    Supply: phenobarbital 15 mg tablets

    Give: _____ tablet(s)

14. Order: **Diabinese 125 mg p.o. daily**

    Supply: Diabinese 100 mg or 250 mg tablets

    Select: _____ mg

    Give: _____ tablet(s)

15. Order: **chlorpromazine 60 mg IM stat**

    Supply: chlorpromazine 25 mg/mL

    Give: _____ mL

16. Order: **Synthroid 0.15 mg p.o. daily**

    Supply: Synthroid 75 mcg tablets

    Give: _____ tablet(s)

17. Order: **elixophyllin elixir 96 mg p.o. q.6h**

    Supply: elixophyllin elixir 80 mg per 15 mL

    Give: _____ mL

18. Order: **Solu-Medrol 100 mg IV q.6h**

    Supply: Solu-Medrol 80 mg/mL

    Give: _____ mL

19. Order: **fluphenazine elixir 8 mg p.o. q.8h**

    Supply: fluphenazine elixir 2.5 mg per 5 mL

    Give: _____ mL

20. Order: **Trimox 350 mg p.o. q.8h**

    Supply: Trimox 250 mg per 5 mL

    Give: _____ mL

After completing these problems, see pages 540–541 to check your answers.

USING DIMENSIONAL ANALYSIS TO CALCULATE DOSAGES

You may prefer to use dimensional analysis as an alternative to either the formula method or ratio-proportion for calculating drug doses. When using the dimensional analysis method, you are not required to memorize formulas and the conversion step, if needed, is part of the calculation.

You should practice with all methods and then select the method that is the easiest and most logical for you. Regardless of which method you prefer, you will have to master knowledge of common equivalents (such as, 1 g = 1,000 mg, 1 mg = 1,000 mcg, 1 L = 1,000 mL, 1 in = 2.5 cm, 1 kg = 2.2 lb).

When using dimensional analysis, you must first determine the unit of measure (tablets, capsules, mL, etc.) that you seek to administer. This is determined by the medication order and the unit provided by the pharmacy.

If a medication is dispensed as a tablet, you would administer 1 tablet, a portion of a tablet, or multiple tablets. If a medication is dispensed as an oral or injection solution, you would usually administer milliliters (mL) of the liquid. The unit of what is to be administered will be the left side of your equation.

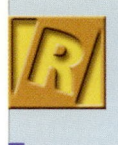

RULE

Step 1	Determine units desired	For dimensional analysis, first write the unknown X and unit of measure desired on the left side of the equation, followed by an equal sign (=).

X (unknown quantity) is written first, followed by the **unit of measure** and then by an equal sign (=). For example,

X tablet =

or

X mL =

EXAMPLE ■

The prescriber orders *digoxin 0.125 mg p.o. daily.* Digoxin 250 mcg (0.25 mg) **tablets** are provided by the pharmacy.

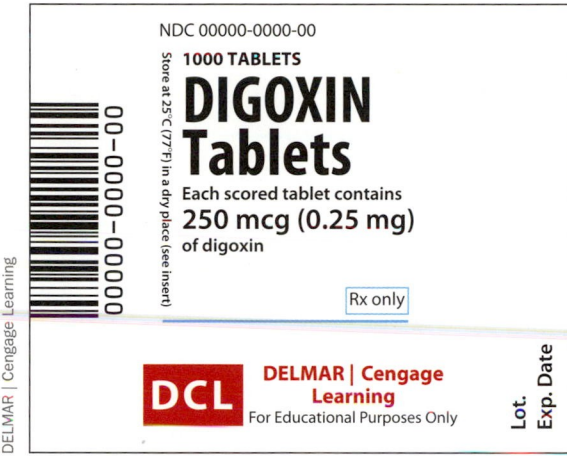

After review of the order and after receiving the medication in tablet form from the pharmacy, you determine that the unit to be administered is a **tablet.** However, the amount to administer is still unknown **(X).** The left side of your equation is ready.

X tablet =

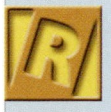

RULE

Step 2	Think	Carefully consider the reasonable amount of the drug that should be administered.

Once you have determined the unit of measure (tablet or mL) that you seek to administer, you must determine the reasonable amount of medication that must be prepared for administration.

In Step 1, you determined that the units are tablets and X tablet is set up to the left of the equal sign. In Step 2, you must consider the reasonable amount of the drug. You must decide whether you are going to administer 1 tablet, a portion of a tablet, or multiple tablets.

Because the pharmacy provided digoxin 0.25 mg tablets, logically, you recognize that the reasonable amount will be less than 1 tablet because 0.125 mg (the ordered dosage) is less than 0.25 mg (the dosage provided). In fact you know that 0.125 is $\frac{1}{2}$ of 0.25, so you reason that you will give $\frac{1}{2}$ tablet.

RULE

Step 3   Calculate   Set up the remainder of your dimensional analysis equation to include all necessary *desired dosage* ratio factors.

Now, you must continue to build your equation to determine the unknown amount (X) of tablets for the dose to administer. The right side of your equation will include all information required to arrive at X.

To determine the unknown (X) amount of tablets to prepare for administration, you must consider the strength and units (supply dosage) dispensed by the pharmacy. A 0.25 mg tablet of Lanoxin was dispensed. Therefore, you have available 0.25 mg per tablet or 0.25 mg/1 tablet.

In this example, 0.25 mg/1 tablet is the same as 1 tablet/0.25 mg. Normally, it does not matter if the tablet is the numerator or denominator because 1 tablet is truly 0.25 mg of the drug Lanoxin that was dispensed. However, the correct ratio to use in your calculations is determined as you continue to build your equation.

To determine whether to use 1 tablet/0.25 mg or to use 0.25 mg/1 tablet, you must look at the units to the left of your equal sign.

X tablet =

X tablets is the same as X tablets/1. Tablet is the numerator; 1 is the denominator. This is the *amount to give ratio.*

$$\frac{\text{X tablet}}{1} =$$

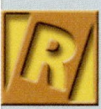

MATH TIP

Dividing or multiplying a number by 1 does not change its value.

Because tablet is in the numerator on the left side of the equal sign, you must match it with tablet in the numerator on the right side of the equal sign. Therefore, you will choose **1 tablet/0.25 mg.** This is the *supply dosage ratio.*

$$\frac{\text{X tablet}}{1} = \frac{\text{1 tablet}}{0.25 \text{ mg}}$$

RULE

For dimensional analysis, the units in the numerator on the left of the equal sign are the same units that are placed in the numerator of the first ratio factor on the right side of the equation.

⚠ **CAUTION**   **THIS IS INCORRECT**

$$\frac{\text{X tablet}}{1} = \frac{0.25 \text{ mg}}{1 \text{ tablet}}$$

THIS IS INCORRECT because tablets do not appear in the numerator on the left and right sides of the equation.

Let's continue; you have not completed setting up this problem. You need one more ratio factor. Because you are looking only for the number of tablets to administer, you must cancel all other units so that only tablet(s) remain in the numerator as a unit of measure on the right side of the equation. The remaining information available to you is the dosage ordered by the physician for the nurse to administer. In this example, it is *Lanoxin 0.125 mg.*

You know that Lanoxin 0.125 mg is the same as Lanoxin 0.125 mg/1 because dividing or multiplying a number by 1 does not change its value. Therefore, **0.125 mg/1** is added to the equation, with mg in the numerator of the second ratio factor so that mg will cancel out leaving the amount of tablets to administer to the patient. This is the *ordered dosage ratio.*

RULE

When the units in a numerator and the units in a denominator are the same, they cancel each other out.

Amount to Give Ratio	=	**Supply Dosage Ratio**	×	**Ordered Dosage Ratio**

$$\frac{X \text{ tablet}}{1} = \frac{1 \text{ tablet}}{0.25 \text{ mg}} \times \frac{\textbf{0.125 mg}}{\textbf{1}}$$

$$\frac{X \text{ tablet}}{1} = \frac{1 \text{ tablet}}{0.25 \text{ m\!\!/g}} \times \frac{0.125 \text{ m\!\!/g}}{1}$$

MATH TIP

When using dimensional analysis and after all cancellations have been made, only the units of measure to be administered remain (such as tablet or mL).

CAUTION   THIS IS INCORRECT

$$\frac{X \text{ tablet}}{1} = \frac{1 \text{ tablet}}{0.25 \text{ mg}} \times \frac{1}{0.125 \text{ mg}}$$

THIS IS INCORRECT because **mg** does not appear in the numerator and the denominator on the right side of the equation. Therefore, **mg** cannot be cancelled out.

As you look at the correct equation and after all units are cancelled, only **tablet** (the unit of measure to administer) remains on the right side of the equation.

$$\frac{X \text{ tablet}}{1} = \frac{1 \textbf{ tablet}}{0.25 \text{ m\!\!/g}} \times \frac{0.125 \text{ m\!\!/g}}{1}$$

Now eliminate everything that was cancelled out and calculate for the **amount of tablets** to give.

$$\frac{X \text{ tablet}}{1} = \frac{0.125}{0.25} \text{ tablet} = \textbf{0.5 tablet}$$

X tablet = 0.5 tablet
X = 0.5
You will administer 0.5 ($\frac{1}{2}$) of a 0.25 mg tablet of Lanoxin to provide 0.125 mg of the drug.

CAUTION

Remember, before dividing a full tablet or caplet you must know whether the formulation provided by the pharmacy may be split. The effect of a drug will be altered if it is split when the drug is provided as an extended release (ER or XL), sustained release (SR), delayed release, or enteric-coated formulation.

CAUTION

If you calculate that a partial *capsule* of medication is to be administered, first stop and think, "Does this make sense?" Recalculate. If you are certain the calculation is correct, you should consult the pharmacist or prescriber for clarification and further direction because capsules are not formulated to be divided.

Let's consider more examples.

EXAMPLE 1 ■

The drug order is for **Lopressor 50 mg p.o. q.12h.** The pharmacy dispenses Lopressor 25 mg tablets.

Step 1	Determine units	tablet (tab)
Step 2	Think	50 mg ordered
		25 mg tab supplied
		Dose will be greater than 1 tab. You will give 2 tab.

Step 3   Calculate $\dfrac{X \text{ tab}}{1} = \dfrac{1 \text{ tab}}{25 \text{ mg}} \times \dfrac{50 \text{ mg}}{1} = \dfrac{50}{25} \text{ tab} = 2 \text{ tab}$

EXAMPLE 2 ■

Order: **Tylenol 240 mg p.o. q.4h p.r.n., pain**

Supply: Tylenol (acetaminophen) 160 mg chewable tablets

Step 1	Determine units	tab
Step 2	Think	240 mg ordered
		160 mg tab supplied
		Dose will be more than 1 tab, but less than 2 tab.

Step 3   Calculate $\dfrac{X \text{ tab}}{1} = \dfrac{1 \text{ tab}}{160 \text{ mg}} \times \dfrac{240 \text{ mg}}{1} = \dfrac{240}{160} \text{ tab} = 1.5 \left(1\tfrac{1}{2}\right) \text{ tab}$

EXAMPLE 3 ■

Order: **cephalexin suspension 250 mg p.o. q.6h**

Supply: cephalexin 100 mg/mL

Step 1	Determine units	mL
Step 2	Think	250 mg ordered
		100 mg/mL supplied
		Dose will be greater than 1 mL and even greater than 2 mL.

Step 3   Calculate $\dfrac{X \text{ mL}}{1} = \dfrac{1 \text{ mL}}{100 \text{ mg}} \times \dfrac{250 \text{ mg}}{1} = \dfrac{250}{100} \text{ mL} = 2.5 \text{ mL}$

Dimensional analysis is a unique method of calculation because converting units of measurement can be included in the calculation on the right side of the equation. Let's consider calculating the proper dose to administer when the ordered units and the supplied units are **not** the same. All calculations and conversions necessary to arrive at your answer will still be included on the right side of the equal sign.

When you correctly set up your equation in dimensional analysis so that all units cancel except for the one you seek (amount to give), you will not be required to memorize formulas or acronyms. In both the formula and ratio-proportion methods, conversions are completed initially and as a separate step. In dimensional analysis, this is not necessary.

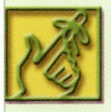

REMEMBER

When using dimensional analysis and after all cancellations have been made, only the units desired remain (such as tablet or mL).

For example, the prescriber orders **Lanoxin (digoxin) 125 mcg p.o. q.AM.** The pharmacy supplies Lanoxin 0.125 mg tablets.

Order: **Lanoxin 125 mcg**

Supply: Lanoxin 0.125 mg tab

Step 1	**Determine units**	tablet
Step 2	**Think**	125 mcg ordered
		0.125 mg supplied
		1 mg = 1,000 mcg
Step 3	**Calculate**	Include the *conversion factor* in the right side of the equation as the second ratio, and then add the ordered dosage as the final ratio. Set it up so that all units cancel except the desired unit (tab). Notice that mg and mcg cancel.

$$\begin{array}{ccccccc} \text{Amount} & & \text{Supply} & & \text{Conversion} & & \text{Ordered} \\ \text{to Give} & = & \text{Dosage} & \times & \text{Factor} & \times & \text{Dosage} \\ \text{Ratio} & & \text{Ratio} & & \text{Ratio} & & \text{Ratio} \end{array}$$

$$\frac{\text{X tab}}{1} = \frac{1 \text{ tab}}{0.125 \text{ mg}} \times \frac{1 \text{ mg}}{1,000 \text{ mcg}} \times \frac{125 \text{ mcg}}{1} = \frac{125}{125} \text{ tab} = 1 \text{ tab}$$

CAUTION   THIS IS INCORRECT

$$\frac{\text{X tab}}{1} = \frac{1 \text{ tab}}{0.125 \text{ mg}} \times \frac{1,000 \text{ mcg}}{1 \text{ mg}} \times \frac{1}{125 \text{ mcg}}$$

THIS IS INCORRECT. All units cannot be cancelled out because mg does not appear in the numerator and the denominator. It appears twice in the denominator. If you continued with this calculation, your result would be 64 tablets instead of 1. Think about the magnitude of such an error. Your common sense would alert you that this is wrong.

As you continue to practice dimensional analysis, you realize you can set up the problems without the added step of placing a 1 under X tablets on the left or under the ordered dosage on the right side of the equation. Consider the same Lanoxin example.

EXAMPLE ■

$$\textbf{X tab} = \frac{1 \text{ tab}}{0.125 \text{ mg}} \times \frac{1 \text{ mg}}{1,000 \text{ mcg}} \times \textbf{125 mcg} = 1 \text{ tab}$$

Let's practice this shortened method of dimensional analysis with more examples.

EXAMPLE 1 ■

Order: *potassium chloride 30 mEq p.o. daily*

Supply: potassium chloride 20 mEq per 15 mL

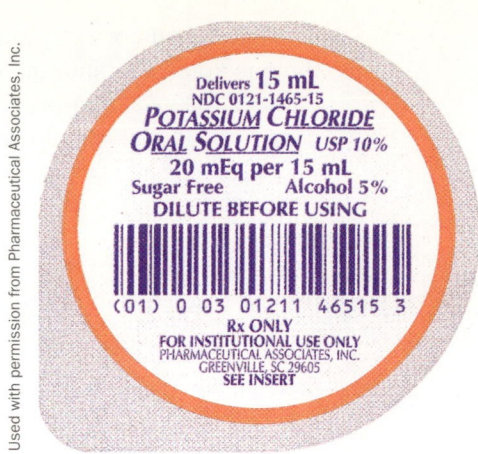

Used with permission from Pharmaceutical Associates, Inc.

Step 1	**Determine units**	mL
Step 2	**Think**	You will administer more than 15 mL because the dosage ordered (30 mEq) is greater than that which is supplied in 15 mL (20 mEq).
Step 3	**Calculate**	$\text{X mL} = \frac{15 \text{ mL}}{20 \text{ mEq}} \times 30 \text{ mEq} = \frac{450}{20} \text{ mL} = 22.5 \text{ mL}$

EXAMPLE 2 ■

Order: *oxycodone HCl 15 mg p.o. q.4h p.r.n., pain*

Supply: oxycodone hydrochloride oral concentrated solution 20 mg/mL

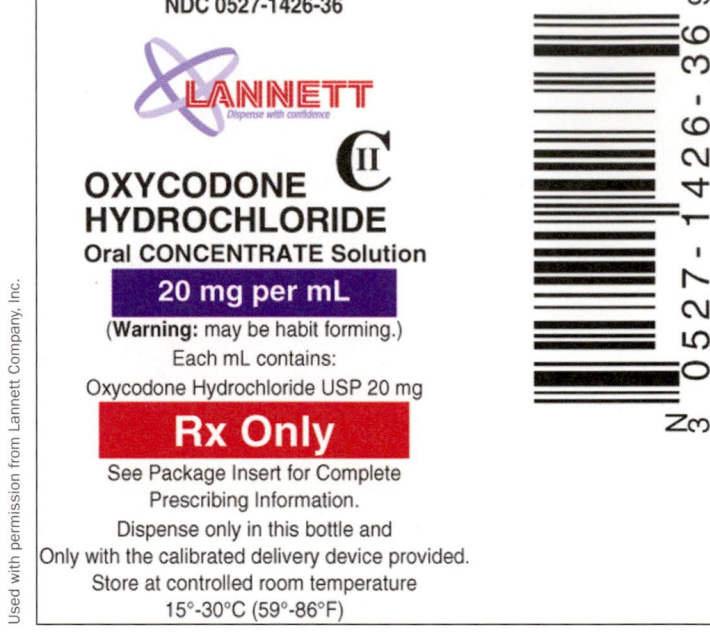

Used with permission from Lannett Company, Inc.

Step 1	**Determine units**	mL
Step 2	**Think**	20 mg in 1 mL
		15 mg is less than 20 mg.
		Dose will be less than 1 mL.
Step 3	**Calculate**	$\text{X mL} = \frac{1 \text{ mL}}{20 \text{ mg}} \times 15 \text{ mg} = \frac{15}{20} \text{ mL} = 0.75 \text{ mL}$

CAUTION

This is a concentrated medication and a small oral dose. It is necessary to administer the exact dose prescribed to avoid medication over- or under-dosing. If a delivery device is supplied with the medication, it must be used. If a delivery device is not supplied, you must clearly label the oral syringe so that the medication is not inadvertently administered by the parenteral route.

EXAMPLE 3 ■

Order: **terbutaline sulfate 10 mg p.o. t.i.d.**

Supply: terbutaline sulfate 5 mg tab

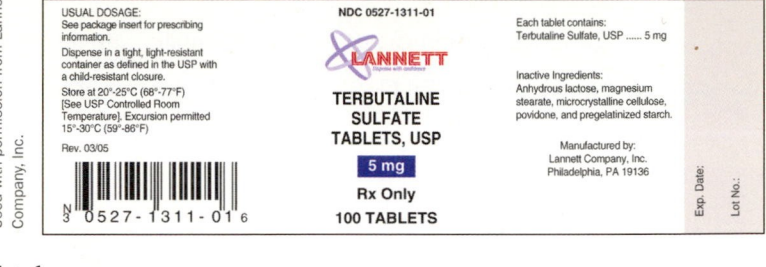

Step 1 **Determine units** tab

Step 2 **Think** 5 mg in 1 tab

10 mg is more than 5 mg.

Dose will be more than 1 tab. You want to give 2 tab.

Step 3 **Calculate** $X \text{ tab} = \frac{1 \text{ tab}}{5 \text{ mg}} \times 10 \text{ mg} = \frac{10}{5} \text{ tab} = 2 \text{ tab}$

EXAMPLE 4 ■

Order: **haloperidol decanoate 0.25 g IM monthly**

Supply: haloperidol decanoate injection 100 mg/mL

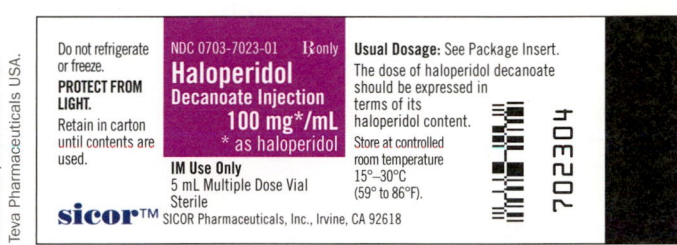

Step 1 **Determine units** mL

Step 2 **Think** 100 mg in 1 mL

1 g = 1,000 mg

Dose will be more than 1 mL.

Step 3 **Calculate** $X \text{ mL} = \frac{1 \text{ mL}}{100 \text{ mg}} \times \frac{1{,}000 \text{ mg}}{1 \text{ g}} \times 0.25 \text{ g} = \frac{250 \text{ mL}}{100} = 2.5 \text{ mL}$

EXAMPLE 5 ■

Order: **dexamethasone 3 mg IV q.6h**

Supply: dexamethasone sodium phosphate injection 4 mg/mL

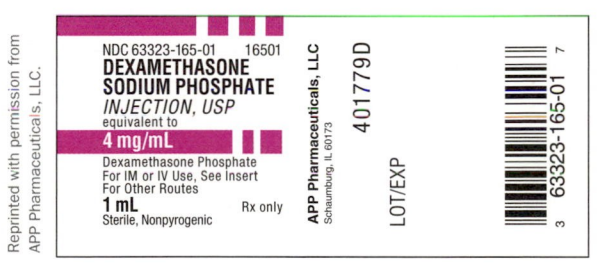

Step 1 **Determine units** mL

Step 2 **Think** 4 mg in 1 mL

3 mg is less than 4 mg.

Dose will be less than 1 mL.

Step 3 **Calculate** $X \text{ mL} = \frac{1 \text{ mL}}{4 \text{ mg}} \times 3 \text{ mg} = \frac{3}{4} \text{ mL} = 0.75 \text{ mL}$

EXAMPLE 6 ■

Order: **levothyroxine 0.075 mg p.o. a.c. breakfast**

Supply: Synthroid (levothyroxine) 25 mcg tablets

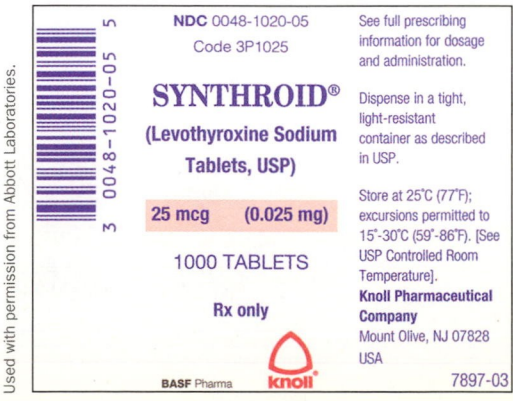

Step 1 **Determine units** tab

Step 2 **Think** Give more than 1 tab; in fact, you will give 3 tab.

Step 3 **Calculate** $X \text{ tab} =$

$\frac{1 \text{ tab}}{25 \text{ mcg}} \times \frac{1{,}000 \text{ mcg}}{1 \text{ mg}} \times 0.075 \text{ mg} = \frac{75}{25} \text{ tab} = 3 \text{ tab}$

EXAMPLE 7 ■

Order: *penicillin G potassium 1.2 million units IM daily*

Supply: penicillin G potassium vial with 5 million units to be reconstituted

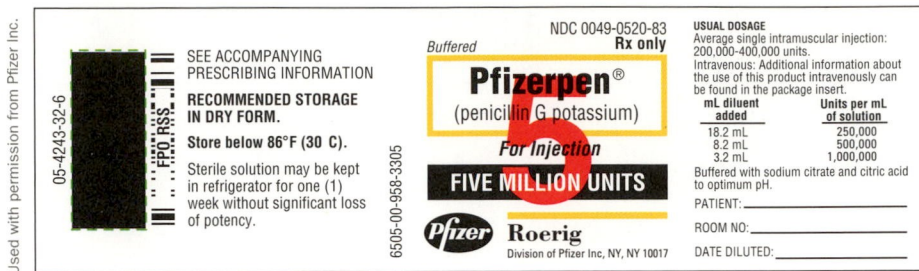

Step 1	Determine units	mL
Step 2	Think	Maximum IM dose volume to be administered to an adult patient is 3 mL. You choose to dilute with 8.2 mL of diluent. Per the label, the concentration is now 500,000 units/mL. You will give more than 1 mL to administer 1,200,000 or 1.2 million units.

Step 3 **Calculate**

$$X \text{ mL} = \frac{1 \text{ mL}}{500,000 \text{ units}} \times 1,200,000 \text{ units} = \frac{1,200,000}{500,000} \text{ mL} = 2.4 \text{ mL}$$

You can also add additional ratios to the right side of the equation to account for additional factors relevant to the patient and required conversions. Examples 8–10 demonstrate dimensional analysis dosage calculations for orders based on body weight (such as mg/kg). Refer to Chapter 14 for more information about medications ordered and recommended according to body weight.

EXAMPLE 8 ■

An elderly patient weighs 50 kg and is diagnosed with methicillin resistant staphylococcus aureas (MRSA) pneumonia.

Order: *vancomycin 15 mg/kg IV q.12h*

Supply: vancomycin 1 g diluted with 20 mL of sterile water for injection

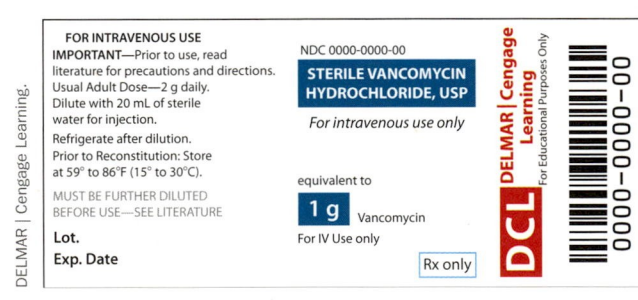

Step 1	Determine units	mL
Step 2	Think	You will need to calculate the dosage for a patient who weighs 50 kg by including an *ordered dosage/kg ratio* and a *body weight ratio*. 1 g = 1,000 mg Supply dosage is 1 g per 20 mL.

Step 3 **Calculate**

Set up the calculation to include all the ratio factors needed to calculate the dose so that g, mg, and kg all cancel leaving mL.

$$\underset{\text{Ratio}}{\underset{\text{to Give}}{\text{Amount}}} = \underset{\text{Ratio}}{\underset{\text{Dosage}}{\text{Supply}}} \times \underset{\text{Ratio}}{\underset{\text{Factor}}{\text{Conversion}}} \times \underset{\text{Ratio}}{\underset{\text{Dosage/kg}}{\text{Ordered}}} \times \underset{\text{Ratio}}{\underset{\text{Weight}}{\text{Body}}}$$

$$X \text{ mL} = \frac{20 \text{ mL}}{1 \text{ g}} \times \frac{1 \text{ g}}{1,000 \text{ mg}} \times \frac{15 \text{ mg}}{1 \text{ kg}} \times 50 \text{ kg} = \frac{20 \times 1 \times 15 \times 50}{1 \times 1,000 \times 1} \text{ mL} = \frac{15,000}{1,000} \text{ mL} = 15 \text{ mL}$$

EXAMPLE 9 ■

An adolescent burn patient weighs 99 lb.

Order: *vancomycin 10 mg/kg IV q.8h*

Supply: vancomycin 500 mg diluted with 10 mL sterile water for injection

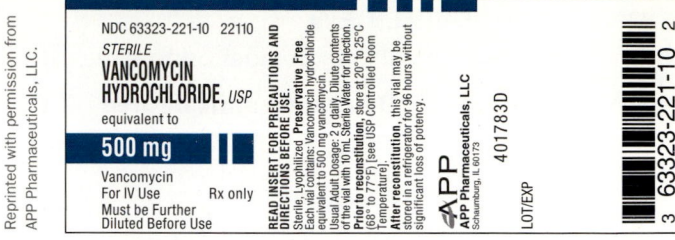

Step 1	**Determine units**	mL
Step 2	**Think**	You will need to calculate the dosage for a patient who weighs 99 lb. To calculate the ordered dosage, you must add a conversion factor ratio to convert the patient's weight to kg.

$$1 \text{ kg} = 2.2 \text{ lb}$$

Supply dosage is 500 mg per 10 mL.

Step 3	**Calculate**	Set up the calculation to include all the ratio factors needed to calculate the dose so that mg, lb, and kg all cancel leaving mL remaining.

Amount to Give Ratio	=	Supply Dosage Ratio	×	Ordered Dosage/kg Ratio	×	Conversion Factor Ratio	×	Body Weight Ratio

$$X \text{ mL} = \frac{10 \text{ mL}}{500 \text{ mg}} \times \frac{10 \text{ mg}}{1 \text{ kg}} \times \frac{1 \text{ kg}}{2.2 \text{ lb}} \times 99 \text{ lb} = \frac{10 \times 10 \times 1 \times 99}{500 \times 1 \times 2.2} \text{ mL} = \frac{9{,}900}{1{,}100} \text{ mL} = 9 \text{ mL}$$

The key to dimensional analysis is to think carefully about all the ratio factors required and to be careful setting up the ratios for your calculations so that all units cancel except the unit of the unknown (X) amount to give. Let's examine one final example that requires two conversions: supply dosage and weight.

EXAMPLE 10 ■

A patient diagnosed with MRSA bacteremia weighs 143 lb.

Order: *vancomycin 15 mg/kg IV q.12h*

Supply: vancomycin 1 g diluted with 20 mL of sterile water for injection

FOR INTRAVENOUS USE
IMPORTANT—Prior to use, read literature for precautions and directions.
Usual Adult Dose—2 g daily. Dilute with 20 mL of sterile water for injection.
Refrigerate after dilution.
Prior to Reconstitution: Store at 59° to 86°F (15° to 30°C).
MUST BE FURTHER DILUTED BEFORE USE—SEE LITERATURE
Lot.
Exp. Date

NDC 0000-0000-00
STERILE VANCOMYCIN HYDROCHLORIDE, USP
For intravenous use only
equivalent to
1 g Vancomycin
For IV Use only
Rx only

Step 1	**Determine units**	mL
Step 2	**Think**	You will need to calculate the dosage for a patient who weighs 143 lb.

$$1 \text{ kg} = 2.2 \text{ lb}$$

Supply dosage is 1 g per 20 mL.

$$1 \text{ g} = 1{,}000 \text{ mg}$$

Step 3	**Calculate**	Set up the calculation to include all the ratio factors needed to calculate the dose so that g, mg, lb, and kg all cancel leaving mL.

Amount to Give Ratio	=	Supply Dosage Ratio	×	Conversion Factor Ratio	×	Ordered Dosage/kg Ratio	×	Conversion Factor Ratio	×	Body Weight Ratio

$$X \text{ mL} = \frac{20 \text{ mL}}{1 \text{ g}} \times \frac{1 \text{ g}}{1{,}000 \text{ mg}} \times \frac{15 \text{ mg}}{1 \text{ kg}} \times \frac{1 \text{ kg}}{2.2 \text{ lb}} \times 143 \text{ lb} = \frac{20 \times 1 \times 15 \times 1 \times 143}{1 \times 1{,}000 \times 1 \times 2.2} \text{ mL}$$

$$= \frac{42{,}900}{2{,}200} \text{ mL} = 19.5 \text{ mL}$$

QUICK REVIEW

When calculating dosages using dimensional analysis:

Step 1   **Determine units desired**   X units = on the left side of the equation.

Step 2   **Think**   Carefully consider the reasonable amount of the drug to give.

Step 3   **Calculate**   Set up the remainder of the dimensional analysis equation to include all necessary *desired dosage* ratio factors.

- When using dimensional analysis, you must first determine units of the medication you seek to administer: tablets, mL, etc.

- The unknown and units are placed on the left side of the equal sign: X tablets =

- The units in the numerator on the left of the equal sign are the same units that are placed in the numerator of the first ratio on the right side of the equation.

- All conversions are entered into the right side of the equation.

- When the units in a numerator and the units in a denominator are the same, they cancel each other out.

- When using dimensional analysis and after all cancellations have been made, only the units (tablets, mL, etc.) of the dose to administer remain.

- Always determine units, then think or reason for the logical answer, set up your equation of ratio factors to cancel units leaving the one you want to give, and calculate.

Review Set 30

Use dimensional analysis to calculate the amount you will prepare for each dose.

1. Order: **heparin 5,000 units subcut stat**

   Supply: heparin 10,000 units/mL

   Give: _____ mL

2. Order: **ketorolac 45 mg IV q.6h p.r.n., pain**

   Supply: ketorolac 15 mg/mL

   Give: _____ mL

3. Order: **phenytoin sodium 15 mg/kg slowly IV drip stat (patient weighs 250 lb)**

   Supply: phenytoin sodium 250 mg per 5 mL.

   Give: _____ mL

4. Order: **hydroxyzine pamoate 60 mg p.o. q.4h p.r.n., nausea**

   Supply: hydroxyzine pamoate 25 mg per 5 mL

   Give: _____ mL

5. Order: **Keflex 0.5 g p.o. q.12h**

   Supply: Keflex (cephalexin) 250 mg per 5 mL

   Give: _____ mL

6. Order: **Depakene 0.01 g/kg p.o. q.12h (patient weighs 143 lb)**

   Supply: Depakene (valproic acid) 250 mg per 5 mL

   Give: _____ mL

7. Order: **DiaBeta 3.75 mg p.o. a.c. breakfast daily**

   Supply: DiaBeta (glyburide) 2.5 mg tablets

   Give: _____ tab

8. Order: **Lopressor 100 mg p.o. daily**

   Supply: Lopressor (metoprolol tartrate) 50 mg tablets

   Give: _____ tab

9. Order: **Lasix 20 mg per GT b.i.d.**

   Supply: Lasix (furosemide) 10 mg/mL

   Give: _____ mL

10. Order: **potassium chloride 24 mEq p.o. daily**

    Supply: Micro-K (potassium chloride) 8 mEq/tablet

    Give: _____ tab

11. Order: **Robinul 4 mcg/kg IM 1 h pre-op** (patient weighs 185 lb)

    Supply: Robinul (glycopyrrolate) 0.2 mg/mL

    Give: _____ mL

12. Order: **Epogen 150 units/kg subcut 3x/week** (patient weighs 133 lb)

    Supply: Epogen (epoetin alfa) 10,000 units/mL

    Give: _____ mL

13. Order: **morphine 50 mcg/kg subcut q.4h p.r.n., pain** (patient weighs 27 lb)

    Supply: morphine 2 mg/mL

    Give: _____ mL

14. Order: **albuterol sulfate 3 mg p.o. t.i.d.**

    Supply: albuterol sulfate syrup 2 mg per 5 mL

    Give: _____ mL

15. Order: **octreotide 150 mcg subcut t.i.d.**

    Supply: Sandostatin (octreotide) 0.2 mg/mL

    Give: _____ mL

16. Order: **phenobarbital 120 mg via GT daily**

    Supply: phenobarbital 20 mg/mL

    Give: _____ mL

17. Order: **midazolam 80 mcg/kg IM stat** (patient weighs 80 kg)

    Supply: midazolam 2 mg/mL

    Give: _____ mL

18. Order: **hydroxyzine hydrochloride 60 mg IM on call to OR**

    Supply: hydroxyzine hydrochloride 50 mg/mL

    Give: _____ mL

19. Order: **cefaclor 990 mg/day total, divided p.o. q.8h**

    Supply: cefaclor 375 mg per 5 mL

    Give: _____ mL (per dose)

20. Order: **tobramycin 62 mg IV q.8h**

    Supply: tobramycin sulfate 20 mg per 2 mL

    Give: _____ mL

After completing these problems, see page 541 to check your answers.

For more practice, recalculate the amount you will prepare for each dose in Review Sets 22 through 26 using the formula and dimensional analysis methods.

CRITICAL THINKING SKILLS

Medications supplied in solution form are labeled with the concentration of the supplied dosage. Errors may occur if the nurse fails to check the quantity of the concentration prior to calculating the dose.

ERROR

Failing to check the concentration carefully on the label and assuming the quantity of the supplied dose is 1 mL.

Possible Scenario

A patient experienced a generalized seizure at work and was medicated with an anticonvulsant and hospitalized for observation overnight. The patient began to seize again, this time the episodes occurred continuously, and an order was given to treat for status epilepticus with *diazepam 5 mg IV stat.* The nurse removed a vial labeled with diazepam 10 mg from the computer dispensing system. Assuming there was 10 mg per mL, the nurse calculated the dose using the dosage calculation formula as follows:

$$\frac{D}{H} \times Q \text{ (quantity)} = \frac{10 \text{ mg}}{5 \text{ mg}} \times 1 \text{ mL} = 0.5 \text{ mL} \quad \textbf{INCORRECT}$$

The nurse administered 0.5 mL of the medication and placed the opened vial on the bedside table. The seizure did not stop, and after 10 minutes the physician ordered a second 5 mg dose. The nurse used the same vial and removed the solution remaining, expecting to have only enough for one more 0.5 mL dose. The nurse was surprised to find that there was actually 1.5 mL remaining in the vial. After examining the vial more carefully the nurse saw the concentration was clearly 10 mg per 2 mL. Realizing the previous calculation error, the nurse recalculated the dose as follows:

$$\frac{D}{H} \times Q \text{ (quantity)} = \frac{10 \text{ mg}}{5 \text{ mg}} \times 2 \text{ mL} = 1 \text{ mL} \quad \textbf{CORRECT}$$

The nurse then administered the correct amount of 1 mL for the second 5 mg dose. A few minutes later the patient's seizures started to subside.

Potential Outcome

Due to a calculation error, the patient received a sub therapeutic dose of medication in a medical emergency. If the nurse did not recognize the error, the patient may have received additional inadequate doses of diazepam and the seizures may have lasted a significantly longer period of time. The longer the continuous seizure activity persists the greater the risk for neurological damage.

Prevention

Many solutions supplied in ampules and vials have a dose concentration expressed per 1 mL. Nurses may become so accustomed to this that eventually they fail to look closely at the information provided on the labels. Use care reading the labels of all medications, even those you administer frequently. Medications supplied by different pharmaceutical companies may be prepared with different concentrations. When using the dosage calculation formula, always check for the Q (quantity of dosage concentration). Don't assume it is 1 mL.

CRITICAL THINKING SKILLS

Medication errors will occur if the right side of the equation is set up improperly when using the dimensional analysis method for dosage calculations.

ERROR

All ratios necessary to arrive at the desired units are not entered correctly into the dimensional analysis equation.

Possible Scenario

The physician ordered **erythromycin ethylsuccinate 20 mg/kg p.o. once prior to a dental procedure** for a child who weighed 45 lb. Six hours after the procedure, the child would receive an additional dosage of 10 mg/kg. The nurse who prepared the initial dose obtained erythromycin ethylsuccinate 200 mg per 5 mL from the pharmacy. The nurse calculated the dose using dimensional analysis and incorrectly set up the problem this way:

$$X \text{ mL} = \frac{5 \text{ ml}}{200 \text{ mg}} \times \frac{20 \text{ mg}}{1 \text{ kg}} \times 45 \text{ lbs} = 22.5 \text{ mL} \quad \textbf{INCORRECT}$$

The nurse who had prepared the drug was having a difficult time administering it to the child, who was experiencing a significant amount of oral pain. As the nurse requested the assistance of another nurse, the second nurse questioned the amount of drug measured in a plastic medicine cup that was being given as the prophylactic therapy before the dental procedure. At this point the two nurses recalculated the dosage together and the correct dose was prepared.

Potential Outcome

Although doses as high as 30 to 50 mg/kg/day of erythromycin are given to children, the specific dose is determined by the severity of the infection. This child, who did not have a diagnosed infection, would have received a dose double of that which was ordered by the physician and then a double dose of the drug ordered to be administered again 6 hours later. Improper administration of antibiotics has been attributed to bacterial mutations and development of strains of bacteria that are resistant to many antibiotics.

Prevention

This type of calculation error occurred because the nurse set up the dimensional analysis problem incorrectly. All necessary calculations were not entered into the right side of the equation. The problem should have been set up and calculated this way:

$$X \text{ mL} = \frac{5 \text{ mL}}{200 \text{ mg}} \times \frac{20 \text{ mg}}{1 \text{ kg}} \times \frac{1 \text{ kg}}{2.2 \text{ lbs}} \times 45 \text{ lbs} = 10.2 \text{ mL} \quad \textbf{CORRECT}$$

Remember, all units of measure must cancel out leaving only the unit you seek to give, in this case, mL. The nurse should have noticed that both mL and lb were remaining in the incorrect equation. That would have been a clue to double check the calculation. It is important to think carefully before you begin your calculations to determine all the ratios necessary and the proper way to set up the dimensional analysis equation.

PRACTICE PROBLEMS—CHAPTER 13

Calculate the amount to prepare 1 dose using both the formula and dimensional analysis methods.

1. Order: lactulose 30 g in 100 mL fluid p.r. t.i.d.

   Supply: lactulose 3.33 g per 5 mL

   Give: _____ mL in 100 mL

2. Order: penicillin G potassium 500,000 units IM q.i.d.

   Supply: penicillin G potassium 5,000,000 units per 20 mL

   Give: _____ mL

3. Order: Keflex 100 mg p.o. q.i.d.

   Supply: Keflex oral suspension 250 mg per 5 mL

   Give: _____ mL

4. Order: **amoxicillin 125 mg p.o. q.i.d.**

   Supply: amoxicillin 250 mg per 5 mL

   NOTE: You are giving home-care instructions.

   Give: _____ t

5. Order: **Benadryl 25 mg IM stat**

   Supply: Benadryl 10 mg/mL

   Give: _____ mL

6. Order: **diphenhydramine 40 mg p.o. stat**

   Supply: diphenhydramine 12.5 mg per 5 mL

   Give: _____ mL

7. Order: **penicillin G potassium 350,000 units IM b.i.d.**

   Supply: penicillin G potassium 500,000 units per 2 mL

   Give: _____ mL

8. Order: **Valium 3.5 mg IM q.6h p.r.n., anxiety**

   Supply: Valium 10 mg per 2 mL

   Give: _____ mL

9. Order: **tobramycin sulfate 90 mg IV q.8h**

   Supply: tobramycin sulfate 80 mg per 2 mL

   Give: _____ mL

10. Order: **heparin 2,500 units subcut b.i.d.**

    Supply: heparin 20,000 units/mL

    Give: _____ mL

11. Order: **Compazine 8 mg IM q.6h p.r.n., nausea**

    Supply: Compazine 10 mg per 2 mL

    Give: _____ mL

12. Order: **gentamicin 60 mg IV q.6h**

    Supply: gentamicin 80 mg per 2 mL

    Give: _____ mL

13. Order: **piperacillin 500 mg IV b.i.d.**

    Supply: piperacillin 1 g per 2.5 mL

    Give: _____ mL

14. Order: **Nilstat Oral Suspension 250,000 units p.o. q.i.d.**

    Supply: Nilstat Oral Suspension 100,000 units/mL

    Give: _____ mL

15. Order: **erythromycin estolate 80 mg p.o. q.4h**

    Supply: erythromycin estolate 250 mg per 5 mL

    Give: _____ mL

16. Order: **potassium chloride 10 mEq p.o. stat**

    Supply: potassium chloride 20 mEq per 15 mL

    Give: _____ mL

17. Order: **nafcillin 400 mg IV q.6h**

    Supply: nafcillin 1 g per 4 mL

    Give: _____ mL

18. Order: **Synthroid 150 mcg p.o. daily**

    Supply: Synthroid 0.075 mg tablets

    Give: _____ tablet(s)

19. Order: **amoxicillin 400 mg p.o. q.8h**

    Supply: amoxicillin 250 mg per 5 mL

    Give: _____ mL

20. Order: **phenytoin 225 mg IV stat**

    Supply: phenytoin 50 mg/mL

    Give: _____ mL

21. Order: **Elixophyllin 160 mg p.o. q.6h**

    Supply: Elixophyllin 80 mg per 15 mL

    Give: _____ mL

22. Order: **chlorpromazine 35 mg IM stat**

    Supply: chlorpromazine 25 mg/mL

    Give: _____ mL

23. Order: **oxycodone hydrochloride 8 mg p.o. q.4h p.r.n., pain**

    Supply: oxycodone hydrochloride 20 mg/mL

    Add: _____ mL

24. Order: **promethazine 25 mg via NG tube h.s.**

    Supply: promethazine 6.25 mg per 5 mL

    Give: _____ mL

25. Order: **cefaclor 300 mg p.o. t.i.d.**

    Supply: cefaclor 125 mg per 5 mL

    Give: _____ mL

26. Describe the strategy you would implement to prevent this medication error.

Possible Scenario

The physician ordered **Amoxil 50 mg p.o. q.i.d.** for a child with an upper respiratory infection. Amoxil is supplied in an oral suspension with 125 mg per 5 mL. The nurse calculated the dose this way:

$$\frac{D}{H} \times Q = \frac{125 \text{ mg}}{50 \text{ mg}} \times 5 \text{ mL} = \frac{625}{50} \text{ mL} = 12.5 \text{ mL} \qquad \text{INCORRECT}$$

Give 12.5 mL orally four times a day.

Potential Outcome

The patient received a large overdose and should have received only 2 mL. The child would likely develop complications from overdosage of amoxicillin. When the physician was notified of the error, she would likely have ordered the medication discontinued and had extra blood lab work done. An incident report would be filed and the family would be notified of the error.

Prevention

_____

_____

After completing these problems, see page 541–542 to check your answers.

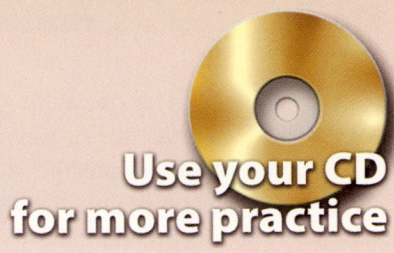
Use your CD
for more practice

14

Pediatric and Adult Dosages Based on Body Weight

OBJECTIVES

Upon mastery of Chapter 14, you will be able to calculate drug dosages based on body weight and verify the safety of medication orders. To accomplish this you will also be able to:

- Convert pounds to kilograms.
- Consult a reputable drug resource to calculate the recommended safe dosage per kilogram of body weight.
- Compare the ordered dosage with the recommended safe dosage.
- Determine whether the ordered dosage is safe to administer.
- Apply body weight dosage calculations to patients across the life span.

O nly a doctor, dentist, physician assistant, or nurse practitioner (in some states) may prescribe the dosage of medications. However, before administering a drug, the nurse should know if the ordered dosage is safe. This is important for all patients, but it is of the utmost importance to infants, children, frail elderly, and critically ill adults.

CAUTION
Those who administer drugs to patients are legally responsible for recognizing incorrect and unsafe dosages and for alerting the prescribing practitioner.

The one who administers a drug is just as responsible for the patient's safety as the one who prescribes it. For the protection of the patient and yourself, you must familiarize yourself with the recommended dosage of drugs or consult a reputable drug reference, such as the *package insert* that accompanies the drug or the *Hospital Formulary*.

Standard adult dosage is determined by the drug manufacturer. Dosage is usually recommended based on the requirements of an average-weight adult. Frequently an adult range is given, listing a minimum and maximum safe dosage, allowing the nurse to simply compare what is ordered to what is recommended.

Dosages for infants and children are based on their unique and changing body differences. The prescribing practitioner must consider the weight, height, body surface area, age, and condition of the child as contributing factors to safe and effective medication dosages. The two methods currently used for calculating safe pediatric dosages are *body weight* (such as mg/kg) and *body surface area* (BSA, measured in square meters, m^2). The body weight method is more common in pediatric situations and is emphasized in this chapter. The BSA method is based on both weight and height. It is used primarily in oncology and critical care situations. BSA is discussed in Chapter 16. Although used most frequently in pediatrics, both the body weight and BSA methods are also used for adults, especially in critical care situations. The calculations are the same.

ADMINISTERING MEDICATIONS TO CHILDREN

Numerically, the infant's or child's dosage appears smaller, but proportionally pediatric dosages are frequently much larger per kilogram of body weight than the usual adult dosage. Infants—birth to 1 year—have a greater percentage of body water and diminished ability to absorb water-soluble drugs, necessitating dosages of oral and some parenteral drugs that are proportionally higher than those given to persons of larger size. Children—age 1 to 12 years—metabolize drugs more readily than adults, which necessitates higher dosages. Both infants and children, however, are growing, and their organ systems are still maturing. Immature physiological processes related to absorption, distribution, metabolism, and excretion put them continuously at risk for overdose, toxic reactions, and even death. Adolescents—age 13 to 18 years—are often erroneously thought of as adults because of their body weight (greater than 110 pounds or 50 kilograms) and mature physical appearance. In fact, they should still be regarded as physiologically immature, with unpredictable growth spurts and hormonal surges. Drug therapy for the pediatric population is further complicated because little detailed pharmacologic research has been done on children and adolescents. The infant or child, therefore, must be frequently evaluated for desired clinical responses to medications, and serum drug levels are needed to help adjust some drug dosages. It is important to remember that administration of an incorrect dosage to adult patients is dangerous, but with a child, the risk is even greater. Therefore, using a reputable drug reference to verify safe pediatric dosages is a critical health care skill.

A well-written drug reference developed especially for pediatrics is MyNursingPDA: *Pediatric Drugs and Nursing Implications* (Bindler, Howry, Wilson, Shannon, & Stang, 2009). There are also a variety of pocket-size pediatric drug handbooks. Two widely used handbooks are *Johns Hopkins Hospital: The Harriet Lane Handbook* (2008) and *Pediatric Dosage Handbook: Including Neonatal Dosing, Drug Administration, & Extemporaneous Preparations* (Taketomo, Kraus & Hodding, 2009).

CONVERTING POUNDS TO KILOGRAMS

The body weight method uses calculations based on the person's weight in kilograms. Recall that the pounds to kilograms conversion was introduced in Chapter 4.

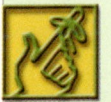

REMEMBER

1 kg = 2.2 lb and 1 lb = 16 oz
Simply stated, weight in pounds is approximately twice (slightly more) the metric weight in kg; or weight in kg is approximately $\frac{1}{2}$ (slightly less) of weight in pounds. You can estimate kg by halving the weight in lb.

MATH TIP

When converting pounds to kilograms, round kilogram weight to one decimal place (tenths).

EXAMPLE 1 ▪

Convert 45 lb to kg

Approximate equivalent: 1 kg = 2.2 lb

Think: $\frac{1}{2}$ of 45 = approximately 23 (answer will be slightly less)

$$\frac{1\ kg}{2.2\ lb} \diagup\!\!\!\!\diagdown \frac{X\ kg}{45\ lb}$$

$$2.2X = 45$$

$$\frac{2.2X}{2.2} = \frac{45}{2.2}$$

$$X = 20.45\ kg = 20.5\ kg$$

EXAMPLE 2 ▪

Convert 10 lb 12 oz to kg

Approximate equivalents: 1 kg = 2.2 lb

                                    1 lb = 16 oz

First convert ounces to pounds.

$$\frac{1\ lb}{16\ oz} \diagup\!\!\!\!\diagdown \frac{X\ lb}{12\ oz}$$

$$16X = 12$$

$$\frac{16X}{16} = \frac{12}{16}$$

$$X = \frac{3}{4}\ lb$$

Now you know that 10 lb 12 oz = $10\frac{3}{4}$ lb

Now you are ready to convert $10\frac{3}{4}$ lb to kg. Because you are converting to the metric system, your answer must be in decimals.

Think: $\frac{1}{2}$ of $10\frac{3}{4}$ = approximately 5

$$10\frac{3}{4} = 10.75$$

$$\frac{1\ kg}{2.2\ lb} \diagup\!\!\!\!\diagdown \frac{X\ kg}{10.75\ lb}$$

$$2.2X = 10.75$$

$$\frac{2.2X}{2.2} = \frac{10.75}{2.2}$$

$$X = 4.88\ kg = 4.9\ kg$$

BODY WEIGHT METHOD FOR CALCULATING SAFE PEDIATRIC DOSAGE

The most common method of prescribing and administering the therapeutic amount of medication for a child is to calculate the amount of drug according to the child's body weight in **kilograms.** The nurse then compares the child's ordered dosage to the recommended safe dosage from a reputable drug resource before administering the medication. The intent is to ensure that the ordered dosage is safe and effective before calculating the amount to give and administering the dose to the patient.

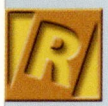

> **RULE**
>
> To verify safe pediatric dosage:
>
> 1. Convert the child's weight from pounds to kilograms (rounded to tenths).
>
> 2. Calculate the safe dosage in mg/kg or mcg/kg (rounded to tenths) for a child of this weight, as recommended by a reputable drug reference: **multiply mg/kg by child's weight in kg.**
>
> 3. Compare the ordered dosage to the recommended dosage, and decide if the dosage is safe.
>
> 4. If safe, calculate the amount to give and administer the dose; if the dosage seems unsafe, consult with the prescribing practitioner before administering the drug.
>
> Note: The dosage per kg may be mg/kg, mcg/kg, g/kg, mEq/kg, unit/kg, milliunit/kg, etc.

For each pediatric medication order, you must ask yourself, "Is this dosage safe?" Let's work through some examples.

Single-Dosage Drugs

Single-dosage drugs are intended to be given once or p.r.n. Dosage ordered by the body weight method is based on **mg/kg/dose, calculated by multiplying the recommended mg by the patient's kg weight for each dose.**

EXAMPLE ■

The physician orders **morphine sulfate 1.8 mg IM stat.** The child weighs 79 lb. You need to determine if this dosage is safe.

1. **Convert lb to kg.** Approximate equivalent: 1 kg = 2.2 lb

   Think: $\frac{1}{2}$ of 79 = approximately 40 (answer will be slightly less)

   $$\frac{1\ kg}{2.2\ lb} \diagdown \diagup \frac{X\ kg}{79\ lb}$$

   $$2.2\ X = 79$$

   $$\frac{2.2X}{2.2} = \frac{79}{2.2}$$

   $$X = 35.90\ kg = 35.9\ kg$$

2. **Calculate mg/kg as recommended by a reputable drug resource.** A reputable drug resource indicates that the usual IM or subcut dosage may be initiated at 0.05 mg/kg/dose.

   Use ratio-proportion to calculate how many mg per dose of the medication should be ordered.

   For each dose: Ratio for recommended mg/kg = Ratio for desired mg/kg

   $$\frac{0.05\ mg}{1\ kg} \diagdown \diagup \frac{X\ mg}{35.9\ kg}$$

   $$X = 0.05 \times 35.9$$

   $$X = 1.79\ mg = 1.8\ mg\ (per\ dose)$$

   Or, you can simply multiply mg/kg/dose by the child's weight in kg.

MATH TIP

Notice that the kg unit of measurement cancels out, leaving the unit as mg/dose.

$\frac{mg/\cancel{kg}}{dose} \times \cancel{kg} = mg/dose$

Or,

$mg/\cancel{kg}/dose \times \cancel{kg} = mg/dose$

Per dose: $0.05 \text{ mg}/\cancel{kg}/dose \times 35.9 \cancel{kg} = 1.79 \text{ mg}/dose = 1.8 \text{ mg}/dose$

3. **Decide if the dosage is safe by comparing ordered and recommended dosages.** For this child's weight, 1.8 mg is the recommended dosage, and 1.8 mg is the ordered dosage. Yes, the dosage is safe.

4. **Calculate one dose.** Apply the three steps of dosage calculation.

   Order: **morphine sulfate 1.8 mg IM stat**

   Supply: morphine sulfate 5 mg/mL (Figure 14-1)

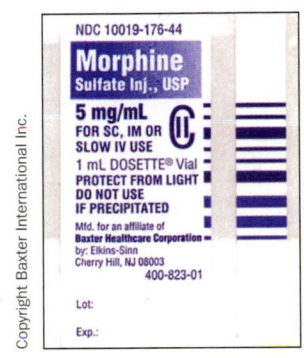

Step 1	**Convert**	No conversion is necessary.
Step 2	**Think**	You want to give less than 1 mL. Estimate that you want to give less than 0.5 mL.

Step 3 **Calculate**

$$\frac{\text{Dosage on hand}}{\text{Amount on hand}} = \frac{\text{Dosage desired}}{X \text{ Amount desired}}$$

$$\frac{5 \text{ mg}}{1 \text{ mL}} \diagdown\!\!\!\!\!\diagup \frac{1.8 \text{ mg}}{X \text{ mL}}$$

$$5X = 1.8$$

$$\frac{5X}{5} = \frac{1.8}{5}$$

$$X = 0.36 \text{ mL}$$

This is a small, child's dose. Measure 0.36 mL in a 1 mL syringe. Route is IM. You may need to change the needle.

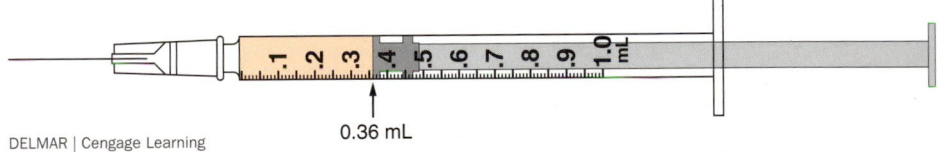

0.36 mL

Single-Dosage Range

Some single-dosage medications indicate a minimum and maximum range, or a safe dosage range.

EXAMPLE ■

The practitioner orders **Vistaril 20 mg IM q.4h p.r.n., nausea.** The child weighs 44 lb. Is this a safe dosage?

1. **Convert lb to kg.** Approximate equivalent: 1 kg = 2.2 lb

   THINK: $\frac{1}{2}$ of 44 = 22 (answer will be slightly less)

   $$\frac{1 \text{ kg}}{2.2 \text{ lb}} \diagdown\!\!\!\!\!\diagup \frac{X \text{ kg}}{44 \text{ lb}}$$

   $$2.2 \, X = 44$$

   $$\frac{2.2 \, X}{2.2} = \frac{44}{2.2}$$

   $$X = 20 \text{ kg}$$

2. **Calculate recommended dosage.** A reputable drug resource indicates that the usual IM dosage is 0.5 mg to 1 mg/kg/dose every 4 hours as needed. Notice that the recommended dosage is represented as a range of "0.5 to 1 mg/kg/dose" for dosing flexibility. Calculate the minimum and maximum safe dosage range.

Use ratio-proportion to calculate mg/kg range for each dose.

Ratio for minimum recommended mg/kg $=$ Ratio for minimum desired mg/kg

$$\frac{0.5 \text{ mg}}{1 \text{ kg}} \quad \times \quad \frac{X \text{ mg}}{20 \text{ kg}}$$

$$X \quad = \quad 0.5 \times 20$$

$$X \quad = \quad 10 \text{ mg (per dose)}$$

Ratio for maximum recommended mg/kg $=$ Ratio for maximum desired mg/kg

$$\frac{1 \text{ mg}}{1 \text{ kg}} \quad \times \quad \frac{X \text{ mg}}{20 \text{ kg}}$$

$$X \quad = \quad 1 \times 20$$

$$X \quad = \quad 20 \text{ mg (per dose)}$$

Or, you can simply multiply mg/kg/dose $\times$ the child's weight in kg.

Minimum per dose: 0.5 mg/kg/dose $\times$ 20 kg $=$ 10 mg/dose

Maximum per dose: 1 mg/kg/dose $\times$ 20 kg $=$ 20 mg/dose

3. **Decide if the ordered dosage is safe.** The recommended dosage range is 10 mg to 20 mg, and the ordered dosage of 20 mg is within this range. Yes, the ordered dosage is safe.

4. **Calculate 1 dose.** Apply the three steps of dosage calculation.

Order: Vistaril 20 mg IM q.4h p.r.n., nausea

Supply: Vistaril 50 mg/mL (Figure 14-2)

FIGURE 14-2   Vistaril 50 mg/mL label

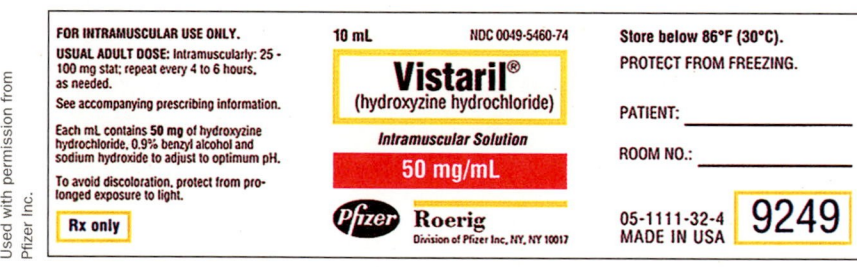

Step 1	Convert	No conversion is necessary.
Step 2	Think	Estimate that you want to give less than 1 mL; in fact, you want to give less than 0.5 mL.
Step 3	Calculate	$\dfrac{\text{Dosage on hand}}{\text{Amount on hand}} = \dfrac{\text{Dosage desired}}{\text{X Amount desired}}$

$$\frac{50 \text{ mg}}{1 \text{ mL}} \quad \times \quad \frac{20 \text{ mg}}{X \text{ mL}}$$

$$50X \quad = \quad 20$$

$$\frac{50X}{50} \quad = \quad \frac{20}{50}$$

$$X \quad = \quad 0.4 \text{ mL}$$

This is a small, child's dose. Measure it in a 1 mL syringe. Route is IM. You may need to change the needle.

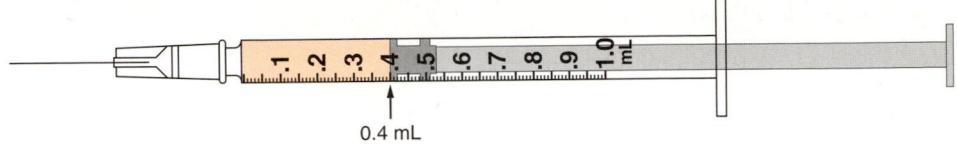

0.4 mL

DELMAR | Cengage Learning

Routine or Round-the-Clock Drugs

Routine or round-the-clock drugs are intended to produce a continuous effect on the body over 24 hours. They are recommended as a *total daily dosage:* **mg/kg/day to be divided into some number of individual doses,** such as "3 divided doses," "4 divided doses," "divided doses every 8 hours," and so on. "Three divided doses" means the drug total daily dosage is divided equally and is administered three times per day, either t.i.d. or q.8h. Likewise, "4 divided doses" means the total daily drug dosage is divided equally and administered four times per day either q.i.d. or q.6h. Recommendations such as "divided doses every 8 hours" specifies that the total daily drug dosage should be divided equally and administered q.8h.

EXAMPLE ▪

The practitioner orders *cefaclor 100 mg p.o. t.i.d.* The child weighs $33\frac{1}{2}$ lb. Is this dosage safe?

1. **Convert lb to kg.** Approximate equivalent: 1 kg = 2.2 lb

   THINK: $\frac{1}{2}$ of 33 = approximately 17 (answer will be slightly less)

   Represent $33\frac{1}{2}$ as 33.5 because you are converting lb to kg (metric measure) and the answer must be in decimals.

   $$\frac{1 \text{ kg}}{2.2 \text{ lb}} \diagup\!\!\!\!\diagdown \frac{X \text{ kg}}{33.5 \text{ lb}}$$

   $$2.2X = 33.5$$

   $$\frac{2.2X}{2.2} = \frac{33.5}{2.2}$$

   $$X = 15.22 \text{ kg} = 15.2 \text{ kg}$$

2. **Calculate recommended dosage.** Figure 14-3 shows the recommended dosage on the drug label, "Usual dose—Children, 20 mg/kg a day . . . in three divided doses." First, calculate the total daily dosage using ratio-proportion or simply multiply: 20 mg/kg/day × 15.2 kg = 304 mg/day. Then, divide this total daily dosage into 3 doses: 304 mg ÷ 3 doses = 101.3 mg/dose.

3. **Decide if the ordered dosage is safe.** Yes, the ordered dosage is safe because this is an *oral* dose and 100 mg is a *reasonably safe* dosage for a recommended single dosage of 101.3 mg.

FIGURE 14-3   cefaclor 125 mg/5 mL label

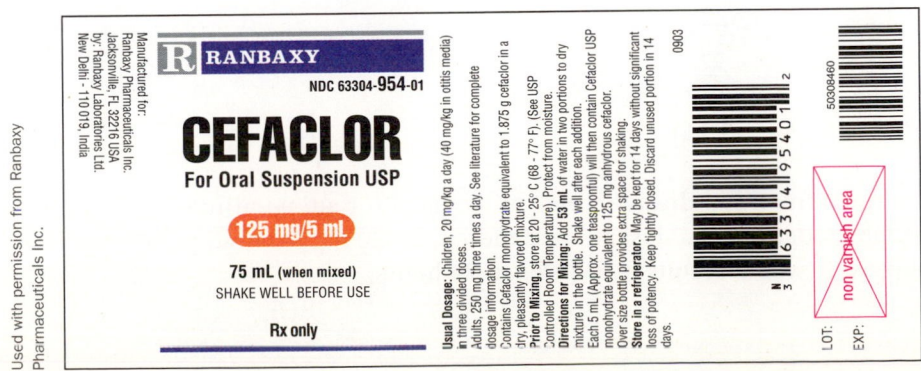

Used with permission from Ranbaxy Pharmaceuticals Inc.

4. **Calculate 1 dose.** Apply the three steps of dosage calculation.

Order: *cefaclor 100 mg p.o. t.i.d.*

Supply: cefaclor 125 mg per 5 mL

Step 1 **Convert**   No conversion is necessary.

Step 2 **Think**   You want to give less than 5 mL. Estimate that you want to give between 2.5 mL and 5 mL.

Step 3 **Calculate**

$$\frac{\text{Dosage on hand}}{\text{Amount on hand}} = \frac{\text{Dosage desired}}{\text{X Amount desired}}$$

$$\frac{125\ mg}{5\ mL} \diagdown \frac{100\ mg}{X\ mL}$$

$$125X = 500$$

$$\frac{125X}{125} = \frac{500}{125}$$

$$X = 4\ mL$$

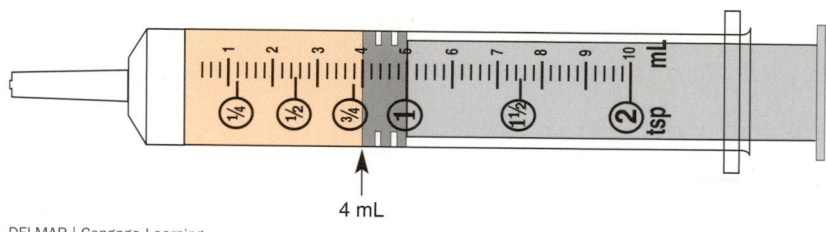

4 mL

DELMAR | Cengage Learning

Total Daily Dosage Range per Kilogram

Many medications are recommended by a minimum and maximum mg/kg range per day to be divided into some number of doses. Amoxicillin is an antibiotic that is used to treat a variety of infections in adults and children. It is often given in divided doses round-the-clock for a total daily dosage.

EXAMPLE ■

Suppose the physician orders **amoxicillin 200 mg p.o. q.8h** for an infant who weighs 22 lb. Is this dosage safe?

1. **Convert lb to kg.** Approximate equivalent: 1 kg = 2.2 lb

   THINK: $\frac{1}{2}$ of 22 = 11 (answer will be slightly less)

   $$\frac{1\ kg}{2.2\ lb} \diagdown \frac{X\ kg}{22\ lb}$$

   $$2.2X = 22$$

   $$\frac{2.2X}{2.2} = \frac{22}{2.2}$$

   $$X = 10\ kg$$

2. **Calculate recommended dosage.** Look at the label for amoxicillin (Figure 14-4). The label describes the recommended dosage for children as "20 mg-40 mg/kg/day in divided doses every eight hours. . . ." which results in 3 doses in 24 hours.

FIGURE 14-4 Amoxicillin 250 mg/5 mL label

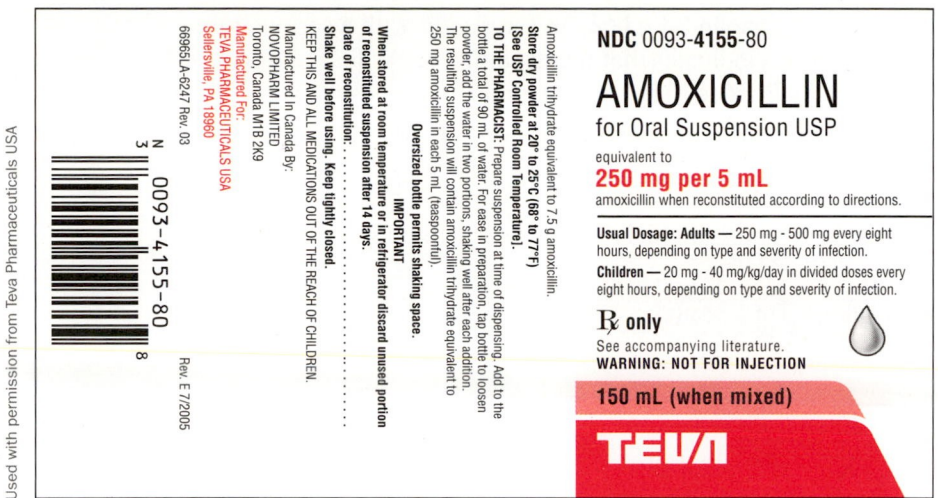

Calculate the minimum and maximum daily dosage using ratio-proportion or simply multiply mg/kg/day × the child's weight in kg then divide by the number of doses per day.

Minimum total daily dosage: 20 mg/kg/day × 10 kg = 200 mg/day

Minimum dosage for each single dose: 200 mg ÷ 3 doses = 66.66 mg/dose = 66.7 mg/dose

Maximum total daily dosage: 40 mg/kg/day × 10 kg = 400 mg/day

Maximum dosage for each single dose: 400 mg ÷ 3 doses = 133.33 mg/dose = 133.3 mg/dose

The single dosage range is 66.7 to 133.3 mg/dose.

3. **Decide if the ordered dosage is safe.** The ordered dosage is 200 mg, and the allowable, safe dosage is 66.7 to 133.3 mg/dose. No, this dosage is too high and is not safe.

4. **Contact the prescriber to discuss the order.**

You can save yourself a calculation step with the following shortcut, based on the total daily dosage.

Calculate recommended minimum and maximum daily dosage range for *this* child.

You know the total daily dosage is divided into 3 doses in 24 hours.

Minimum total daily dosage: 20 mg/kg/day × 10 kg = 200 mg/day

Maximum total daily dosage: 40 mg/kg/day × 10 kg = 400 mg/day

Daily dosage per this order: 200 mg/dose × 3 doses/day = 600 mg/day

Decide if the ordered daily dosage is safe. The ordered daily dosage is 600 mg, and the allowable safe daily dosage is 200 to 400 mg/day. No, the dosage ordered is too high and is not safe. It could result in serious harm to the infant, including renal damage, especially if this is continued for the full course of therapy. Further, the nurse who administered the dosage would be liable for any patient harm.

Total Daily Dosage Range per Kilogram with Maximum Daily Allowance

Some medications have a range of mg/kg/day recommended, with a maximum allowable total amount per day also specified.

EXAMPLE ■

The physician orders *cefazolin 2.1 g IV q.8h* for a child with a serious joint infection. The child weighs 95 lb. The drug reference indicates that the usual IM or IV dosage of cefazolin for infants and children is 50 to 100 mg/kg/day divided every 8 hours; maximum dosage is 6 g/day. This means that regardless of how much the child weighs, the maximum safe allowance of this drug is 6 g per 24 hours.

1. **Convert lb to kg.** Approximate equivalent: 1 kg = 2.2 lb

    THINK: $\frac{1}{2}$ of 95 = approximately 48 (answer will be slightly less)

    $$\frac{1 \text{ kg}}{2.2 \text{ lb}} \quad \diagdown\!\!\!\!\diagup \quad \frac{X \text{ kg}}{95 \text{ lb}}$$

    $$2.2 \text{ X} = 95$$

    $$\frac{2.2 \text{ X}}{2.2} = \frac{95}{2.2}$$

    $$X = 43.18 \text{ kg} = 43.2 \text{ kg}$$

2. **Calculate recommended dosage.**

    Minimum mg/kg/day: 50 mg/kg/day × 43.2 kg = 2,160 mg/day

    Minimum mg/dose: 2,160 mg ÷ 3 doses = 720 mg/dose or 0.72 g/dose (1 g = 1,000 mg)

    Maximum mg/kg/day: 100 mg/kg/day × 43.2 kg = 4,320 mg/day, which is still below the maximum allowable per day dosage of 6 g or 6,000 mg.

    Maximum mg/dose: 4,320 mg ÷ 3 doses = 1,440 mg/dose or 1.44 g/dose

3. **Decide if the dosage is safe.** No, the dosage is too high. It exceeds both the highest mg/kg/dose extreme of the range (1,440 mg/dose), and it exceeds the maximum allowable dosage. At 6 g/day, no more than 2 g/dose would be allowed. The ordered dosage of 2.1 g is not safe because 3 doses/day would deliver 6.3 g of the drug (2.1 g × 3 = 6.3 g). This example points out the importance of carefully reading all dosage recommendations.

4. **Contact the prescriber to discuss the order.**

Underdosage

Underdosage, as well as overdosage, can be a hazard. If the medication is necessary for the treatment or comfort of the patient, then giving too little can be just as hazardous as giving too much. Dosage that is less than the recommended therapeutic amount is also considered unsafe because it may be ineffective.

EXAMPLE ■

The nurse notices a baby's fever has not come down below 102.6°F in spite of several doses of ibuprofen that the physician ordered as an antipyretic (fever reducer). The order reads *ibuprofen 40 mg p.o. q.6h p.r.n., temp 101.6°F and above.* The 7-month-old baby weighs $17\frac{1}{2}$ lb.

1. **Convert lb to kg.** Approximate equivalent: 1 kg = 2.2 lb.

    THINK: $\frac{1}{2}$ of $17\frac{1}{2}$ = approximately 9 (answer will be slightly less)

    Represent $17\frac{1}{2}$ as 17.5 because you are converting lb to kg; kg is metric measured in decimals.

    $$\frac{1 \text{ kg}}{2.2 \text{ lb}} \quad \diagdown\!\!\!\!\diagup \quad \frac{X \text{ kg}}{17.5 \text{ lb}}$$

    $$2.2\text{X} = 17.5$$

    $$\frac{2.2\text{X}}{2.2} = \frac{17.5}{2.2}$$

    $$X = 8 \text{ kg}$$

2. **Calculate safe dosage.** The drug reference states "Usual dosage . . . oral: Children: . . . Antipyretic: 6 months to 12 years: Temperature less than 102.5°F (39°C) 5 mg/kg/dose; temperature greater than 102.5°F: 10 mg/kg/dose; given every 6 to 8 hr; Maximum daily dose: 40 mg/kg/day."

   The recommended safe mg/kg dosage to treat this child's fever of 102.6°F is based on 10 mg/kg/dose. For the 8 kg child, per dose, 10 mg/kg/dose × 8 kg = 80 mg/dose

3. **Decide if the dosage is safe.** The nurse realizes that the dosage as ordered is insufficient to lower the child's fever. Because it is below the recommended therapeutic dosage, it is unsafe.

4. **Contact the physician.** Upon discussion with the physician, the doctor agrees and revises the order to *ibuprofen 80 mg p.o. q.6h p.r.n., fever greater than 102.5°F and ibuprofen 40 mg p.o. q.6h p.r.n., fever less than 102.5°F.* Underdosage with an antipyretic may result in serious complications of hyperthermia. Likewise, consider how underdosage with an antibiotic may lead to a superinfection and underdosage of a pain reliever may be inadequate to effectively treat the patient's pain, delaying recovery. Remember, the information in the drug reference provides important details related to specific use of medications and appropriate dosages for certain age groups to provide safe, therapeutic dosing. Both the physician and nurse must work together to ensure accurate and safe dosages that are within the recommended parameters as stated by the manufacturer on the label, in a drug insert, or in a reputable drug reference.

CAUTION

Once an adolescent attains a weight of 50 kg (110 lb) or greater, the standard adult dosage is frequently prescribed instead of a calculated dosage by weight. The health care professional must carefully verify that the order for a child's dosage does not exceed the maximum adult dosage recommended by the manufacturer.

CAUTION

Many over-the-counter preparations, such as fever reducers and cold preparations, have printed dosing instructions that show the recommended child dose per pound (Figure 14-5). Manufacturers understand that most parents in the United States measure their child's weight in pounds and are most familiar with household measurement. The recommended dosage is measured in teaspoons. Recall that pounds and teaspoons are primarily used for measurement in the home setting. In the clinical setting, you should measure body weight in kg and calculate dosage by the body weight method, using recommended dosage in mg/kg, not mg/lb.

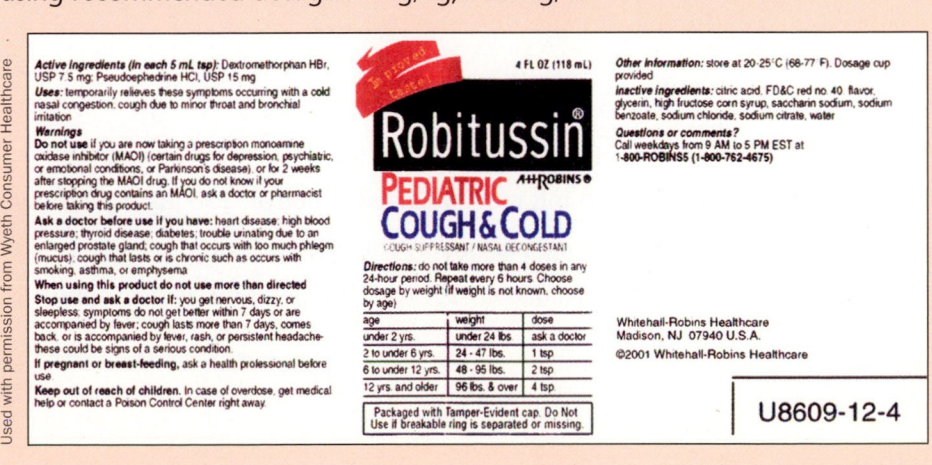

FIGURE 14-5
Label with dosage instructions per pound

COMBINATION DRUGS

Some medications contain two drugs combined into one solution or suspension. To calculate the safe dosage of these medications, the nurse should consult a pediatric drug reference. Often the nurse will need to calculate the safe dosage for each of the medications combined in the solution or suspension. Combination drugs are usually ordered by the amount to give or dose volume of the concentration desired.

EXAMPLE 1 ■

The physician orders Pediazole 6 mL (erythromycin 200 mg and sulfisoxazole 600 mg per 5 mL) p.o. q.6h for a child weighing 44 lb. The pediatric drug reference states that Pediazole is a combination drug containing 200 mg of erythromycin ethylsuccinate with 600 mg of sulfisoxazole acetyl in every 5 mL oral suspension. The usual dosage for Pediazole is 50 mg erythromycin and 150 mg sulfisoxazole/kg/day in equally divided doses administered every 6 hours. Is the order safe?

Because this is a combination drug, notice that the order is for the dose volume (6 mL). To verify that the dose is safe, you must calculate the recommended dosage and the recommended quantity to give to supply that dosage for each drug component.

1. **Convert lb to kg.** Approximate equivalent: 1 kg = 2.2 lb

   THINK: $\frac{1}{2}$ of 44 = 22 (answer will be slightly less)

   $$\frac{1 \text{ kg}}{2.2 \text{ lb}} \diagdown\!\!\!\!\!\diagup \frac{X \text{ kg}}{44 \text{ lb}}$$

   $$2.2X = 44$$

   $$\frac{2.2X}{2.2} = \frac{44}{2.2}$$

   $$X = 20 \text{ kg}$$

2. **Calculate the safe dosage for each drug component.**

   erythromycin per day: 50 mg/kg/day × 20 kg = 1,000 mg/day; divided into 4 doses/day
   1,000 mg ÷ 4 doses = 250 mg/dose

   sulfisoxazole per day: 150 mg/kg/day × 20 kg = 3,000 mg/day; divided into 4 doses/day
   3,000 mg ÷ 4 doses = 750 mg/dose

3. **Calculate the volume of medication recommended for 1 dose for each drug component.**

   erythromycin: 250 mg is the recommended dosage; the supply has 200 mg per 5 mL.

   $$\frac{\text{Dosage on hand}}{\text{Amount on hand}} = \frac{\text{Dosage desired}}{\text{X Amount desired}}$$

   $$\frac{200 \text{ mg}}{5 \text{ mL}} \diagdown\!\!\!\!\!\diagup \frac{250 \text{ mg}}{\text{X mL}}$$

   $$200X = 1,250$$

   $$\frac{200X}{200} = \frac{1,250}{200}$$

   $$X = 6.25 \text{ mL} = 6 \text{ mL recommended to deliver 250 mg erythromycin}$$

   As this is an oral dosage, it is safely and reasonably rounded to 6 mL.

   sulfisoxazole: 750 mg is the recommended dosage; 600 mg per 5 mL is the supply.

   $$\frac{\text{Dosage on hand}}{\text{Amount on hand}} = \frac{\text{Dosage desired}}{\text{X Amount desired}}$$

   $$\frac{600 \text{ mg}}{5 \text{ mL}} \diagdown\!\!\!\!\!\diagup \frac{750 \text{ mg}}{\text{X mL}}$$

   $$600X = 3,750$$

   $$\frac{600X}{600} = \frac{3,750}{600}$$

   $$X = 6.25 \text{ mL} = 6 \text{ mL recommended to deliver 750 mg sulfisoxazole}$$

4. **Decide if the dose ordered is safe.** The ordered dose is 6 mL, and the appropriate dose based on the recommended dosage for each component is 6 mL. The dose is safe. **Realize that because this is a combination product; 6 mL contains *both* medications delivered in this suspension.** Therefore, 6 mL is given, not 6 mL plus 6 mL.

EXAMPLE 2 ■

The physician orders Septra suspension (co-trimoxazole) 7.5 mL ($1\frac{1}{2}$t) of TMP 40 mg per 5 mL p.o. q.12h for a child who weighs 22 lb. The drug reference states that Septra is a combination drug containing trimethoprim (TMP) 40 mg and sulfamethoxazole 200 mg in 5 mL oral suspension. It further states that the usual dosage of Septra is based on the TMP component, which is 6 to 12 mg/kg/day p.o. in divided doses q.12h for a mild to moderate infection. Is this dose volume safe?

1. **Convert lb to kg.** Approximate equivalent: 1 kg = 2.2 lb

   THINK: $\frac{1}{2}$ of 22 = 11 (answer will be slightly less)

   $$\frac{1 \text{ kg}}{2.2 \text{ lb}} \quad \diagup\!\!\!\!\diagdown \quad \frac{X \text{ kg}}{22 \text{ lb}}$$

   $$2.2X \;=\; 22$$

   $$\frac{2.2X}{2.2} \;=\; \frac{22}{2.2}$$

   $$X \;=\; 10 \text{ kg}$$

2. **Calculate the safe dose for the TMP range.**

   TMP minimum daily dosage: 6 mg/kg/day × 10 kg = 60 mg/day

   Divided into 2 doses/day: 60 mg ÷ 2 doses = 30 mg/dose

   TMP maximum daily dosage: 12 mg/kg/day × 10 kg = 120 mg/day

   Divided into 2 doses/day: 120 mg ÷ 2 doses = 60 mg/dose

3. **Calculate the volume of medication for the dosage range.**

   Minimum dose volume: $\dfrac{\text{Dosage on hand}}{\text{Amount on hand}} = \dfrac{\text{Dosage desired}}{X \text{ Amount desired}}$

   $$\frac{40 \text{ mg}}{5 \text{ mL}} \quad \diagup\!\!\!\!\diagdown \quad \frac{30 \text{ mg}}{X \text{ mL}}$$

   $$40X \;=\; 150$$

   $$\frac{40X}{40} \;=\; \frac{150}{40}$$

   $$X \;=\; 3.75 \text{ mL, minimum per dose}$$

   Maximum dose volume: $\dfrac{\text{Dosage on hand}}{\text{Amount on hand}} = \dfrac{\text{Dosage desired}}{X \text{ Amount desired}}$

   $$\frac{40 \text{ mg}}{5 \text{ mL}} \quad \diagup\!\!\!\!\diagdown \quad \frac{60 \text{ mg}}{X \text{ mL}}$$

   $$40X \;=\; 300$$

   $$\frac{40X}{40} \;=\; \frac{300}{40}$$

   $$X \;=\; 7.5 \text{ mL, maximum per dose}$$

4. **Decide if the dose volume is safe.** Because the physician ordered 7.5 mL, the dosage falls within the safe range and is a safe dose.

   What dosage of TMP did the physician actually order per dose for this child?

   Use ratio-proportion: Ratio for dosage on hand = Ratio for desired dosage

Notice that the unknown X is now in the numerator; but the known is still on the left and the unknown is on the right. You are not calculating the amount of dose volume to give (mL desired); you are calculating the dosage (X) to determine if the dosage ordered is safe.

$$\frac{\text{Dosage on hand}}{\text{Amount on hand}} = \frac{\text{X Dosage desired}}{\text{Amount desired}}$$

$$\frac{40 \text{ mg}}{5 \text{ mL}} \quad\times\quad \frac{\text{X mg}}{7.5 \text{ mL}} \qquad \text{The unknown "X" is the desired dosage.}$$

$$5X = 300$$

$$\frac{5X}{5} = \frac{300}{5}$$

$$X = 60 \text{ mg}$$

The patient receives 60 mg of TMP in each 7.5 mL dose.
This is the dosage of TMP you would give in one 7.5 mL dose, which matches the upper limit of the safe dosage range.

EXAMPLE 3 ■

The pediatric oral surgeon orders **Tylenol and codeine suspension 10 mL (acetaminophen 120 mg with codeine 12 mg per 5 mL) p.o. q.4h p.r.n., pain** for a child weighing 42 lb, who had two teeth repaired. The drug reference states that Tylenol and codeine is a combination drug containing 120 mg of acetaminophen and 12 mg of codeine phosphate per 5 mL. Safe dosage is based on the codeine component, which is 0.5 to 1 mg/kg/dose every 4 to 6 hours as needed. Is this dose volume safe?

1. **Convert lb to kg.** Approximate equivalent: 1 kg = 2.2 lb

   THINK: $\frac{1}{2}$ of 42 = 21 (answer will be slightly less)

   $$\frac{1 \text{ kg}}{2.2 \text{ lb}} \quad\times\quad \frac{\text{X kg}}{42 \text{ lb}}$$

   $$2.2X = 42$$

   $$\frac{2.2X}{2.2} = \frac{42}{2.2}$$

   $$X = 19.09 \text{ kg} = 19.1 \text{ kg}$$

2. **Calculate the safe dosage range for the codeine.**

   codeine minimum per dose: 0.5 mg/k̶g̶/dose × 19.1 k̶g̶ = 9.55 mg/dose = 9.6 mg/dose

   codeine maximum per dose: 1 mg/k̶g̶/dose × 19.1 k̶g̶ = 19.1 mg/dose

3. **Calculate the volume of medication for the minimum and maximum dose.**

   Minimum dose volume: $\quad\dfrac{\text{Dosage on hand}}{\text{Amount on hand}} = \dfrac{\text{Dosage desired}}{\text{X Amount desired}}$

   $$\frac{12 \text{ mg}}{5 \text{ mL}} \quad\times\quad \frac{9.6 \text{ mg}}{\text{X mL}}$$

   $$12X = 48$$

   $$\frac{12X}{12} = \frac{48}{12}$$

   $$X = 4 \text{ mL, minimum per dose}$$

   Maximum dose volume: $\quad\dfrac{\text{Dosage on hand}}{\text{Amount on hand}} = \dfrac{\text{Dosage desired}}{\text{X Amount desired}}$

   $$\frac{12 \text{ mg}}{5 \text{ mL}} \quad\times\quad \frac{19.1 \text{ mg}}{\text{X mL}}$$

   $$12X = 95.5$$

   $$\frac{12X}{12} = \frac{95.5}{12}$$

   $$X = 7.95 \text{ mL} = 8 \text{ mL, maximum per dose}$$

4. **Decide if the dose volume is safe.** The ordered dose of 10 mL exceeds the maximum safe dose range; the dose is not safe. Contact the physician to discuss the order.

Be sure to take the time to double-check pediatric dosage. The health care provider who administers the medication has the last opportunity to ensure safe drug therapy.

ADULT DOSAGES BASED ON BODY WEIGHT

Some adult dosage recommendations are based on body weight, too, although less frequently than for children. The information you learned about calculating and verifying children's body weight dosages can be applied to adults. It is important that you become familiar and comfortable with reading labels, drug inserts, and drug reference books to check any order that appears questionable.

Let's look at information that would be found in a drug reference book about the adult dosage recommendations for the drug gentamicin (Figure 14-6). Notice that the adult dosage is recommended by body weight and varies depending on the frequency of administration.

FIGURE 14-6   Gentamicin 80 mg/2 mL label with adult dosing instructions from drug reference

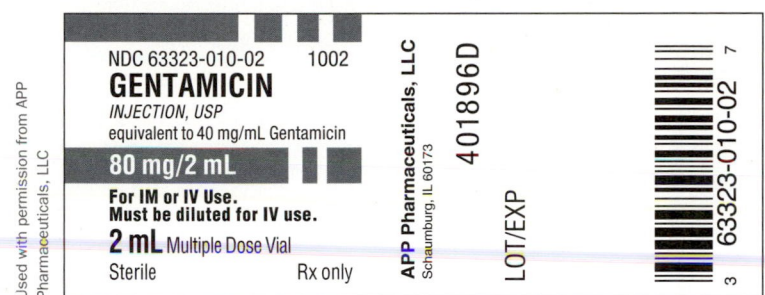

EXAMPLE ■

Order: gentamicin 100 mg IV q.8h for a patient with bacterial septicemia

Supply: gentamicin 80 mg per 2 mL

Recommended adult dosage from drug reference 1 to 1.7 mg/kg q.8h

Patient's weight: 150 lb

Convert lb to kg. Approximate equivalent: 1 kg = 2.2 lb.

THINK: $\frac{1}{2}$ of 150 = 75 (answer will be slightly less)

$$\frac{1\text{ kg}}{2.2\text{ lb}} \quad \diagdown\hspace{-0.9em}\diagup \quad \frac{X\text{ kg}}{150\text{ lb}}$$

$$2.2X \quad = \quad 150$$

$$\frac{2.2X}{2.2} \quad = \quad \frac{150}{2.2}$$

$$X \quad = \quad 68.18\text{ kg} = 68.2\text{ kg}$$

Minimum per dose: 1 mg/kg/dose × 68.2 kg = 68.2 mg/dose

Maximum per dose: 1.7 mg/kg/dose × 68.2 kg = 115.94 mg/dose = 115.9 mg/dose

The ordered dosage of gentamicin 100 mg given intravenously every 8 hours is within the recommended range and is safe.

Calculate the amount to give for 1 dose.

Step 1	Convert	No conversion needed.

Step 2 Think 100 mg is a little larger than 80 mg so you want to give a little more than 2 mL

Step 3 Calculate

$$\frac{80 \text{ mg}}{2 \text{ mL}} \times \frac{100 \text{ mg}}{X \text{ mL}}$$

$$80X = 200$$
$$\frac{80X}{80} = \frac{200}{80}$$
$$X = 2.5 \text{ mL, given intravenously every 8 hours}$$

QUICK REVIEW

To use the body weight method to verify the safety of pediatric and adult dosages:

- Convert body weight from pounds and ounces to kilograms: 1 kg = 2.2 lb; 1 lb = 16 oz.

- Calculate the recommended safe dosage in mg/kg.

- Compare the ordered dosage with the recommended dosage to decide if the dosage is safe.

- If the dosage is safe, calculate the amount to give for 1 dose; if not safe, notify the prescriber.

- Combination drugs are ordered by dose volume. Check a reputable drug reference to be sure the dose ordered contains the safe amount of each drug as recommended.

Review Set 31

Calculate 1 dose of safe pediatric dosages.

1. Order: **dicloxacillin sodium 125 mg p.o. q.6h** for a child who weighs 55 lb. The recommended dosage of dicloxacillin sodium for children weighing less than 40 kg is 12.5 to 25 mg/kg/day p.o. in equally divided doses q.6h for moderate to severe infections.

   Child's weight: _____ kg

   Recommended minimum daily dosage for this child: _____ mg/day

   Recommended minimum single dosage for this child: _____ mg/dose

   Recommended maximum daily dosage for this child: _____ mg/day

   Recommended maximum single dosage for this child: _____ mg/dose

   Is the dosage ordered safe? _____

2. Dicloxacillin sodium is available as an oral suspension of 62.5 mg per 5 mL. If the dosage ordered in question 1 is safe, give _____ mL. If not safe, explain why not and describe what you should do. _____

   _____

3. Order: **Chloromycetin 55 mg IV q.12h** for an 8-day-old infant who weighs 2,200 g. The recommended dosage of Chloromycetin (chloramphenicol) for neonates less than 2 kg is 25 mg/kg once daily, and for neonates more than 2 kg and older than 7 days of age is 50 mg/kg/day divided q.12h.

   Child's weight: _____ kg

   Recommended daily dosage for this child: _____ mg/day

   Recommended single dosage for this child: _____ mg/dose

   Is the dosage ordered safe? _____

4. Chloramphenicol is available as a solution for injection of 1 g per 10 mL. If the dosage ordered in question 3 is safe, give _____ mL. If not safe, explain why not and describe what you should do. _____

_____

5. Order: **Suprax 120 mg p.o. daily** for a child who weighs 33 lb. The recommended dosage of Suprax (cefixime) for children who weigh less than 50 kg is 8 mg/kg p.o. once daily or 4 mg/kg q.12h.

   Child's weight: _____ kg

   Recommended single dosage for this child: _____ mg/dose

   Is the dosage ordered safe? _____

6. Suprax is available as a suspension of 100 mg per 5 mL in a 50 mL bottle. If the dosage ordered in question 5 is safe, give _____ mL. If not safe, explain why not and describe what you should do. _____

_____

   How many full doses are available in the bottle of Suprax? _____ dose(s)

7. Order: **Panadol 480 mg p.o. q.4h p.r.n. for temperature 101.6°F or greater.** The child's weight is 32 kg. The recommended child's dosage of Panadol (acetaminophen) is 10 to 15 mg/kg/dose p.o. q.4h p.r.n. for fever.

   Child's weight: _____ kg

   Recommended minimum single dosage for this child: _____ mg/dose

   Recommended maximum single dosage for this child: _____ mg/dose

   Is the dosage ordered safe? _____

8. Panadol is available as a suspension of 160 mg per 5 mL. If the dosage ordered in question 7 is safe, give _____ mL. If not safe, explain why not and describe what you should do. _____

_____

9. Order: **Keflex 125 mg p.o. q.6h** for a child who weighs 44 lb. The recommended pediatric dosage of Keflex (cephalexin) is 25 to 50 mg/kg/day in 4 equally divided doses.

   Child's weight: _____ kg

   Recommended minimum daily dosage for this child: _____ mg/day

   Recommended minimum single dosage for this child: _____ mg/dose

   Recommended maximum daily dosage for this child: _____ mg/day

   Recommended maximum single dosage for this child: _____ mg/dose

   Is the dosage ordered safe? _____

10. Keflex is available in a suspension of 125 mg per 5 mL. If the dosage ordered in question 9 is safe, give _____ mL. If not safe, explain why not and describe what you should do.

_____

_____

The labels provided represent the drugs available to answer questions 11 through 25. Verify safe dosages, indicate the amount to give, and draw an arrow on the accompanying measuring device. Explain unsafe dosages and describe the appropriate action to take.

11. Order: **tobramycin 8 mg IV q.6h** for an infant who weighs 5,000 g. The recommended pediatric dosage of tobramycin is 2 to 2.5 mg/kg q.8h or 1.5 to 1.9 mg/kg q.6h.

Infant's weight: _____ kg

Recommended minimum single dosage for this infant: _____ mg/dose

Recommended maximum single dosage for this infant: _____ mg/dose

Is the dosage ordered safe? _____

Reprinted with permission from APP Pharmaceuticals, LLC

NDC 63323-305-02   300502
TOBRAMYCIN
INJECTION, USP
PEDIATRIC
20 mg/2 mL
(10 mg/mL)
For IM or IV Use
Must dilute for IV use.
2 mL Multiple Dose Vial

APP Pharmaceuticals, LLC
Schaumburg, IL 60173

402101B   LOT/EXP

3 63323-305-02 4

12. If the dosage ordered in question 11 is safe, give _____ mL. If not safe, explain why not and describe what you should do. _____

_____

½   1   1½   ②   2½   3 mL

DELMAR | Cengage Learning

13. Order: **Kantrex 34 mg IV q.8h** for an infant who weighs 7 lb 8 oz. The recommended dosage of Kantrex (kanamycin sulfate) for adults and children is 15 mg/kg/day in 2 or 3 equal doses, not to exceed 1.5 g/day.

Child's weight: _____ kg

Recommended daily dosage for this child: _____ mg/day

Recommended single dosage for this child: _____ mg/dose

Is the dosage ordered safe? _____

Used with permission from Bristol-Myers Squibb Company. All rights reserved.

NDC 0015-3512-20
EQUIVALENT TO   NSN 6505-00-926-9202
75 mg KANAMYCIN per 2 mL
KANTREX®
Kanamycin Sulfate Injection, USP
Pediatric Injection
FOR I.M. OR I.V. USE
CAUTION: Federal law prohibits dispensing without prescription.

0.099% sodium bisulfite added as an antioxidant, buffered with 0.33% sodium citrate. • Adjusted to pH 4.5 with H₂SO₄. • Kantrex Pediatric Injection should not be physically mixed with other antibacterial agents.
READ ACCOMPANYING CIRCULAR
Distributed by APOTHECON®
A Bristol-Myers Squibb Co.
Princeton, NJ 08540
Made in USA   3512200RL-1

MAXIMUM DOSE: 15 MG/KG/DAY

Cont:
Exp. Date:

14. If the dosage ordered in question 13 is safe, give _____ mL. If not safe, explain why not and describe what you should do. _____

_____

.1   .2   .3   .4   .5   .6   .7   .8   .9   1.0 mL

DELMAR | Cengage Learning

15. Order: **co-trimoxazole suspension 7.5 mL of trimethoprim 40 mg per 5 mL p.o. q.12h** for a child who weighs 15 kg and has an urinary tract infection. The recommended dosage of co-trimoxazole (trimethoprim and sulfamethoxazole) for such infections in children is based on the trimethoprim at 8 mg/kg/day in 2 equal doses.

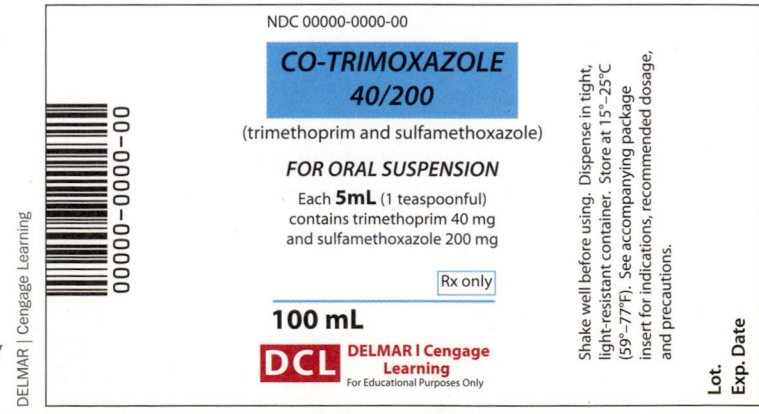

NDC 00000-0000-00

**CO-TRIMOXAZOLE
40/200**
(trimethoprim and sulfamethoxazole)

FOR ORAL SUSPENSION

Each **5mL** (1 teaspoonful) contains trimethoprim 40 mg and sulfamethoxazole 200 mg

Rx only

100 mL

DCL DELMAR I Cengage Learning
For Educational Purposes Only

Shake well before using. Dispense in tight, light-resistant container. Store at 15°–25°C (59°–77°F). See accompanying package insert for indications, recommended dosage, and precautions.

Lot.
Exp. Date

Recommended daily trimethoprim dosage for this child: _____ mg/day

Recommended single trimethoprim dosage for this child: _____ mg/dose

Recommended single dose for this child: _____ mL/dose

Is the dose ordered safe? _____

16. If the dose ordered in question 15 is safe, give _____ mL. If not safe, explain why not and describe what you should do. _____

_____

The dose ordered is equivalent to _____ teaspoons.

DELMAR | Cengage Learning

17. Order: **gentamicin 40 mg IV q.8h** for a premature neonate who is 5 days old and weighs 1,800 g. The recommended dosage of gentamicin for children is 2 to 2.5 mg/kg q.8h; for neonates, it is 2.5 mg/kg q.8h; and for premature neonates less than 1 week of age, it is 2.5 mg/kg q.12h.

Neonate's weight:

_____ kg

Recommended single dosage for this neonate:

_____ mg/dose

Is the ordered dosage safe? _____

NDC 63323-010-20   1020
GENTAMICIN
INJECTION, USP
equivalent to
40 mg/mL
Gentamicin   Rx only
For IM or IV Use.
Must be diluted for IV use.
20 mL Multiple Dose Vial

Reprinted with permission from APP Pharmaceuticals, LLC

APP Pharmaceuticals, LLC
Schaumburg, IL 60173

401897D

LOT/EXP

18. If the dosage ordered in question 17 is safe, give _____ mL. If not safe, explain why not and describe what you should do. _____

_____

DELMAR | Cengage Learning

19. Order: **ampicillin 400 mg IM q.6h** for a 10-year-old child who weighs 72 lb. Recommended dosage: See label.

Child's weight: _____ kg

Recommended minimum daily dosage for this child: _____ mg/day

Recommended minimum single dosage for this child: _____ mg/dose

Recommended maximum daily dosage for this child: _____ mg/day

Recommended maximum single dosage for this child: _____ mg/dose

Is the dosage ordered safe? _____

NDC 00000-0000-00
AMPICILLIN
For Injection, USP
ampicillin sodium equivalent to
500 mg ampicillin
For IM or IV Use
Rx only

For IM Use: add 1.7 mL diluent. The resulting solution provides 250 mg ampicillin per mL. IM or IV Injection: USE SOLUTION WITHIN 1 HOUR. IV Infusion: See package insert. Usual dosage: Children: 25 to 50 mg/kg/day in equally divided doses at 6 hour intervals. Adults: 250 to 500 mg every 6 hours. Package insert includes detailed precautions and indications. Store at controlled room temperature 15°–30°C (59°–86°F).

DELMAR | Cengage Learning
For Educational Purposes Only

DCL

DELMAR | Cengage Learning

20. If the dosage ordered in question 19 is safe, give _____ mL. If not safe, explain why not and describe what you should do. _____

_____

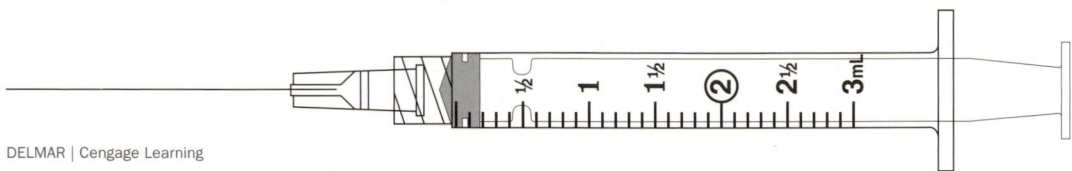

DELMAR | Cengage Learning

21. Order: **amoxicillin oral suspension 100 mg p.o. q.8h** for a child who weighs 39 lb. Recommended dosage: See label.

Child's weight: _____ kg

Recommended
minimum
daily dosage
for this child:
_____ mg/day

Recommended
minimum
single dosage
for this child:
_____ mg/dose

Recommended
maximum
daily dosage for this
child: _____ mg/day

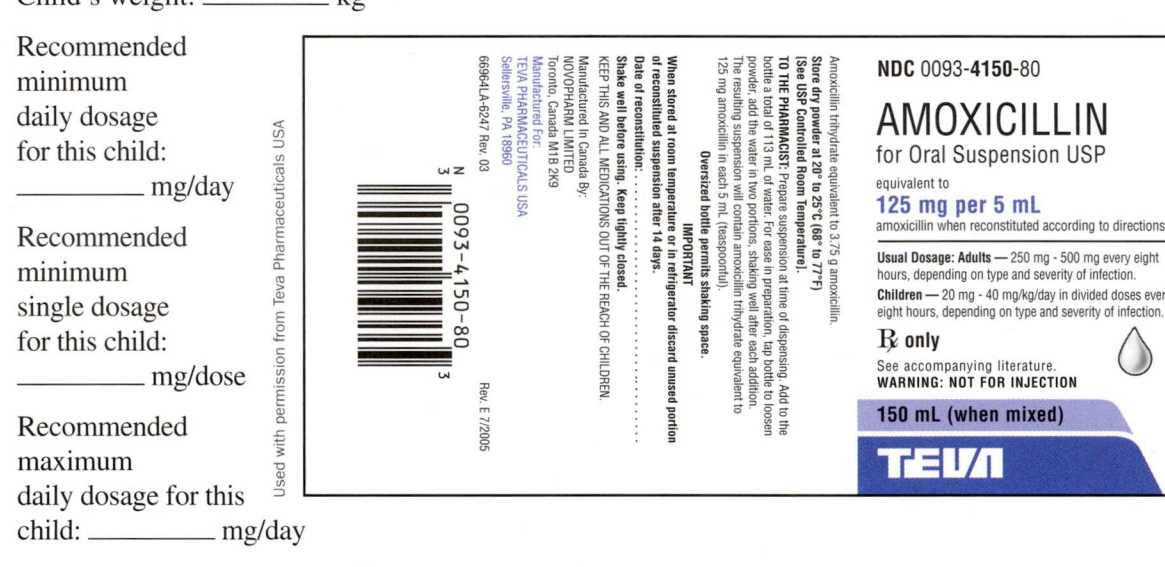

Recommended maximum single dosage for this child: _____ mg/dose

Is the dosage ordered safe? _____

22. If the dosage ordered in question 21 is safe, give _____ mL. If not safe, explain why not and describe what you should do. _____

_____

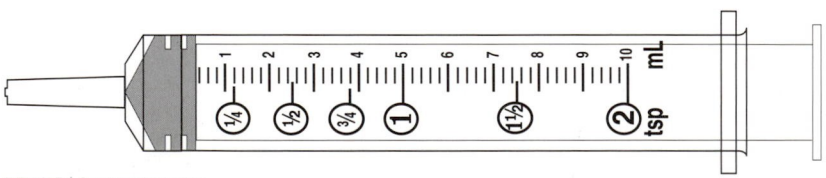

DELMAR | Cengage Learning

23. Order: **Terramycin 100 mg IM q.8h** for a 9-year-old child who weighs 55 lb. Recommended pediatric dosage: See label.

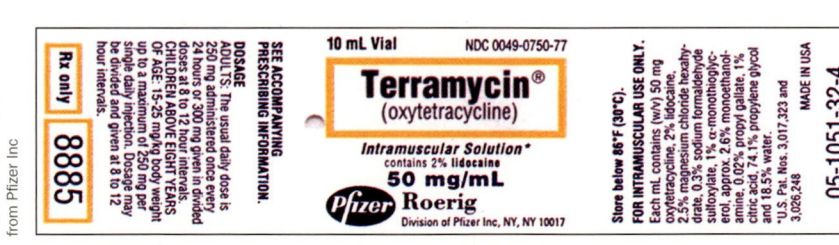

Child's weight: _____ kg

Recommended minimum daily dosage for this child: _____ mg/day

Recommended minimum single dosage for this child: _____ mg/dose

Recommended maximum daily dosage for this child: _____ mg/day

Recommended maximum single dosage for this child: _____ mg/dose

Is the dosage ordered safe? _____

24. If the dosage ordered in question 23 is safe, give _____ mL. If not safe, explain why not and describe what you should do. _____

_____

DELMAR | Cengage Learning

25. Order: **Terramycin 275 mg IM daily** for a 7-year-old child who weighs 21 kg. Recommended pediatric dosage: See label for question 23.

Is the ordered dosage safe? _____ Explain: _____

_____

Refer to the following drug label information from a drug reference book for gentamicin to answer questions 26 through 30.

26. What is the recommended adult dosage of gentamicin for conventional interval dosing?

_____

27. What is the recommended adult dosage of gentamicin for extended interval dosing?

_____

28. What single dosage range of gentamicin administered q.8h should you expect for an adult who weighs 130 lb? _____ mg to _____ mg/dose

29. What single dosage range of gentamicin administered q.24h should you expect for an adult who weighs 130 lb? _____ mg to _____ mg/dose

30. Would an order for **gentamicin 300 mg IV q.24h** for an adult who weighs 130 lb be a safe dosage? If not, explain why.

_____

After completing these problems, see pages 543–545 to check your answers.

CRITICAL THINKING SKILLS

Medication errors in pediatrics often occur when the nurse fails to properly identify the child before administering the dose.

ERROR

Failing to identify the child before administering a medication.

Possible Scenario

Suppose the physician ordered *ampicillin 500 mg IV q.6h* for a child with pneumonia. The nurse calculated the dosage to be safe, checked to be sure the child had no allergies, and prepared the medication. The child had been assigned to a semiprivate room. The nurse entered the room and noted only one child in the room and administered the IV ampicillin to that child, without checking the identification of the child. Within an hour of the administered ampicillin the child began to break out in hives and had signs of respiratory distress. The nurse asked the child's mother, "Does Johnny have any known allergies?" The mother replied, "This is James, not Johnny, and yes, James is allergic to penicillin. His roommate, Johnny, is in the playroom." At this point the nurse realized the ampicillin was given to the wrong child, who was allergic to penicillin.

Potential Outcome

James's physician would have been notified, and he would likely have ordered epinephrine subcut stat (given for anaphylactic reactions), steroids, and an antihistamine, followed by close monitoring of the child. Anaphylactic reactions can range from mild to severe. Ampicillin is a derivative of penicillin and would not have been prescribed for a child such as James.

Prevention

This error could easily have been avoided had the nurse remembered the cardinal rule of *identifying the child* before administering *any* medication. Children are mobile, and you cannot assume the identity of a child simply because he or she is in a particular room. The correct method of identifying the child is to check the wrist or ankle band and compare it to the medication administration record with the child's name and ID number. Finally, remember that the first of the *Six Rights* of medication administration is the *right patient.*

CRITICAL THINKING SKILLS

When the recommended dosage of a medication is given with a high and low range, the minimum and maximum doses must be calculated to determine the safety of a drug order. This is the only way to assure that the drug to be administered is not an overdose or an underdose.

ERROR

Calculating only the maximum recommended dose of an ordered medication to determine safety.

Possible Scenario

The physician ordered *tobramycin 9.5 mg IV q.8h* for a 2-week-old infant who weighed 11 pounds and who had a serious infection. The recommended dosage for children and infants greater than 1 week old is 1.5 to 1.9 mg/kg q.6h or 2 to 2.5 mg/kg q.8h. The nurse calculated a safe dosage range prior to administering what would be the third dose of this medication, although it was administered two previous times by other nurses. First the nurse correctly converted the infant's weight from pounds to kilograms by dividing 11 by 2.2 to equal 5 kg. Then the nurse correctly calculated the minimum and maximum recommended doses by multiplying the recommended dosage by the infant's weight.

Minimum single q.8h dose: 2 mg/kg × 5 kg = 10 mg
Maximum single q.8h dose: 2.5 mg/kg × 5 kg = 12.5 mg

The nurse recognized that the ordered dose fell below the minimum recommended dose for tobramycin to be administered every 8 hours. Considering the serious infection the infant had, the nurse doubted the physician planned to give such a low dose and notified the physician. The physician realized that the dose was mistakenly calculated according to the q.12h recommendation and wrote a new order.

Potential Outcome

The first 2 dosages of tobramycin fell slightly below the minimum recommended dose for the frequency ordered. This situation was discussed with the nurse manager of the pediatric unit along with the other two staff nurses involved. One staff nurse admitted to administering medication occasionally without actually calculating a safe dose if it looked like it was the correct dose. The other nurse always checked to see that ordered medications were not overdoses but didn't usually worry about checking for underdoses. The nurse manager emphasized the importance of always verifying doses on pediatric patients, especially infants. In this situation the mistake was caught early and corrected but could have caused significant harm to the infant by inadequately treating a severe infection.

Prevention

When reading drug reference guides, make sure you read all the dosage recommendations thoroughly. It is easy to see how, when in a hurry, a physician or nurse might have missed seeing some of the information provided in the scenario and thought it read 1.5 to 1.9 mg/kg q.8h. Don't hurry or take shortcuts when administering medications. Always calculate the minimum and maximum recommended doses when a dosage range is given.

PRACTICE PROBLEMS—CHAPTER 14

Convert the following weights to kilograms. Round to one decimal place.

1. 12 lb = _____ kg

2. 8 lb 4 oz = _____ kg

3. 1,570 g = _____ kg

4. 2,300 g = _____ kg

5. 34 lb = _____ kg

6. 6 lb 10 oz = _____ kg

7. 52 lb = _____ kg

8. 890 g = _____ kg

9. The recommended dosage of tobramycin for adults with serious infections that are not life-threatening is 3 mg/kg/day in 3 equally divided doses q.8h. What should you expect the total daily dosage of tobramycin to be for an adult with a serious infection who weighs 80 kg? _____ mg/day

10. What should you expect the single dosage of tobramycin to be for the adult described in question 9? _____ mg/dose

The labels provided represent the drugs available to answer questions 11 through 42. Verify safe dosages and indicate the amount to give and draw an arrow on the accompanying measuring device. Explain unsafe dosages and describe the appropriate action to take.

11. Order: **gentamicin 40 mg IV q.8h** for a child who weighs 43 lb. The recommended dosage for children is 2 to 2.5 mg/kg q.8h.

    Child's weight: _____ kg

    Recommended minimum single dosage for this child: _____ mg/dose

Reprinted with permission from APP Pharmaceuticals, LLC

NDC 63323-010-02   1002
GENTAMICIN
INJECTION, USP
equivalent to 40 mg/mL Gentamicin
80 mg/2 mL
For IM or IV Use.
Must be diluted for IV use.
2 mL Multiple Dose Vial
Sterile   Rx only
APP Pharmaceuticals, LLC
Schaumburg, IL 60173
401896D
LOT/EXP
63323-010-02

Recommended maximum single dosage for this child: _____ mg/dose

Is the ordered dosage safe? _____

12. If the dosage ordered in question 11 is safe, give _____ mL. If not safe, explain why not and describe what you should do. _____

_____

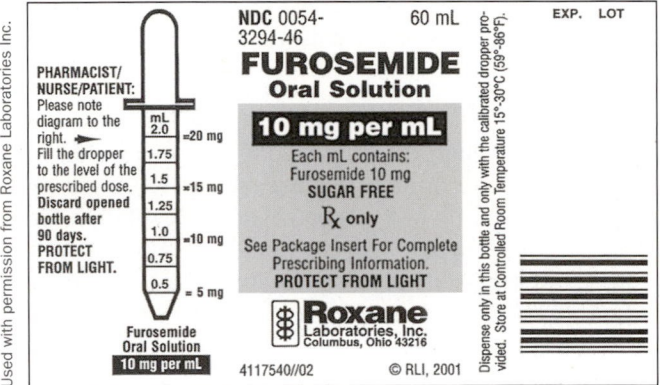

DELMAR | Cengage Learning

13. Order: **furosemide oral solution 10 mg p.o. b.i.d.** for a child who weighs 16 lb. The recommended pediatric dosage is 0.5 to 2 mg/kg b.i.d.

Child's weight: _____ kg

Recommended minimum single dosage for this child: _____ mg/dose

Recommended maximum single dosage for this child: _____ mg/dose

Is the ordered dosage safe? _____

Used with permission from Roxane Laboratories Inc.

PHARMACIST/
NURSE/PATIENT:
Please note
diagram to the
right. ➡
Fill the dropper
to the level of the
prescribed dose.
Discard opened
bottle after
90 days.
PROTECT
FROM LIGHT.

mL 2.0 = 20 mg
1.75
1.5 = 15 mg
1.25
1.0 = 10 mg
0.75
0.5 = 5 mg

Furosemide
Oral Solution
10 mg per mL

NDC 0054-3294-46   60 mL   EXP. LOT

FUROSEMIDE
Oral Solution

10 mg per mL

Each mL contains:
Furosemide 10 mg
SUGAR FREE

R_x only

See Package Insert For Complete
Prescribing Information.
PROTECT FROM LIGHT

Roxane
Laboratories, Inc.
Columbus, Ohio 43216

4117540//02   © RLI, 2001

Dispense only in this bottle and only with the calibrated dropper provided. Store at Controlled Room Temperature 15°-30°C (59°-86°F).

14. If the dosage ordered in question 13 is safe, give _____ mL. If not safe, explain why not and describe what you should do. _____

_____

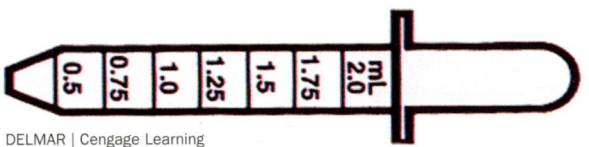

DELMAR | Cengage Learning

0.5 0.75 1.0 1.25 1.5 1.75 mL 2.0

15. Order: **carbamazepine 150 mg p.o. b.i.d.** for a child who is 5 years old and weighs 40 lb. The recommended dosage for children under 6 years of age is 10 to 20 mg/kg/day in 2 to 4 divided doses per day, not to exceed 400 mg/day.

Child's weight: _____ kg

Recommended minimum daily dosage for this child: _____ mg/day

Recommended minimum single dosage for this child: _____ mg/dose

Recommended maximum daily dosage for this child: _____ mg/day

Recommended maximum single dosage for this child: _____ mg/dose

Is the dosage ordered safe? _____

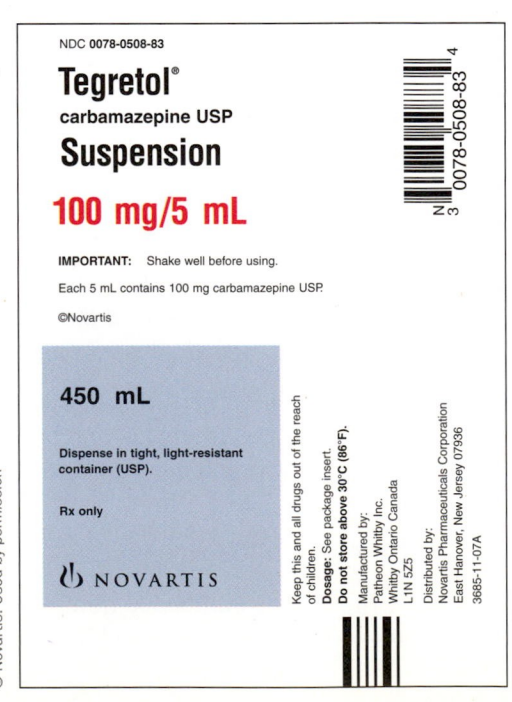

© Novartis. Used by permission

NDC 0078-0508-83

Tegretol®
carbamazepine USP
Suspension

100 mg/5 mL

IMPORTANT: Shake well before using.

Each 5 mL contains 100 mg carbamazepine USP.

©Novartis

450 mL

Dispense in tight, light-resistant container (USP).

Rx only

ὓ NOVARTIS

Keep this and all drugs out of the reach of children.
Dosage: See package insert.
Do not store above 30°C (86°F).

Manufactured by:
Patheon Whitby Inc.
Whitby Ontario Canada
L1N 5Z5

Distributed by:
Novartis Pharmaceuticals Corporation
East Hanover, New Jersey 07936

3685-11-07A

16. If the dosage ordered in question 15 is safe, give _____ mL. If not safe, explain why not and describe what you should do. _____

_____

17. Order: **Depakene 150 mg p.o. b.i.d.** for a child who is 10 years old and weighs 64 lb. The recommended dosage for adults and children 10 years and older is 10 to 15 mg/kg/day up to a maximum of 60 mg/kg/day. If the total daily dosage exceeds 250 mg, divide the dose.

Child's weight: _____ kg

Recommended minimum daily dosage for this child: _____ mg/day

Recommended minimum single dosage for this child: _____ mg/dose

Recommended maximum daily dosage for this child: _____ mg/day

Recommended maximum single dosage for this child: _____ mg/dose

Is the dosage ordered safe? _____

Do not accept if band on cap is broken or missing.

Each 5 mL contains equivalent of 250 mg valproic acid as the sodium salt.

See enclosure for prescribing information.

©Abbott
Abbott Laboratories
North Chicago,
IL 60064, U.S.A.
Exp.
Lot

NDC 0074-5682-16
16 fl oz Syrup

DEPAKENE®

VALPROIC ACID
SYRUP, USP

**250 mg
per 5 mL**

6505-01-094-9241
Dispense in the original container or a glass, USP tight container.
Store below 86°F (30°C).

Caution: Federal (U.S.A.) law prohibits dispensing without prescription.

02-7538-2/R12

18. If the dosage ordered in question 17 is safe, give _____ mL. If not safe, explain why not and describe what you should do. _____

_____

19. Order: **penicillin G sodium 125,000 units IV daily** for an infant who weighs 2,500 g. The recommended dosage for infants is 50,000 units/kg/day in a single dose.

Child's weight: _____ kg

Recommended daily dosage for this child: _____ units/day

Recommended single dosage for this child: _____ units/dose

Is the ordered dosage safe? _____

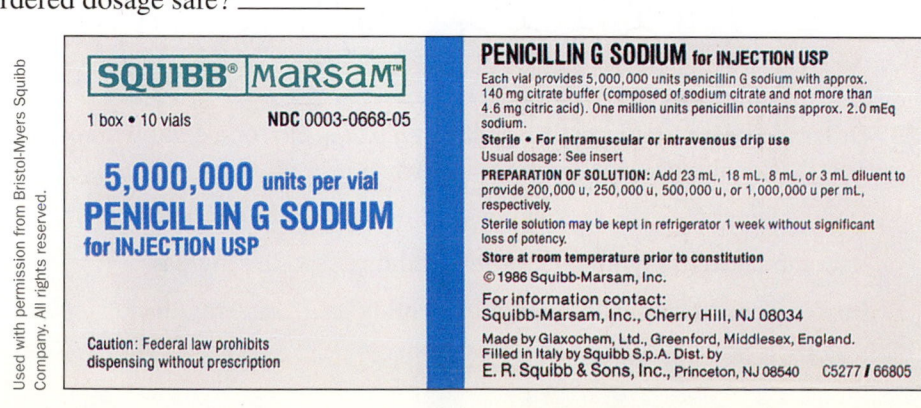

SQUIBB® MARSAM™

1 box • 10 vials   NDC 0003-0668-05

**5,000,000 units per vial
PENICILLIN G SODIUM
for INJECTION USP**

Caution: Federal law prohibits dispensing without prescription

PENICILLIN G SODIUM for INJECTION USP
Each vial provides 5,000,000 units penicillin G sodium with approx. 140 mg citrate buffer (composed of sodium citrate and not more than 4.6 mg citric acid). One million units penicillin contains approx. 2.0 mEq sodium.
Sterile • For intramuscular or intravenous drip use
Usual dosage: See insert
PREPARATION OF SOLUTION: Add 23 mL, 18 mL, 8 mL, or 3 mL diluent to provide 200,000 u, 250,000 u, 500,000 u, or 1,000,000 u per mL, respectively.
Sterile solution may be kept in refrigerator 1 week without significant loss of potency.
Store at room temperature prior to constitution
© 1986 Squibb-Marsam, Inc.
For information contact:
Squibb-Marsam, Inc., Cherry Hill, NJ 08034
Made by Glaxochem, Ltd., Greenford, Middlesex, England.
Filled in Italy by Squibb S.p.A. Dist. by
E. R. Squibb & Sons, Inc., Princeton, NJ 08540   C5277 / 66805

20. If the dosage ordered in question 19 is safe, reconstitute with _____ mL diluent for a total solution volume of _____ mL with a concentration of _____ units/mL. Give _____ mL. If not safe, explain why not and describe what you should do. _____

_____

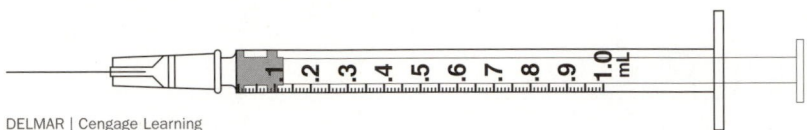

DELMAR | Cengage Learning

21. Order: **amoxicillin oral suspension 150 mg p.o. q.8h** for a child who weighs 41 lb. Recommended dosage: See label below.

Child's weight: _____ kg

Recommended minimum daily dosage for this child: _____ mg/day

Recommended minimum single dosage for this child: _____ mg/dose

Recommended maximum daily dosage for this child: _____ mg/day

Recommended maximum single dosage for this child: _____ mg/dose

Is the dosage ordered safe? _____

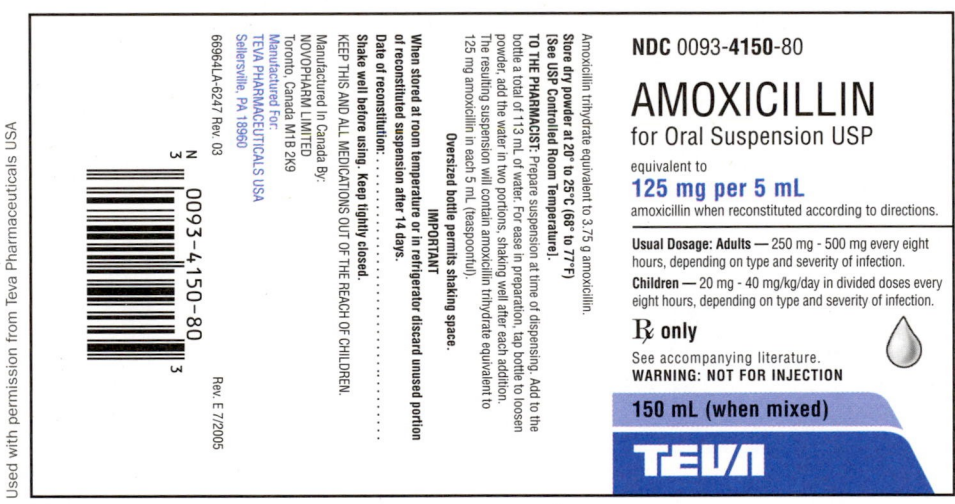

NDC 0093-4150-80

AMOXICILLIN
for Oral Suspension USP

equivalent to
125 mg per 5 mL
amoxicillin when reconstituted according to directions.

Usual Dosage: Adults — 250 mg - 500 mg every eight hours, depending on type and severity of infection.
Children — 20 mg - 40 mg/kg/day in divided doses every eight hours, depending on type and severity of infection.

℞ only
See accompanying literature.
WARNING: NOT FOR INJECTION

150 mL (when mixed)

TEVA

22. If the dosage ordered in question 21 is safe, give _____ mL. If not safe, explain why not and describe what you should do. _____

_____

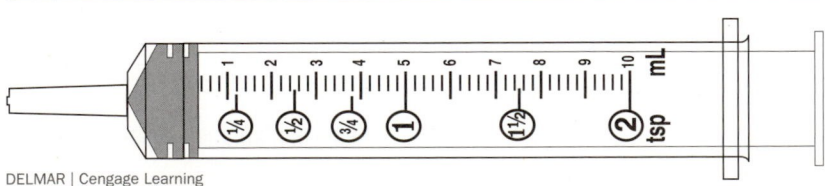

DELMAR | Cengage Learning

23. Order: **cefaclor oral suspension 187 mg p.o. q. 8h** for a child with otitis media who weighs $30\frac{1}{2}$ lb. Recommended dosage: See label.

Child's weight: _____ kg

Recommended daily dosage for this child: _____ mg/day

Recommended single dosage for this child: _____ mg/dose

Is the dosage ordered safe? _____

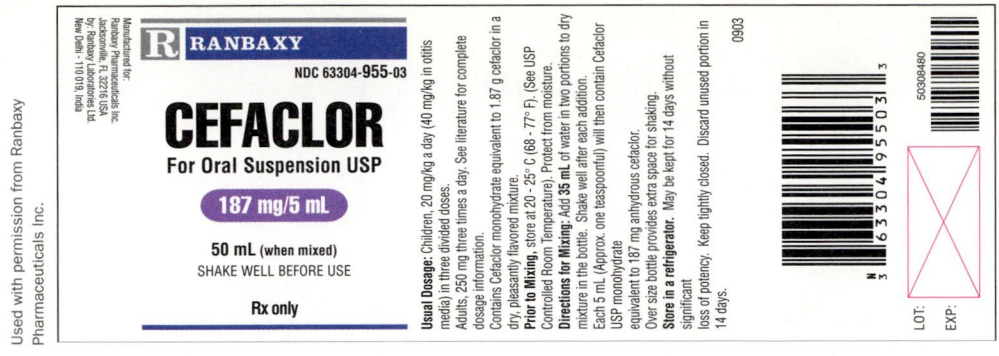

24. If the dosage ordered in question 23 is safe, give _____ mL. If not safe, explain why not and describe what you should do. _____

_____

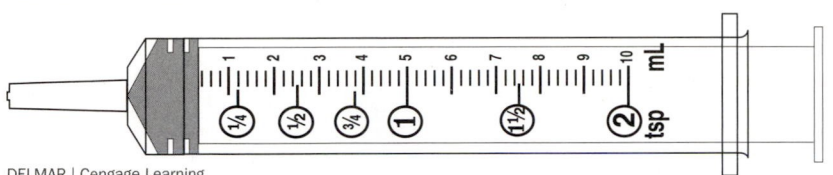

DELMAR | Cengage Learning

25. Order: **Narcan 100 mcg subcut stat** for a child who weighs 22 lb. Recommended pediatric dosage: 0.01 mg/kg/dose.

   Child's weight: _____ kg

   Recommended single dosage for this child: _____ mg/dose

   Is the dosage ordered safe? _____

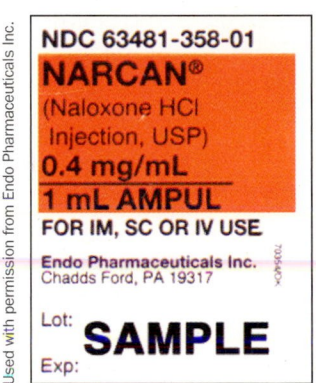

26. If the dosage ordered in question 25 is safe, give _____ mL. If not safe, explain why not and describe what you should do.

   _____

_____

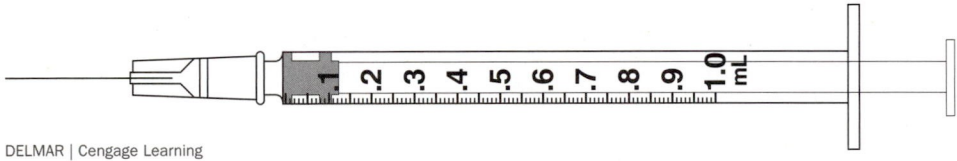

DELMAR | Cengage Learning

27. Order: **tobramycin 35 mg IV q.8h** for a child who weighs 14 kg. The recommended pediatric dosage of tobramycin is 2 to 2.5 mg/kg q.8h or 1.5 to 1.9 mg/kg q.6h.

   Recommended minimum single dosage for this child: _____ mg/dose

   Recommended maximum single dosage for this child: _____ mg/dose

   Is the dosage ordered safe? _____

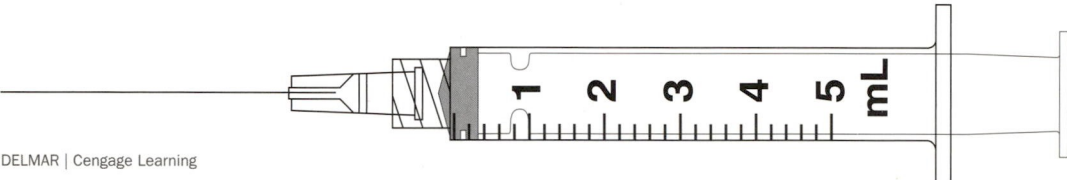

Reprinted with permission from APP Pharmaceuticals, LLC

NDC 63323-305-02   300502

TOBRAMYCIN
INJECTION, USP
PEDIATRIC

20 mg/2 mL
(10 mg/mL)
For IM or IV Use
Must dilute for IV use.
2 mL Multiple Dose Vial

APP Pharmaceuticals, LLC
Schaumburg, IL 60173

402101B

LOT/EXP

3 63323-305-02 4

28. If the dosage ordered in question 27 is safe, give _____ mL. If not safe, explain why not and describe what you should do. _____

_____

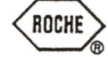

DELMAR | Cengage Learning

29. Order: **Rocephin 1 g IV q.12h** for a child with a serious infection who weighs 20 lb. The recommended pediatric dosage of Rocephin (ceftriaxone sodium) is a total daily dosage of 50 to 75 mg/kg, given once a day (or in equally divided doses twice a day), not to exceed 2 g/day.

Child's weight: _____ kg

Recommended minimum daily dosage for this child: _____ mg/day

Recommended minimum single dosage for this child: _____ mg/dose

Recommended maximum daily dosage for this child: _____ mg/day

Recommended maximum single dosage for this child: _____ mg/dose

Is the dosage ordered safe? _____

ROCEPHIN® ◇ ROCHE ◇   **1 g**
(ceftriaxone injection)

Galaxy®   **50 mL**   NDC 0004-2002-78
Single Dose   Iso-osmotic   Code 2G3524
Container   Sterile Nonpyrogenic

Each 50 mL contains: ceftriaxone sodium equivalent to 1 g ceftriaxone with approx. 1.9 g dextrose hydrous, USP, added to adjust osmolality. pH may have been adjusted with sodium hydroxide and/or hydrochloric acid. pH range 6 to 8.
Usual dosage: See accompanying literature.
Cautions: Administer IV using sterile equipment. Must not be used in series connections. Do not add supplementary medication. Check for minute leaks and solution clarity. Rx only.
Store at or below -20°C (-4°F). Thaw at room temperature (25°C/77°F) or under refrigeration (5°C/41°F). DO NOT FORCE THAW BY IMMERSION IN WATER BATHS OR BY MICROWAVE IRRADIATION. The thawed solution is stable for 21 days under refrigeration or 72 hours at room temperature. Do not refreeze.
U.S. Pat. Nos. 4,686,125; 4,779,997   PL 2040 Plastic
Roche and Rocephin are registered trademarks of Hoffmann-La Roche Inc.
Galaxy is a registered trademark of Baxter International Inc.
Manufactured for Roche Laboratories Inc., Nutley, NJ 07110   7-34-2-327
By Baxter Healthcare Corporation, Deerfield, IL 60015 USA   7-34-2-327

Copyright Baxter International Inc.

30. If the dosage ordered in question 29 is safe, give _____ mL. If not safe, explain why not and describe what you should do. _____

_____

31. Order: **Robinul 50 mcg IM 60 minutes pre-op** for a child who weighs 11.4 kg. The recommended pediatric pre-anesthesia dosage of Robinul (glycopyrrolate) is 0.002 mg/lb of body weight given intramuscularly.

Child's weight: _____ lb

Recommended single dosage for this child: _____ mg/dose

Is the dosage ordered safe? _____

Copyright Baxter International Inc.

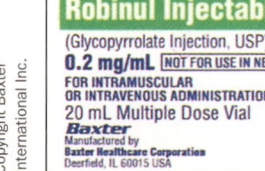

NDC 60977-155-63

Robinul Injectable
(Glycopyrrolate Injection, USP)   Rx only
0.2 mg/mL [NOT FOR USE IN NEWBORNS]
FOR INTRAMUSCULAR
OR INTRAVENOUS ADMINISTRATION
20 mL Multiple Dose Vial
Baxter
Manufactured by
Baxter Healthcare Corporation
Deerfield, IL 60015 USA

Water for Injection, USP q.s./Benzyl Alcohol, NF (preservative) 0.9%.
pH adjusted, when necessary, with hydrochloric acid and/or sodium hydroxide.
Usual Dosage:
See accompanying descriptive literature.
Store at 20°C-25°C (68°F-77°F) [See USP Controlled Room Temperature].
462-182-00

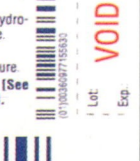

VOID

32. If the dosage ordered in question 31 is safe, give _____ mL. If not safe, explain why not and describe what you should do. _____

33. Order: **ceftriaxone 600 mg IV q.12h** for a 6-month-old infant with a serious infection who weighs 18 lb. For the treatment of serious miscellaneous infections other than meningitis, the recommended total daily dosage of ceftriaxone for pediatric patients is 50 to 75 mg/kg given in divided doses every 12 hours. The total daily dose should not exceed 2 grams.

    Child's weight: _____ kg

    The total daily dosage ordered for this infant:
    _____ mg/day or _____ g/day

    Recommended minimum single dosage for this child: _____ mg/dose

    Recommended maximum single dosage for this child: _____ mg/dose

    Is the dosage ordered safe? _____

    TEVA

    NDC 0703-0335-01 ℞only

    Ceftriaxone for Injection, USP

    1 gram

    For I.M. or I.V. Use
    Single Use Vial

    Each vial contains: ceftriaxone sodium powder equivalent to 1 gram ceftriaxone.
    For I.M. Administration : Reconstitute with 2.1 mL 1% Lidocaine Hydrochloride Injection (USP) or Sterile Water for Injection (USP). Each 1 mL of solution contains approximately 350 mg equivalent of ceftriaxone.
    For I.V. Administration : See Package Insert
    Usual Dosage: See Package Insert

    Storage Prior to Reconstitution: Store powder at 20° to 25°C (68° to 77°F) [See USP Controlled Room Temperature].
    Protect from Light.
    Storage After Reconstitution: See Package Insert
    Mfd for: Teva Parenteral Medicines Irvine, CA 92618

    Iss. 9/2007
    39C1701450907

    Package Insert for IV: "Add 9.6 mL to 1 g vial. After reconstitution, each 1 mL of solution contains approximately 100 mg equivalent of ceftriaxone."

34. If the dosage ordered in question 33 is safe, reconstitute with _____ mL diluent for a total solution volume of _____ mL with a concentration of _____ mg/mL. Give _____ mL. If not safe, explain why not and describe what you should do. _____

35. Order: **amoxicillin/clavulanate 200 mg p.o. q.12h** for a 5-year-old child who weighs 45 lb. The recommended dosage of this combination drug is based on the amoxicillin at 25 mg/kg/day in divided doses q.12h or 20 mg/kg/day in divided doses q.8h.

    Child's weight:
    _____ kg

    Recommended daily dosage for this child:
    _____ mg/day

    Recommended single dosage for this child:
    _____ mg/dose

    Is the dosage ordered safe? _____

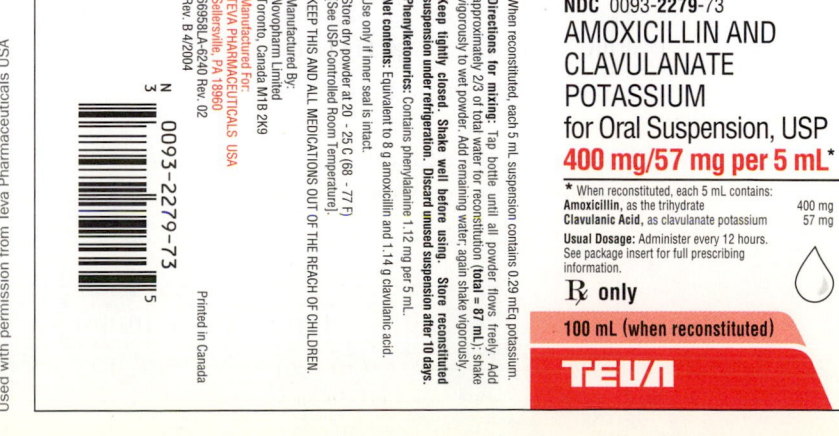

Manufactured For:
TEVA PHARMACEUTICALS USA
Sellersville, PA 18960
6695BLA-6240 Rev. 02
Rev. B 4/2004

Manufactured By:
Novopharm Limited
Toronto, Canada M1B 2K9

When reconstituted, each 5 mL suspension contains 0.29 mEq potassium.
Directions for mixing: Tap bottle until all powder flows freely. Add approximately 2/3 of total water for reconstitution (**total = 87 mL**); shake vigorously to wet powder. Add remaining water; again shake vigorously.
Keep tightly closed. Shake well before using. Store reconstituted suspension under refrigeration. Discard unused suspension after 10 days.
Phenylketonurics: Contains phenylalanine 1.12 mg per 5 mL.
Net contents: Equivalent to 8 g amoxicillin and 1.14 g clavulanic acid.
Use only if inner seal is intact.
Store dry powder at 20 - 25 C (68 - 77 F) [See USP Controlled Room Temperature].
KEEP THIS AND ALL MEDICATIONS OUT OF THE REACH OF CHILDREN.

N 3
0093-2279-73

Printed in Canada

NDC 0093-2279-73
AMOXICILLIN AND CLAVULANATE POTASSIUM
for Oral Suspension, USP
400 mg/57 mg per 5 mL*

* When reconstituted, each 5 mL contains:
Amoxicillin, as the trihydrate .... 400 mg
Clavulanic Acid, as clavulanate potassium ..... 57 mg
Usual Dosage: Administer every 12 hours. See package insert for full prescribing information.

℞ only

100 mL (when reconstituted)

TEVA

36. If the dosage ordered in question 35 is safe, give _____ mL. If not safe, explain why not and describe what you should do. _____

_____

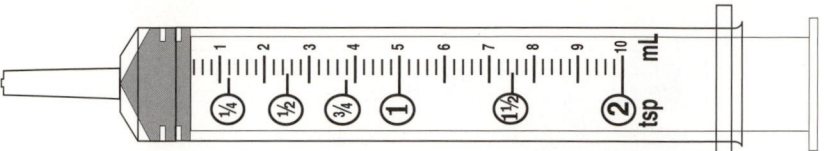

37. Order: **cefaclor oral suspension 75 mg p.o. t.i.d.** for a child with an upper respiratory infection who weighs 18 lb. Recommended dosage: See label.

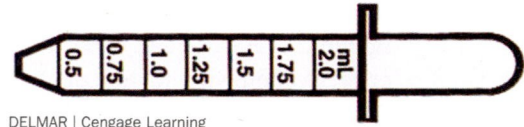

Child's weight: _____ kg

Recommended daily dosage for this child: _____ mg/day

Recommended single dosage for this child: _____ mg/dose

Is the dosage ordered safe? _____

38. If the dosage ordered in question 37 is safe, give _____ mL. If not safe, explain why not and describe what you should do. _____

39. Order: **Vantin 100 mg p.o. q.i.d. × 10 days** for a 4-year-old child with tonsillitis who weighs 45 lb. Recommended dosage for children 5 months to 12 years: 5 mg/kg (maximum of 100 mg/dose) q.12h (maximum daily dosage: 200 mg) for 5 to 10 days.

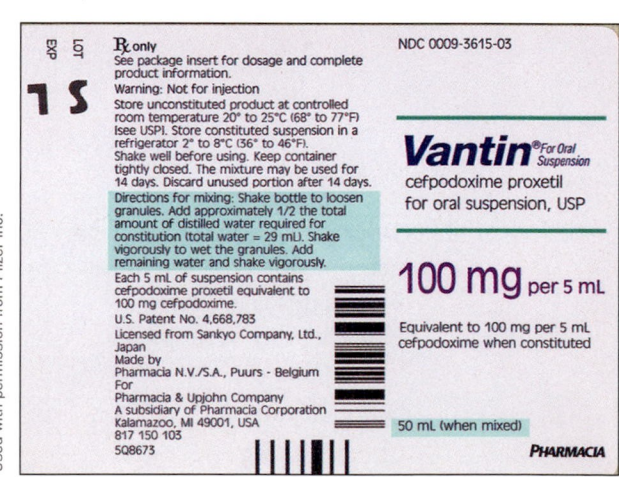

Child's weight: _____ kg

Recommended daily dosage for this child: _____ mg/day

The total daily dosage ordered for this child: _____ mg/day

Is the dosage ordered safe? _____

40. If the dosage ordered in question 39 is safe, give _____ mL. If not safe, explain why not and describe what you should do. _____

_____

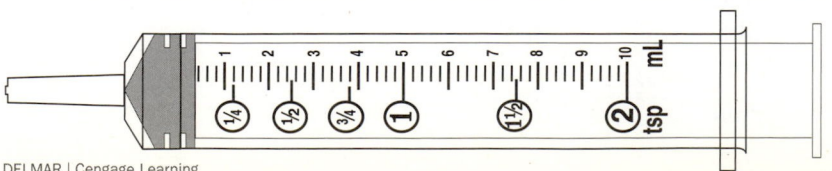

41. Order: **Biaxin 175 mg p.o. q.12h** for a child who weighs 51 lb. Recommended pediatric dosage: See label.

    Child's weight:

    _____ kg

    Recommended daily dosage for this child:

    _____ mg/day

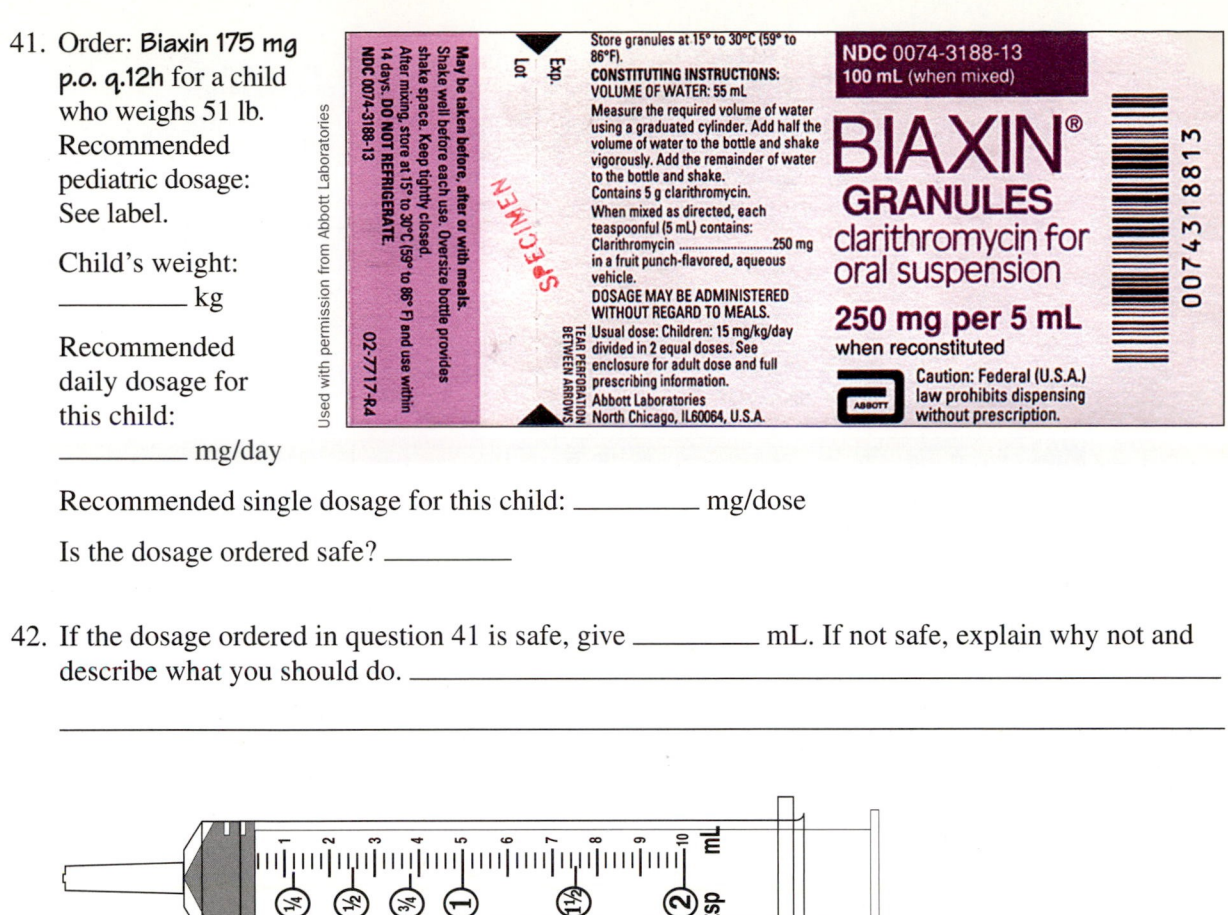

Recommended single dosage for this child: _____ mg/dose

Is the dosage ordered safe? _____

42. If the dosage ordered in question 41 is safe, give _____ mL. If not safe, explain why not and describe what you should do. _____

_____

DELMAR | Cengage Learning

Questions 43 through 48 ask you to apply the steps on your own to determine safe dosages, just as you would do in the clinical setting. Calculate the amount to give and mark an arrow on the measuring device, or explain unsafe dosages and describe the appropriate action. Note if a reconstitution label is required (see question 49).

43. Order: **methylprednisolone 10 mg IV q.6h** for a child who weighs 95 lb. Recommended pediatric dosage: Not less than 0.5 mg/kg/day.

    If the dosage ordered is safe, give _____ mL. If not safe, explain why not and describe what you should do. _____

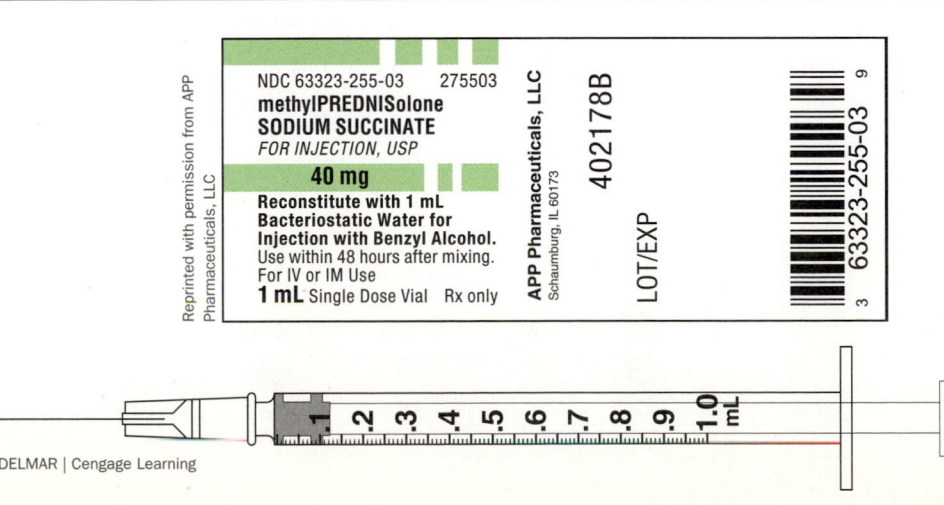

DELMAR | Cengage Learning

44. Order: **albuterol 1.4 mg p.o. t.i.d.** for a 2-year-old child who weighs 31 lb. Recommended pediatric dosage: 0.1 mg/kg, not to exceed 2 mg t.i.d.

    If the dosage ordered is safe, give _____ mL. If not safe, explain why not and describe what you should do. _____

    _____

    _____

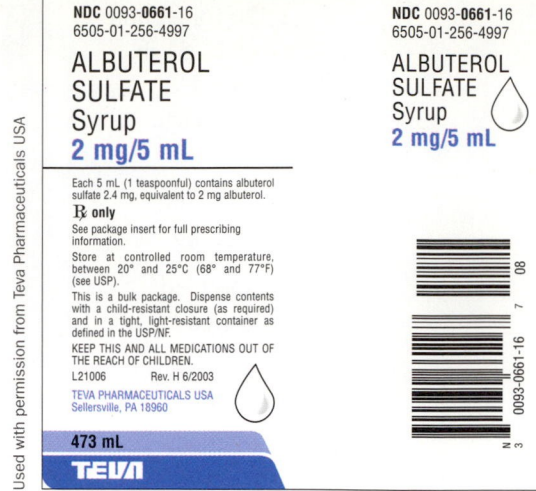

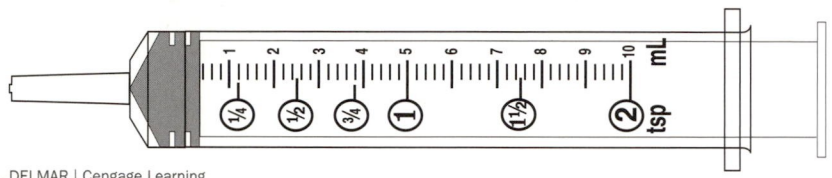

45. Order: **penicillin G potassium 450,000 units IV q.6h** for a child with a streptococcal infection who weighs 12 kg. Recommended pediatric dosage for streptococcal infections is 150,000 units/kg/day given in equal doses q.4 to 6h.

    If the dosage ordered is safe, reconstitute to a dosage supply of _____ units/mL and give _____ mL. If not safe, explain why not and describe what you should do. _____

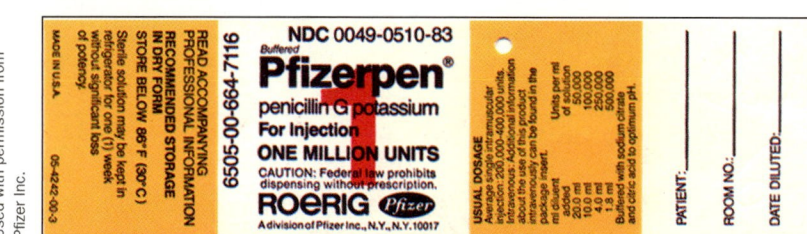

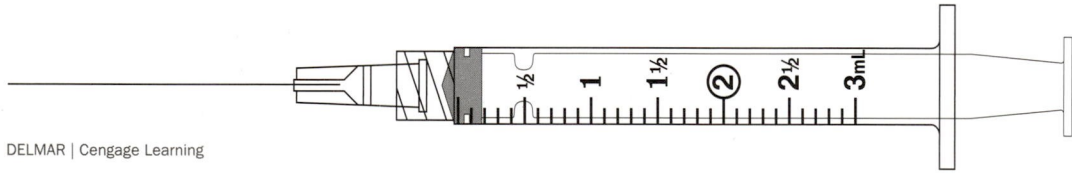

46. Order: **Klonopin 1 mg p.o. b.i.d.** for a 9-year-old child on initial therapy who weighs 56 lb. The recommended initial pediatric dosage of Klonopin (clonazepam) for children up to 10 years or 30 kg is 0.01 to 0.03 mg/kg/day in 2 to 3 divided doses up to a maximum of 0.05 mg/kg/day.

    If the dosage ordered is safe, give _____ tablet(s). If not safe, explain why not and describe what you should do. _____

    _____

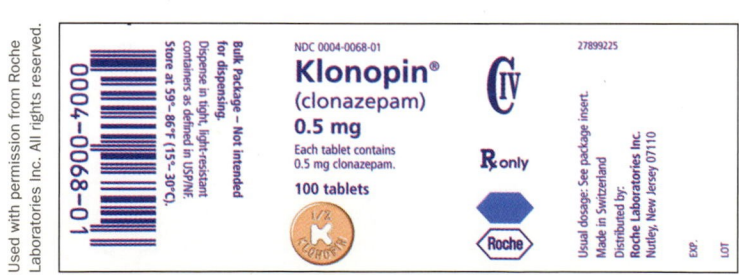

47. Order: **morphine sulfate 1 mg IM stat** for a child who weighs 18 lb. Recommended pediatric dosage: IM or subcut dosage may be initiated at 0.05 mg/kg/dose.

    If the dosage ordered is safe, give _____ mL. If not safe, explain why not and describe what you should do. _____

    _____

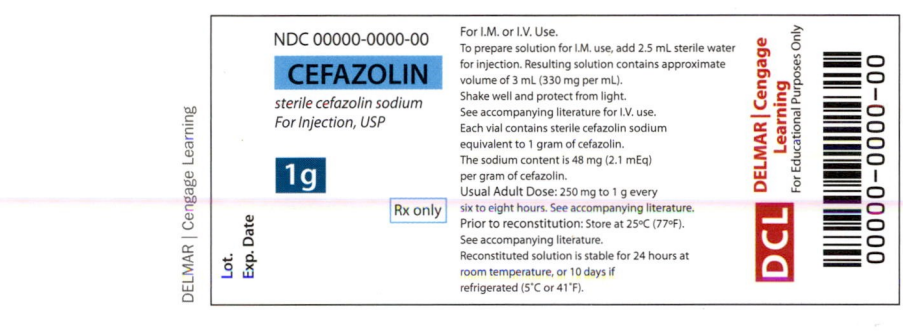

DELMAR | Cengage Learning

48. Order: **cefazolin 250 mg IM q.8h** for a 3-year-old child who weighs 35 lb. The recommended pediatric dosage of cefazolin sodium for children over 1 month: 25 to 50 mg/kg/day in 3 to 4 divided doses.

    If the dosage ordered is safe, give _____ mL. If not safe, explain why not and describe what you should do. _____

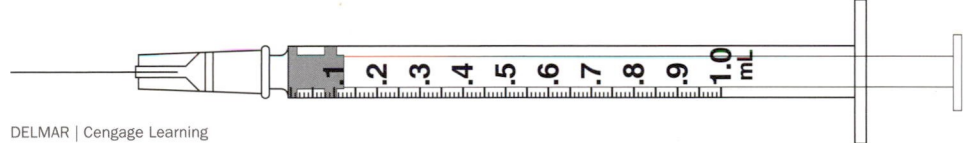

DELMAR | Cengage Learning

49. Refer to questions 43 through 48. Identify which drugs require a reconstitution label.

    _____

    _____

50. Describe the strategy or strategies you would implement to prevent this medication error.

    Possible Scenario
    Suppose the family practice resident ordered **tobramycin 110 mg IV q.8h** for a child with cystic fibrosis who weighs 10 kg. The pediatric reference guide states that the safe dosage of tobramycin for a child with severe infections is 7.5 mg/kg/day in 3 equally divided doses. The nurse received five admissions the evening of this order and thought, "I'm too busy to calculate the safe dosage this time." The pharmacist prepared and labeled the medication in a syringe and the nurse administered the first dose of the medication. An hour later the resident arrived on the pediatric unit and inquired if the nurse had given the first dose. When the nurse replied "yes," the resident replied with concern, "I just realized that I ordered an adult dose of tobramycin. I had hoped you hadn't given the medication yet."

Potential Outcome

The resident's next step would likely have been to discontinue the tobramycin and order a stat tobramycin level. The level would most likely have been elevated, and the child would have required close monitoring for renal damage and hearing loss.

Prevention

_____

_____

After completing these problems, see pages 545–551 to check your answers.

REFERENCES

Bindler, R. M., Howry, L., Wilson, B. A., Shannon, M. T., & Stang, C. L. (2009). MyNursingPDA: *Pediatric drug guide with nursing implications.* Upper Saddle River, NJ: Prentice Hall.

Johns Hopkins Hospital. (2008). *The Harriet Lane handbook* (18th ed.). St. Louis: Mosby-Year Book, Inc.

Taketomo, C. K., Hodding, J. H. & Kraus, D. M., (2009). *Pediatric dosage handbook: Including neonatal dosing, drug administration, & extemporaneous preparations* (15th ed.). Cleveland: LEXI-COMP.

SECTION 3 SELF-EVALUATION

Chapter 10—Oral Dosage of Drugs

The following labels (A–N) represent the drugs you have available on your medication cart for the orders in questions 1 through 10. Select the correct label and identify the corresponding letter for filling these medication orders. Calculate the amount to give.

1. Order: Neurontin 0.2 g p.o. daily

   Select label _____ and give _____ capsule(s)

2. Order: atomoxetine 40 mg p.o. daily

   Select label _____ and give _____ capsule(s)

3. Order: Aricept 10 mg p.o. daily

   Select label _____ and give _____ tablet(s)

4. Order: valporic acid 100 mg p.o. b.i.d.

   Select label _____ and give _____ mL

5. Order: potassium chloride 16 mEq p.o. daily

   Select label _____ and give _____ mL

6. Order: nitroglycerin 13 mg p.o. t.i.d.

   Select label _____ and give _____ capsule(s)

7. Order: Synthroid 0.05 mg p.o. daily

   Select label _____ and give _____ tablet(s)

8. Order: codeine gr $\frac{1}{4}$ p.o. q.6h p.r.n., cough

   Select label _____ and give _____ tablet(s)

9. Order: furosemide 12.5 mg p.o. b.i.d.

   Select label _____ and give _____ mL

10. Order: albuterol sulfate 3 mg p.o. t.i.d.

    Select label _____ and give _____ mL

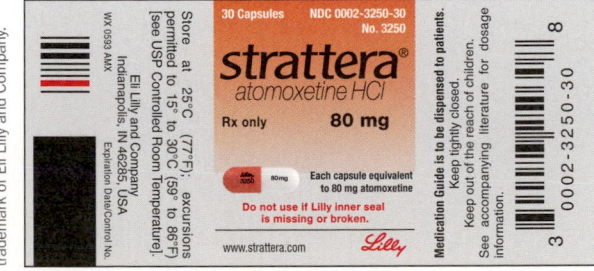

A

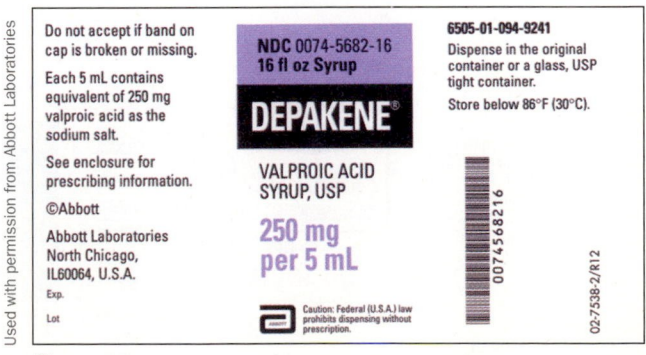

B

Store at controlled room temperature 15°- 30ºC (59º - 86ºF).

DOSAGE AND USE
See package insert for full prescribing information.

Each capsule contains 100 mg of gabapentin.

Manufactured by:
Pfizer Pharmaceuticals Ltd.
Vega Baja, PR 00694

NDC 0071-0803-24
100 Capsules   **Rx only**

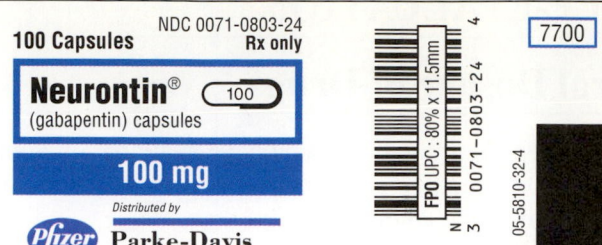

Neurontin®   100
(gabapentin) capsules

100 mg

Distributed by
Pfizer **Parke-Davis**
Division of Pfizer Inc, NY, NY 10017

N 3 0071-0803-24 4
FPO UPC : 80% x 11.5mm
05-5810-32-4

7700

C

N 3 58177-006-03 6

Each extended-release capsule contains:

Nitroglycerin. . . . . 9 mg

KEEP THIS AND ALL DRUGS OUT OF THE REACH OF CHILDREN.

NDC 58177-006-03

Nitroglycerin

Extended-release Capsules

9 mg

Manufactured by:
Time-Caps Labs Inc. for
ETHEX Corporation
St. Louis, MO 63043-2413

60 Capsules

Dispense in a tight container as defined in the USP/NF.

Store at controlled room temperature 15°-30°C (59°-86°F).

USUAL DOSAGE: See package insert for dosage, including nitrate-free intervals.

Rx Only

P2062-7 6/98

ETHEX ETHEX ETHEX ETHEX ETHEX

D

---

3 0048-1020-05 5

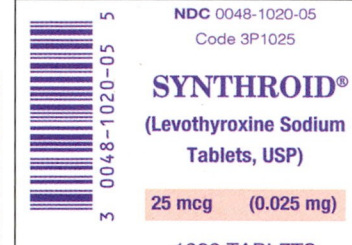

NDC 0048-1020-05
Code 3P1025

SYNTHROID®

(Levothyroxine Sodium Tablets, USP)

25 mcg   (0.025 mg)

1000 TABLETS

Rx only

BASF Pharma   **knoll®**

See full prescribing information for dosage and administration.

Dispense in a tight, light-resistant container as described in USP.

Store at 25°C (77°F); excursions permitted to 15°-30°C (59°-86°F). [See USP Controlled Room Temperature].

Knoll Pharmaceutical Company
Mount Olive, NJ 07828
USA

7897-03

E

WW 8734 AMX

Eli Lilly and Company
Indianapolis, IN 46285, USA

Expiration Date/Control No.

Store at 25°C (77°F); excursions permitted to 15° to 30°C (59° to 86°F) [see USP Controlled Room Temperature].

30 Capsules   NDC 0002-3229-30
                No. 3229

strattera®
atomoxetine HCl

Rx only   **40 mg**

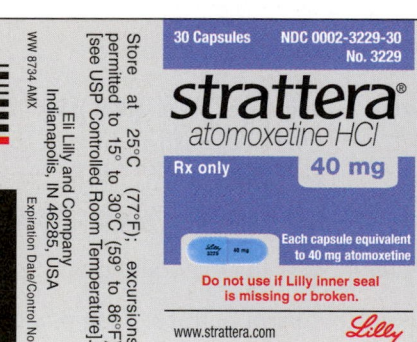

Each capsule equivalent to 40 mg atomoxetine

Do not use if Lilly inner seal is missing or broken.

www.strattera.com   **Lilly**

Medication Guide is to be dispensed to patients.
Keep tightly closed.
Keep out of the reach of children.
See accompanying literature for dosage information.

3 0002-3229-30 4

F

Store at controlled room temperature 59° to 86°F (15° to 30°C).

Dispense in tight containers (USP).

DOSAGE AND USE
See accompanying prescribing information.
Each tablet contains 5 mg donepezil hydrochloride.

200316

NDC 62856-245-90

ARICEPT® ⑤
(donepezil HCl tablets)

5 mg
90 Tablets

Manufactured and Marketed by
Eisai **Eisai Inc.**
Teaneck, NJ 07666

Marketed by
Pfizer Pfizer Inc
NY, NY 10017

3 N 62856-245-90 2

7012

Rx only

©2003 Eisai Inc.

G

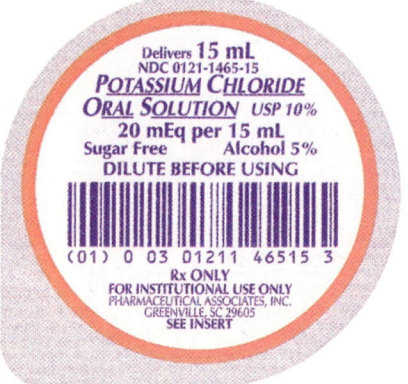

Delivers **15 mL**
NDC 0121-1465-15
**POTASSIUM CHLORIDE
ORAL SOLUTION** USP 10%
20 mEq per 15 mL
Sugar Free   Alcohol 5%
DILUTE BEFORE USING

(01) 0 03 01211 46515 3

Rx ONLY
FOR INSTITUTIONAL USE ONLY
PHARMACEUTICAL ASSOCIATES, INC.
GREENVILLE, SC 29605
SEE INSERT

H

NDC 58177-005-03

Nitroglycerin
Extended-release Capsules

6.5 mg

Each extended-release capsule contains:

Nitroglycerin . . . . 6.5 mg

KEEP THIS AND ALL DRUGS OUT OF THE REACH OF CHILDREN.

Manufactured by
Time-Cap Labs Inc. for
ETHEX Corporation
St. Louis, MO 63043-2413

Dispense in a tight container as defined in the USP/NF.

Store at controlled room temperature 15°-30°C (59°-86°F).

USUAL DOSAGE: See package insert for dosage, including nitrate-free intervals.

℞ Only

60 Capsules

P3806 11/01

ETHEX ETHEX ETHEX ETHEX ETHEX

I

Store at controlled room temperature 59° to 86°F (15° to 30°C).

Dispense in tight containers (USP).

DOSAGE AND USE
See accompanying prescribing information.

Each tablet contains 10 mg donepezil hydrochloride.

NDC 62856-246-90

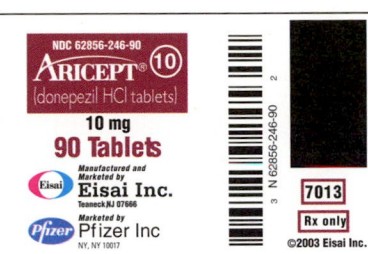

ARICEPT® 10
(donepezil HCl tablets)

10 mg
90 Tablets

Manufactured and Marketed by
Eisai Inc.
Teaneck, NJ 07666

Marketed by
Pfizer Pfizer Inc
NY, NY 10017

3 N 62856-246-90 2

7013

Rx only

©2003 Eisai Inc.

200317

J

See Package Insert for Complete Prescribing Information.

Store at Controlled Room Temperature 15°-30°C (59°-86°F).

PROTECT FROM MOISTURE.

Dispense in a well-closed container as defined in the USP/NF.

TABLETS IDENTIFIED 54 783

(Side One) ⊖⊖ 54/783 (Side Two)

DO NOT USE UNLESS TABLETS CARRY THIS IDENTIFICATION

NDC 0054-4156-25   100 Tablets   EXP. LOT

30 mg C II

CODEINE
Sulfate
Tablets USP

Each tablet contains
Codeine Sulfate 30 mg

℞ only.

Roxane
Laboratories, Inc.
Columbus, Ohio 43216

4151001
039
© RLI, 1999

3 0054-4156-25 7

K

NDC 0093-0661-16
6505-01-256-4997

ALBUTEROL SULFATE
Syrup

2 mg/5 mL

Each 5 mL (1 teaspoonful) contains albuterol sulfate 2.4 mg, equivalent to 2 mg albuterol.

℞ only

See package insert for full prescribing information.

Store at controlled room temperature, between 20° and 25°C (68° and 77°F) (see USP).

This is a bulk package. Dispense contents with a child-resistant closure (as required) and in a tight, light-resistant container as defined in the USP/NF.

KEEP THIS AND ALL MEDICATIONS OUT OF THE REACH OF CHILDREN.

L21006   Rev. H 6/2003

TEVA PHARMACEUTICALS USA
Sellersville, PA 18960

473 mL

TEVA

NDC 0093-0661-16
6505-01-256-4997

ALBUTEROL SULFATE
Syrup

2 mg/5 mL

08
7
0093-0661-16
N 3

L

PHARMACIST/ NURSE/PATIENT:
Please note diagram to the right.
Fill the dropper to the level of the prescribed dose.
Discard opened bottle after 90 days.
PROTECT FROM LIGHT.

mL
2.0 =20 mg
1.75
1.5 =15 mg
1.25
1.0 =10 mg
0.75
0.5 = 5 mg

Furosemide
Oral Solution
10 mg per mL

NDC 0054-3294-46   60 mL   EXP. LOT

FUROSEMIDE
Oral Solution

10 mg per mL

Each mL contains:
Furosemide 10 mg
SUGAR FREE

℞ only

See Package Insert For Complete Prescribing Information.
PROTECT FROM LIGHT.

Roxane
Laboratories, Inc.
Columbus, Ohio 43216

4117540//02   © RLI, 2001

Dispense only in this bottle and only with the calibrated dropper provided. Store at Controlled Room Temperature 15°-30°C (59°-86°F).

M

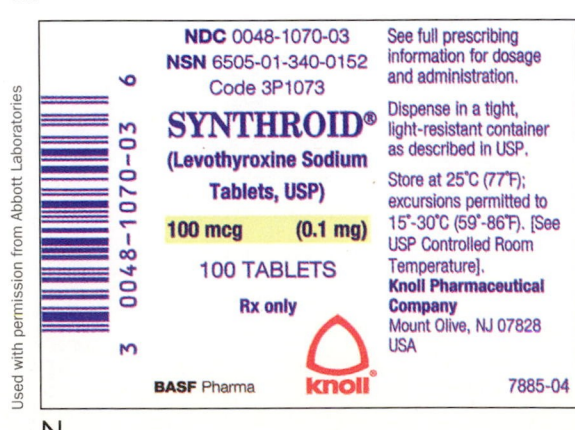

NDC 0048-1070-03
NSN 6505-01-340-0152
Code 3P1073

SYNTHROID®
(Levothyroxine Sodium Tablets, USP)

100 mcg   (0.1 mg)

100 TABLETS

Rx only

See full prescribing information for dosage and administration.

Dispense in a tight, light-resistant container as described in USP.

Store at 25°C (77°F); excursions permitted to 15°-30°C (59°-86°F). [See USP Controlled Room Temperature].

Knoll Pharmaceutical Company
Mount Olive, NJ 07828 USA

BASF Pharma   **knoll**   7885-04

3 0048-1070-03 6

N

Chapter 11—Parenteral Dosage of Drugs

The following labels (A–H) represent the drugs you have available on your medication cart for the orders in questions 11 through 18. Select the correct label and identify the corresponding letter for filling these parenteral medication orders. Calculate the amount to give.

11. Order: clindamycin 0.6 g IV q.12h

    Select label _____ and give _____ mL

12. Order: phenytoin 175 mg IV stat

    Select label _____ and give _____ mL

13. Order: epinephrine 200 mcg subcut stat

    Select label _____ and give _____ mL

14. Order: furosemide 8 mg IV daily

    Select label _____ and give _____ mL

15. Order: gentamicin 60 mg IV q.8h

    Select label _____ and give _____ mL

16. Order: heparin 750 units subcut stat

    Select label _____ and give _____ mL

17. Order: morphine gr $\frac{1}{10}$ subcut q.4h pr.n., pain

    Select label _____ and give _____ mL

18. Order: Narcan 0.3 mg IM stat

    Select label _____ and give _____ mL

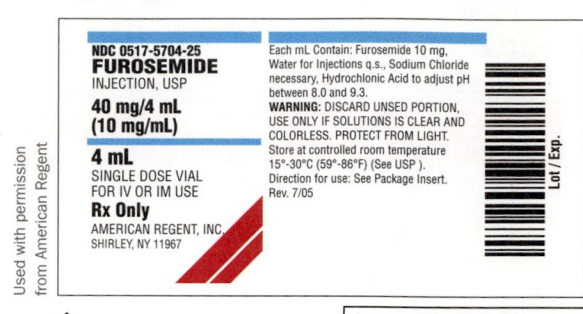

A

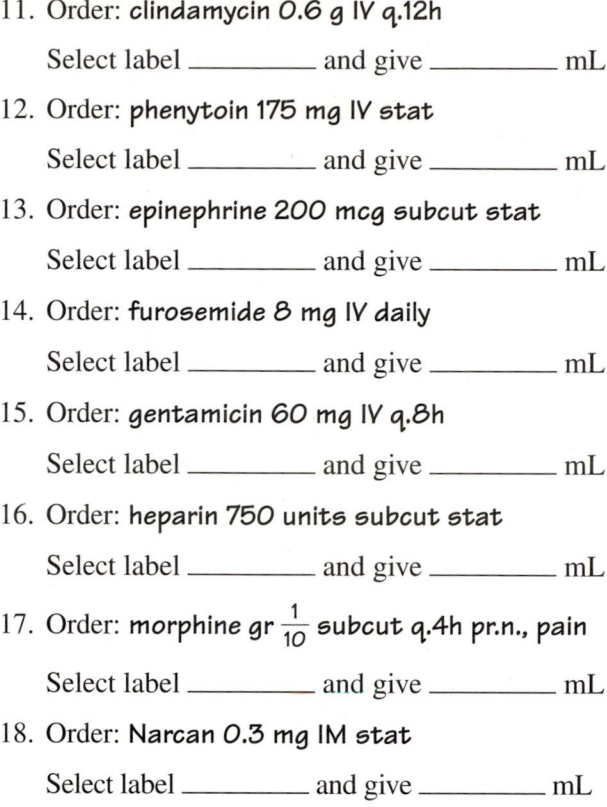

B

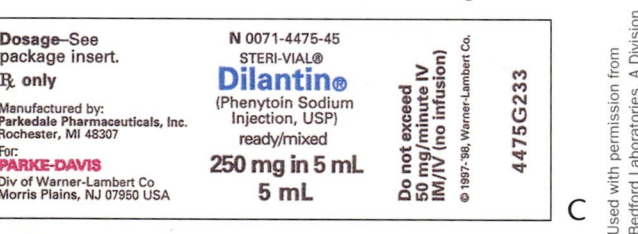

C

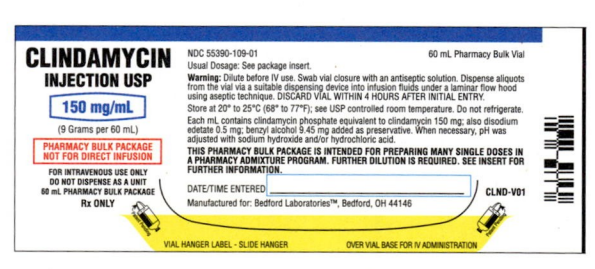

E

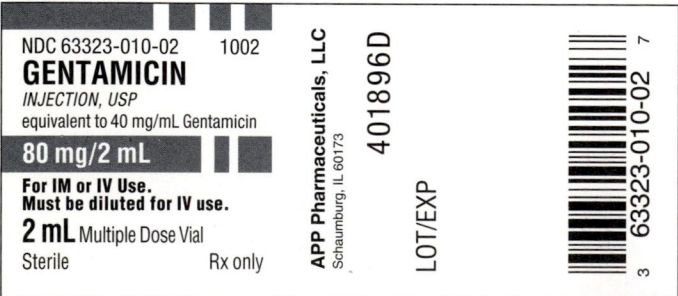

D

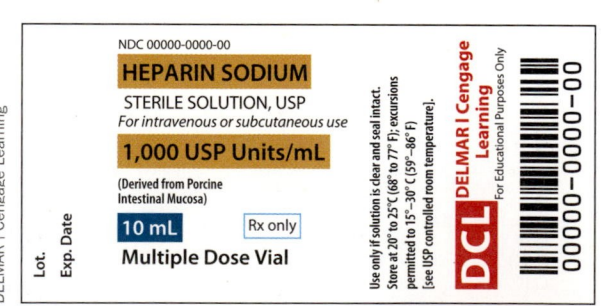

F

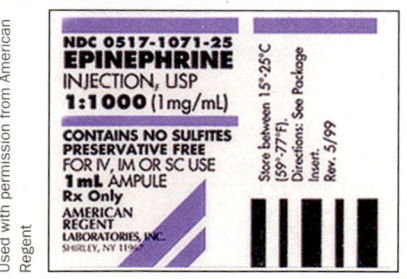

G

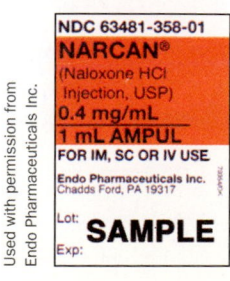

H

For questions 19 and 20, select and mark the amount to give on the correct syringe.

19. Order: Humulin-N NPH U-100 insulin 48 units subcut 30 min ā breakfast

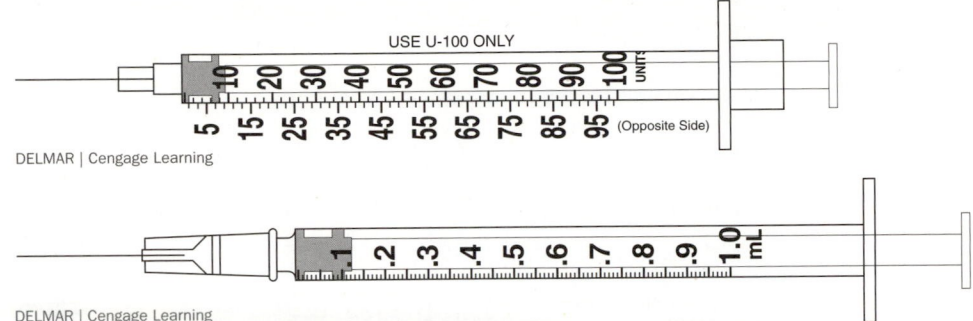

20. Order: Novolin R Regular U-100 insulin 12 units c̄ Novolin N NPH U-100 insulin 28 units subcut 30 min ā dinner

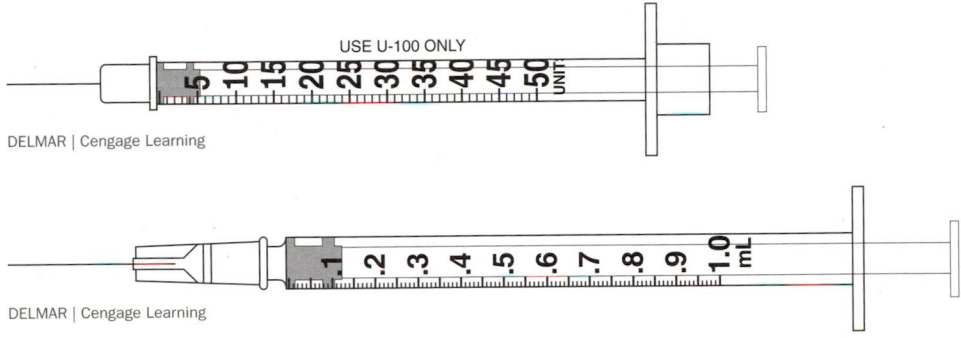

Chapter 12—Reconstitution of Solutions

For questions 21 through 26, specify the amount of diluent to add and the resulting solution concentration. Calculate the amount to give and indicate the dose with an arrow on the accompanying syringe. Finally, make a reconstitution label, if required.

21. Order: Zithromax 500 mg IV daily

Reconstitute with _____ mL diluent for a total solution volume of _____ mL with a concentration of _____ mg/mL.

Give: _____ mL

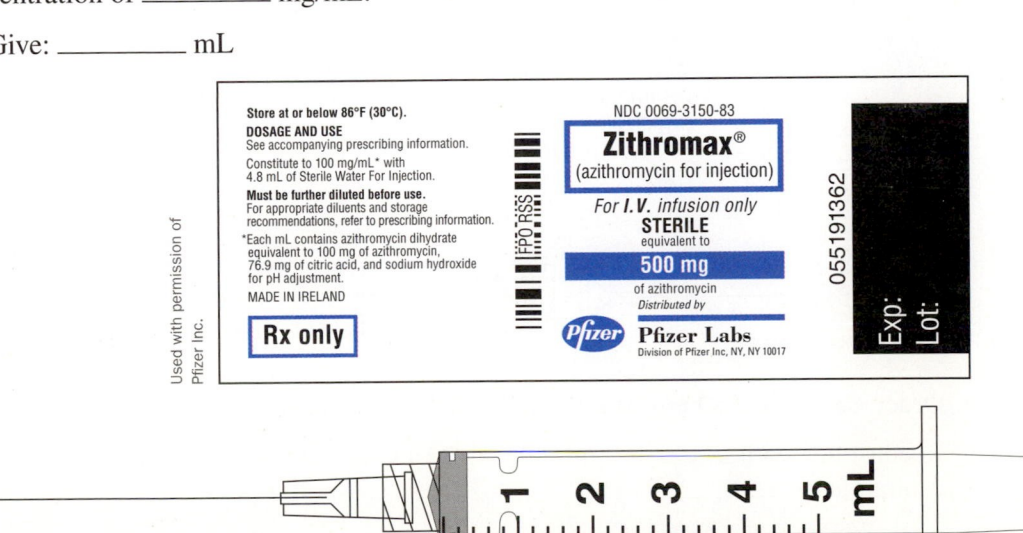

22. Order: **vancomycin 400 mg IV q.6h**

Reconstitute with _____ mL diluent for a total solution volume of _____ mL with a concentration of _____ mg/_____ mL.

Give: _____ mL. There are _____ full doses available in this vial.

NDC 63323-221-10   22110

STERILE

VANCOMYCIN HYDROCHLORIDE, *USP*

equivalent to

500 mg

Vancomycin
For IV Use   Rx only
Must be Further
Diluted Before Use

READ INSERT FOR PRECAUTIONS AND DIRECTIONS BEFORE USE.
Sterile. Lyophilized. **Preservative Free**
Each vial contains: Vancomycin hydrochloride equivalent to 500 mg vancomycin.
Usual Adult Dosage: 2 g daily. Dilute contents of the vial with 10 mL Sterile Water for Injection. **Prior to reconstitution,** store at 20° to 25°C (68° to 77°F) [See USP Controlled Room Temperature].
After reconstitution, this vial may be stored in a refrigerator for 96 hours without significant loss of potency.

APP
APP Pharmaceuticals, LLC
Schaumburg, IL 60173

401783D

LOT/EXP

3 63323-221-10 2

DELMAR | Cengage Learning

23. Order: **ceftriaxone 150 mg IV q.12h**

Reconstitute with _____ mL diluent for a total solution volume of _____ mL with a concentration of _____ mg/mL.

Give: _____ mL

TEVA

NDC 0703-0315-01   Rx only

Ceftriaxone
for Injection, USP

250 mg

For I.M. or I.V. Use
Single Use Vial

Each vial contains: ceftriaxone sodium powder equivalent to 250 mg ceftriaxone.
For I.M. Administration : See Package Insert
A 350 mg/mL concentration is not recommended for the 250 mg vial since it may not be possible to withdraw the entire contents.
For I.V. Administration : See Package Insert
Usual Dosage: See Package Insert

Iss. 9/2007
39C1302450907

Storage Prior to Reconstitution:
Store powder at 20° to 25°C (68° to 77°F) [See USP Controlled Room Temperature].
Protect from Light.
Storage After Reconstitution:
See Package Insert
Mfd for: Teva Parenteral Medicines, Irvine, CA 92618

Package Insert instructions for IV administration: *"Add 2.4 mL diluent to 250 mg vial. After reconstitution, each 1 mL of solution contains approximately 100 mg equivalent of ceftriaxone. Reconstituted solution is stable at room temperature for 24 hours and refrigerated for 3 days."*

DELMAR | Cengage Learning

24. Order: **cefazolin 750 mg IM q.8h** (See label on next page.)

Reconstitute with _____ mL diluent for a total solution volume of _____ mL with a concentration of _____ mg/mL.

Give: _____ mL

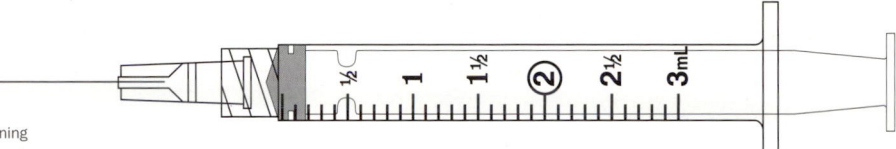

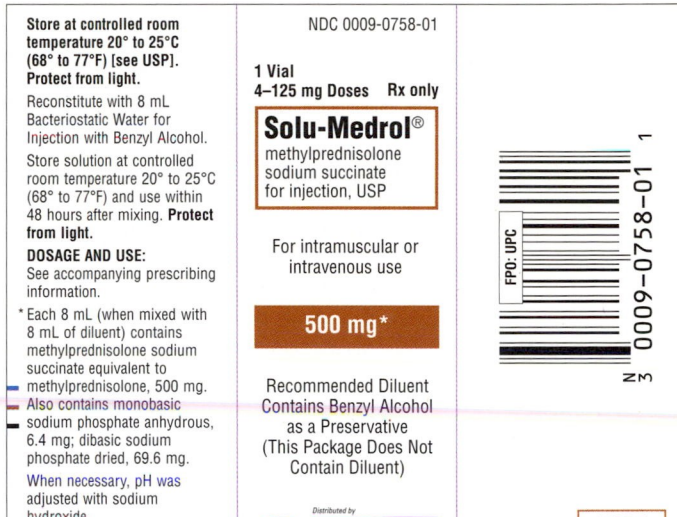

25. Order: **Solu-Medrol 250 mg IV q.6h**
Reconstitute with _____ mL
diluent for a total solution volume of
_____ mL with a concentration
of _____ mg/mL.
Give: _____ mL. There are
_____ full doses available in
this vial.

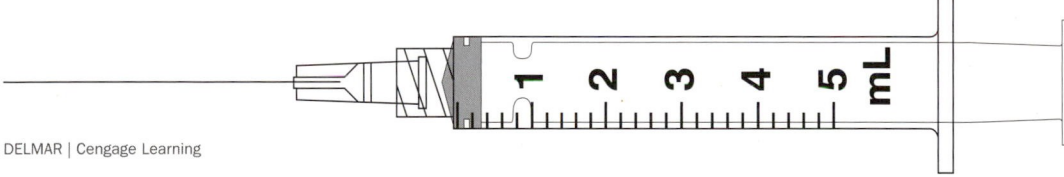

26. Order: **Vantin 100 mg p.o. q.12h**

Reconstitute with _____ mL diluent for a total solution volume of _____ mL with a concentration of _____ mg per _____ mL or _____ mg/mL.
Give: _____ mL

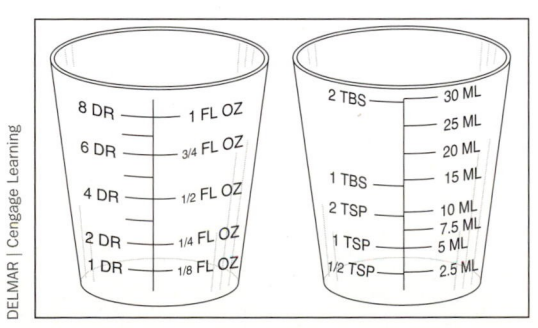

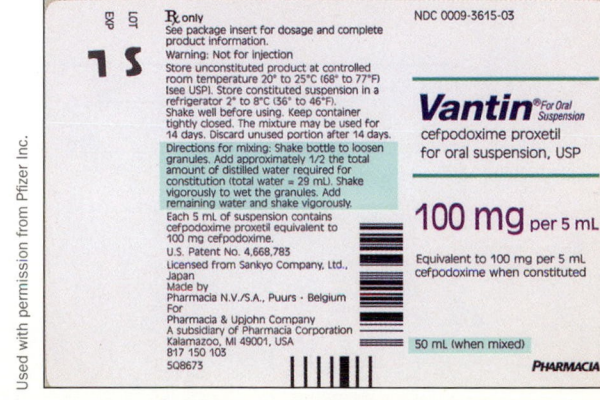

27. How many full doses are available of the medication supplied for question 26? _____ dose(s)

28. Will the medication supplied expire before it is used up for the order in question 26? _____

    Explain: _____

Prepare the following therapeutic solutions.

29. 360 mL of $\frac{1}{3}$ strength hydrogen peroxide diluted with normal saline

    Supply: 60 mL bottles of stock hydrogen peroxide solution

    Add _____ mL solute and _____ mL solvent

30. 240 mL $\frac{3}{4}$ strength Ensure

    Supply: 8 fl oz can of Ensure

    Add _____ mL Ensure and _____ mL water

Refer to the following order for questions 31 and 32.

Order: Give $\frac{2}{3}$ strength Ensure 240 mL via NG tube q.3h

Supply: Ready-to-use Ensure 8 fl oz can and sterile water.

31. How much sterile water would you add to the 8 fl oz can of Ensure? _____ mL

32. How many complete feedings would this make? _____ feeding(s)

Use the following information to answer questions 33 and 34.

You will prepare formula to feed nine infants in the nursery. Each infant has an order for **4 fl oz** of $\frac{1}{2}$ **strength Isomil formula q.3h.** You have 8 fl oz cans of ready-to-use Isomil and sterile water.

33. How many cans of formula will you need to open to prepare the reconstituted formula for all nine infants for one feeding each? _____ can(s)

34. How many mL of sterile water will you add to the Isomil to reconstitute the formula for one feeding for all nine infants? _____ mL

Chapter 13—Alternative Dosage Calculation Methods: Formula and Dimensional Analysis

Use the conversion factor method in questions 35 through 38 to convert each of the following amounts to the unit indicated. Indicate the approximate equivalent used in the conversion.

	Equivalent			Equivalent
35. 15 mg = gr _____	_____	37. 625 mg = _____ mcg	_____
36. 115 lb = _____ kg	_____	38. 0.3 g = _____ mg	_____

Medication Cart Exercise: Formula Method and Dimensional Analysis

You are to prepare medicines for patients assigned to your medication cart. The following labels represent the drugs you have available for questions 39 through 44. Use both the formula and dimensional analysis methods to calculate the dosages.

39. Order: **methotrexate 175 mg IV stat**

    Give: _____ mL

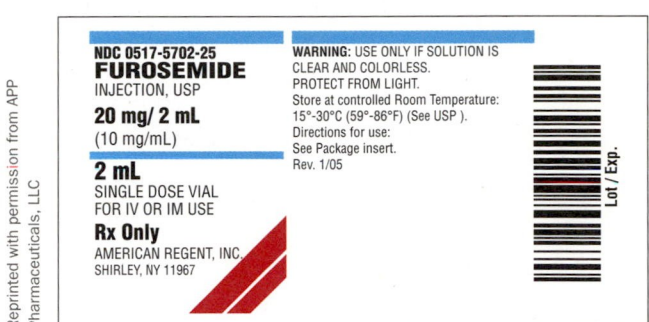

40. Order: **furosemide 15 mg IM stat**

    Give: _____ mL

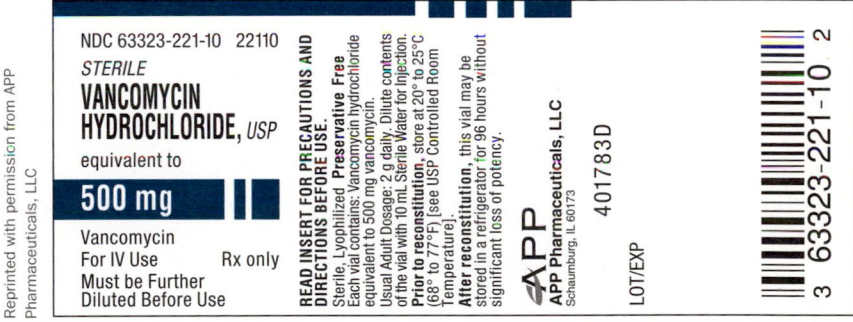

41. Order: **vancomycin hydrochloride 500 mg IV q.6h**

    Give: _____ mL

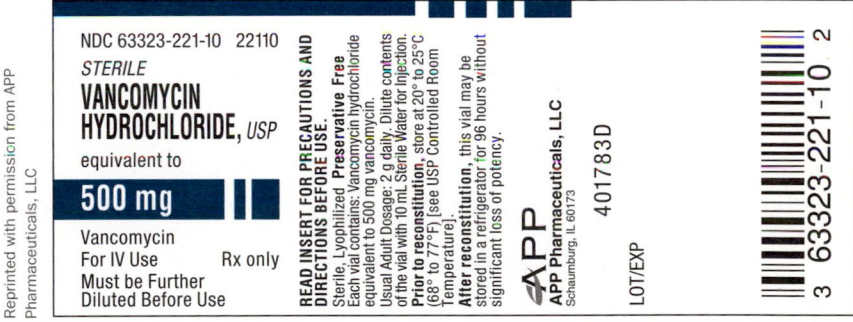

42. Order: **Nitrostat gr $\frac{1}{100}$ SL p.r.n., angina**

    Give: _____ tablet(s)

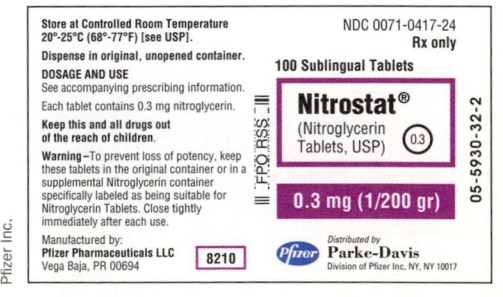

43. Order: **metoclopramide 15 mg IV q.3h × 3 doses**

    Give: _____ mL

44. Order: **levothyroxine 0.15 mg IV daily**

    Give: _____ mL

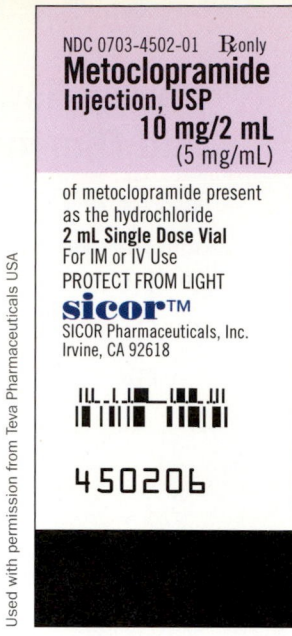

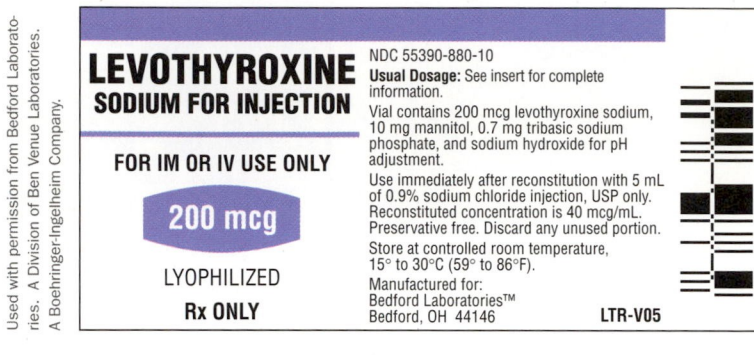

Chapter 14—Pediatric and Adult Dosages Based on Body Weight

Calculate and assess the safety of the following dosages. Mark safe dosages on the measuring device supplied.

45. Order: **morphine gr $\frac{1}{10}$ subcut q.4h p.r.n. severe pain** for a child who weighs 67 lb. Recommended pediatric dosage: 100 to 200 mcg/kg q.4h, up to a maximum of 15 mg/dose.

    If the dosage ordered is safe, give _____ mL. If not safe, explain why not and describe what you should do. _____

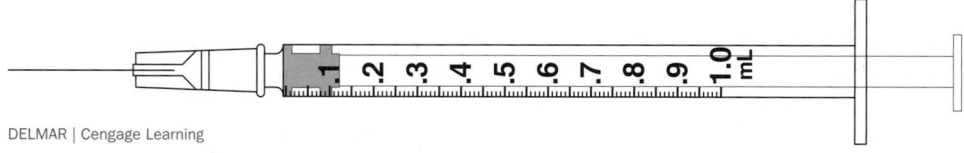

DELMAR | Cengage Learning

46. Order: **amoxicillin 75 mg p.o. q.8h** for a 15 lb infant. Recommended dosage: See label.

    If the dosage ordered is safe, reconstitute with _____ mL diluent for a total solution volume of _____ mL and a concentration of _____ mg/mL and give _____ mL. If not safe, explain why not and describe what you should do. _____

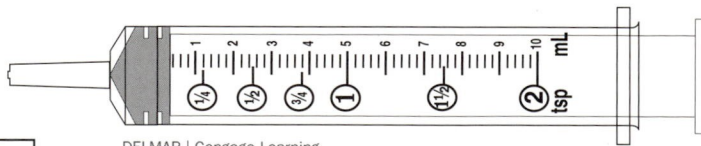

DELMAR | Cengage Learning

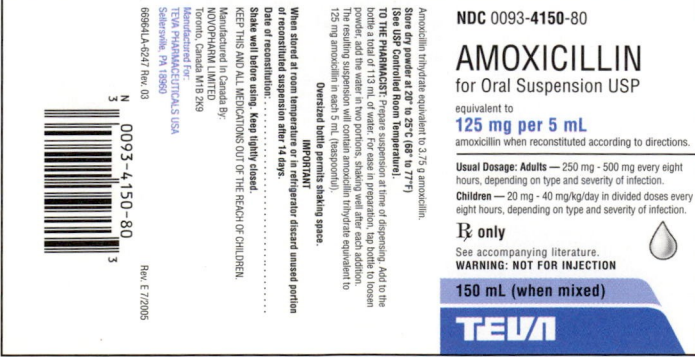

47. Order: **phenytoin 100 mg IV t.i.d.** for a child who weighs 20 kg. Recommended pediatric dosage: 5 mg/kg/day in 2 to 3 divided doses. If the dosage ordered is safe, give _____ mL. If not safe, explain why not and describe what you should do. _____

Used with permission from Pfizer Inc.

Dosage–See package insert. **℞ only** Manufactured by: **Parkedale Pharmaceuticals, Inc.** Rochester, MI 48307 For: **PARKE-DAVIS** Div of Warner-Lambert Co Morris Plains, NJ 07950 USA	N 0071-4475-45 STERI-VIAL® **Dilantin®** (Phenytoin Sodium Injection, USP) ready/mixed **250 mg in 5 mL** **5 mL**

Do not exceed 50 mg/minute IV IM/IV (no infusion)

© 1997-'98, Warner-Lambert Co.

4475G233

DELMAR | Cengage Learning

48. Order: **cefaclor 187 mg p.o. q.i.d.** for a child with otitis media who weighs 16 lb. Recommended dosage: See label.

If the dosage ordered is safe, reconstitute with _____ mL diluent for a total solution volume of _____ mL and a concentration of _____ mg/mL. Give _____ mL. If not safe, explain why not and describe what you should do. _____

Used with permission from Ranbaxy Pharmaceuticals Inc.

Manufactured for: Ranbaxy Pharmaceuticals Inc. Jacksonville, FL 32216 USA by: Ranbaxy Laboratories Ltd. New Delhi - 110 019, India

℞ RANBAXY

NDC 63304-**957**-03

CEFACLOR

For Oral Suspension USP

375 mg/5 mL

50 mL (when mixed)

SHAKE WELL BEFORE USE

Rx only

Usual Dosage: Children, 20 mg/kg a day (40 mg/kg in otitis media) in three divided doses.
Adults, 250 mg three times a day. See literature for complete dosage information.
Contains Cefaclor monohydrate equivalent to 3.75 g cefaclor in a dry, pleasantly flavored mixture.
Prior to Mixing, store at 20 - 25° C (68 - 77° F). (See USP Controlled Room Temperature). Protect from moisture.
Directions for Mixing: Add **35 mL** of water in two portions to dry mixture in the bottle. Shake well after each addition.
Each 5 mL (Approx. one teaspoonful) will then contain Cefaclor USP monohydrate equivalent to 375 mg anhydrous cefaclor.
Over size bottle provides extra space for shaking.
Store in a refrigerator. May be kept for 14 days without significant loss of potency. Keep tightly closed. Discard unused portion in 14 days.

0903

50308530

non varnish area

LOT:
EX

DELMAR | Cengage Learning

49. a) Order: **Kantrex 60 mg IV q.8h** for a child who weighs 16 lb. The recommended dosage of Kantrex for adults and children is 15 mg/kg/day in 2 to 3 divided doses, not to exceed 1.5 g/day.

If the ordered dosage is safe, give _____ mL. If not safe, explain why not and describe what you should do. _____

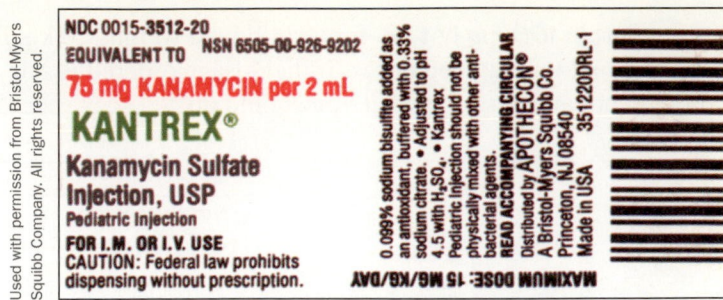

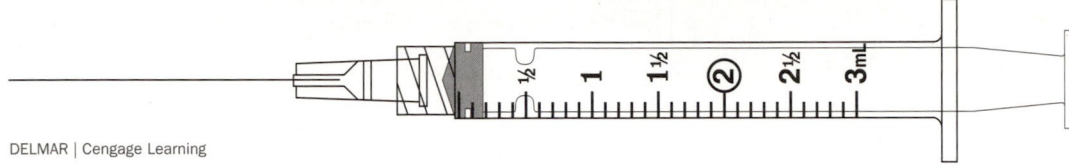

DELMAR | Cengage Learning

b) Refer to the recommended dosage of Kantrex given in question 49(a). What would you expect the single q.8h dosage of Kantrex to be for an adult who weighs 275 lb?

_____ mg/dose

50. Describe the strategy you would implement to prevent this medication error.

Possible Scenario

The physician ordered *amoxicillin 50 mg p.o. q.i.d.* for a child with an upper respiratory infection. Amoxicillin is supplied in an oral suspension with 125 mg per 5 mL. The nurse calculated the dose this way:

$$\frac{125 \text{ mg}}{50 \text{ mg}} = \frac{X \text{ mL}}{5 \text{ mL}}$$

$$50X = 625 \qquad \textbf{INCORRECT}$$

$$\frac{50X}{50} = \frac{625}{50}$$

$$X = 12.5 \text{ mL}$$

Potential Outcome

The patient received a large overdose and should have received only 2 mL. The child would likely develop complications from the overdose of amoxicillin. When the physician was notified of the error, she would likely have ordered the medication discontinued and had extra blood lab work done. An incident report would be filed and the family would be notified of the error.

Prevention

_____

_____

After completing these problems, see pages 551–556 to check your answers. Give yourself 2 points for each correct answer.

Perfect score = 100   My score = _____

Minimum mastery score = 86 (43 correct)

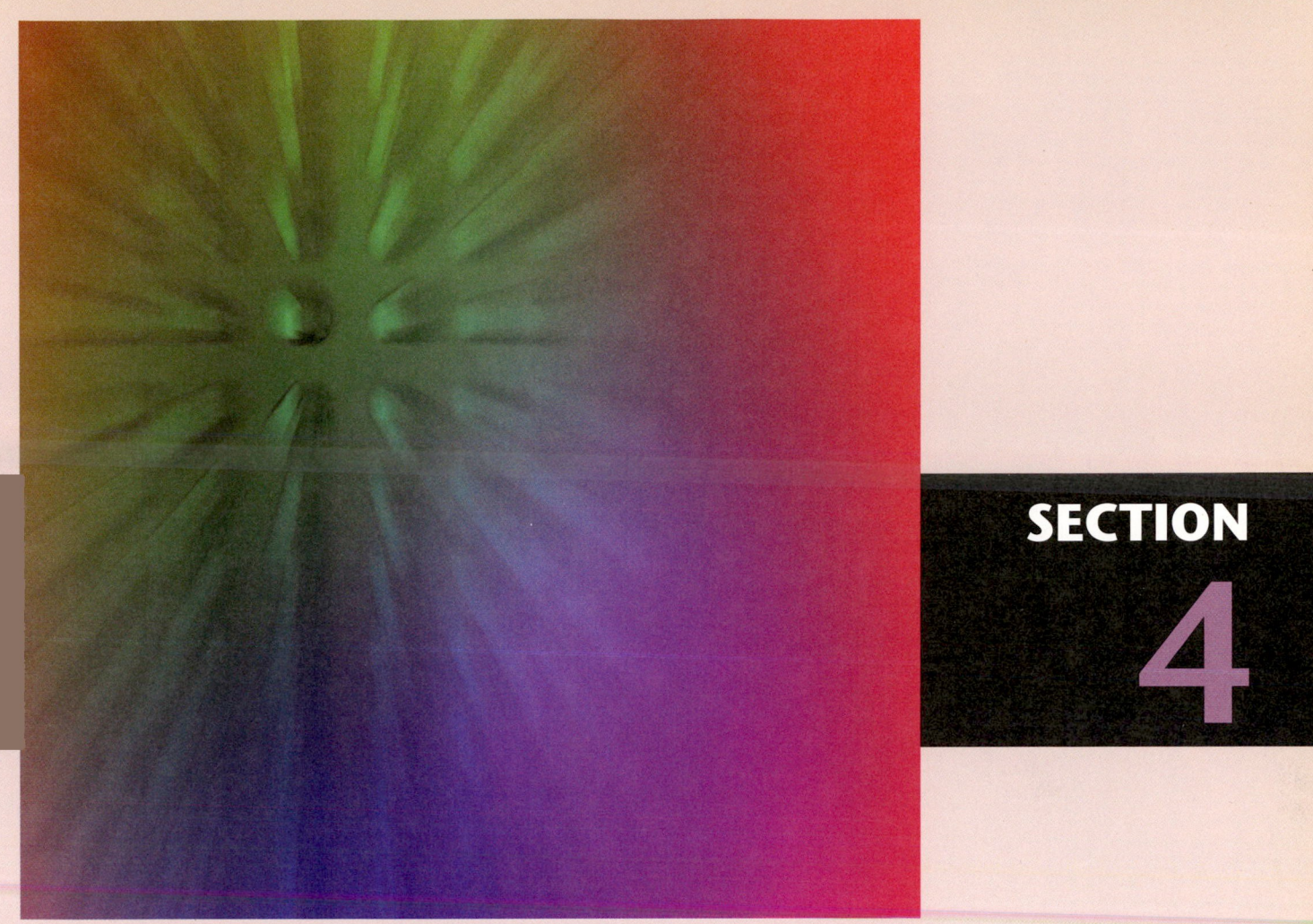

4

Advanced Calculations

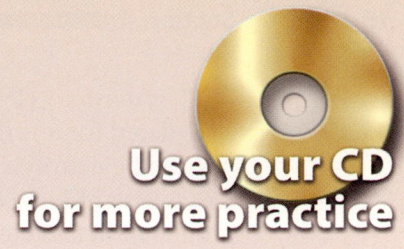
Use your CD for more practice

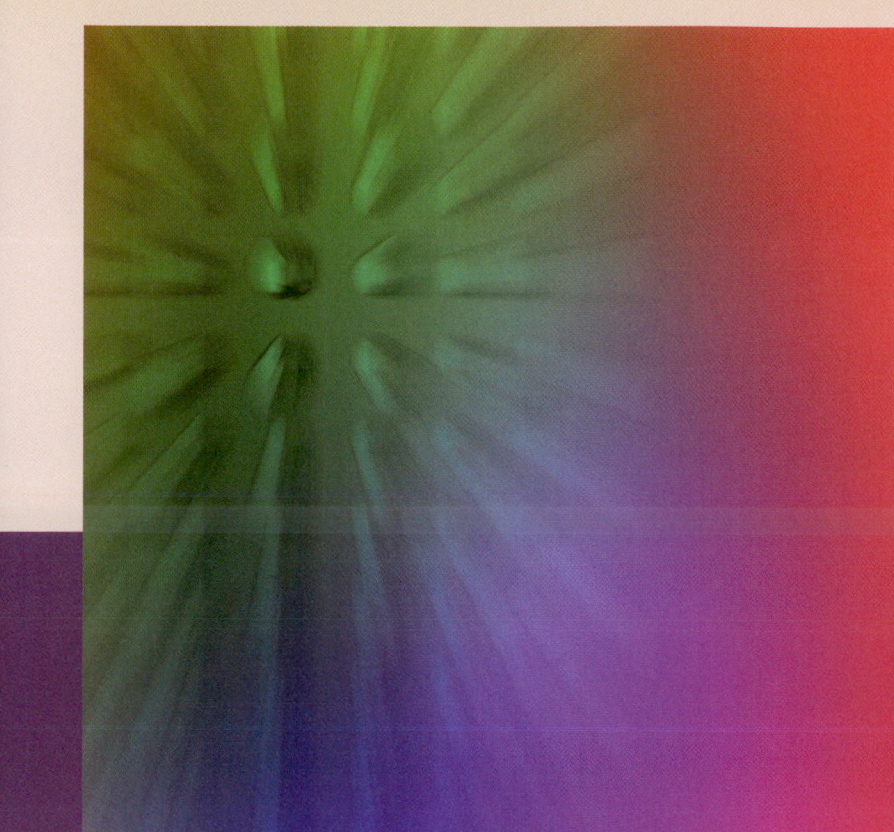

15

Intravenous Solutions, Equipment, and Calculations

OBJECTIVES

Upon mastery of Chapter 15, you will be able to calculate intravenous (IV) solution flow rates for electronic or manual infusion systems. To accomplish this you will also be able to:

- Identify common IV solutions and equipment.
- Calculate the amount of specific components in common IV fluids.
- Define the following terms: IV, peripheral line, central line, primary IV, secondary IV, saline/heparin locks, IV piggyback (IV PB), and IV push.
- Calculate milliliters per hour: mL/h.
- Recognize the calibration or drop factor in gtt/mL as stated on the IV tubing package.
- Apply the formula method to calculate IV flow rate in gtt/min:

$$\frac{V \text{ (volume)}}{T \text{ (time in min)}} \times C \text{ (drop factor calibration)} = R \text{ (rate of flow)}$$

- Apply the shortcut method to calculate IV flow rate in gtt/min:

$$\frac{mL/h}{\text{drop factor constant}} = gtt/min$$

- Recalculate the flow rate when the IV is off schedule.
- Calculate small-volume IV PB.
- Calculate rate for IV push medications.
- Calculate IV infusion time.
- Calculate IV infusion volume.

*I*ntravenous (IV) means the administration of fluids or medication through a vein. IV fluids are ordered for a variety of reasons. They may be ordered for replacement of lost fluids, to maintain fluid and electrolyte balance, or to administer IV medications. *Replacement fluids* are often ordered because of losses that may occur from hemorrhage, vomiting, or diarrhea. *Maintenance fluids* sustain normal fluid and electrolyte balance. They may be used for the patient who is not yet depleted but is beginning to show symptoms of depletion. They may also be ordered for the patient who has the potential to become depleted, such as the patient who is allowed nothing by mouth (NPO) for surgery.

IV fluids and drugs may be administered by two methods: *continuous* and *intermittent* infusion. Continuous IV infusions replace or maintain fluid and electrolytes and serve as a vehicle for drug administration. Intermittent, such as IV PB and IV push, infusions are used for IV administration of drugs and supplemental fluids. Intermittent peripheral infusion devices, also known as saline or heparin locks, are used to maintain venous access without continuous fluid infusion.

IV therapy is an important and challenging nursing role. This chapter covers the essential information and presents step-by-step calculations to help you gain a thorough understanding and mastery of this subject. Let's begin by analyzing IV solutions.

IV SOLUTIONS

IV solutions are ordered by a physician or prescribing practitioner; however, they are administered and monitored by the nurse. It is the responsibility of the nurse to ensure that the correct IV fluid is administered to the correct patient at the prescribed rate, following the same six rights for medication administration. IV fluids can be supplied in plastic solution bags or glass bottles with the volume of the IV fluid container typically varying from 50 mL to 1,000 mL. Some IV bags may even contain more than 1,000 mL. Solutions used for total parenteral nutrition usually contain 2,000 mL or more in a single bag. The IV solution bag or bottle will be labeled with the exact components and amount of the IV solution. Health care practitioners often use abbreviations when communicating about the IV solution. Therefore, it is important for the nurse to know the common IV solution components and the solution concentration strengths represented by such abbreviations.

Solution Components

Glucose (dextrose), water, saline (sodium chloride or NaCl), and selected electrolytes and salts are found in IV fluids. Dextrose and sodium chloride are the two most common solute components. Learn these common IV component abbreviations.

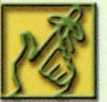

REMEMBER
Common IV Component Abbreviations

Abbreviation	Solution Component
D	Dextrose
W	Water
S	Saline
NS	Normal Saline (0.9% NaCl)
NaCl	Sodium Chloride
RL	Ringer's Lactate
LR	Lactated Ringer's

Solution Strength

The abbreviation letters indicate the solution components, and the numbers indicate the solution strength or concentration of the components (as shown in the examples that follow, such as, D_5W). The numbers may be written as subscripts in the medical order.

FIGURE 15-1   IV solution label: D_5W

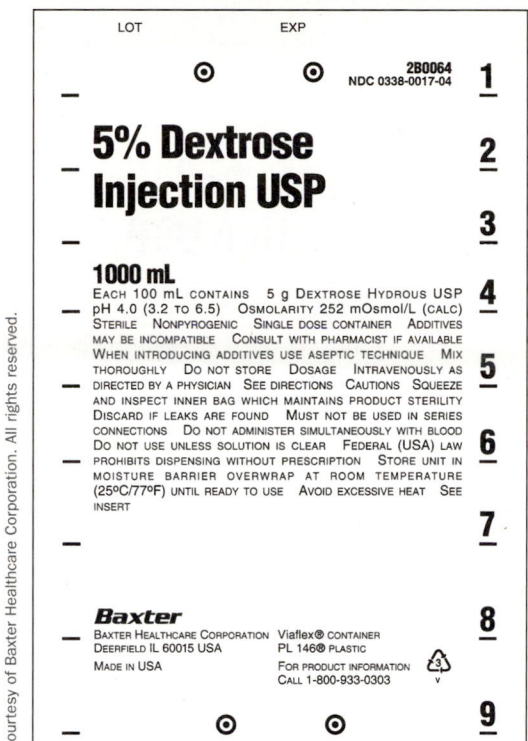

LOT   EXP

2B0064
NDC 0338-0017-04

5% Dextrose Injection USP

1000 mL
EACH 100 mL CONTAINS   5 g DEXTROSE HYDROUS USP
pH 4.0 (3.2 TO 6.5)   OSMOLARITY 252 mOsmol/L (CALC)
STERILE   NONPYROGENIC   SINGLE DOSE CONTAINER   ADDITIVES
MAY BE INCOMPATIBLE   CONSULT WITH PHARMACIST IF AVAILABLE
WHEN INTRODUCING ADDITIVES USE ASEPTIC TECHNIQUE   MIX
THOROUGHLY   DO NOT STORE   DOSAGE   INTRAVENOUSLY AS
DIRECTED BY A PHYSICIAN   SEE DIRECTIONS   CAUTIONS   SQUEEZE
AND INSPECT INNER BAG WHICH MAINTAINS PRODUCT STERILITY
DISCARD IF LEAKS ARE FOUND   MUST NOT BE USED IN SERIES
CONNECTIONS   DO NOT ADMINISTER SIMULTANEOUSLY WITH BLOOD
DO NOT USE UNLESS SOLUTION IS CLEAR   FEDERAL (USA) LAW
PROHIBITS DISPENSING WITHOUT PRESCRIPTION   STORE UNIT IN
MOISTURE BARRIER OVERWRAP AT ROOM TEMPERATURE
(25ºC/77ºF) UNTIL READY TO USE   AVOID EXCESSIVE HEAT   SEE
INSERT

Baxter
BAXTER HEALTHCARE CORPORATION   VIAFLEX® CONTAINER
DEERFIELD IL 60015 USA   PL 146® PLASTIC
MADE IN USA   FOR PRODUCT INFORMATION
                                CALL 1-800-933-0303

1 2 3 4 5 6 7 8 9

FIGURE 15-2   IV solution label: D_5LR

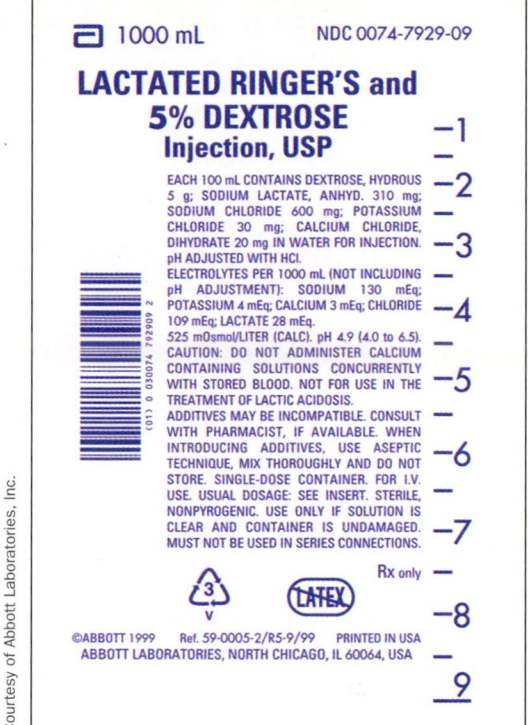

1000 mL   NDC 0074-7929-09

LACTATED RINGER'S and 5% DEXTROSE Injection, USP

EACH 100 mL CONTAINS DEXTROSE, HYDROUS
5 g; SODIUM LACTATE, ANHYD. 310 mg;
SODIUM CHLORIDE 600 mg; POTASSIUM
CHLORIDE 30 mg; CALCIUM CHLORIDE,
DIHYDRATE 20 mg IN WATER FOR INJECTION.
pH ADJUSTED WITH HCl.
ELECTROLYTES PER 1000 mL (NOT INCLUDING
pH ADJUSTMENT): SODIUM   130 mEq;
POTASSIUM 4 mEq; CALCIUM 3 mEq; CHLORIDE
109 mEq; LACTATE 28 mEq.
525 mOsmol/LITER (CALC). pH 4.9 (4.0 to 6.5).
CAUTION: DO NOT ADMINISTER CALCIUM
CONTAINING SOLUTIONS CONCURRENTLY
WITH STORED BLOOD. NOT FOR USE IN THE
TREATMENT OF LACTIC ACIDOSIS.
ADDITIVES MAY BE INCOMPATIBLE. CONSULT
WITH PHARMACIST, IF AVAILABLE. WHEN
INTRODUCING ADDITIVES, USE ASEPTIC
TECHNIQUE, MIX THOROUGHLY AND DO NOT
STORE. SINGLE-DOSE CONTAINER. FOR I.V.
USE. USUAL DOSAGE: SEE INSERT. STERILE,
NONPYROGENIC. USE ONLY IF SOLUTION IS
CLEAR AND CONTAINER IS UNDAMAGED.
MUST NOT BE USED IN SERIES CONNECTIONS.

Rx only

©ABBOTT 1999   Ref. 59-0005-2/R5-9/99   PRINTED IN USA
ABBOTT LABORATORIES, NORTH CHICAGO, IL 60064, USA

1 2 3 4 5 6 7 8 9

EXAMPLE 1 ▪

Suppose an order includes D_5W. This abbreviation means *dextrose 5% in water* and is supplied as 5% Dextrose Injection, as in Figure 15-1. This means that the solution strength of the solute (dextrose) is 5%. The solvent is water. Recall from Chapter 8 that parenteral solutions expressed in a percent indicate X g per 100 mL. Read the IV bag label and notice that "each 100 mL contains 5 g dextrose. . . ." For every 100 mL of solution, there are 5 g of dextrose.

EXAMPLE 2 ▪

Suppose a nurse writes D_5LR in the nurse's notes. This abbreviation means *dextrose 5% in Lactated Ringer's* and is supplied as Lactated Ringer's and 5% Dextrose Injection, as in Figure 15-2.

EXAMPLE 3 ▪

An order states D_5NS **1,000 mL IV q.8h.** This order means *administer 1,000 mL 5% dextrose in normal saline intravenously every 8 hours* and is supplied as 5% Dextrose and 0.9% Sodium Chloride (NaCl), as in Figure 15-3. *Normal saline* is the common term for 0.9% NaCl because it has the same concentration of sodium chloride normally present in the blood. Another name is *physiologic saline*. The concentration of sodium chloride in normal saline is 0.9 g (or 900 mg) per 100 mL of solution.

Another common saline IV concentration is 0.45% NaCl, as in Figure 15-4. Notice that 0.45% NaCl is $\frac{1}{2}$ the strength of 0.9% NaCl, which is normal saline. Thus, it is usually written as $\frac{1}{2}$ NS for $\frac{1}{2}$ normal saline. Another saline solution strength is 0.225% NaCl (also abbreviated as $\frac{1}{4}$ NS).

The goal of intravenous therapy, achieved through fluid infusion, is to maintain or regain fluid and electrolyte balance. When dextrose or saline *(solute)* is diluted in water for injection *(solvent)*, the result is *an IV solution* that can be administered to maintain or approximate the normal blood plasma. Blood or

FIGURE 15-3   IV solution label: D₅NS

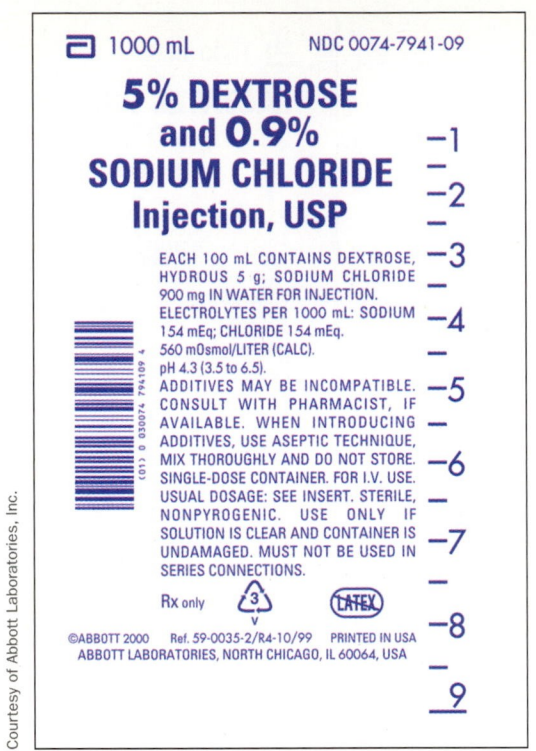

FIGURE 15-4   IV solution label: 0.45% NaCl

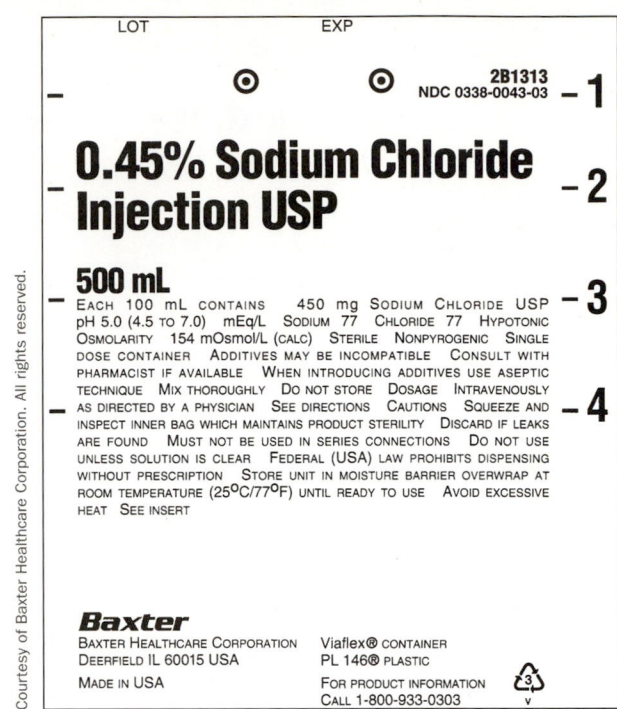

serum concentration is described in terms of *tonicity* or *osmolarity* and is measured in milliOsmols per liter, or mOsm/L. IV fluids are concentrated and classified as *isotonic* (the same tonicity or osmolarity as blood and other body serums), *hypotonic* (lower tonicity or osmolarity than blood and other body serums), or *hypertonic* (higher tonicity or osmolarity than blood and other body serums). Normal saline (0.9% NaCl or physiologic saline) is an isotonic solution. The osmolarity of a manufactured solution is detailed on the printed label. Look for the mOsm/L in the fine print under the solution name in Figures 15-1 through 15-4.

Figure 15-5 compares the three solution concentrations to normal serum osmolarity. Parenteral therapy is determined by unique patient needs, and these basic factors must be considered when ordering and infusing IV solutions.

FIGURE 15-5 Comparison of IV solution concentrations by osmolarity

Normal Serum Osmolarity
(Normal Average Tonicity—All Ages)
280–320 mOsm/L

Hypotonic (<250 mOsm/L) *Solvent exceeds solute*—used to dilute excess serum electrolytes, as in hyperglycemia	**Isotonic** (250–375 mOsm/L) *Solvent and solutes are balanced*—used to expand volume and maintain normal tonicity	**Hypertonic** (>375 mOsm/L) *Solutes exceed solvent*— used to correct electrolyte imbalances, as in loss from excess vomiting and diarrhea
Example of IV solution: *0.45% Saline* (154 mOsm/L)	Examples of IV solution: *0.9% Saline* (308 mOsm/L) *Lactated Ringer's* (273 mOsm/L) *5% Dextrose in Water* (252 mOsm/L)	Example of IV solution: *5% Dextrose and 0.9% NaCl* (560 mOsm/L) *5% Dextrose and Lactated Ringer's* (525 mOsm/L)

Solution Additives

Electrolytes also may be added to the basic IV fluid. Potassium chloride (KCl) is a common IV additive and is measured in *milliequivalents* (mEq). The order is usually written to indicate the amount of milliequivalents per liter (1,000 mL) to be added to the IV fluid.

EXAMPLE ▪

The physician orders D₅NS 1,000 mL IV c̄ 20 mEq KCl/L q.8h. This means to infuse 1,000 mL 5% dextrose and 0.9% sodium chloride IV solution with 20 milliequivalents potassium chloride added per liter every 8 hours.

QUICK REVIEW

- Pay close attention to IV abbreviations: *letters* indicate the solution components and *numbers* indicate the concentration or solution strength.

- Dextrose and sodium chloride (NaCl) are common IV solutes.

- Solution strength expressed as a percent (%) indicates the number of g per 100 mL.

- Normal Saline is 0.9% sodium chloride: 0.9 g NaCl per 100 mL solution.

- IV solution tonicity or osmolarity is measured in mOsm/L.

- D₅W and normal saline are common isotonic solutions.

Review Set 32

For each of the following IV solutions labeled A through H:
  a. Specify the *letter* of the illustration corresponding to the fluid abbreviation.

  b. List the *solute(s)* of each solution, and identify the *strength (g/mL)* of each solute.

  c. Identify the *osmolarity (mOsm/L)* of each solution.

  d. Identify the *tonicity (isotonic, hypotonic, or hypertonic)* of each solution.

	a. Letter of matching illustration	b. Components and strength	c. Osmolarity (mOsm/L)	d. Tonicity
1. NS	_____	_____	_____	_____
2. D₅W	_____	_____	_____	_____
3. D₅NS	_____	_____	_____	_____
4. D₅ ½NS	_____	_____	_____	_____
5. D₅ ¼NS	_____	_____	_____	_____
6. D₅LR	_____	_____	_____	_____
7. D₅ ½NS c̄ 20 mEq KCl/L	_____	_____	_____	_____
8. ½NS	_____	_____	_____	_____

After completing these problems, see page 556 to check your answers.

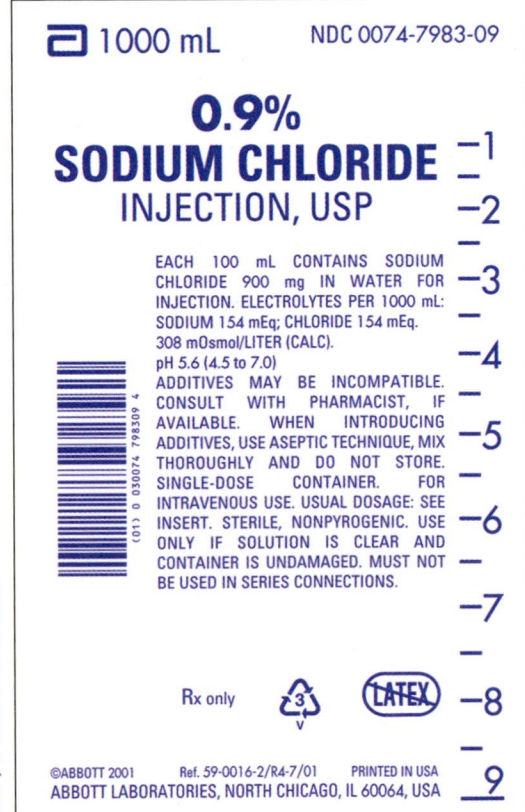

A

Courtesy of Abbott Laboratories, Inc.

500 mL   NDC 0074-7924-03

5% DEXTROSE and 0.225% SODIUM CHLORIDE
Injection, USP

—1

EACH 100 mL CONTAINS DEXTROSE, HYDROUS 5 g; SODIUM CHLORIDE 225 mg IN WATER FOR INJECTION. ELECTROLYTES PER 1000 mL: SODIUM 38.5 mEq; CHLORIDE 38.5 mEq.

—2

329 mOsmol/LITER (CALC).   pH 4.3 (3.5 to 6.5). ADDITIVES MAY BE INCOMPATIBLE. CONSULT WITH PHARMACIST, IF AVAILABLE. WHEN INTRODUCING ADDITIVES, USE ASEPTIC TECHNIQUE, MIX THOROUGHLY AND DO NOT STORE. SINGLE-DOSE CONTAINER. FOR I.V. USE. USUAL DOSAGE: SEE INSERT. STERILE, NONPYROGENIC. USE ONLY IF SOLUTION IS CLEAR AND CONTAINER IS UNDAMAGED. MUST NOT BE USED IN SERIES CONNECTIONS.

—3

Rx only

©ABBOTT 2000   Ref. 59-0023-2/R4-10/99   PRINTED IN USA
ABBOTT LABORATORIES, NORTH CHICAGO, IL 60064, USA

—4

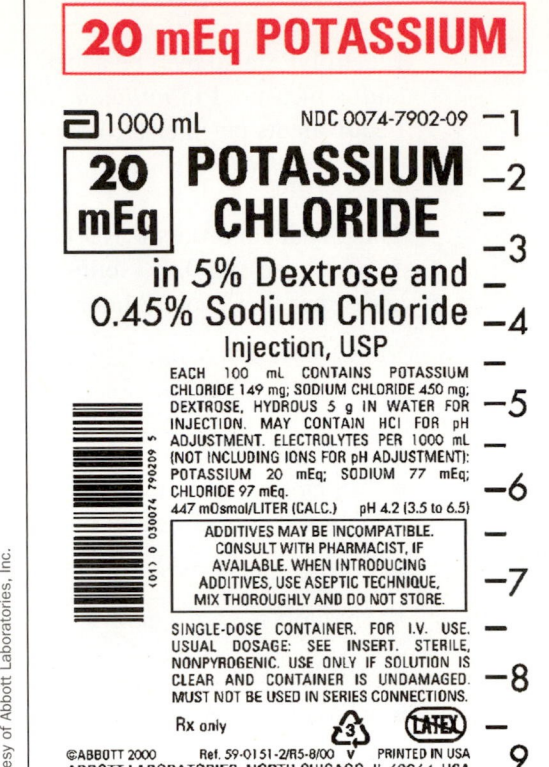

B

Courtesy of Abbott Laboratories, Inc.

20 mEq POTASSIUM

1000 mL   NDC 0074-7902-09 —1

20 mEq **POTASSIUM CHLORIDE**
in 5% Dextrose and 0.45% Sodium Chloride
Injection, USP

—2
—3
—4

EACH 100 mL CONTAINS POTASSIUM CHLORIDE 149 mg; SODIUM CHLORIDE 450 mg; DEXTROSE, HYDROUS 5 g IN WATER FOR INJECTION. MAY CONTAIN HCl FOR pH ADJUSTMENT. ELECTROLYTES PER 1000 mL (NOT INCLUDING IONS FOR pH ADJUSTMENT): POTASSIUM 20 mEq; SODIUM 77 mEq; CHLORIDE 97 mEq.
447 mOsmol/LITER (CALC.)   pH 4.2 (3.5 to 6.5)

—5
—6

ADDITIVES MAY BE INCOMPATIBLE. CONSULT WITH PHARMACIST, IF AVAILABLE. WHEN INTRODUCING ADDITIVES, USE ASEPTIC TECHNIQUE, MIX THOROUGHLY AND DO NOT STORE.

—7

SINGLE-DOSE CONTAINER. FOR I.V. USE. USUAL DOSAGE: SEE INSERT. STERILE, NONPYROGENIC. USE ONLY IF SOLUTION IS CLEAR AND CONTAINER IS UNDAMAGED. MUST NOT BE USED IN SERIES CONNECTIONS.

—8

Rx only

©ABBOTT 2000   Ref. 59-0151-2/R5-8/00   PRINTED IN USA
ABBOTT LABORATORIES, NORTH CHICAGO, IL 60064, USA

9

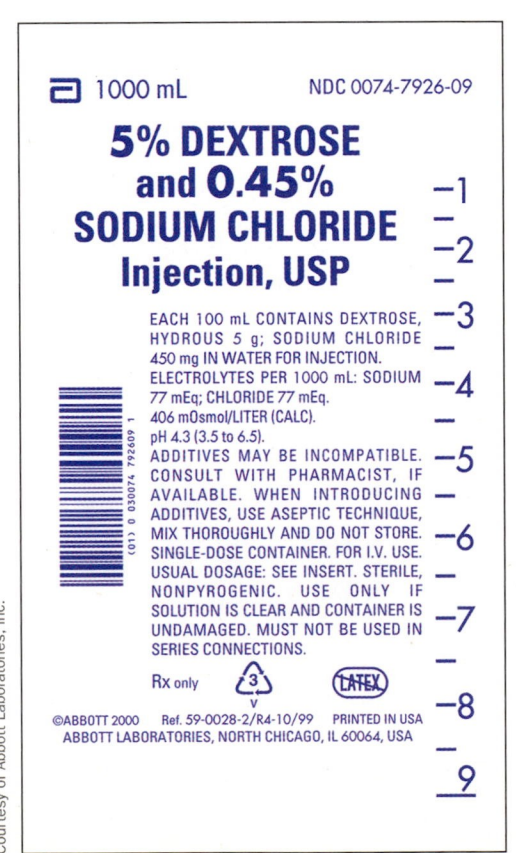

C

Courtesy of Abbott Laboratories, Inc.

1000 mL   NDC 0074-7983-09

0.9% SODIUM CHLORIDE
INJECTION, USP

—1
—2

EACH 100 mL CONTAINS SODIUM CHLORIDE 900 mg IN WATER FOR INJECTION. ELECTROLYTES PER 1000 mL: SODIUM 154 mEq; CHLORIDE 154 mEq.
308 mOsmol/LITER (CALC).
pH 5.6 (4.5 to 7.0)

—3
—4

ADDITIVES MAY BE INCOMPATIBLE. CONSULT WITH PHARMACIST, IF AVAILABLE. WHEN INTRODUCING ADDITIVES, USE ASEPTIC TECHNIQUE, MIX THOROUGHLY AND DO NOT STORE. SINGLE-DOSE CONTAINER. FOR INTRAVENOUS USE. USUAL DOSAGE: SEE INSERT. STERILE, NONPYROGENIC. USE ONLY IF SOLUTION IS CLEAR AND CONTAINER IS UNDAMAGED. MUST NOT BE USED IN SERIES CONNECTIONS.

—5
—6
—7

Rx only

—8

©ABBOTT 2001   Ref. 59-0016-2/R4-7/01   PRINTED IN USA
ABBOTT LABORATORIES, NORTH CHICAGO, IL 60064, USA

9

D

Courtesy of Abbott Laboratories, Inc.

1000 mL   NDC 0074-7926-09

5% DEXTROSE and 0.45% SODIUM CHLORIDE
Injection, USP

—1
—2
—3

EACH 100 mL CONTAINS DEXTROSE, HYDROUS 5 g; SODIUM CHLORIDE 450 mg IN WATER FOR INJECTION. ELECTROLYTES PER 1000 mL: SODIUM 77 mEq; CHLORIDE 77 mEq.
406 mOsmol/LITER (CALC).
pH 4.3 (3.5 to 6.5).

—4

ADDITIVES MAY BE INCOMPATIBLE. CONSULT WITH PHARMACIST, IF AVAILABLE. WHEN INTRODUCING ADDITIVES, USE ASEPTIC TECHNIQUE, MIX THOROUGHLY AND DO NOT STORE. SINGLE-DOSE CONTAINER. FOR I.V. USE. USUAL DOSAGE: SEE INSERT. STERILE, NONPYROGENIC. USE ONLY IF SOLUTION IS CLEAR AND CONTAINER IS UNDAMAGED. MUST NOT BE USED IN SERIES CONNECTIONS.

—5
—6
—7

Rx only

—8

©ABBOTT 2000   Ref. 59-0028-2/R4-10/99   PRINTED IN USA
ABBOTT LABORATORIES, NORTH CHICAGO, IL 60064, USA

9

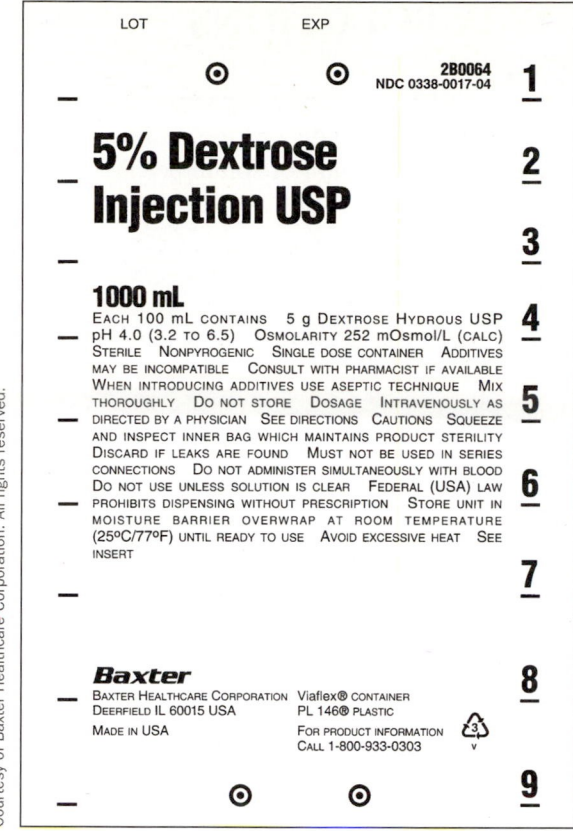

LOT   EXP

NDC 0338-0017-04   **2B0064**   **1**

5% Dextrose Injection USP   **2**

3

1000 mL   **4**

EACH 100 mL CONTAINS   5 g DEXTROSE HYDROUS USP pH 4.0 (3.2 TO 6.5) OSMOLARITY 252 mOsmol/L (CALC) STERILE NONPYROGENIC SINGLE DOSE CONTAINER ADDITIVES MAY BE INCOMPATIBLE CONSULT WITH PHARMACIST IF AVAILABLE WHEN INTRODUCING ADDITIVES USE ASEPTIC TECHNIQUE MIX THOROUGHLY DO NOT STORE DOSAGE INTRAVENOUSLY AS DIRECTED BY A PHYSICIAN SEE DIRECTIONS CAUTIONS SQUEEZE AND INSPECT INNER BAG WHICH MAINTAINS PRODUCT STERILITY DISCARD IF LEAKS ARE FOUND MUST NOT BE USED IN SERIES CONNECTIONS DO NOT ADMINISTER SIMULTANEOUSLY WITH BLOOD DO NOT USE UNLESS SOLUTION IS CLEAR FEDERAL (USA) LAW PROHIBITS DISPENSING WITHOUT PRESCRIPTION STORE UNIT IN MOISTURE BARRIER OVERWRAP AT ROOM TEMPERATURE (25ºC/77ºF) UNTIL READY TO USE AVOID EXCESSIVE HEAT SEE INSERT   **5** **6** **7**

Baxter   **8**
BAXTER HEALTHCARE CORPORATION   VIAFLEX® CONTAINER
DEERFIELD IL 60015 USA   PL 146® PLASTIC
MADE IN USA   FOR PRODUCT INFORMATION
CALL 1-800-933-0303   ♲

9

E

LOT   EXP

NDC 0338-0043-03   **2B1313**   **1**

0.45% Sodium Chloride Injection USP   **2**

500 mL   **3**

EACH 100 mL CONTAINS   450 mg SODIUM CHLORIDE USP pH 5.0 (4.5 TO 7.0) mEq/L SODIUM 77 CHLORIDE 77 HYPOTONIC OSMOLARITY 154 mOsmol/L (CALC) STERILE NONPYROGENIC SINGLE DOSE CONTAINER ADDITIVES MAY BE INCOMPATIBLE CONSULT WITH PHARMACIST IF AVAILABLE WHEN INTRODUCING ADDITIVES USE ASEPTIC TECHNIQUE MIX THOROUGHLY DO NOT STORE DOSAGE INTRAVENOUSLY AS DIRECTED BY A PHYSICIAN SEE DIRECTIONS CAUTIONS SQUEEZE AND INSPECT INNER BAG WHICH MAINTAINS PRODUCT STERILITY DISCARD IF LEAKS ARE FOUND MUST NOT BE USED IN SERIES CONNECTIONS DO NOT USE UNLESS SOLUTION IS CLEAR FEDERAL (USA) LAW PROHIBITS DISPENSING WITHOUT PRESCRIPTION STORE UNIT IN MOISTURE BARRIER OVERWRAP AT ROOM TEMPERATURE (25ºC/77ºF) UNTIL READY TO USE AVOID EXCESSIVE HEAT SEE INSERT   **4**

Baxter
BAXTER HEALTHCARE CORPORATION   VIAFLEX® CONTAINER
DEERFIELD IL 60015 USA   PL 146® PLASTIC
MADE IN USA   FOR PRODUCT INFORMATION
CALL 1-800-933-0303   ♲

F

🄰 1000 mL   NDC 0074-7941-09

5% DEXTROSE and 0.9% SODIUM CHLORIDE Injection, USP

–1
–2
–3

EACH 100 mL CONTAINS DEXTROSE, HYDROUS 5 g; SODIUM CHLORIDE 900 mg IN WATER FOR INJECTION. ELECTROLYTES PER 1000 mL: SODIUM 154 mEq; CHLORIDE 154 mEq. 560 mOsmol/LITER (CALC). pH 4.3 (3.5 to 6.5). ADDITIVES MAY BE INCOMPATIBLE. CONSULT WITH PHARMACIST, IF AVAILABLE. WHEN INTRODUCING ADDITIVES, USE ASEPTIC TECHNIQUE, MIX THOROUGHLY AND DO NOT STORE. SINGLE-DOSE CONTAINER. FOR I.V. USE. USUAL DOSAGE: SEE INSERT. STERILE, NONPYROGENIC. USE ONLY IF SOLUTION IS CLEAR AND CONTAINER IS UNDAMAGED. MUST NOT BE USED IN SERIES CONNECTIONS.   –4 –5 –6 –7

Rx only   ♲   ⬭LATEX⬭   –8

©ABBOTT 2000   Ref. 59-0035-2/R4-10/99   PRINTED IN USA
ABBOTT LABORATORIES, NORTH CHICAGO, IL 60064, USA   –9

(01) 0 030074 794109 4

G

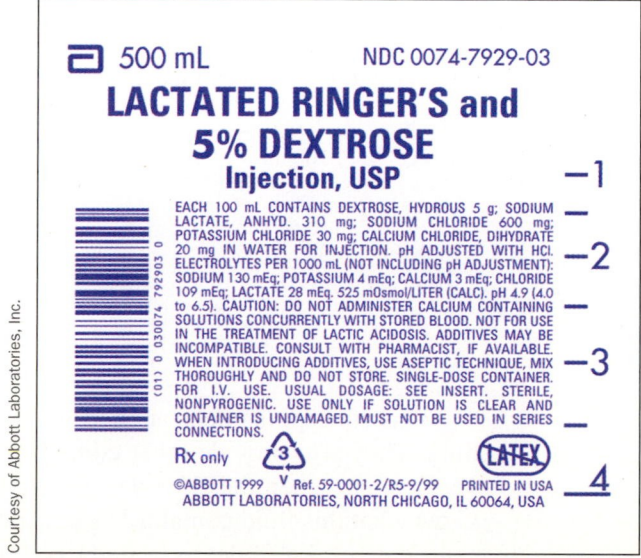

🄰 500 mL   NDC 0074-7929-03

LACTATED RINGER'S and 5% DEXTROSE Injection, USP

–1

EACH 100 mL CONTAINS DEXTROSE, HYDROUS 5 g; SODIUM LACTATE, ANHYD. 310 mg; SODIUM CHLORIDE 600 mg; POTASSIUM CHLORIDE 30 mg; CALCIUM CHLORIDE, DIHYDRATE 20 mg IN WATER FOR INJECTION. pH ADJUSTED WITH HCl. ELECTROLYTES PER 1000 mL (NOT INCLUDING pH ADJUSTMENT): SODIUM 130 mEq; POTASSIUM 4 mEq; CALCIUM 3 mEq; CHLORIDE 109 mEq; LACTATE 28 mEq. 525 mOsmol/LITER (CALC). pH 4.9 (4.0 to 6.5). CAUTION: DO NOT ADMINISTER CALCIUM CONTAINING SOLUTIONS CONCURRENTLY WITH STORED BLOOD. NOT FOR USE IN THE TREATMENT OF LACTIC ACIDOSIS. ADDITIVES MAY BE INCOMPATIBLE. CONSULT WITH PHARMACIST, IF AVAILABLE. WHEN INTRODUCING ADDITIVES, USE ASEPTIC TECHNIQUE, MIX THOROUGHLY AND DO NOT STORE. SINGLE-DOSE CONTAINER. FOR I.V. USE. USUAL DOSAGE: SEE INSERT. STERILE, NONPYROGENIC. USE ONLY IF SOLUTION IS CLEAR AND CONTAINER IS UNDAMAGED. MUST NOT BE USED IN SERIES CONNECTIONS.   –2 –3

Rx only   ♲   ⬭LATEX⬭

©ABBOTT 1999   Ref. 59-0001-2/R5-9/99   PRINTED IN USA
ABBOTT LABORATORIES, NORTH CHICAGO, IL 60064, USA   –4

(01) 0 030074 792903 0

H

CALCULATING COMPONENTS OF IV SOLUTIONS WHEN EXPRESSED AS A PERCENT

Recall from Chapter 8 that solution strength expressed as a percent (%) indicates the number of g per 100 mL. Understanding this concept allows you to calculate the total amount of solute per IV order.

EXAMPLE 1 ▪

Order: D_5W 1,000 mL IV q.8h

Calculate the amount of dextrose in 1,000 mL D_5W.

This can be calculated using ratio-proportion.

Recall that % indicates g per 100 mL; therefore, D_5 5% dextrose or 5 g dextrose per 100 mL of solution.

$$\frac{5 \text{ g}}{100 \text{ mL}} \diagup\!\!\!\!\diagdown \frac{X \text{ g}}{1,000 \text{ mL}}$$

$$100X = 5,000$$
$$\frac{100X}{100} = \frac{5,000}{100}$$
$$X = 50 \text{ g}$$

1,000 mL of D_5W contains 50 g of dextrose.

EXAMPLE 2 ▪

Order: $D_5\frac{1}{4}NS$ 500 mL IV q.6h

Calculate the amount of dextrose and sodium chloride in 500 mL.

D_5 = Dextrose 5% = 5 g dextrose per 100 mL

$$\frac{5 \text{ g}}{100 \text{ mL}} \diagup\!\!\!\!\diagdown \frac{X \text{ g}}{500 \text{ mL}}$$

$$100X = 2,500$$
$$\frac{100X}{100} = \frac{2,500}{100}$$
$$X = 25 \text{ g (dextrose)}$$

$\frac{1}{4}NS$ = 0.225% NaCl = 0.225 g NaCl per 100 mL

(Recall that NS or normal saline is 0.9% NaCl; therefore, $\frac{1}{4}$ NS is $\frac{1}{4} \times 0.9\% = 0.225\%$ NaCl.)

$$\frac{0.225 \text{ g}}{100 \text{ mL}} \diagup\!\!\!\!\diagdown \frac{X \text{ g}}{500 \text{ mL}}$$

$$100X = 112.5$$
$$\frac{100X}{100} = \frac{112.5}{100}$$
$$X = 1.125 \text{ g (NaCl)}$$

500 mL $D_5\frac{1}{4}$ NS contains 25 g dextrose and 1.125 g sodium chloride.

This concept is important because it helps you understand that IV solutions provide much more than fluid. They also provide other components. For example, now you know what you are administering to your patient when the IV order prescribes D_5W. Think, "I am hanging D_5W intravenous solution. Do I know what this fluid contains? Yes, it contains dextrose as the solute and water as the solvent in the concentration of 5 g of dextrose in every 100 mL of solution." Regular monitoring and careful understanding of intravenous infusions cannot be stressed enough.

Review Set 33

Calculate the amount of dextrose and/or sodium chloride in each of the following IV solutions.

1. 1,000 mL of D_5NS

   dextrose _____ g

   sodium chloride _____ g

2. 500 mL of $D_5 \frac{1}{2}NS$

   dextrose _____ g

   sodium chloride _____ g

3. 250 mL of $D_{10}W$

   dextrose _____ g

4. 750 mL of NS

   sodium chloride _____ g

5. 500 mL of D_5 0.225% NaCl

   dextrose _____ g

   sodium chloride _____ g

6. 3 L of D_5NS

   dextrose _____ g

   sodium chloride _____ g

7. 0.5 L of $D_{10} \frac{1}{4}NS$

   dextrose _____ g

   sodium chloride _____ g

8. 300 mL of D_{12} 0.9% NaCl

   dextrose _____ g

   sodium chloride _____ g

9. 2 L of D_5 0.225% NaCl

   dextrose _____ g

   sodium chloride _____ g

10. 0.75 L of 0.45% NaCl

   sodium chloride _____ g

After completing these problems, see page 557 to check your answers.

IV SITES

IV fluids may be ordered via a *peripheral line,* such as a vein in the arm, leg, or sometimes a scalp vein for infants, if other sites are inaccessible. Blood flowing through these veins can usually dilute the components in IV fluids. Glucose or dextrose is usually concentrated between 5% and 10% for short-term IV therapy. Peripheral veins can accommodate a maximum glucose concentration of 12%. The rate of infusion in peripheral veins should not exceed 200 mL in 1 hour.

IV fluids that are transparent flow smoothly into relatively small peripheral veins. When blood transfusion or replacement is needed, a larger vein is preferred to facilitate ease of blood flow. Whole blood or its components, especially packed cells, can be viscous and must be infused within a short period of time.

IV fluids may also be ordered via a *central line,* in which a special catheter is inserted to access a large vein, for example, in the chest. The subclavian vein, for example, may be used for a central line. Central lines may be accessed either directly through the chest wall or indirectly via a neck vein or peripheral vein in the arm. If a peripheral vein is used to access a central vein, you may see the term *peripherally inserted central catheter* or *PICC line.* Larger veins can accommodate higher concentrations of glucose (up to 35%) and other nutrients and faster rates of IV fluids (greater than 200 mL in 1 hour). They are often utilized if the patient is expected to need IV therapy for an extended period.

MONITORING IVs

The nurse is responsible for monitoring the patient regularly during an IV infusion.

CAUTION

Generally the IV site and infusion should be checked at least every 30 minutes to 1 hour (according to hospital policy) for volume of remaining fluids, correct infusion rate, and signs of complications.

The major complications associated with IV therapy are phlebitis, infiltration, and infection at the IV site. *Phlebitis* occurs when the vein becomes irritated, red, or painful. (THINK: *warm and cordlike vein.*) *Infiltration* is when the IV catheter becomes dislodged from the vein and IV fluid escapes into the sub-cutaneous tissue. (THINK: *cool and puffy skin.*) Should phlebitis or infiltration occur, the IV is discontinued and another IV site is chosen to restart the IV. The patient should be instructed to notify the nurse of any pain or swelling.

PRIMARY AND SECONDARY IVs

Primary IV tubing packaging and set are shown in Figures 15-6 and 15-7(a). This IV set is used for a typical or *primary IV*. Primary IV tubing includes a drip chamber, one or more injection ports, and a roller clamp and is long enough to be attached to the hub of the IV catheter positioned in the patient's vein. The drip chamber is squeezed until it is half full of IV fluid, and IV fluid is run through the tubing prior to attaching it to the IV catheter to ensure that no air is in the tubing. The nurse can either regulate the rate manually using the roller clamp (Figure 15-7(a)) or place the tubing in an electronic infusion pump (Figures 15-13 through 15-15).

Secondary IV tubing is used when giving medications. Secondary tubing is "piggybacked" into the primary line (Figure 15-8). This type of tubing generally is shorter and also contains a drip chamber and roller clamp. This gives access to the primary IV catheter without having to start another IV. You will notice that in this type of setup, the *secondary IV* set or *piggyback* is hung higher than the primary IV to allow the secondary set of medication to infuse first. When administering primary IV fluids, choose primary IV tubing; when hanging piggybacks, select secondary IV tubing. IV piggybacks are discussed further at the end of this chapter.

FIGURE 15-6 Primary intravenous infusion set package label

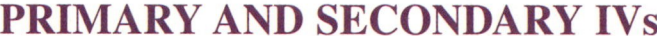

Courtesy of Abbott Laboratories, Inc.

CLEARLINK System   **2C8541s**

CONTINU-FLO Solution Set
with DUO-VENT Spike
105" (2.7 m)
3 Luer Activated Valves
Male Luer Lock Adapter

10
10 drops/mL
Approx.

FIGURE 15-7(a) Standard straight gravity flow IV system

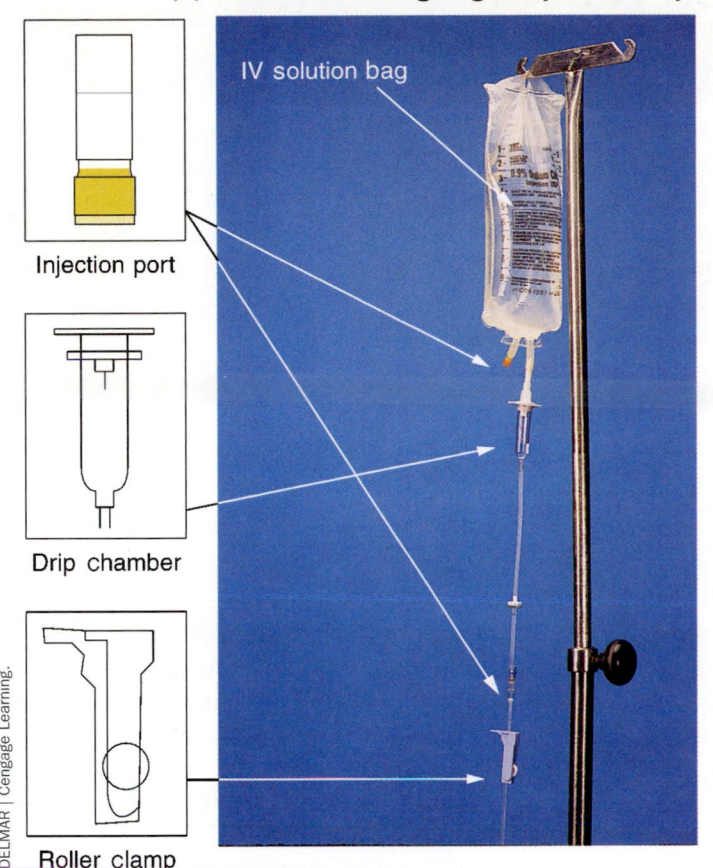

Injection port

Drip chamber

Roller clamp

DELMAR | Cengage Learning.

FIGURE 15-7(b) 1 liter IV solution bag: The numerals 1-9 indicate 100 mL each: 1 = 100 mL, 2 = 200 mL . . . 9 = 900 mL for a total IV solution volume of 1,000 mL.

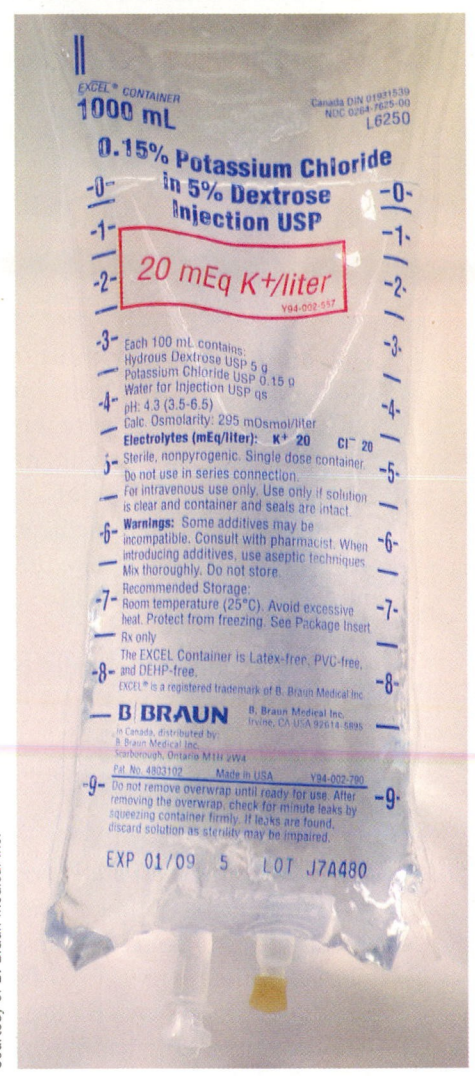

Courtesy of B. Braun Medical Inc.

FIGURE 15-8 IV with piggyback (IV PB)

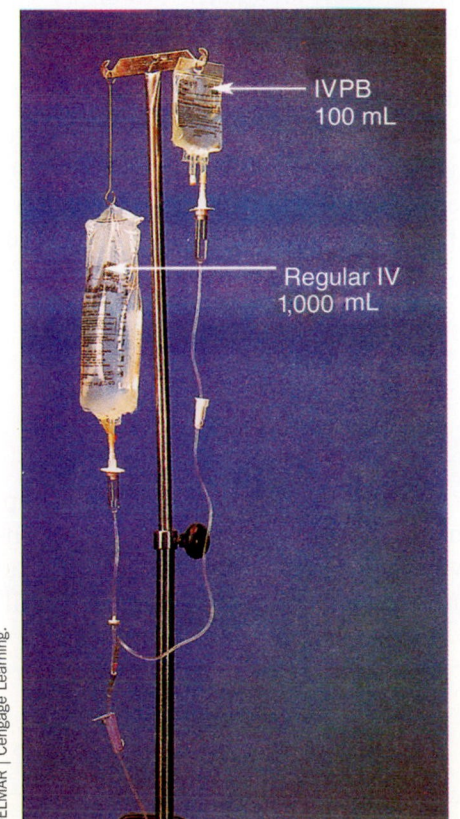

DELMAR | Cengage Learning.

BLOOD ADMINISTRATION TUBING

When blood is administered, a standard blood set (Figure 15-9) or a Y-type blood set (Figure 15-10) is commonly used. The "Y" refers to the two spikes that are attached above the drip chamber. One spike is attached to the blood container, and the other spike is attached to normal saline. Normal saline is used to dilute packed cells and to flush the IV tubing at the beginning and at the end of the transfusion. Blood is usually infused manually by gravity, and the roller clamp on the line is used to adjust the rate. Some electronic pumps may also be used for infusion of blood. In such cases, the nurse would program the pump in mL/h and then the pump would regulate the blood infusion. Blood infusion is calculated the same as any other IV fluid.

IV FLOW RATE

The *flow rate* of an IV infusion is ordered by the physician. It is usually prescribed in mL/h and measured in mL/h or gtt/min. Later sections of this chapter will describe these calculations. It is the nurse's responsibility to regulate, monitor, and maintain this flow rate. Regulation of intravenous therapy is a critical skill in nursing. Because the fluids administered are infusing directly into the patient's circulatory system, careful monitoring is essential to be sure the patient does not receive too much or too little IV fluid and medication. It is also important for the nurse to accurately set and maintain the flow rate to administer the prescribed volume of the IV solution within the specified time period. The nurse records the IV fluids administered and IV flow rates on the IV administration record (IVAR) (Figure 15-11).

IV solutions are usually ordered for a certain volume to run for a stated period of time, such as *125 mL/h* or *1,000 mL per 8 h*. The nurse will use electronic or manual regulating equipment to monitor the flow rate. The calculations you must perform to set the flow rate will depend on the equipment used to administer the IV solutions.

Nurses often label IV bags with a tape marking the infusion times (Figure 15-12), which provides a quick visual check if the IV is infusing on time as prescribed. These labels are attached to the IV bag and indicate the start and stop times of the infusion, as well as how the IV should be progressing. Each hour, from the start time to the stop time, the nurse should mark the label at the level where the solution should be. As a convenience, stock IV bags may be supplied with custom labels with pre-marked time intervals (Figure 15-12(a)). The hourly intervals are marked for liter bags infusing over 6, 8, 10, and 12 hours. Nurses may also use plain tape and mark the hourly time intervals manually (Figure 15-12(b)). The example in Figure 15-12 demonstrates an infusion tape adhered to a liter IV bag (1,000 mL) with a flow rate to be set at 25 gtt/min. The nurse intends to infuse the 1 L in 10 hours at 100 mL/h. Each hour is marked on the tape beginning at 0700 (7:00 AM) when the IV started and 1700 (5:00 PM) when the IV should be complete.

ELECTRONICALLY REGULATED IVs

Frequently, IV solutions are regulated electronically by an infusion device, such as a controller or pump. The use of an electronic infusion device will be determined by the need to strictly regulate the IV. Manufacturers supply special volumetric tubing that must be used with their infusion devices. This special tubing ensures accurate, consistent IV infusions. Each device can be set for a specific flow rate and will set off an alarm if this rate is interrupted. Electronic units today are powered by direct current (from a wall outlet) as well as an internal rechargeable battery. The battery takes over when the unit is unplugged to allow for portability and patient ambulation.

FIGURE 15-9 Standard blood set

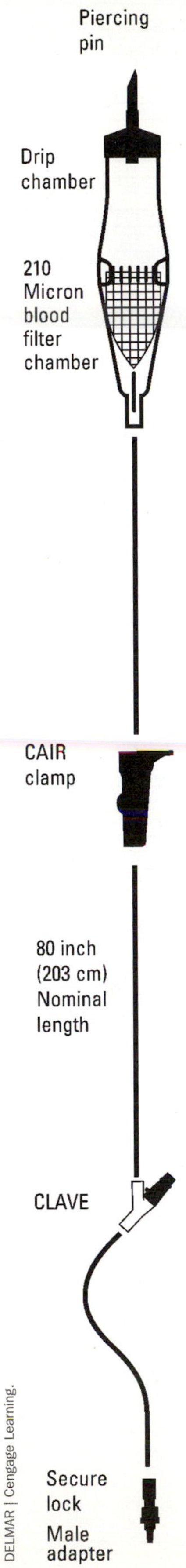

Piercing pin

Drip chamber

210 Micron blood filter chamber

CAIR clamp

80 inch (203 cm) Nominal length

CLAVE

Secure lock

Male adapter

DELMAR | Cengage Learning.

FIGURE 15-10 Y-type blood set

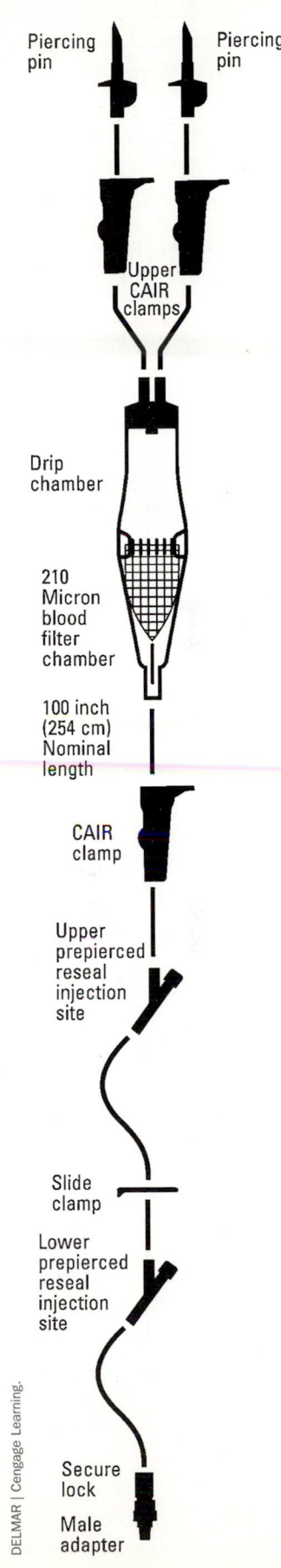

Piercing pin   Piercing pin

Upper CAIR clamps

Drip chamber

210 Micron blood filter chamber

100 inch (254 cm) Nominal length

CAIR clamp

Upper prepierced reseal injection site

Slide clamp

Lower prepierced reseal injection site

Secure lock

Male adapter

DELMAR | Cengage Learning.

FIGURE 15-11 Intravenous Administration Record

Page: 1 of 1		DATE: 11/10/xx through					
Correct	I.V. Order	Rate	Time	Initial	Site / Infusion Port	Pump / Other	Tubing Change
✓	$D_5 \frac{1}{2}$ NS	100 mL/hr	0900	GP	LH / PIV	☑	✓

CIRCULATORY ACCESS SITE

Time	Gauge	Length	Type	Site	# Attempts	Dressing Change	Site Condition	IV Lock	Initial	Time Catheter D/C Intact	Site Condition	Reason Code	Initial
0800	22	1 1/4	I	LH	1	✓	0	☐	GP				
								☐					
								☐					
								☐					

Type:	Site:		Reason Code:	Infusion Port:	Site Condition:
I - Insyte	L - Left	A - Antecubital	1 - Infiltrate	PIV - Peripheral IV	0
B - Butterfly	R - Right	F - Femoral	2 - Physician Order	CVC - CVC	1+
C - Cathlon	H - Hand	J - Jugular	3 - Patient Removed	SG - Swan Ganz	2+
CVC - CVC	FA - Forearm	FT - Foot	4 - Clotted	D - Distal	3+
T - Tunnelled	UA - Upper Arm	S - Scalp	5 - Phlebitis	M - Middle	4+
IP - Implanted Port	SC - Subclavian	U - Umbilical	6 - Site Rotation	P - Proximal	5+
PICC - PICC	C - Chest	RA - Radial	7 - Leaking	R - Red	
A - Arterial Line	**Dressing Change:**		8 - Positional	BL - Blue	**Tubing Change:**
SG - Swan Ganz	T - Transparent		9 - Not Patent	V - Venous	P - Primary
DL - Dual Lumen Peripheral	A - Air Occlusive		10 - Family Refused	S - Sideport	S - Secondary
UAC - UAC	B - Bandaid		**Other:**	AN - Access Needle	E - Extension
UVC - UVC	PR - Pressure Dressing		D - Dial-a-flow	A - Arterial	T - 3 Way Stopcock
					H - Hemodynamic

ALLERGIES: NKA

Initial / Signature - Circulatory Access Site(s) checked hourly.

GP / G. Pickar, R.N. ___ / ___
___ / ___ ___ / ___
___ / ___ ___ / ___
Reconciled by: ___

Smith, James   43y   M

Dr. Jones   Medical Service

Admitted   01-01-xx   Rm 237-1

Adm. # 6634297

IV ADMINISTRATION RECORD

FIGURE 15-12(a) Section of 1 liter (1,000 mL) IV bag labeled with pre-marked custom tape

FIGURE 15-12(b) Section of 1 liter (1,000 mL) IV bag labeled with plain tape

Follow the marking in the white column to infuse 1 liter in 10 h

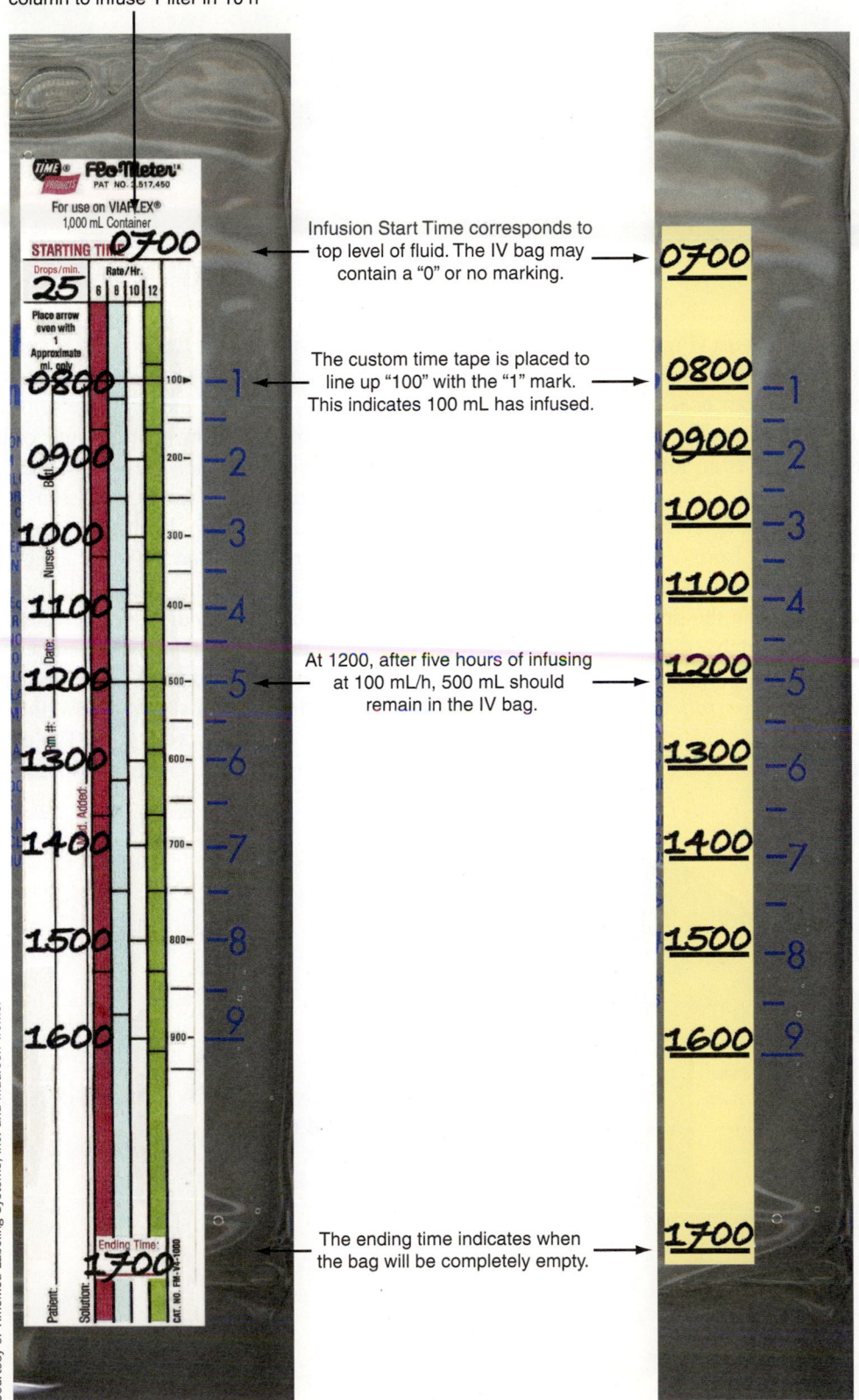

Infusion Start Time corresponds to top level of fluid. The IV bag may contain a "0" or no marking.

The custom time tape is placed to line up "100" with the "1" mark. This indicates 100 mL has infused.

At 1200, after five hours of infusing at 100 mL/h, 500 mL should remain in the IV bag.

The ending time indicates when the bag will be completely empty.

FIGURE 15-13   Alaris PC System

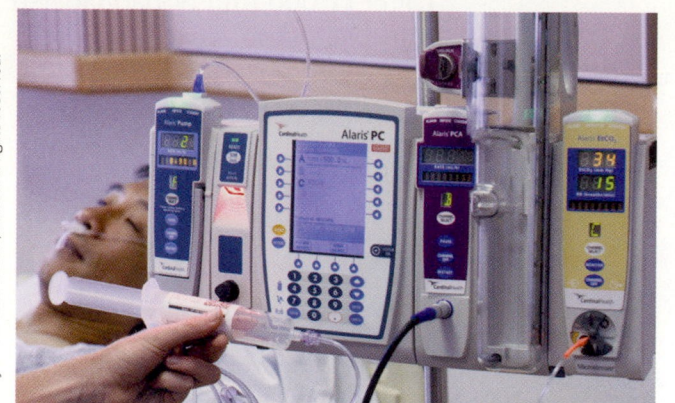

FIGURE 15-14   Syringe pump

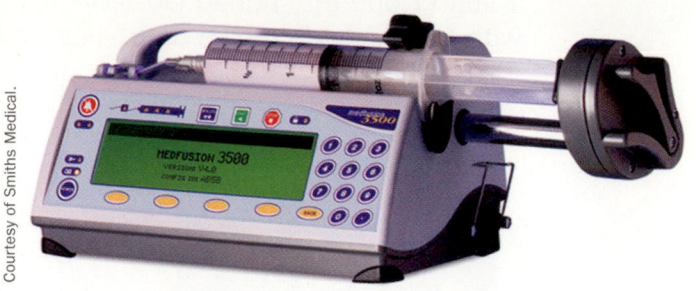

Infusion pumps (Figure 15-13) do not rely on gravity but maintain the flow by displacing fluid at the prescribed rate. Resistance to flow within the system causes positive pressure in relation to the flow rate. The nurse or other user may preset a pressure alarm threshold. When the pressure sensed by the device reaches this threshold, the device stops pumping and sets off an alarm. The amount of change in pressure that results from infiltration or phlebitis may be insufficient to reach the alarm threshold. Therefore, users should not expect the device to stop infusing in the presence of these conditions.

A *syringe pump* (Figure 15-14) is a type of electronic infusion pump. It is used to infuse fluids or medications directly from a syringe. It is most often used in the neonatal and pediatric areas when small volumes of medication are delivered at low rates. It is also used in anesthesia, hospice, labor and delivery, and critical care when the drug cannot be mixed with other solutions or medications or to reduce the volume of diluent fluid delivered to the patient. Syringe pumps can deliver in up to 16 different modes, including mL/h, volume/time, dose or body weight modes, mass modes such as units/h, and other specialty modes.

A *patient-controlled analgesia (PCA) pump* (Figure 15-15) is used to allow the patient to self-administer IV medication to control postoperative and other types of severe pain. The physician or other prescribing practitioner orders the pain medication, which is contained in a prefilled syringe locked

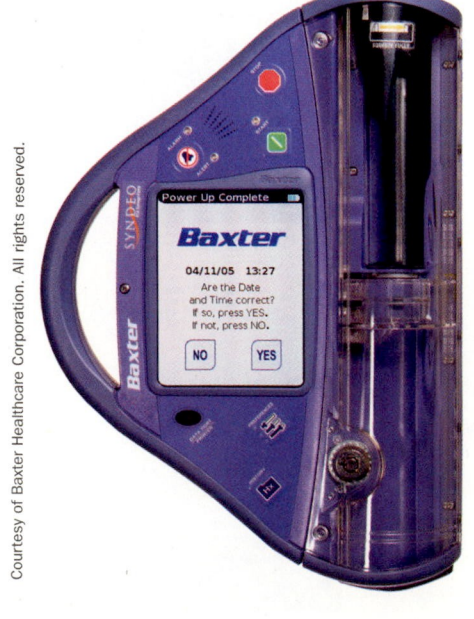

FIGURE 15-15   Syndeo PCA (patient-controlled analgesia) syringe pump

securely in the IV pump. The patient presses the control button and receives the pain medication immediately rather than waiting for someone to bring it. The dose, frequency, and a safety "lock out" time are ordered and programmed into the pump, which delivers an individual therapeutic dose. The pump stores information about the frequency and dosage of the drug requested by and delivered to the patient. The nurse can display this information to document and evaluate pain management effectiveness.

CAUTION

All electronic infusion devices must be monitored frequently (at least every 30 minutes to 1 hour) to ensure proper and safe functioning. Check the policy in your facility.

CALCULATING FLOW RATES FOR ELECTRONIC REGULATORS IN mL/h

When an electronic infusion regulator is used, the IV volume is ordered by the physician and programmed into the device by the nurse. These devices are regulated in mL/h. Usually the physician orders the IV volume to be delivered in mL/h. If not, the nurse must calculate it.

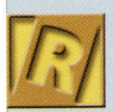

RULE

To regulate an IV volume by electronic infusion pump calibrated in mL/h, calculate:

$$\frac{\text{Total mL ordered}}{\text{Total h ordered}} = \text{mL/h (rounded to a whole number)}$$

or use ratio-proportion: $\dfrac{\text{Total mL}}{\text{Total h}} = \dfrac{\text{X mL}}{1\text{ h}}$

EXAMPLE ■

Order reads: D₅W 250 mL IV over the next 2 h by infusion pump

Step 1 **Think** The pump is set by the rate of mL per hour. So, if 250 mL is to be infused in 2 hours, how much will be infused in 1 hour? Yes, 125 mL will be infused in 1 hour. You would set the pump at 125 mL per hour.

Step 2 **Calculate** Use the formula:

$$\frac{\text{Total mL ordered}}{\text{Total h ordered}} = \text{mL/h}$$

$$\frac{\overset{125}{\cancel{250}}\text{ mL}}{\underset{1}{\cancel{2}}\text{ h}} = \frac{125\text{ mL}}{1\text{ h}} = 125\text{ mL/h}$$

Therefore, set the pump at 125 mL per hour (125 mL/h).

This can also be solved using a ratio-proportion. In fact, the formula *is* a ratio-proportion. Let's look at this more closely.

The ratio-proportion to calculate mL/h looks almost the same as the formula.

$$\frac{\text{Total mL}}{\text{Total h}} = \frac{\text{X mL}}{1\text{ h}}$$

$$\frac{250\text{ mL}}{2\text{ h}} \diagup\!\!\!\!\diagdown \frac{\text{X mL}}{1\text{ h}}$$

$$2\text{X} = 250$$

$$\frac{2\text{X}}{250} = \frac{250}{250}$$

$$\text{X} = 125\text{ mL (per 1 hour)}$$

But, the formula to divide *total mL* by *total h* is quite simple. You can use either formula or ratio-proportion.

In most cases it is easy to calculate mL/h by dividing total mL by total h. However, an IV with medication added or an IV PB may be ordered to be administered in *less than 1 hour* by an electronic infusion device, but the pump must still be set in mL/h.

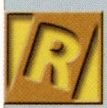

RULE

$$\frac{\text{Total mL ordered}}{\text{Total min ordered}} = \frac{\text{X mL/h}}{60 \text{ min/h}}$$

X = mL/h (rounded to a whole number)

EXAMPLE ■

Order: Ampicillin 500 mg IV in 50 mL D$_5$ $\frac{1}{2}$NS in 30 min by infusion pump

Step 1   Think   The pump is set by the rate of mL per hour. If 50 mL is to be infused in 30 minutes, then 100 mL will be infused in 60 minutes because 100 mL is twice as much as 50 mL and 60 minutes is twice as much as 30 minutes. Set the rate of the controller at 100 mL/h to infuse 50 mL per 30 min.

Step 2   Calculate

$$\frac{\text{Total mL ordered}}{\text{Total min ordered}} = \frac{\text{X mL/h}}{60 \text{ min/h}}$$

$$\frac{50 \text{ mL}}{30 \text{ min}} \times \frac{\text{X mL/h}}{60 \text{ min/h}}$$

$$30X = 3{,}000$$
$$\frac{30X}{30} = \frac{3{,}000}{30}$$
$$X = 100 \text{ mL/h}$$

CAUTION

Typical values of mL/h to expect for IV flow rate calculations are in the range of 50 to 200 mL/h. Use this guideline as part of checking for reasonable answers.

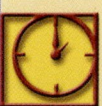

QUICK REVIEW

For electronic infusion regulators:

- $\dfrac{\text{Total mL ordered}}{\text{Total h ordered}}$ = mL/h

- If the infusion time is less than 1 hour, then

  $$\frac{\text{Total mL ordered}}{\text{Total min ordered}} = \frac{\text{X mL/h}}{60 \text{ min/h}}$$

- Round mL/h to a whole number.

Review Set 34

Calculate the flow rate at which you will program the electronic infusion regulator for the following IV orders.

1. D_5W 1 L IV to infuse in 10 h

   Flow rate: _____ mL/h

2. NS 1,800 mL IV to infuse in 15 h

   Flow rate: _____ mL/h

3. D_5W 2,000 mL IV in 24 h

   Flow rate: _____ mL/h

4. NS 100 mL IV PB in 30 min

   Flow rate: _____ mL/h

5. Antibiotic in 30 mL D_5W IV in 15 min

   Flow rate: _____ mL/h

6. NS 2.5 L IV in 20 h

   Flow rate: _____ mL/h

7. D_5LR 500 mL IV in 4 h

   Flow rate: _____ mL/h

8. 0.45% NaCl 600 mL IV in 3 h

   Flow rate: _____ mL/h

9. Antibiotic in 150 mL D_5W IV in 2 h

   Flow rate: _____ mL/h

10. NS 3 L IV in 24 h

    Flow rate: _____ mL/h

11. LR Injection 1.5 L IV in 24 h

    Flow rate: _____ mL/h

12. $D_{10}W$ 240 mL IV in 10 h

    Flow rate: _____ mL/h

13. D_5W 750 mL IV in 5 h

    Flow rate: _____ mL/h

14. D_5NS 1.5 L IV in 12 h

    Flow rate: _____ mL/h

15. D_5 0.45% NaCl 380 mL IV in 9 h

    Flow rate: _____ mL/h

After completing these problems, see page 557 to check your answers.

MANUALLY REGULATED IVs

When an electronic infusion device is not used, the nurse manually regulates the IV rate. To do this, the nurse must calculate the ordered IV rate based on a certain *number of drops per minute (gtt/min)*. This actually represents the ordered milliliters per hour, as you will shortly see in the calculation.

The number of drops dripping per minute into the IV drip chamber (Figures 15-7(a) and 15-16) are counted and regulated by opening or closing the roller clamp. You actually place your digital or analog watch with a second hand at the level of the drip chamber and count the drops as they fall during a 1-minute period or fraction thereof (referred to as the *watch count*). This manual, gravity flow rate depends on the IV tubing calibration called the *drop factor*.

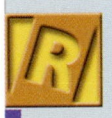

RULE

Drop factor = gtt/mL

The drop factor is the number of drops per milliliter (gtt/mL) a particular IV tubing set will deliver. It is determined by the size of the tubing or needle releasing the drops into the drip chamber (Figure 15-16). The drop factor is stated on the IV tubing package and varies according to the manufacturer of the IV equipment. For example, the tubing depicted in Figure 15-6 delivers 10 gtt/mL. The wider tubing delivers larger drops (macrodrops), therefore there are fewer drops in 1 mL (Figure 15-16(a)). The small needle

FIGURE 15-16   Intravenous drip chambers; comparison of (a) macrodrops and (b) microdrops

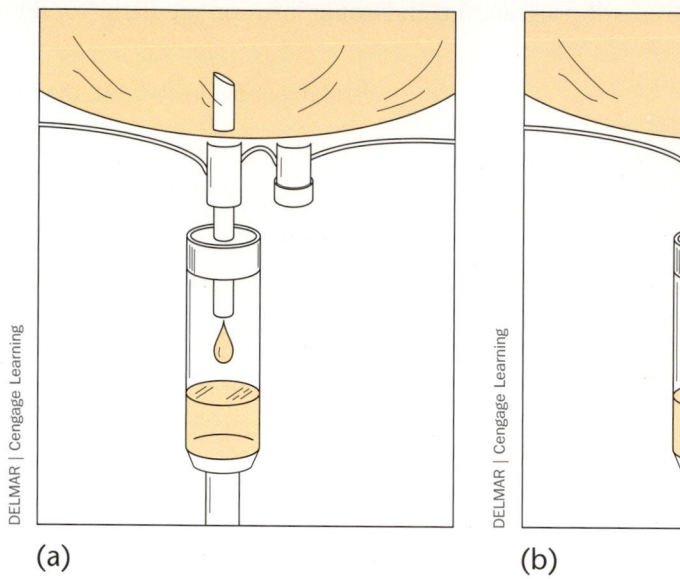

(a)   (b)

FIGURE 15-17   Comparison of calibrated drop factors

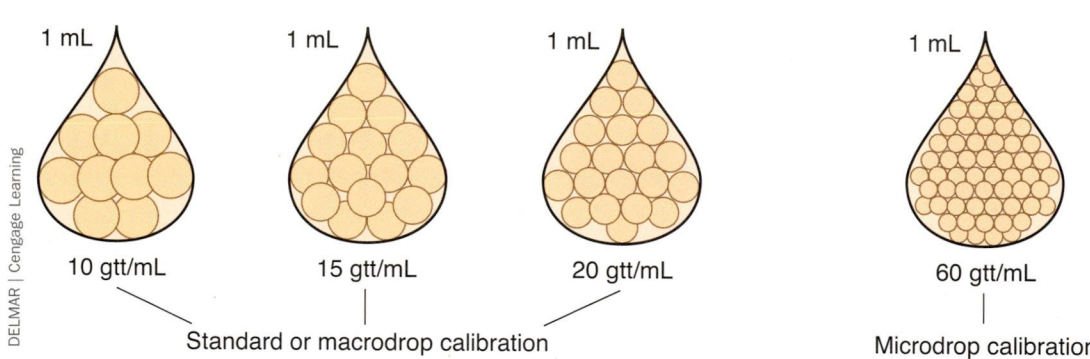

1 mL   1 mL   1 mL   1 mL

10 gtt/mL   15 gtt/mL   20 gtt/mL   60 gtt/mL

Standard or macrodrop calibration   Microdrop calibration

delivers very small drops therefore there are many drops in 1 mL (Figure 15-16(b)). The standard macrodrop IV tubing is available in various sizes that deliver 10, 15, or 20 drops per mL (gtt/mL). The microdrip tubing delivers 60 gtt/mL. Hospitals typically stock one macrodrop tubing for routine adult IV administration and the microdrip tubing for situations requiring more exact measurement or to manage a very slow infusion rate.

Figure 15-16 compares macrodrops and microdrops. Figure 15-17 illustrates the size and number of drops in 1 mL for each drop factor. Notice that the fewer the number of drops per milliliter, the larger the actual drop size.

QUICK REVIEW

- Drop factor = gtt/mL
- The drop factor is stated on the IV tubing package.
- Macrodrop factors: 10, 15, or 20 gtt/mL
- Microdrop factor: 60 gtt/mL

Review Set 35

Identify the drop factor calibration of the IV tubing pictured.

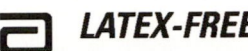 **LATEX-FREE**

No. 4967

PRIMARY I.V. SET,
Convertible Pin, 80 Inch
with Backcheck Valve
and 2 Injection Sites
Piggyback

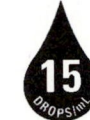

1. _____ gtt/mL

LifeShield® **LATEX-FREE**   No. 11409

HEMA® II Y-TYPE BLOOD SET,
Nonvented, 100 Inch
with 2 Prepierced Injection Sites
and Secure Lock

2. _____ gtt/mL

CLEARLINK System
2C8546s

Continu-Flo Solution Set
60

60 drops/mL
Approx.

106" (2.7 m)
3 Luer Activated Valves
Male Luer Lock Adapter

3. _____ gtt/mL

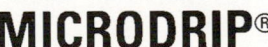   No. 1883

PRIMARY I.V. SET,
Vented, 70 Inch
with Y-Injection Site
MICRODRIP®

4. _____ gtt/mL

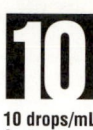

CLEARLINK System   **2C8541s**

CONTINU-FLO Solution Set with DUO-VENT Spike
105" (2.7 m)
3 Luer Activated Valves
Male Luer Lock Adapter

10
10 drops/mL
Approx.

5. _____ gtt/mL

After completing these problems, see page 557 to check your answers.

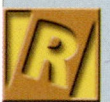

CALCULATING FLOW RATES FOR MANUALLY REGULATED IVs IN gtt/min

In this section you will learn two methods to calculate IV flow rate for manually regulated IVs: the formula method and the shortcut method.

Formula Method

The formula method can be used to determine the flow rate in drops per minute (gtt/min).

> **RULE**
>
> The formula method to calculate IV flow rate for manually regulated IVs ordered in mL/h or for a prescribed number of minutes is:
>
> $$\frac{V}{T} \times C = R$$
>
> $$\frac{\text{Volume (mL)}}{\text{Time (min)}} \times \text{Calibration or drop factor (gtt/mL)} = \text{Rate (gtt/min)}$$

In this formula:

V: *volume to be infused* designated in mL; ordered by the prescriber (primary infusion) or recommended by pharmacist or drug reference guide (such as for an IV PB medication)

T: *time required to infuse V,* converted to minutes; ordered by the prescriber (primary infusion) or recommended by pharmacist or drug reference guide (such as for an IV PB medication)

C: *calibration of tubing* (drop factor) in gtt/mL; noted on package

R: *rate of flow* in gtt/min. THINK: The unknown is the watch count

The rate of IV fluid and IV medications is expressed as a specific volume to be infused in a certain time period. Most IV fluid orders are written as X mL/h, which means X mL in 60 minutes. However, some IV medications are to be administered in less than 1 hour—for example, over 30 minutes.

> **MATH TIP**
>
> Carry calculations to one decimal place. Round gtt/min to the nearest whole number because you can watch-count only whole drops.

Let's look at some examples of how to calculate the flow rate or watch count in gtt/min.

EXAMPLE 1 ■

The physician orders D_5W IV at 125 mL/h. The infusion set is calibrated for a drop factor of 10 gtt/mL. Calculate the IV flow rate in gtt/min. Notice that the mL cancel out, leaving gtt/min.

$$\frac{V}{T} \times C = \frac{125 \text{ mL}}{60 \text{ min}} \times 10 \text{ gtt/mL} = \frac{125 \cancel{\text{mL}}}{\underset{6}{\cancel{60} \text{ min}}} \times \frac{\overset{1}{\cancel{10} \text{ gtt}}}{1 \cancel{\text{mL}}} = \frac{125 \text{ gtt}}{6 \text{ min}} = 20.8 \text{ gtt/min} = 21 \text{ gtt/min}$$

Use your watch to count the drops and adjust the roller clamp to deliver 21 gtt/min.

EXAMPLE 2 ■

Order: **Lactated Ringer's IV at 150 mL/h.** The drop factor is 15 gtt/mL.

$$\frac{V}{T} \times C = \frac{150 \cancel{\text{mL}}}{\underset{4}{\cancel{60} \text{ min}}} \times \overset{1}{\cancel{15}} \text{ gtt/}\cancel{\text{mL}} = \frac{150 \text{ gtt}}{4 \text{ min}} = 37.5 \text{ gtt/min} = 38 \text{ gtt/min}$$

EXAMPLE 3 ■

Order: **Ampicillin 500 mg IV in 100 mL of NS, infuse over 45 min**

The drop factor is 20 gtt/mL. Notice that the time is less than 1 hour. Also notice that the 500 mg does not figure into the calculations because it is the dosage of ampicillin dissolved in the IV fluid. Only the *total volume of 100 mL* is needed to complete the calculations.

$$\frac{V}{T} \times C = \frac{100 \cancel{\text{mL}}}{45 \text{ min}} \times 20 \text{ gtt/}\cancel{\text{mL}} = \frac{2,000 \text{ gtt}}{45 \text{ min}} = 44.4 \text{ gtt/min} = 44 \text{ gtt/min}$$

MATH TIP

When the IV drop factor is 60 gtt/mL (microdrip sets), then the flow rate in gtt/min is the same as the volume ordered in mL/h.

EXAMPLE 4 ■

Order: **D_5W NS IV at 50 mL/h.** The drop factor is 60 gtt/mL.

$$\frac{V}{T} \times C = \frac{50 \cancel{\text{mL}}}{\cancel{60} \text{ min}} \times \cancel{60} \text{ gtt/}\cancel{\text{mL}} = 50 \text{ gtt/min}$$

Notice that the order of 50 mL/h is the *same* as the flow rate of 50 gtt/min when the drop factor is 60 gtt/mL. This will always be the rule when the drop factor is 60 gtt/mL.

Sometimes the prescriber will order a total IV volume to be infused over a total number of hours. In such cases, first calculate the mL/h (rounded to tenths), then calculate gtt/min (rounded to a whole number).

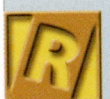

RULE

The formula method to calculate IV flow rate for manually regulated IVs ordered in total volume and total hours is:

Step 1 $\dfrac{\text{Total mL}}{\text{Total hours}}$ = mL/h (round result to tenths)

Step 2 $\dfrac{V}{T} \times C = R$ (round result to a whole number)

EXAMPLE ■

Order: NS IV 3,000 mL per 24 h. Drop factor is 15 gtt/min.

Step 1   **Convert** $\dfrac{\text{Total mL}}{\text{Total h}} = \dfrac{3,000 \text{ mL}}{24 \text{ h}} = 125 \text{ mL/h}$

Step 2   **Think** $\dfrac{V}{T} \times C = R: \dfrac{125 \text{ mL}}{60 \text{ min}} \times 15 \text{ gtt/mL} = \dfrac{125 \text{ mL}}{\underset{4}{\cancel{60} \text{ min}}} \times \dfrac{\overset{1}{\cancel{15}} \text{ gtt}}{1 \cancel{\text{ mL}}} = \dfrac{125 \text{ gtt}}{4 \text{ min}} = 31.2 \text{ gtt/min}$

$= 31 \text{ gtt/min}$

CAUTION

Typical values of gtt/min to expect in calculations are in the range of 20 to 100 gtt/min. Use this guideline as part of checking for reasonable answers.

QUICK REVIEW

- The formula method to calculate the flow rate, or watch count, in gtt/min for manually regulated IV rates ordered in mL/h or mL/min is:

  $\dfrac{V}{T} \times C = R: \dfrac{\text{Volume (mL)}}{\text{Time (min)}} \times$ Calibration or drop factor (gtt/mL) = Rate (gtt/min)

- When total volume and total hours are ordered, first calculate mL/h.

- When the drop factor calibration is 60 (microdrop sets), then the flow rate in gtt/min is the same as the ordered volume in mL/h.

- Round gtt/min to a whole number.

Review Set 36

1. State the rule for the formula method to calculate IV flow rate in gtt/min when mL/h are known.

_____

Calculate the flow rate or watch count in gtt/min.

2. Order: D₅W 3,000 mL IV at 125 mL/h

   Drop factor: 10 gtt/mL

   _____ gtt/min

3. Order: LR 250 mL IV at 50 mL/h

   Drop factor: 60 gtt/mL

   _____ gtt/min

4. Order: NS 100 mL bolus IV to infuse in 60 min

   Drop factor: 20 gtt/mL

   _____ gtt/min

5. Order: D₅ ½ NS IV with 20 mEq KCl per liter to run at 25 mL/h

   Drop factor: 60 gtt/mL

   _____ gtt/min

6. Order: Two 500 mL units of whole blood IV to be infused in 4 h

   Drop factor: 20 gtt/mL

   _____ gtt/min

7. Order: $D_5 \frac{1}{4}$ NS 1 L to infuse in 6 h

    Drop factor: 15 gtt/mL

    _____ gtt/min

8. Order: D_5NS IV at 150 mL/h

    Drop factor: 20 gtt/mL

    _____ gtt/min

9. Order: NS 150 mL bolus IV to infuse in 45 min

    Drop factor: 15 gtt/mL

    _____ gtt/min

10. Order: D_5W antibiotic solution 80 mL IV to infuse in 60 min

    Drop factor: 60 gtt/mL

    _____ gtt/min

11. Order: Packed red blood cells 480 mL IV to infuse in 4 h

    Drop factor: 10 gtt/mL

    _____ gtt/min

12. Order: D_5W IV at 120 mL/h

    Drop factor: 15 gtt/mL

    _____ gtt/min

13. Order: D_5 0.45% NaCl IV at 50 mL/h

    Drop factor: 20 gtt/mL

    _____ gtt/min

14. Order: LR 2,500 mL IV at 165 mL/h

    Drop factor: 20 gtt/mL

    _____ gtt/min

15. Order: D_5LR 3,500 mL IV to run at 160 mL/h

    Drop factor: 15 gtt/mL

    _____ gtt/min

After completing these problems, see pages 557–558 to check your answers.

Shortcut Method

By converting the volume and time in the formula method to mL per h (or mL per 60 min), you can use a shortcut to calculate flow rate. This shortcut is derived from the drop factor (C), which cancels out each time and reduces the 60 minutes (T). You are left with the *drop factor constant*. Look at these examples.

EXAMPLE 1 ■

Administer Normal Saline 1,000 mL IV at 125 mL/h with a microdrop infusion set calibrated for 60 gtt/mL. Use the formula $\frac{V}{T} \times C = R$.

$$\frac{V}{T} \times C = \frac{125 \cancel{mL}}{\cancel{60} \text{ min}} \times \overset{1}{\cancel{60}} \text{ gtt}/\cancel{mL} = \frac{125 \text{ gtt}}{\textcircled{1} \text{ min}} = 125 \text{ gtt/min}$$

The drop factor constant for an infusion set with 60 gtt/mL is 1. Therefore, to administer 125 mL/h, set the flow rate at 125 gtt/min. Recall that when the drop factor is 60, then gtt/min = mL/h.

EXAMPLE 2 ■

Administer NS 1,000 mL IV at 125 mL/h with 20 gtt/mL infusion set.

$$\frac{V}{T} \times C = \frac{125 \cancel{mL}}{\underset{3}{\cancel{60}} \text{ min}} \times \overset{1}{\cancel{20}} \text{ gtt}/\cancel{mL} = \frac{125 \text{ gtt}}{\textcircled{3} \text{ min}} = 41.6 \text{ gtt/min} = 42 \text{ gtt/min}$$

Drop factor constant = 3

Each drop factor constant is obtained by dividing 60 by the drop factor calibration from the infusion set.

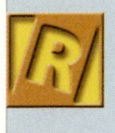

REMEMBER

Drop Factor	Drop Factor Constant
10 gtt/mL	$\frac{60}{10} = 6$
15 gtt/mL	$\frac{60}{15} = 4$
20 gtt/mL	$\frac{60}{20} = 3$
60 gtt/mL	$\frac{60}{60} = 1$

Most hospitals consistently use infusion equipment manufactured by one company. Each manufacturer typically supplies one macrodrop and one microdrop system. You will become familiar with the supplier used where you work; therefore, the shortcut method is practical, quick, and simple to use.

RULE

The shortcut method to calculate IV flow rate is:

$$\frac{mL/h}{Drop\ factor\ constant} = gtt/min$$

Let's examine four examples using the shortcut method.

EXAMPLE 1 ■

The IV order reads: **D₅W 1,000 mL IV at 125 mL/h.** The infusion set is calibrated for a drop factor of 10 gtt/mL. Drop factor constant: 6

$$\frac{mL/h}{Drop\ factor\ constant} = gtt/min$$

$$\frac{125\ mL/h}{6} = 20.8\ gtt/min = 21\ gtt/min$$

EXAMPLE 2 ■

Order reads: **LR 1,000 mL IV at 150 mL/h.** The drop factor is 15 gtt/mL. Drop factor constant: 4

$$\frac{mL/h}{Drop\ factor\ constant} = gtt/min$$

$$\frac{150\ mL/h}{4} = 37.5\ gtt/min = 38\ gtt/min$$

EXAMPLE 3 ■

Order reads: **D₅ ½NS 200 mL IV in 2 h.** The drop factor is 20 gtt/mL. Drop factor constant: 3

Step 1 $\frac{Total\ mL}{Total\ h} = mL/h$

$$\frac{200}{2} = 100\ mL/h$$

Step 2 $\frac{mL/h}{Drop\ factor\ constant} = gtt/min$

$$\frac{100\ mL/h}{3} = 33.3\ gtt/min = 33\ gtt/min$$

EXAMPLE 4 ■

Order reads: **D₅W NS 500 mL IV at 50 mL/h.** The drop factor is 60 gtt/mL. Drop factor constant: 1

$$\frac{mL/h}{Drop\ factor\ constant} = gtt/min$$

$$\frac{50\ mL/h}{1} = 50\ gtt/min$$

Remember, when the drop factor is 60 (microdrop), set the flow rate at the same gtt/min as the mL/h.

CAUTION

For the shortcut method to work, the rate has to be written in mL/h. The shortcut method will not work if the time is less than 1 hour or is calculated in minutes, such as 30 or 90 minutes.

QUICK REVIEW

■ The drop factor constant is 60 divided by the drop factor.

Drop Factor	Drop Factor Constant
10 gtt/mL	6
15 gtt/mL	4
20 gtt/mL	3
60 gtt/mL	1 → Set the flow rate at the same number of gtt/min as the number of mL/h.

■ $\dfrac{\text{mL/h}}{\text{Drop factor constant}}$ = gtt/min

Review Set 37

1. The drop factor constant is derived by dividing _____ by the drop factor calibration.

Determine the drop factor constant for each of the following infusion sets.

2. 60 gtt/mL _____

3. 20 gtt/mL _____

4. 15 gtt/mL _____

5. 10 gtt/mL _____

6. State the rule for the shortcut method to calculate the IV flow rate in gtt/min. _____

_____

Calculate the IV flow rate in gtt/min using the shortcut method.

7. Order: D₅W 1,000 mL IV to infuse at 200 mL/h

   Drop factor: 15 gtt/mL

   Flow rate: _____ gtt/min

8. Order: D₅W 750 mL IV to infuse at 125 mL/h

   Drop factor: 20 gtt/mL

   Flow rate: _____ gtt/min

9. Order: D₅W 0.45% Saline 500 mL IV to infuse at 165 mL/h

   Drop factor: 10 gtt/mL

   Flow rate: _____ gtt/min

10. Order: NS 2 L IV to infuse at 60 mL/h

    Drop factor: microdrop infusion set

    Flow rate: _____ gtt/min

11. Order: D₅W 400 mL IV to infuse at 50 mL/h

    Drop factor: 10 gtt/mL

    Flow rate: _____ gtt/min

12. Order: NS 3 L IV to infuse at 125 mL/h

    Drop factor: 15 gtt/mL

    Flow rate: _____ gtt/min

13. Order: D₅LR 500 mL IV to infuse in 6 h

    Drop factor: 20 gtt/mL

    Flow rate: _____ gtt/min

14. Order: 0.45% NaCl 0.5 L IV to infuse in 20 h

    Drop factor: 60 gtt/mL

    Flow rate: _____ gtt/min

15. Order: D_5 0.9% NaCl 650 mL IV to infuse in 10 h

   Drop factor: 10 gtt/mL

   Flow rate: ＿＿＿＿＿ gtt/min

After completing these problems, see page 558 to check your answers.

SUMMARY

Calculating mL/h to program infusion devices and gtt/min to watch-count manually regulated IVs are two major IV calculations you need to know. Further, you have learned to calculate the supply dosage of certain IV solutes. These important topics warrant additional reinforcement and review.

QUICK REVIEW

■ Solution strength expressed as a percent (%) indicates the number of g of solute per 100 mL of solution.

■ When regulating IV flow rate for an electronic infusion device, calculate mL/h.

■ When calculating IV flow rate to regulate an IV manually, calculate mL/h; then find the drop factor, and calculate gtt/min by using the:

Formula Method

$$\frac{V}{T} \times C = R$$

or Shortcut Method: $\dfrac{mL/h}{Drop\ factor\ constant} = gtt/min$

■ Carefully monitor patients receiving IV fluids at least hourly.

   ■ Check remaining IV fluids.

   ■ Check IV flow rate.

   ■ Observe IV site for complications.

Review Set 38

Calculate the IV flow rate for these manually regulated IV administrations.

1. Order: 0.45% NaCl 3,000 mL IV for 24 h

   Drop factor: 15 gtt/mL

   Flow rate: ＿＿＿＿＿ mL/h

   Flow rate: ＿＿＿＿＿ gtt/min

2. Order: D_5W 200 mL IV to run at 100 mL/h

   Drop factor: Microdrop, 60 gtt/mL

   Flow rate: ＿＿＿＿＿ gtt/min

3. Order: $D_5 \frac{1}{2}$ NS 800 mL IV for 8 h

   Drop factor: 20 gtt/mL

   Flow rate: ＿＿＿＿＿ mL/h

   Flow rate: ＿＿＿＿＿ gtt/min

4. Order: NS 1,000 mL IV at 50 mL/h

   Drop factor: 60 gtt/mL

   Flow rate: ＿＿＿＿＿ gtt/min

5. Order: D_5W 1,500 mL IV for 12 h

   Drop factor: 15 gtt/mL

   Flow rate: ＿＿＿＿＿ mL/h

   Flow rate: ＿＿＿＿＿ gtt/min

6. Order: theophylline 0.5 g IV in 250 mL D_5W to run for 2 h by infusion pump

   Drop factor: 60 gtt/mL

   Flow rate: ＿＿＿＿＿ mL/h

   Flow rate: ＿＿＿＿＿ gtt/min

7. Order: D_5 0.45% NaCl 2,500 mL IV at 105 mL/h

   Drop factor: 20 gtt/mL

   Flow rate: ＿＿＿＿＿ gtt/min

8. Order: D$_5$ 0.45% NaCl 500 mL IV at 100 mL/h

   Drop factor: 10 gtt/mL

   Flow rate: _____ gtt/min

9. Order: NS 1,200 mL IV at 150 mL/h

   Drop factor: 10 gtt/mL

   Flow rate: _____ gtt/min

Calculate the IV flow rate for these electronically regulated IV administrations.

10. Order: D$_5$ 0.45% NaCl 1,000 mL IV to infuse over 8 h

    Flow rate: _____ mL/h

11. Order: D$_5$NS 2,000 mL IV to infuse over 24 h

    Flow rate: _____ mL/h

12. Order: LR 500 mL IV to infuse over 4 h

    Flow rate: _____ mL/h

13. Order: 100 mL IV antibiotic to infuse in 30 min

    Flow rate: _____ mL/h

14. Order: 50 mL IV antibiotic to infuse in 20 min

    Flow rate: _____ mL/h

15. Order: 150 mL IV antibiotic to infuse in 45 min

    Flow rate: _____ mL/h

What is the total dosage of the solute(s) the patient will receive for each of the following IV solutions?

16. 3,000 mL $\frac{1}{2}$ NS   NaCl: _____ g

17. 200 mL D$_{10}$ NS   D: _____ g   NaCl: _____ g

18. 2,500 mL NS   NaCl: _____ g

19. 650 mL D$_5$ 0.45% NaCl   D: _____ g   NaCl: _____ g

20. 1,000 mL D$_5$ $\frac{1}{4}$ NS   D: _____ g   NaCl: _____ g

After completing these problems, see pages 558–559 to check your answers.

ADJUSTING IV FLOW RATE

IV fluids, especially those with medicines added (called additives), are viewed as medications with specific dosages (rates of infusion, in this case). It is the responsibility of the nurse to maintain this rate of flow through careful calculations and close observation at regular intervals. Various circumstances, such as gravity, condition, and movement of the patient, can alter the set flow rate of an IV, causing the IV to run ahead of or behind schedule.

CAUTION

It is not the discretion of the nurse to arbitrarily speed up or slow down the flow rate to catch up the IV. This practice can result in serious conditions of overhydration or underhydration and electrolyte imbalance. Avoid off-schedule IV flow rates by regularly monitoring IVs at least every 30 minutes to 1 hour. Check your agency policy.

During your regular monitoring of the IV, if you find that the rate is not progressing as scheduled or is significantly ahead of or behind schedule, the physician may need to be notified as warranted by the patient's condition, hospital policy, or good nursing judgment. Some hospital policies allow the flow rate per minute to be adjusted a certain percentage of variation. A safe rule is that the flow rate per minute may be adjusted by *up to 25 percent more or less* than the original prescribed rate depending on the condition of the patient. In such cases, assess the patient. If the patient is stable, recalculate the flow rate to administer the total milliliters remaining over the number of hours remaining of the original order.

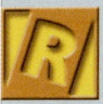

RULE

- Check for institutional policy regarding correcting off-schedule IV rates and the percentage of variation. This variation should not exceed 25 percent.
- If adjustment is permitted, use the following formula to recalculate the mL/h and gtt/min for the time remaining and the percentage of variation.

Step 1 $\dfrac{\text{Remaining volume}}{\text{Remaining hours}} = \text{Recalculated mL/h}$

Step 2 $\dfrac{V}{T} \times C = R \text{ (gtt/min)}$

Step 3 $\dfrac{\text{Adjusted rate (gtt/min or mL/h)} - \text{Ordered rate (gtt/min or mL/h)}}{\text{Ordered rate (gtt/min or mL/h)}} = \% \text{ variation}$

The percent variation will be positive (+) if the administration is slow and the rate has to be increased and negative (−) if the administration is too fast and the rate has to be decreased.

EXAMPLE 1 ▪

The order reads **D₅W 1,000 mL IV at 125 mL/h for 8 h.** The drop factor is 10 gtt/mL, and the IV is correctly set at 21 gtt/min. You would expect that after 4 hours, one-half of the total, or 500 mL, of the solution would be infused (125 mL/h × 4 h = 500 mL). However, when you check the IV bag the fourth hour after starting the IV, you find 600 milliliters remaining. The rate of flow is *behind schedule*, and the hospital allows a 25% IV flow variation with careful patient assessment and if the patient's condition is stable. The patient is stable, so you decide to compute a new flow rate for the remaining 600 milliliters to complete the IV fluid order in the remaining 4 hours.

Step 1   **Convert** $\dfrac{\text{Remaining volume}}{\text{Remaining hours}} = \text{Recalculated mL/h}$

$$\dfrac{600 \text{ mL}}{4 \text{ h}} = 150 \text{ mL/h}$$

Step 2   **Think** $\dfrac{V}{T} \times C = \dfrac{150 \text{ mL}}{\overset{6}{\cancel{60} \text{ min}}} \times \overset{1}{\cancel{10}} \text{ gtt/mL} = \dfrac{150 \text{ gtt}}{6 \text{ min}} = 25 \text{ gtt/min (Adjusted flow rate)}$

You could also use the shortcut method.

$$\dfrac{\text{mL/h}}{\text{Drop factor constant}} = \text{gtt/min}$$

$$\dfrac{150 \text{ mL/h}}{6} = 25 \text{ gtt/min}$$

Step 3   **Calculate** $\dfrac{\text{Adjusted gtt/min} - \text{Ordered gtt/min}}{\text{Ordered gtt/min}} = \% \text{ of variation}$

$$\dfrac{25 - 21}{21} = \dfrac{4}{21} = 0.19 = 19\%; \text{ within the acceptable 25\% of variation}$$

depending on policy and patient's condition

    Compare 25 gtt/min (in the last example) with the starting flow rate of 21 gtt/min. You can see that adjusting the total remaining volume over the total remaining hours changes the flow rate only 4 gtt/min. Most patients can tolerate this small amount of increase per minute over several hours. However, trying to catch up the lost 100 milliliters in 1 hour can be dangerous. To infuse an extra 100 milliliters in 1 hour, with a drop factor of 10, you would need to speed up the IV to a much faster rate. Let's see what that rate would be.

$$\dfrac{V}{T} \times C = \dfrac{100 \text{ mL}}{\overset{6}{\cancel{60} \text{ min}}} \times \overset{1}{\cancel{10}} \text{ gtt/mL} = \dfrac{100 \text{ gtt}}{6 \text{ min}} = 16.6 \text{ gtt/min} = 17 \text{ gtt/min more than the original rate}$$

To catch up the IV over the next hour, the flow rate would have to be 17 drops per minute faster than the original 21 drops per minute rate. The infusion would have to be set at $17 + 21 = 38$ gtt/min for 1 hour and then slowed to the original rate. Such an increase would be $\frac{38 - 21}{21} = \frac{17}{21} = 81\%$ greater than the ordered rate. This could present a serious problem. **Do not do it! If permitted by hospital policy, the flow rate for the remainder of the order must be recalculated when the IV is off-schedule and should not exceed a 25 percent adjustment, unless instructed otherwise by a physician.**

EXAMPLE 2 ■

The order reads: **LR 500 mL IV to run over 10 h at 50 mL/h.** The drop factor is 60 gtt/mL and the IV is correctly infusing at 50 gtt/min. After $2\frac{1}{2}$ hours, you find 300 mL remaining. Almost half of the total volume has already infused in about one-quarter the time. This IV infusion is *ahead of schedule*. You would compute a new flow rate of 300 mL to complete the IV fluid order in the remaining $7\frac{1}{2}$ hours. The patient would require close assessment for fluid overload.

Step 1   Convert
$$\frac{\text{Remaining volume}}{\text{Remaining hours}} = \text{Recalculated mL/h}$$

$$\frac{300 \text{ mL}}{7.5 \text{ h}} = 40 \text{ mL/h}$$

Time remaining is $7\frac{1}{2}$ h (10 h $- 2\frac{1}{2}$ h)

Step 2   Think
$$\frac{V}{T} \times C = \frac{40 \text{ mL}}{60 \text{ min}} \times 60 \text{ gtt/mL} = 40 \text{ gtt/min (Adjusted flow rate)}$$

Or, you know when drop factor is 60, then mL/h = gtt/min.

Step 3   Calculate
$$\frac{\text{Adjusted gtt/min} - \text{Ordered gtt/min}}{\text{Ordered gtt/min}} = \% \text{ of variation}$$

$$\frac{40 - 50}{50} = \frac{-10}{50} = -0.2 = -20\% \text{ within the acceptable 25\% of variation}$$

Remember, the negative percent of variation (–20%) indicates that the adjusted flow rate will be decreased.

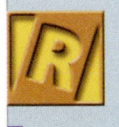

RULE

Shortcut for IV Rate Adjustment Check (Step 3):

Ordered IV Rate ± (Ordered IV Rate ÷ 4) = Acceptable IV Adjustment Range

You know that you can adjust the flow rate by as much as ±25 percent, and you know that $25\% = \frac{1}{4}$. Therefore, after recalculating the adjusted flow rate, you can check the safety of the recalculated rate by using a shortcut that does not include percents. To do this you divide the ordered rate by 4 and add or subtract the result from the ordered rate to determine the acceptable range of adjustment.

In the *first* example, the ordered rate is 21 gtt/min, and the recalculated rate is 25 gtt/min. Is this within the safe range? Use the shortcut to calculate the acceptable range.

Ordered IV Rate ± (Ordered IV Rate ÷ 4) = Acceptable IV Adjustment Range

$$21 + (21 \div 4) = 21 + 5.25 = 26.25 = 26 \text{ gtt/min}$$

$$21 + (21 \div 4) = 21 - 5.25 = 15.75 = 16 \text{ gtt/min}$$

The safe range is 16 to 26 gtt/min. Yes, 25 gtt/min is within the safe ±25% range.

This may be an easier calculation for you than working with percents. Let's look at the *second* example. The ordered rate is 50 gtt/min and the recalculated rate is 40 gtt/min. What is the acceptable range?

Ordered IV Rate ± (Ordered IV Rate ÷ 4) = Acceptable IV Adjustment Range

$$50 + (50 \div 4) = 50 + 12.5 = 62.5 = 63 \text{ gtt/min}$$

$$50 - (50 \div 4) = 50 - 12.5 = 37.5 = 38 \text{ gtt/min}$$

The safe range is 38 to 63 gtt/min. Yes, it is safe to slow the rate to 40 gtt/min, which is within the safe ±25% range.

A safe rule is that the recalculated flow rate should not vary from the ordered rate by more than 25 percent. If the recalculated rate does vary from the order by more than 25 percent, contact your supervisor or the doctor for further instructions. The original order may have to be revised. Regular monitoring helps to prevent or minimize this problem.

Patients who require close monitoring for IV fluids will most likely have the IV regulated by an electronic infusion device. Because of the nature of their condition, "catching up" these IVs, if off-schedule, is not recommended. If an IV regulated by an electronic infusion pump is off-schedule or inaccurate, suspect that the infusion pump may need recalibration. Consult with your supervisor, as appropriate.

QUICK REVIEW

- Regular IV monitoring and patient assessment at least every 30 minutes to 1 hour is important to maintain prescribed IV flow rate.

- Do not arbitrarily speed up or slow down IV flow rates that are off-schedule.

- Check hospital policy regarding adjustment of off-schedule IV flow rates and the percentage of variation allowed. If permitted, a safe rule is a maximum 25 percent variation for patients in stable condition.

- Use the remaining time and the remaining IV fluid volume to recalculate off-schedule IV flow rate:

Step 1 $\dfrac{\text{Remaining volume}}{\text{Remaining hours}} = \text{Recalculated mL/h}$

Step 2 $\dfrac{V}{T} \times C = R \text{ (gtt/min)}$

Step 3 $\dfrac{\text{Adjusted gtt/min} - \text{Ordered gtt/min}}{\text{Ordered gtt/min}} = \% \text{ variation}$

- Contact the prescribing health care professional for a new IV fluid order if the recalculated IV flow rate variation exceeds the allowed variation or if the patient's condition is unstable.

Review Set 39

Compute the flow rate in drops per minute. Hospital policy permits recalculation of IVs when off-schedule, with a maximum variation in rate of 25 percent for patients who are stable. Compute the percent of variation.

1. Order: **Lactated Ringer's 1,500 mL IV for 12 h at 125 mL/h**

   Drop factor: 20 gtt/mL

   Original flow rate: _____ gtt/min

   After 6 hours, there are 850 mL remaining; describe your action now.

   Time remaining: _____ h

   Recalculated flow rate: _____ mL/h

   Recalculated flow rate: _____ gtt/min

   Variation: _____ %

   Action: _____

2. Order: **Lactated Ringer's 1,000 mL IV for 6 h at 167 mL/h**

   Drop factor: 15 gtt/mL

   Original flow rate: _____ gtt/min

   After 4 hours, there are 360 mL remaining; describe your action now.

   Time remaining: _____ h

   Recalculated flow rate: _____ mL/h

   Recalculated flow rate: _____ gtt/min

   Variation: _____ %

   Action: _____

3. Order: **D$_5$W 1,000 mL IV for 8 h at 125 mL/h**

   Drop factor: 20 gtt/mL

   Original flow rate: _____ gtt/min

   After 4 hours, there are 800 mL remaining; describe your action now.

   Time remaining: _____ h

   Recalculated flow rate: _____ mL/h

   Recalculated flow rate: _____ gtt/min

   Variation: _____ %

   Action: _____

4. Order: **NS 2,000 mL IV for 12 h at 167 mL/h**

   Drop factor: 10 gtt/mL

   Original flow rate: _____ gtt/min

   After 8 hours, there are 750 mL remaining; describe your action now.

   Time remaining: _____ h

   Recalculated flow rate: _____ mL/h

   Recalculated flow rate: _____ gtt/min

   Variation: _____ %

   Action: _____

5. Order: **NS 1,000 mL IV for 8 h at 125 mL/h**

   Drop factor: 10 gtt/mL

   Original flow rate: _____ gtt/min

   After 4 hours, there are 750 mL remaining; describe your action now.

   Time remaining: _____ h

   Recalculated flow rate: _____ mL/h

   Recalculated flow rate: _____ gtt/min

   Variation: _____ %

   Action: _____

6. Order: **NS 2,000 mL IV for 16 h at 125 mL/h**

   Drop factor: 15 gtt/mL

   Original flow rate: _____ gtt/min

   After 6 hours, 650 mL of fluid have infused; describe your action now.

   Solution remaining: _____ mL   Time remaining: _____ h

   Recalculated flow rate: _____ mL/h

   Recalculated flow rate: _____ gtt/min

   Variation: _____ %

   Action: _____

7. Order: **NS 900 mL IV for 6 h at 150 mL/h**

   Drop factor: 20 gtt/mL

   Original flow rate: _____ gtt/min

   After 3 hours, there are 700 mL remaining; describe your action now.

   Time remaining: _____ h

   Recalculated flow rate: _____ mL/h

   Recalculated flow rate: _____ gtt/min

   Variation: _____ %

   Action: _____

8. Order: **D₅NS 500 mL IV for 5 h at 100 mL/h**

   Drop factor: 20 gtt/mL

   Original flow rate: _____ gtt/min

   After 2 hours, there are 250 mL remaining; describe your action now.

   Time remaining: _____ h

   Recalculated flow rate: _____ mL/h

   Recalculated flow rate: _____ gtt/min

   Variation: _____ %

   Action: _____

9. Order: **NS 1 L IV for 20 h at 50 mL/h**

   Drop factor: 15 gtt/mL

   Original flow rate: _____ gtt/min

   After 10 hours, there are 600 mL remaining; describe your action now.

   Time remaining: _____ h

   Recalculated flow rate: _____ mL/h

   Recalculated flow rate: _____ gtt/min

   Variation: _____ %

   Action: _____

10. Order: D₅W 1,000 mL IV for 10 h at 100 mL/h

   Drop factor: 60 gtt/mL

   Original flow rate: _____ gtt/min

   After 5 hours, there are 500 mL remaining; describe your action now.

   Time remaining: _____ h

   Recalculated flow rate: _____ mL/h

   Recalculated flow rate: _____ gtt/min

   Variation: _____ %

   Action: _____

After completing these problems, see pages 559–560 to check your answers.

INTERMITTENT IV INFUSIONS

Sometimes the patient needs to receive supplemental fluid therapy and/or IV medications but does not need continuous replacement or maintenance IV fluids. Several intermittent IV infusion systems are available to administer IV drugs. These include IV PB, IV locks for IV push drugs, the ADD-Vantage system, and volume control sets (such as Buretrol). Volume control sets are discussed in Chapter 16.

IV Piggybacks

A medication may be ordered to be dissolved in a small amount of IV fluid (usually 50 to 100 mL) and run piggyback to the regular IV fluids (Figure 15-8). Recall that the IV PB (or secondary IV) requires a secondary IV set.

   The IV PB medication may come premixed by the manufacturer or pharmacy, or the nurse may need to prepare it. Whichever the case, it is always the responsibility of the nurse to accurately and safely administer the medication. The infusion time may be less than 60 minutes, so it is important to carefully read the order and recommended infusion time.

   Sometimes the physician's order for the IV PB medication will not include an infusion time or rate. It is understood, when this is the case, that the nurse will follow the manufacturer's guidelines for infusion rates, keeping in mind the amount of fluid accompanying the medication and any standing orders that limit fluid amounts or rates. Appropriate infusion times are readily available in many drug reference books. Reference books are usually available on most nursing units, or you can consult with a hospital pharmacist.

EXAMPLE 1 ■

Order: **cefazolin 0.5 g in 100 mL D₅W IV PB to run over 30 min**

Drop factor: 20 gtt/mL

What is the flow rate in gtt/min?

$$\frac{V}{T} \times C = \frac{100 \text{ mL}}{\underset{3}{30 \text{ min}}} \times \overset{2}{20} \text{ gtt/mL} = \frac{200 \text{ gtt}}{3 \text{ min}} = 66.6 \text{ gtt/min} = 67 \text{ gtt/min}$$

EXAMPLE 2 ■

If an electronic infusion pump is used to administer the same order as in Example 1, remember that you would need to program the device in mL/h.

Step 1   **Think**   If 100 mL will be administered in 30 minutes or one-half hour, then 200 mL will be administered in twice this time or 60 minutes.

Step 2   **Calculate**   Use ratio-proportion to calculate mL/h.

$$\frac{100\ \text{mL}}{30\ \text{min}} \searrow \swarrow \frac{X\ \text{mL/h}}{60\ \text{min/h}}$$

$$30X = 6,000$$

$$\frac{30X}{30} = \frac{6,000}{30}$$

$$X = 200\ \text{mL/h}$$

Set the electronic IV PB regulator to 200 mL/h. Remember, though, that the actual volume of 100 mL will be infused in 30 minutes.

Saline and Heparin IV Locks for IV Push Drugs

IV locks can be attached to the hub of the IV catheter that is positioned in the vein. The lock may be referred to as a *saline lock,* meaning that saline is used to flush or maintain the IV catheter patency, or a *heparin lock* if heparin is used to maintain the IV catheter patency. Sometimes a more general term, such as *intermittent peripheral infusion device,* may be used. Medications can be given *IV push,* meaning that a syringe is attached to the lock and medication is pushed in. An *IV bolus,* usually a quantity of IV fluid, can be run in over a specified period of time through an IV setup that is attached to the lock. Using either a saline or heparin lock allows for intermittent medication and fluid infusion. Heparin and saline locks are also being used for outpatient and home care medication therapy. Refer to the policy at your hospital or health care agency regarding the frequency, volume, and concentration of saline or heparin to be used to maintain the IV lock.

 **CAUTION**
Heparin lock flush solution is usually concentrated to 10 units/mL or 100 units/mL. Much higher concentrations of heparin are given IV or subcut, so carefully check the concentration.

Dosage calculations for IV push injections are the same as calculations for intramuscular (IM) injections. The IV push route of administration is often preferred when immediate onset of action is desired for persons with small or wasted muscle mass or poor circulation or for drugs that have limited absorption from body tissues. The IV route of administration is also generally preferred over IM when IV access is available because repeated IM injections can be painful. Therefore, when a peripheral IV is in place, an IM route is avoided.

Drug literature and institutional guidelines recommend an acceptable rate (per minute or per incremental amount of time) for IV push drug administration. Most timed IV push administration recommendations are for 1 to 5 minutes or more. For smooth manual administration of IV push drugs, calculate the incremental volume to administer over 15-second intervals. You should time the administration with a digital or sweep second-hand watch or clock.

 **CAUTION**
IV drugs are potent and rapid acting. Never infuse IV push drugs more rapidly than recommended by agency policy or pharmacology literature. Some drugs require further dilution after reconstitution for IV push administration. Carefully read package inserts and reputable drug resources for minimum dilution and minimum time for IV administration.

EXAMPLE 1 ■

Order: **Ativan 3 mg IV push 20 min preoperatively**

Supply: Ativan 4 mg/mL with drug literature guidelines of *IV infusion not to exceed 2 mg/min*

How much Ativan should you prepare?

Step 1 Convert   No conversion is necessary.

Step 2 Think   You want to give less than 1 mL.

Step 3 Calculate
$$\frac{\text{Dosage on hand}}{\text{Amount on hand}} = \frac{\text{Dosage desired}}{\text{X Amount desired}}$$

$$\frac{4\ \text{mg}}{1\ \text{mL}} \diagdown \frac{3\ \text{mg}}{\text{X mL}}$$

$$4\,X = 3$$
$$\frac{4\,X}{4} = \frac{3}{4}$$
$$X = 0.75\ \text{mL}$$

What is a safe infusion time?

Use ratio-proportion to calculate the time required to administer the drug dosage as ordered.

$$\frac{\text{Dosage recommended}}{\text{Time recommended}} = \frac{\text{Dosage desired}}{\text{X Time desired}}$$

$$\frac{2\ \text{mg}}{1\ \text{min}} \diagdown \frac{3\ \text{mg}}{\text{X min}}$$

$$2X = 3$$
$$\frac{2X}{2} = \frac{3}{2}$$
$$X = 1\tfrac{1}{2}\ \text{min}$$

Administer 0.75 mL over $1\tfrac{1}{2}$ min.

How much should you infuse every 15 seconds?

Convert: 1 min = 60 sec; $1\tfrac{1}{2}$ min × 60 sec/min = 90 sec

$$\frac{0.75\ \text{mL}}{90\ \text{sec}} \diagdown \frac{\text{X mL}}{15\ \text{sec}}$$

$$90X = 11.25$$
$$\frac{90X}{90} = \frac{11.25}{90}$$

X = 0.125 mL = 0.13 mL of Ativan 4 mg/mL infused IV push every 15 seconds will deliver 3 mg of Ativan

This is a small amount. Use a 1 mL syringe to prepare 0.75 mL and slowly administer 0.13 mL every 15 seconds.

EXAMPLE 2 ■

Order: **Cefizox 1,500 mg IV push q.8h**

Supply: Cefizox 2 g powder with directions, *For direct IV administration, reconstitute each 1 g in 10 mL sterile water and give slowly over 3 to 5 minutes.*

How much Cefizox should you prepare?

Step 1 Convert   2 g = 2.000. = 2,000 mg

Step 2 Think   If 1 g (or 1,000 mg) requires 10 mL for dilution, then 2 g (or 2,000 mg) requires twice this amount or 20 mL for dilution. Therefore, to administer 1,500 mg, you will prepare more than 10 mL and less than 20 mL.

Step 3   Calculate $\dfrac{\text{Dosage on hand}}{\text{Amount on hand}} = \dfrac{\text{Dosage desired}}{\text{X Amount desired}}$

$$\dfrac{2{,}000 \text{ mg}}{20 \text{ mL}} \quad\diagdown\diagup\quad \dfrac{1{,}500 \text{ mg}}{\text{X mL}}$$

$$2{,}000\text{X} \quad=\quad 30{,}000$$

$$\dfrac{2{,}000\text{X}}{2{,}000} = \dfrac{30{,}000}{2{,}000}$$

$$\text{X} \quad=\quad 15 \text{ mL}$$

What is a safe infusion time?

This amount is larger than the Ativan dosage from Example 1, so you should use the longer infusion time recommendation (1 g per 5 min). Remember the unknown X is the time to infuse the dosage desired.

$$\dfrac{\text{Dosage recommended}}{\text{Time recommended}} = \dfrac{\text{Dosage desired}}{\text{X Time desired}}$$

$$\dfrac{1{,}000 \text{ mg}}{5 \text{ min}} \quad\diagdown\diagup\quad \dfrac{1{,}500 \text{ mg}}{\text{X min}}$$

$$\dfrac{1{,}000\text{X}}{1{,}000} = \dfrac{7{,}500}{1{,}000}$$

$$\text{X} \quad=\quad 7.5 \text{ min}$$

Administer 15 mL over 7.5 min.

How much should you infuse every 15 seconds?

Convert: 1 min = 60 sec

7.5 m̶i̶n̶ × 60 sec/m̶i̶n̶ = 450 sec

$$\dfrac{15 \text{ mL}}{450 \text{ sec}} \quad\diagdown\diagup\quad \dfrac{\text{X mL}}{15 \text{ sec}}$$

$$450\text{X} = 225$$

$$\dfrac{450\text{X}}{450} = \dfrac{225}{450}$$

$$\text{X} = 0.5 \text{ mL}$$ (of Cefizox 2 g per 20 mL infused IV push every 15 seconds to deliver 1,500 mg of Cefizox)

Use a 20 mL syringe to prepare 15 mL and slowly infuse 0.5 mL every 15 seconds.

ADD-Vantage System

Another type of IV medication setup commonly used in hospitals is the ADD-Vantage system by Abbott Laboratories (Figure 15-18). This system uses a specially designed IV bag with a medication vial port. The medication vial comes with the ordered dosage and medication prepared in a powder form. The medication vial is attached to the special IV bag, and together they become the IV PB container. The powder is dissolved by the IV fluid and used within a specified time. This system maintains asepsis and eliminates the extra time and equipment (syringe and diluent vials) associated with reconstitution of powdered medications. Several drug manufacturers market many common IV antibiotics using products similar to the ADD-Vantage system.

QUICK REVIEW

- Intermittent IV infusions usually require more or less than 60 minutes of infusion time.
- Calculate IV PB flow rate in gtt/min: $\dfrac{V}{T} \times C = R$.
- Use a proportion to calculate IV PB flow rate in mL/h for an electronic infusion device.
- Use the three-step dosage calculation method to calculate the amount to give for IV push medications: convert, think, calculate.
- Use ratio-proportion to calculate safe IV push time in minutes and seconds as recommended by reputable drug reference.

FIGURE 15-18 ADD-Vantage system: Medications can be added to another solution being infused

1 ASSEMBLE — USE ASEPTIC TECHNIQUE

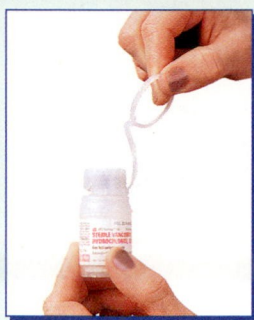

Swing the pull ring over the top of the vial and pull down far enough to start the opening. Then pull straight up to remove the cap. Avoid touching the rubber stopper and vial threads.

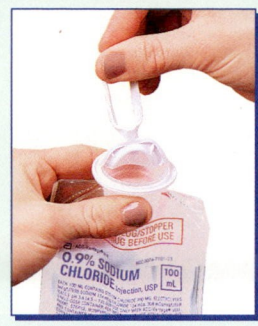

Hold diluent container and gently grasp the tab on the pull ring. Pull up to break the tie membrane. Pull back to remove the cover. Avoid touching the inside of the vial port.

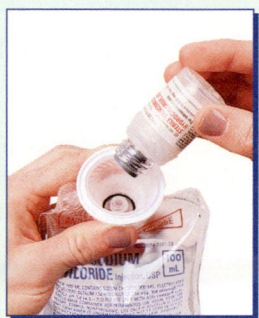

Screw the vial into the vial port until it will go no further. **Recheck the vial to assure that it is tight.** Label appropriately.

2 ACTIVATE — PULL PLUG/STOPPER TO MIX DRUG WITH DILUENT

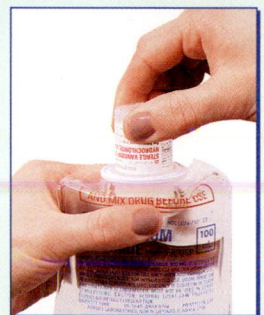

Hold the vial as shown. Push the drug vial down into container and grasp the inner cap of the vial through the walls of the container.

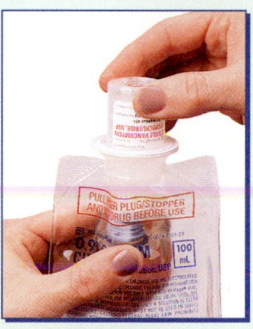

Pull the inner cap from the drug vial: allow drug to fall into diluent container for fast mixing. Do not force stopper by pushing on one side of inner cap at a time.

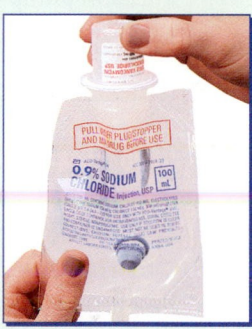

Verify that the plug and rubber stopper have been removed from the vial. The floating stopper is an indication that the system has been activated.

3 MIX AND ADMINISTER — WITHIN THE SPECIFIED TIME

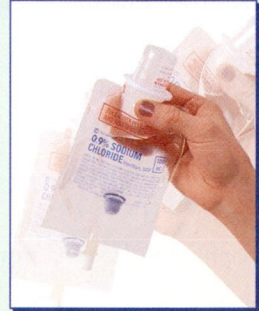

Mix container contents thoroughly to assure complete dissolution. Look through bottom of vial to verify complete mixing. Check for leaks by squeezing container firmly. If leaks are found, discard unit.

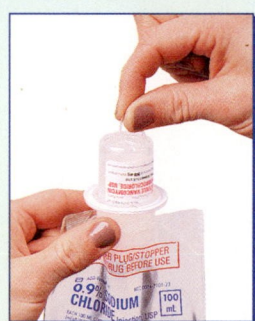

Pull up hanger on the vial.

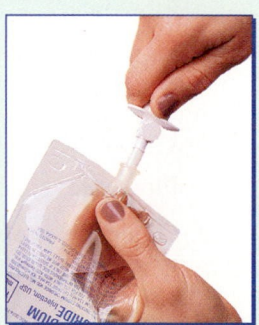

Remove the white administration port cover and spike (pierce) the container with the piercing pin. Administer within the specified time.

Courtesy of Abbott Laboratories, Inc.

Review Set 40

Calculate the IV PB or IV push flow rate.

1. Order: Ancef 1 g in 100 mL D₅W IV PB to be infused over 45 min

   Drop factor: 60 gtt/mL

   Flow rate: _____ gtt/min

2. Order: Ancef 1 g in 100 mL D₅W IV PB to be administered by electronic infusion pump to infuse in 45 min

   Flow rate: _____ mL/h

3. Order: cefazolin 500 mg IV PB diluted in 50 mL D₅W to infuse in 15 min

   Drop factor: 15 gtt/mL

   Flow rate: _____ gtt/min

4. Order: cefazolin 500 mg IV PB diluted in 50 mL D₅W to infuse in 15 min by an electronic infusion pump

   Flow rate: _____ mL/h

5. Order: 50 mL IV PB antibiotic solution to infuse in 30 min

   Drop factor: 60 gtt/mL

   Flow rate: _____ gtt/min

6. Order: Zosyn 3 g in 100 mL D₅W IV PB to be infused over 40 min

   Drop factor: 10 gtt/mL

   Flow rate: _____ gtt/min

7. Order: Unasyn 1.5 g in 50 mL D₅W IV PB to be infused over 15 min

   Drop factor: 15 gtt/mL

   Flow rate: _____ gtt/min

8. Order: Merrem 1 g in 100 mL D₅W IV PB to be infused over 30 min

   Use electronic infusion pump.

   Flow rate: _____ mL/h

9. Order: cefoxitin 750 mg in 50 mL NS IV PB to be infused over 20 min

   Use electronic infusion pump.

   Flow rate: _____ mL/h

10. Order: oxacillin sodium 900 mg in 125 mL D₅W IV PB to be infused over 45 min

    Use electronic infusion pump.

    Flow rate: _____ mL/h

11. Order: Unasyn 0.5 g in 100 mL D₅W IV PB to be infused over 15 min

    Drop factor: 20 gtt/mL

    Flow rate: _____ gtt/min

12. Order: cefotetan 500 mg in 50 mL NS IV PB to be infused over 20 min

    Drop factor: 10 gtt/mL

    Flow rate: _____ gtt/min

13. Order: Merrem 1 g in 100 mL D₅W IV PB to be infused over 50 min

    Use electronic infusion pump.

    Flow rate: _____ mL/h

14. Order: oxacillin sodium 900 mg in 125 mL D₅W IV PB to be infused over 45 min

    Drop factor: 20 gtt/mL

    Flow rate: _____ gtt/min

15. Order: Zosyn 1.3 g in 100 mL D₅W IV PB to be infused over 30 min

    Drop factor: 60 gtt/mL

    Flow rate: _____ gtt/min

16. Order: Lasix 120 mg IV push stat

    Supply: Lasix 10 mg/mL with drug insert, which states, *IV injection not to exceed 40 mg/min.*

    Give: _____ mL per _____ min or _____ mL per 15 sec

17. Order: phenytoin 150 mg IV push stat

    Supply: phenytoin 250 mg per 5 mL with drug insert, which states, *IV infusion not to exceed 50 mg/min.*

    Give: _____ mL per _____ min or _____ mL per 15 sec

18. Order: morphine sulfate 6 mg IV push q.3h p.r.n., pain

    Supply: morphine sulfate 10 mg/mL with drug reference recommendation, which states, *IV infusion not to exceed 2.5 mg/min.*

    Give: _____ mL per _____ min and _____ seconds or _____ mL per 15 sec

19. Order: **cimetidine 300 mg IV push stat**

    Supply: cimetidine 300 mg per 2 mL

    Package insert instructions: *For direct IV injection, dilute 300 mg in 0.9% NaCl to a total volume of 20 mL. Inject over at least 2 minutes.*

    Prepare _____ mL cimetidine

    Dilute with _____ mL 0.9% NaCl for a total of 20 mL of solution.

    Administer _____ mL/min or _____ mL per 15 sec

20. Order: **midazolam hydrochloride 1.5 mg IV push stat**

    Supply: midazolam hydrochloride 1 mg/mL

    Instructions: *Slowly titrate to the desired effect using no more than 1.5 mg initially given over 2-min period.*

    Prepare _____ mL midazolam hydro-chloride

    Give _____ mL/min or _____ mL per 15 sec

After completing these problems, see pages 560–561 to check your answers.

CALCULATING IV INFUSION TIME

Intravenous solutions are usually ordered to be administered at a prescribed number of milliliters per hour, such as **Lactated Ringer's 1,000 mL IV to run at 125 mL/h.** You may need to calculate the total infusion time so that you can anticipate when to add a new bag or bottle or when to discontinue the IV.

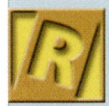

RULE

To calculate IV infusion time:

$$\frac{\text{Total volume}}{\text{mL/h}} = \text{Total hours}$$

Or use ratio-proportion: Ratio for prescribed flow rate in mL/h = Ratio for total mL per X total hours

$$\frac{\text{mL}}{\text{h}} = \frac{\text{Total mL}}{\text{X Total h}}$$

EXAMPLE 1 ■

LR 1,000 mL IV to run at 125 mL/h. How long will this IV last?

$$\frac{\overset{8}{\cancel{1,000}\text{ mL}}}{\underset{1}{\cancel{125}\text{ mL/h}}} = 8\text{ h}$$

Or, use ratio-proportion.

$$\frac{125\text{ mL}}{1\text{ h}} \times \frac{1,000\text{ mL}}{X\text{ h}}$$

$$125X = 1,000$$

$$\frac{125X}{125} = \frac{1,000}{125}$$

$$X = 8\text{ h}$$

MATH TIP

Use fractions for hours that are not whole numbers. They are more exact than decimals, which often have to be rounded. Rounded decimals are harder to use for time.

EXAMPLE 2 ■

D₅W 1,000 mL IV to infuse at 60 mL/h to begin at 0600. At what time will this IV be complete?

$$\frac{1,000 \text{ mL}}{60 \text{ mL/h}} = 16.6 \text{ h} = 16\frac{2}{3} \text{ h}; \frac{2}{3} \text{ h} \times 60 \text{ min/h} = 40 \text{ min}; \text{ Total time: 16 h and 40 min}$$

Or, use ratio-proportion:

$$\frac{60 \text{ mL}}{1 \text{ h}} \quad \times \quad \frac{1,000 \text{ mL}}{\text{X h}}$$

$$60 \text{ X} = 1,000$$

$$\frac{60\text{X}}{60} = \frac{1,000}{60}$$

$$X = 16.6 \text{ h} = 16\frac{2}{3} \text{ h} = 16 \text{ h and 40 min}$$

The IV will be complete at $0600 + 1640 = 2240$ (or 10:40 PM).

You can also determine the infusion time if you know the volume, flow rate in gtt/min, and drop factor. Calculate the infusion time by using the $\frac{V}{T} \times C = R$ formula; T, time in minutes, is unknown.

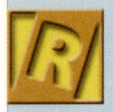

RULE

Use the formula method to calculate time (T):

$$\frac{V}{T} \times C = R$$

EXAMPLE ■

D₅W 80 mL IV at 20 microdrops/min

The drop factor is 60 gtt/mL. Calculate the infusion time.

Step 1 $\quad \frac{V}{T} \times C = R: \frac{80 \text{ mL}}{\text{T min}} \times 60 \text{ gtt/mL} = 20 \text{ gtt/min}$

$$\frac{80 \text{ mL}}{\text{T min}} \times \frac{60 \text{ gtt}}{1 \text{ mL}} = \frac{20 \text{ gtt}}{1 \text{ min}}$$

$$\frac{4,800 \text{ gtt}}{\text{T min}} = \frac{20 \text{ gtt}}{1 \text{ min}}$$

Then you apply ratio-proportion.

$$\frac{4,800}{\text{T}} \quad \times \quad \frac{20}{1}$$

$$20\text{T} = 4,800$$

$$\frac{20\text{T}}{20} = \frac{4,800}{20}$$

$$\text{T} = 240 \text{ min}$$

Step 2 Convert minutes to hours

$$\frac{1 \text{ h}}{60 \text{ min}} \quad \times \quad \frac{\text{X h}}{240 \text{ min}}$$

$$60 \text{ X} = 240$$

$$\frac{60 \text{ X}}{60} = \frac{240}{60}$$

$$\text{X} = 4 \text{ h}$$

Or, simply divide 240 by 60.

$$240 \text{ min} \div 60 \text{ min/h} = 4 \text{ h}$$

CALCULATING IV FLUID VOLUME

If you have an IV that is regulated at a particular flow rate (gtt/min) and you know the drop factor (gtt/mL) and the amount of time, you can determine the volume to be infused.

Apply the flow rate formula; V, volume, is unknown.

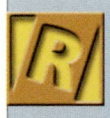

RULE

To calculate IV volume (V):

$$\frac{V}{T} \times C = R$$

EXAMPLE ■

When you start your shift at 7 AM, there is an IV bag of D_5W infusing at the rate of 25 gtt/min. The infusion set is calibrated for a drop factor of 15 gtt/mL. How much can you anticipate that the patient will receive during your 8 hour shift?

$$8 \text{ h} \times 60 \text{ min/h} = 480 \text{ min}$$

$$\frac{V}{T} \times C = R: \frac{V \text{ mL}}{480 \text{ min}} \times 15 \text{ gtt/mL} = 25 \text{ gtt/min}$$

$$\frac{V \text{ mL}}{480 \text{ min}} \times \frac{15 \text{ gtt}}{1 \text{ mL}} = \frac{25 \text{ gtt}}{1 \text{ min}}$$

$$\frac{15V \text{ gtt}}{480 \text{ min}} = \frac{25 \text{ gtt}}{1 \text{ min}}$$

$$\frac{15V}{480} \diagdown \frac{25}{1}$$

$$15V = 12{,}000$$

$$\frac{15V}{15} = \frac{12{,}000}{15}$$

$$V = 800 \text{ mL (to be infused in 8 h)}$$

If the IV is regulated in mL/h, you can also calculate the total volume that will infuse over a specific time.

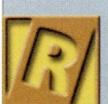

RULE

To calculate IV volume:

Total hours × mL/h = Total volume

Or use ratio-proportion: Ratio for ordered mL/h = Ratio for X total volume per total hours

$$\frac{mL}{h} = \frac{X \text{ Total mL}}{\text{Total h}}$$

EXAMPLE ■

Your patient's IV is running on an infusion pump set at the rate of 100 mL/h. How much will be infused during the next 8 hours?

$$8 \text{ h} \times 100 \text{ mL/h} = 800 \text{ mL}$$

Or, use ratio-proportion:

$$\frac{100 \text{ mL}}{1 \text{ h}} \diagdown \frac{X \text{ mL}}{8 \text{ h}}$$

$$X = 800 \text{ mL}$$

QUICK REVIEW

- The formula to calculate IV infusion time, when mL is known:

$$\frac{\text{Total volume}}{\text{mL/h}} = \text{Total hours}$$

or use ratio-proportion: $\frac{\text{mL}}{\text{h}} = \frac{\text{Total mL}}{\text{X total h}}$

- The formula to calculate IV infusion time, when flow rate in gtt/min, drop factor, and volume are known: $\frac{V}{T} \times C = R$; T is the unknown.

- The formula to calculate total infusion volume, when mL/h are known:

Total hours $\times$ mL/h = Total volume

Or, use ratio-proportion: $\frac{\text{mL}}{\text{h}} = \frac{\text{X total mL}}{\text{Total h}}$

- The formula to calculate IV volume, when flow rate (gtt/min), drop factor, and time are known:

$\frac{V}{T} \times C = R$; V is the unknown.

Review Set 41

Calculate the infusion time and rate (as requested) for the following IV orders:

1. Order: **D₅W 500 mL IV at 30 gtt/min**

   Drop factor: 20 gtt/mL

   Time: _____ h and _____ min

2. Order: **Lactated Ringer's 1,000 mL IV at 25 gtt/min**

   Drop factor: 10 gtt/mL

   Time: _____ h and _____ min

3. Order: **D₅ Lactated Ringer's 800 mL IV at 25 gtt/min**

   Drop factor: 15 gtt/mL

   Time: _____ h

4. Order: **Normal Saline 120 mL IV to run at 20 mL/h**

   Drop factor: 60 microdrops/mL

   Time: _____ h

   Flow rate: _____ gtt/min

5. Order: **D₅W 80 mL IV to run at 20 mL/h**

   Drop factor: 60 microdrops/mL

   Time: _____ h

   Flow rate: _____ gtt/min

Calculate the completion time for the following IVs.

6. At 1600 hours the nurse started **D₅W 1,200 mL IV at 27 gtt/min.** The infusion set used is calibrated for a drop factor of 15 gtt/mL.

   Infusion time: _____ h

   Completion time: _____

7. At 1530 hours the nurse starts **D₅W 2,000 mL IV to run at 125 mL/h.** The infusion set used is calibrated for a drop factor of 10 gtt/mL.

   Infusion time: _____ h

   Completion time: _____

Calculate the total volume (mL) to be infused per 24 hours.

8. An IV of D_5 Lactated Ringer's is infusing on an electronic infusion pump at 125 mL/h.

   Total volume: _____ mL per 24 h

9. An IV is flowing at 12 gtt/min and the infusion set has a drop factor of 15 gtt/mL.

   Total volume: _____ mL per 24 h

10. An IV of D_5W is flowing at 21 gtt/min and the infusion set has a drop factor of 10 gtt/mL.

    Total volume: _____ mL per 24 h

Calculate total volume and time (if requested) for the following IV orders.

11. Order: *0.9% sodium chloride IV infusing at 65 mL/h for 4 h*

    Volume: _____ mL

12. Order: *D_5W IV infusing at 150 mL/h for 2 h*

    Volume: _____ mL

13. Order: *D_5LR IV at 75 mL/h for 8 h*

    Volume: _____ mL

14. Order: *D_5 0.225% NaCl IV at 40 gtt/min for 8 h*

    Drop factor: 60 gtt/mL

    Infusion time: _____ min

    Volume: _____ mL

15. Order: *0.45% NaCl IV at 45 gtt/min for 4 h*

    Drop factor: 20 gtt/mL

    Infusion time: _____ min

    Volume: _____ mL

After completing these problems, see pages 561–562 to check your answers.

CRITICAL THINKING SKILLS

Drug reference guides provide recommendations for the rate at which IV push medications should be administered. Nurses should calculate the volume to be administered over short intervals of time to prevent the medication from being administered too quickly. If the volume of medication is very small, it may need to be diluted further to give the nurse more control over the rate.

ERROR

Not being able to push the plunger of a syringe slowly enough and administering an IV push medication too rapidly.

Possible Scenario

A patient who had recently undergone abdominal surgery was complaining of severe incisional pain. The postoperative orders included **hydromorphone 1 mg IV slow push q.2h for moderate to severe pain.** The supply of hydromorphone available on the surgical unit was 2 mg/mL. The nurse correctly calculated the dose and drew up 0.5 mL into a 3 mL syringe. According to a drug reference guide, it is recommended that the solution be diluted with at least 5 mL of sterile water or 0.9% NaCl for injection and administered slowly at a rate not to exceed 2 mg over 3 to 5 minutes. The nurse did not review the administration guidelines but did intend to give the medication as slowly as possible. Unfortunately, when administering the medication, the plunger moved too quickly, infusing the entire 0.5 mL dose immediately. The nurse was very concerned and remained with the patient for 10 minutes to assess for any adverse effects. The patient felt relief of pain, fell asleep, and did not display any notable adverse consequences.

Potential Outcome

Hydromorphone is an opioid analgesic and is considered a high-alert drug. Two potential serious adverse effects include respiratory depression and confusion. Infusing an IV push medication too rapidly places the patient at greater risk for these serious and other adverse effects.

Prevention

The nurse would have had more control if the volume of solution in the syringe was larger. The 3 mL syringe will not hold a volume of 5 mL and most larger syringes do not have a marking to accurately measure 0.5 mL. The medication can be diluted by first drawing up 0.5 mL of hydromorphone into a 1 mL or 3 mL syringe. Then, using a 10 mL syringe, the 5 mL of the recommended diluent can be drawn up. The needle may be removed and the plugger may be pulled back to leave at least 0.5 mL of air. The nurse can then add the small volume of hydromorphone into the larger syringe by inserting the needle of the smaller syringe directly into the barrel. The excess air should be removed, leaving the resulting 5.5 volume of diluted solution. A new sterile needle or protective cap should then be placed on the 10 mL syringe until it is inserted into the IV tubing. There will now be 5.5 mL to infuse over the recommended 3 to 5 minutes. In order to determine the minimum rate of the IV push injection, divide total volume (5.5 mL) by time (3 min) to calculate mL/min.

$$5.5 \text{ mL} \div 3 \text{ min} = 1.83 \text{ mL/min} = 1.8 \text{ mL/min}$$

The nurse may also push a slightly smaller amount per minute for the slower rate of 5 minutes.

$$5.5 \text{ mL} \div 5 \text{ min} = 1.1 \text{ mL/min}$$

Therefore, the nurse may safely administer the IV push dose of hydromorphone by using a watch and slowly injecting a diluted volume of 1.1 to 1.8 mL (approximately 1 to 2 mL) per min or 0.275 to 0.45 mL (approximately 0.3 to 0.5 mL) per 15 sec.

CRITICAL THINKING SKILLS

It is important to know the equipment you are using. Let's look at an example in which the nurse was unfamiliar with the IV PB setup.

ERROR

Failing to follow manufacturer's directions when using a new IV PB system.

Possible Scenario

Suppose the physician ordered *Rocephin* 1 *g* IV q.12h for an elderly patient with streptococcus pneumonia. The medication was sent to the unit by a pharmacy utilizing the ADD-Vantage system. Rocephin 1 gram was supplied in a powder form and attached to a 50 mL IV bag of D_5W. The directions for preparing the medication were attached to the label. The nurse assigned to the day shift, who was unfamiliar with the new ADD-Vantage system, hung the IV medication, calculated the drip rate, and infused the 50 mL of fluid. The nurse cared for the patient for 3 days. During walking rounds on the third day, the oncoming nurse noticed that the Rocephin powder remained in the vial and never was diluted in the IV bag. The nurse realized that the vial stopper inside of the IV bag was not open. Therefore, the medication powder was not mixed in the IV fluid during this shift for the past 3 days.

Potential Outcome

The omission by the nurse resulted in the patient missing 3 doses of the ordered IV antibiotic. The delay in the medication administration could have serious consequences for the patient, such as worsening of the pneumonia, septicemia, and even death, especially in the elderly. The patient received only one-half of the daily dosage ordered by the physician for 3 days. The physician would be notified of the error and likely order additional diagnostic studies, such as chest X-ray, blood cultures, and an additional one-time dose of Rocephin.

Prevention

This error could easily have been avoided had the nurse read the directions for preparing the medication or consulted with another nurse who was familiar with the system.

PRACTICE PROBLEMS—CHAPTER 15

Compute the flow rate in drops per minute or milliliters per hour as requested. For these situations, hospital policy permits recalculating IVs when off-schedule with a maximum variation in rate of 25 percent.

1. Order: Ampicillin 500 mg dissolved in 100 mL D_5W IV to run for 1 h

   Drop factor: 10 gtt/mL

   Flow rate: _____ gtt/min

2. Order: D_5W 1,000 mL IV per 24h

   Drop factor: 60 gtt/mL

   Flow rate: _____ gtt/min

3. Order: D_5LR 1,500 mL IV to run for 12 h

   Drop factor: 20 gtt/mL

   Flow rate: _____ gtt/min

4. Order: D_5RL 200 mL IV for 24 h

   Drop factor: 60 gtt/mL

   Flow rate: _____ gtt/min

5. Order: $D_{10}W$ 1 L IV to run from 1000 to 1800

   Drop factor: On electronic infusion pump

   Flow rate: _____ mL/h

6. See question 5. At 1100 there are 800 mL remaining. Describe your nursing action now. _____

   _____

7. Order: NS 1,000 mL followed by D_5W 2,000 mL IV to run for 24 h

   Drop factor: 15 gtt/mL

   Flow rate: _____ gtt/min

8. Order: NS 2.5 L IV to infuse at 125 mL/h

   Drop factor: 20 gtt/mL

   Flow rate: _____ gtt/min

9. Order: D_5W 1,000 mL IV for 6 h

   Drop factor: 15 gtt/mL

   After 2 hours, 800 mL remain. Describe your nursing action now. _____

   _____

The IV tubing package in the accompanying figure is the IV system available in your hospital for manually regulated, straight gravity flow IV administration with macrodrop. The patient has an order for D₅W 500 mL IV q.4h written at 1515, and you start the IV at 1530. Questions 10 through 20 refer to this situation.

Courtesy of Abbott Laboratories, Inc.

> a **LATEX-FREE**   No. 4967
>
> # PRIMARY I.V. SET,
> Convertible Pin, 80 Inch   15
> with Backcheck Valve   DROPS/mL
> and 2 Injection Sites
> **Piggyback**
>
> **Abbott Laboratories, Inc.**

10. How much IV fluid will the patient receive in 24 hours? _____ mL

11. Who is the manufacturer of the IV infusion set tubing? _____

12. What is the drop factor calibration for the IV infusion set tubing? _____

13. What is the drop factor constant for the IV infusion set tubing? _____

14. Using the shortcut (drop factor constant) method, calculate the flow rate of the IV as ordered. Show your work.

    Shortcut method calculation: _____

    Flow rate: _____ gtt/min

15. Using the formula method, calculate the flow rate of the IV as ordered. Show your work.

    Formula method calculation: _____

    Flow rate: _____ gtt/min

16. At what time should you anticipate the first IV bag of 500 mL D₅W will be completely infused?

    _____

17. How much IV fluid should be infused by 1730? _____ mL

18. At 1730 you notice that the IV has 210 mL remaining. After assessing your patient and confirming that his or her condition is stable, what should you do? _____

    _____

19. After consulting the physician, you decide to use an electronic infusion pump to better regulate the flow rate. The physician orders that the pump be set to infuse 500 mL every 4 hours. You should set the pump for _____ mL/h

20. The next day the physician adds the order Amoxicillin 250 mg in 50 mL D₅W IV PB to infuse in 30 min q.6h. The patient is still on the IV pump. To infuse the IV PB, set the pump for _____ mL/h

21. List the components and concentration strengths of the IV fluid $D_{2.5} \frac{1}{2}$ NS.

    _____

22. Calculate the amount of dextrose and sodium chloride in D₅NS 500 mL.

    dextrose _____ g

    NaCl _____ g

23. Define a central line. _____

_____

24. Define a primary line. _____

_____

25. Describe the purpose of a saline or heparin lock. _____

_____

26. A safe IV push infusion rate of protamine sulfate is 5 mg/min. What is a safe infusion time to administer 50 mg? _____ min

Protamine sulfate is available in a supply dosage of 10 mg/mL. To administer 50 mg IV push, prepare _____ mL and inject slowly IV at the rate of _____ mL/min or _____ mL per 15 sec.

27. Describe the purpose of the PCA pump. _____

_____

28. Identify two advantages of the syringe pump. _____

_____

29. List two complications of IV sites. _____

_____

30. How often should the IV site be monitored? _____

_____

31. Describe the purpose of the Y-set IV system. _____

_____

For each IV order in questions 32 through 47, use the drop factor to calculate the flow rate in gtt/min.

Order: D_5W 1 L IV to infuse in 12 h

32. Drop factor 10 gtt/mL   Flow rate: _____ gtt/min

33. Drop factor 15 gtt/mL   Flow rate: _____ gtt/min

34. Drop factor 20 gtt/mL   Flow rate: _____ gtt/min

35. Drop factor 60 gtt/mL   Flow rate: _____ gtt/min

Order: D_5NS 2 L IV to infuse in 20 h

36. Drop factor 10 gtt/mL   Flow rate: _____ gtt/min

37. Drop factor 15 gtt/mL   Flow rate: _____ gtt/min

38. Drop factor 20 gtt/mL   Flow rate: _____ gtt/min

39. Drop factor 60 gtt/mL   Flow rate: _____ gtt/min

Order: 0.45% NaCl 1,000 mL IV at 200 mL/h

40. Drop factor 10 gtt/mL   Flow rate: _____ gtt/min

41. Drop factor 15 gtt/mL   Flow rate: _____ gtt/min

42. Drop factor 20 gtt/mL   Flow rate: _____ gtt/min

43. Drop factor 60 gtt/mL   Flow rate: _____ gtt/min

Order: D₅ 0.9% NaCl 500 mL IV at 45 mL/h

44. Drop factor 10 gtt/mL   Flow rate: _____ gtt/min

45. Drop factor 15 gtt/mL   Flow rate: _____ gtt/min

46. Drop factor 20 gtt/mL   Flow rate: _____ gtt/min

47. Drop factor 60 gtt/mL   Flow rate: _____ gtt/min

48. You make rounds before your lunch break and find that a patient has 150 mL of IV fluid remaining. The flow rate is 25 gtt/min. The drop factor is 10 gtt/mL. What volume will be infused during the hour that you are at lunch? _____ mL
    What should you alert your relief nurse to watch for while you are off the unit? _____

    _____

49. Your shift is 0700 to 1500. You make rounds at 0730 and find an IV of D₅ 0.45% NaCl is regulated on an electronic infusion pump at the ordered rate of 75 mL/h with 400 mL remaining. The order specifies a continuous infusion. At what time should you anticipate hanging the next IV bag? _____

50. Describe the strategy you would implement to prevent this medication error.

    Possible Scenario
    Suppose the physician ordered D₅LR 1,000 mL IV at 125 mL/h for an elderly patient just returning from the OR following abdominal surgery. The nurse gathered the IV solution and IV tubing, which had a drop factor of 20 gtt/mL. The nurse did not check the package for the drop factor and assumed it was 60 gtt/mL. The manual rate was calculated this way:

    $$\frac{125 \text{ mL}}{60 \text{ min}} \times 60 \text{ gtt/mL} = 125 \text{ gtt/min} \quad \textbf{INCORRECT}$$

    The nurse infused the D₅LR at 125 gtt/min for 8 hours. During shift report, the patient called for the nurse, complaining of shortness of breath. On further assessment the nurse heard crackles in the patient's lungs and noticed that the patient's third 1,000 mL bottle of D₅LR this shift was nearly empty already. At this point the nurse realized the IV rate was in error. The nurse was accustomed to using the 60 gtt/mL IV set up and therefore calculated the drip rate using the 60 gtt/mL (microdrop) drop factor. However, the tubing used delivered 20 gtt/mL (macrodrop) drop factor. The nurse never looked at the drop factor on the IV set package and assumed it was a 60 gtt/mL set.

    Potential Outcome
    The patient developed signs of fluid overload and could have developed congestive heart failure due to the excessive IV rate. The physician would have been notified and likely ordered Lasix (a diuretic) to help eliminate the excess fluid. The patient likely would have been transferred to the ICU for closer monitoring.

    Prevention

    _____

    _____

Upon completion of these problems, see pages 562–564 to check your answers.

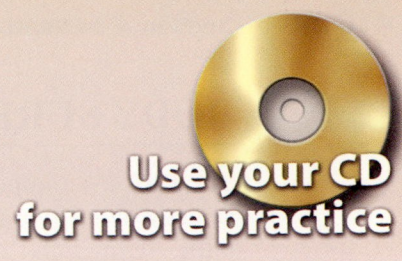
Use your CD for more practice

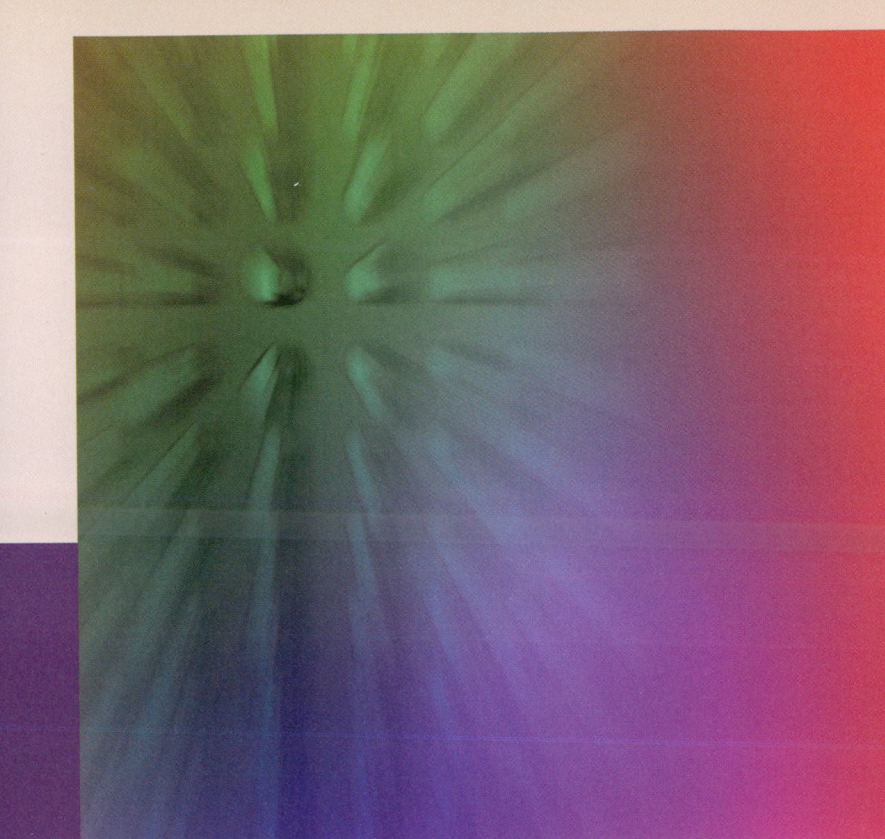

16

Body Surface Area and Advanced Pediatric Calculations

OBJECTIVES

Upon mastery of Chapter 16, you will be able to perform advanced calculations for children and apply these advanced concepts across the life span. To accomplish this you will also be able to:

- Determine the body surface area (BSA) using a calculation formula or a nomogram scale.
- Compute the safe amount of drug to be administered when ordered according to the BSA.
- Calculate intermittent intravenous (IV) medications administered with IV infusion control sets.
- Calculate the minimal and maximal dilution in which an IV medication can be safely prepared and delivered, such as via a syringe pump.
- Calculate pediatric IV maintenance fluids.

This chapter will focus on additional and more advanced calculations used frequently by pediatric nurses. It will help you understand the unique drug and fluid management required by a growing child. Further, these concepts, which are most commonly related to children, are also applied to adults in special situations. Let's start by looking at the BSA method of calculating a dosage and checking for accuracy and safety of a particular drug order.

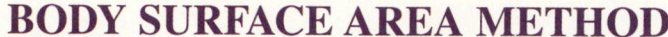

BODY SURFACE AREA METHOD

The BSA is an important measure in calculating dosages for infants and children. BSA is also used for selected adult populations, such as those undergoing open-heart surgery or radiation therapy, severe burn victims, and those with renal disease. Regardless of age, antineoplastic agents (chemotherapy drugs) and an increasing number of other highly potent drug classifications are being prescribed based on BSA.

BSA is a mathematical estimate using the patient's *height* and *weight*. BSA is expressed in square meters (**m²**). BSA can be determined by formula calculation or by using a chart, referred to as a *nomogram,* that estimates the BSA. Because drug dosages recommended by BSA measurement are potent, and because the formula calculation is the most accurate, we will begin with the formulas. In most situations, the prescribing practitioner will compute the BSA for drugs ordered by this method. However, the nurse who administers the drug is responsible for verifying safe dosage, which may require calculating the BSA.

BSA Formula

One BSA formula is based on metric measurement of height in centimeters and weight in kilograms. The other is based on household measurement of height in inches and weight in pounds. Either is easy to compute using the square root function on a calculator. BSA calculators are also readily available on the Internet.

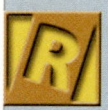

RULE

To calculate BSA in m² based on metric measurement of height and weight:

- $\text{BSA (m}^2) = \sqrt{\dfrac{\text{ht (cm)} \times \text{wt (kg)}}{3{,}600}}$

To calculate BSA in m² based on household measurement of height and weight:

- $\text{BSA (m}^2) = \sqrt{\dfrac{\text{ht (in)} \times \text{wt (lb)}}{3{,}131}}$

Let's apply both formulas, and see how the BSA measurements compare.

MATH TIP

Notice that in addition to metric versus household measurement, the other difference between the two BSA formulas is in the denominators of the fraction within the square root sign.

EXAMPLE 1 ■

Use the metric formula to calculate the BSA of an infant whose length is 50 cm (20 in) and weight is 3.2 kg (7 lb).

$$\text{BSA (m}^2) = \sqrt{\dfrac{\text{ht (cm)} \times \text{wt (kg)}}{3{,}600}} = \sqrt{\dfrac{50 \times 3.2}{3{,}600}} = \sqrt{\dfrac{160}{3{,}600}} = \sqrt{0.044\ldots} = 0.210 = 0.21 \text{ m}^2$$

MATH TIP

To perform BSA calculations using the metric formula on most calculators, follow this sequence: multiply height in cm by weight in kg, divide by 3,600, press =, then press $\sqrt{}$ to arrive at m². Round m² to hundredths (two decimal places). For Example 1, enter 50 × 3.2 ÷ 3,600 = 0.044..., and press $\sqrt{}$ to arrive at 0.210, rounded to 0.21 m².

Or use the BSA formula based on household measurement.

$$\text{BSA (m}^2) = \sqrt{\frac{\text{ht (in)} \times \text{wt (lb)}}{3{,}131}} = \sqrt{\frac{20 \times 7}{3{,}131}} = \sqrt{\frac{140}{3{,}131}} = \sqrt{0.044...} = 0.211 = 0.21 \text{ m}^2$$

MATH TIP

To use the calculator, follow this sequence: multiply height in inches by weight in pounds, divide by 3131, press =, then press $\sqrt{}$ to arrive at the m². Round m² to hundredths (two decimal places). For Example 1, enter 20 × 7 ÷ 3,131 = 0.044..., and press $\sqrt{}$ to arrive at 0.211, rounded to 0.21 m².

EXAMPLE 2 ▪

Calculate the BSA of a child whose height is 105 cm (42 inches) and weight is 31.8 kg (70 lb).

Metric:

$$\text{BSA (m}^2) = \sqrt{\frac{\text{ht (cm)} \times \text{wt (kg)}}{3{,}600}} = \sqrt{\frac{105 \times 31.8}{3{,}600}} = \sqrt{\frac{3{,}339}{3{,}600}} = \sqrt{0.927...} = 0.963 \text{ m}^2 = 0.96 \text{ m}^2$$

Household:

$$\text{BSA (m}^2) = \sqrt{\frac{\text{ht (in)} \times \text{wt (lb)}}{3{,}131}} = \sqrt{\frac{42 \times 70}{3{,}131}} = \sqrt{\frac{2{,}940}{3{,}131}} = \sqrt{0.938...} = 0.969 \text{ m}^2 = 0.97 \text{ m}^2$$

MATH TIP

There is a slight variation in m² calculated by the metric and household methods because of the rounding used to convert centimeters and inches; 1 in = 2.54 cm, which is rounded to 2.5 cm. The results of the two methods are practically equivalent.

EXAMPLE 3 ▪

Calculate the BSA of an adult whose height is 173 cm (69 inches) and weight is 88.6 kg (195 lb).

Metric:

$$\text{BSA (m}^2) = \sqrt{\frac{\text{ht (cm)} \times \text{wt (kg)}}{3{,}600}} = \sqrt{\frac{173 \times 88.6}{3{,}600}} = \sqrt{\frac{15{,}327.8}{3{,}600}} = \sqrt{4.257...} = 2.063 \text{ m}^2 = 2.06 \text{ m}^2$$

Household:

$$\text{BSA (m}^2) = \sqrt{\frac{\text{ht (in)} \times \text{wt (lb)}}{3{,}131}} = \sqrt{\frac{69 \times 195}{3{,}131}} = \sqrt{\frac{13{,}455}{3{,}131}} = \sqrt{4.297...} = 2.073 \text{ m}^2 = 2.07 \text{ m}^2$$

These examples show that either metric or household measurements of height and weight result in essentially the same calculated BSA value.

BSA Nomogram

Some practitioners use a chart called a *nomogram* that *estimates* the BSA by plotting the height and weight and simply connecting the dots with a straight line. Figure 16-1 shows the most well-known BSA chart, the West Nomogram (Kliegman, Behrman, Jenson, & Stanton, 2007). It is used for both children and adults for heights up to 240 cm and 90 inches and weights up to 80 kg and 180 lb.

CAUTION

Notice that the increments of measurement and the spaces on the BSA nomogram are not consistent. Be sure you correctly read the numbers and the calibration values between them.

FIGURE 16-1   Body surface area (BSA) is determined by drawing a straight line from the patient's height (1) in the far left column to his or her weight (2) in the far right column. Intersection of the line with surface area (SA) column (3) is the estimated BSA (m²). For infants and children of normal height and weight, BSA may be estimated from weight alone by referring to the enclosed area.

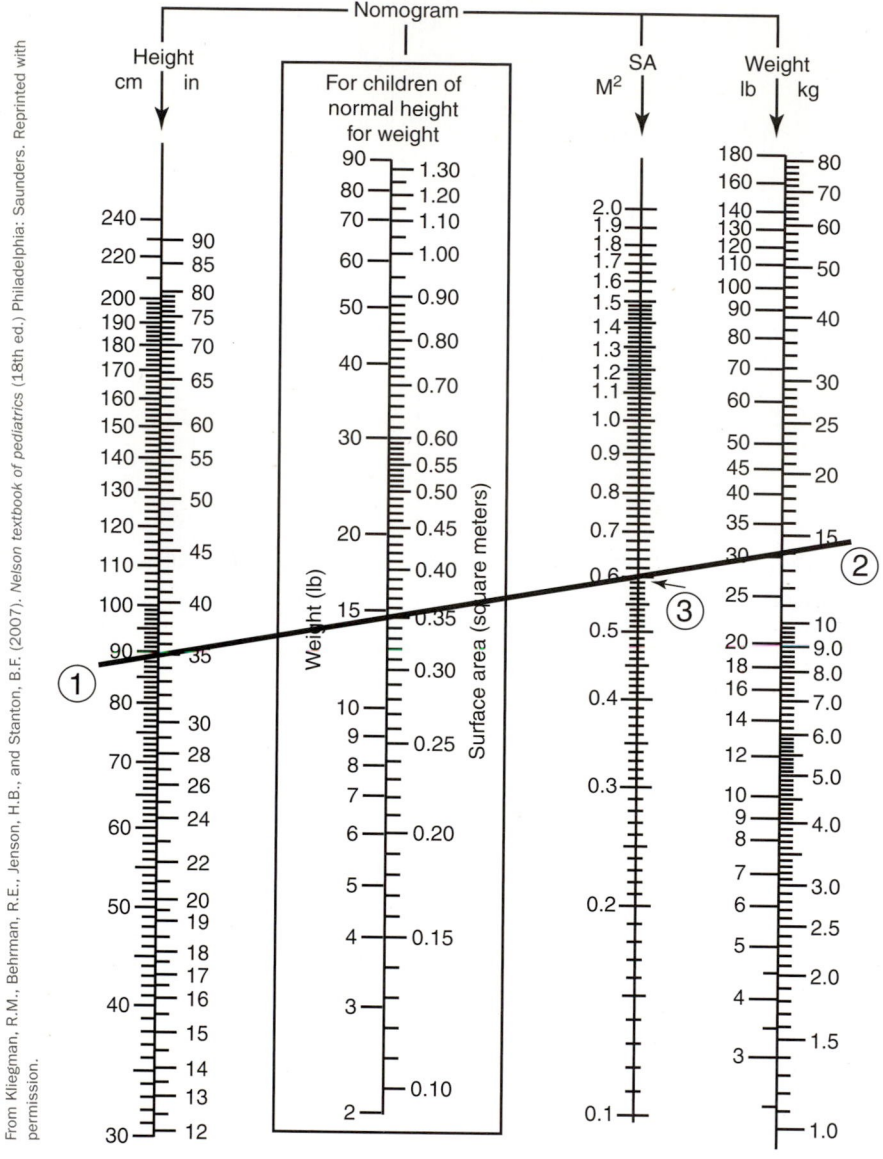

From Kliegman, R.M., Behrman, R.E., Jenson, H.B., and Stanton, B.F. (2007). *Nelson textbook of pediatrics* (18th ed.) Philadelphia: Saunders. Reprinted with permission.

For a child of normal height for weight, the BSA can be determined on the West Nomogram using the weight alone. Notice the enclosed column to the center left. Normal height and weight standards can be found on pediatric growth and development charts.

CAUTION

To use the normal column on the West Nomogram, you must be familiar with normal height and weight standards for children. If you are unsure, use both height and weight to estimate BSA. Do not guess.

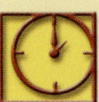

QUICK REVIEW

- BSA is used to calculate select dosages across the life span, most often for children.

- BSA is calculated by height and weight and expressed in m².

- The following metric and household formulas are the preferred methods of calculating BSA:

Metric: BSA (m²) = $\sqrt{\dfrac{ht\ (cm) \times wt\ (kg)}{3,600}}$

Household: BSA (m²) = $\sqrt{\dfrac{ht\ (in) \times wt\ (lb)}{3,131}}$

- Nomograms can be used to estimate BSA, by correlating height and weight measures to m².

Review Set 42

Use the formula method to determine the BSA. Round to 2 decimal places.

1. A child measures 36 inches tall and weighs 40 lb. _____ m²

2. An adult measures 190 cm tall and weighs 105 kg. _____ m²

3. A child measures 94 cm tall and weighs 18 kg. _____ m²

4. A teenager measures 153 cm tall and weighs 46 kg. _____ m²

5. An adult measures 175 cm tall and weighs 85 kg. _____ m²

6. A child measures 41 inches tall and weighs 76 lb. _____ m²

7. An adult measures 62 inches tall and weighs 140 lb. _____ m²

8. A child measures 28 inches tall and weighs 18 lb. _____ m²

9. A teenager measures 160 cm tall and weighs 64 kg. _____ m²

10. A child measures 65 cm tall and weighs 15 kg. _____ m²

11. A child measures 55 inches tall and weighs 70 lb. _____ m²

12. A child measures 92 cm tall and weighs 24 kg. _____ m²

Find the BSA on the West Nomogram (Figure 16-1) for a child of normal height and weight.

13. 4 lb _____ m²   14. 42 lb _____ m²   15. 17 lb _____ m²

Find the BSA on the West Nomogram (Figure 16-1) for children with the following height and weight.

16. 41 inches and 32 lb _____ m²

17. 21 inches and 8 lb _____ m²

18. 140 cm and 30 kg _____ m²

19. 80 cm and 11 kg _____ m²

20. 106 cm and 25 kg _____ m²

After completing these problems, see page 565 to check your answers.

BSA Dosage Calculations

Once the BSA is obtained, the drug dosage can be verified by consulting a reputable drug resource for the recommended dosage. Package inserts, the *Hospital Formulary,* or other dosage handbooks contain pediatric and adults dosages. Remember to carefully read the reference to verify if the drug dosage is calculated in *m² per dose* or *m² per day.*

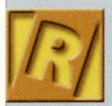

RULE

To verify safe pediatric dosage based on BSA:

1. Determine BSA in m².

2. Calculate the safe dosage based on **BSA: mg/m² × m² = X mg**

3. Compare the ordered dosage to the recommended dosage, and decide if the dosage is safe.

4. If the dosage is safe, calculate the amount to give and administer the dose. If the dosage seems unsafe, consult with the ordering practitioner before administering the drug.

Note: Recommended dosage may specify mg/m², mcg/m², g/m², units/m², milliunits/m², or mEq/m².

EXAMPLE 1 ▰

A child is 126 cm tall and weighs 23 kg. The drug order reads: **Vincasar 1.8 mg IV at 10 AM.** Is this dosage safe for this child? The recommended dosage as noted on the package insert is 2 mg/m². Supply: See label, Figure 16-2.

1. **Determine BSA.** The child's BSA is 0.9 m² (using the metric BSA formula).

$$\text{BSA (m}^2) = \sqrt{\frac{\text{ht (cm)} \times \text{wt (kg)}}{3{,}600}} = \sqrt{\frac{126 \times 23}{3{,}600}} = \sqrt{\frac{2{,}898}{3{,}600}} = \sqrt{0.805} = 0.897 \text{ m}^2 = 0.9 \text{ m}^2$$

2. **Calculate recommended dosage.** mg/m² × m² = 2 mg/m² × 0.9 m² = 1.8 mg

3. **Decide if the dosage is safe.** The dosage ordered is 1.8 mg and 1.8 mg is the amount recommended by BSA. The dosage is safe. How much should you give?

4. **Calculate 1 dose.**

Step 1   **Convert**   No conversion is necessary.

Step 2   **Think**   You want to give more than 1 mL and less than 2 mL. At 1 mg per mL, it is obvious you want to give 1.8 mL.

Step 3   **Calculate**
$$\frac{\text{Dosage on hand}}{\text{Amount on hand}} = \frac{\text{Dosage desired}}{\text{X Amount desired}}$$

$$\frac{1 \text{ mg}}{1 \text{ mL}} \diagdown\!\!\!\!\!\diagup \frac{1.8 \text{ mg}}{\text{X mL}}$$

$$X = 1.8 \text{ mL}$$

FIGURE 16-2   Vincasar 1 mg/mL label

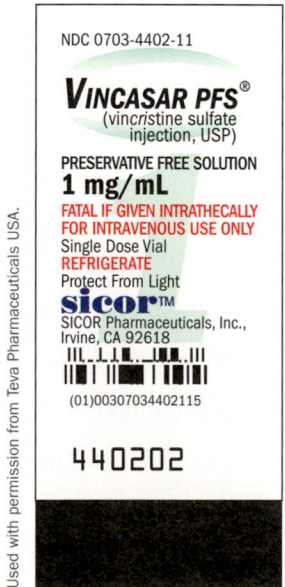

NDC 0703-4402-11

VINCASAR PFS®
(vincristine sulfate injection, USP)

PRESERVATIVE FREE SOLUTION
1 mg/mL
FATAL IF GIVEN INTRATHECALLY
FOR INTRAVENOUS USE ONLY
Single Dose Vial
REFRIGERATE
Protect From Light

sicor™
SICOR Pharmaceuticals, Inc.,
Irvine, CA 92618

(01)00307034402115

440202

Used with permission from Teva Pharmaceuticals USA.

EXAMPLE 2 ■

A 2-year-old child with herpes simplex is 35 inches tall and weighs 30 lb. The drug order reads *acyclovir 100 mg IV b.i.d.* Is this order safe? The drug reference recommends 250 mg/m² q.8h for children younger than 12 years and older than 6 months. Acyclovir is supplied as Zovirax 500 mg injection with directions to reconstitute with 10 mL sterile water for injection for a concentration of 50 mg/mL.

1. **Determine BSA.** The child's BSA is 0.6 m² (using the West Nomogram, Figure 16-1).

2. **Calculate recommended dosage.** mg/m² × m² = 250 mg/m² × 0.6 m² = 150 mg

3. **Decide if the dosage is safe.** The dosage of 100 mg b.i.d. is not safe—the single dosage is too low. Further, the drug should be administered 3 times per day q.8h, not b.i.d. or 2 times per day.

4. **Confer with the prescriber.**

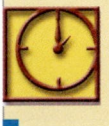

QUICK REVIEW

Safe dosage based on BSA: mg/m² × m², compared to recommended dosage.

Review Set 43

1. What is the dosage of 1 dose of interferon alpha-2b required for a child with a BSA of 0.82 m² if the recommended dosage is 2 million units/m²? _____ units

2. What is the total daily dosage range of mitomycin required for a child with a BSA of 0.59 m² if the recommended dosage range is 10 to 20 mg/m²/day? _____ mg/day to _____ mg/day

3. What is the dosage of calcium EDTA required for an adult with a BSA of 1.47 m² if the recommended dosage is 500 mg/m²? _____ mg

4. What is the total daily dosage of thiotepa required for a adult with a BSA of 2.64 m² if the recommended dosage is 6 mg/m²/day? _____ mg. After 4 full days of therapy, this patient will have received a total of _____ mg of thiotepa.

5. What is the dosage of acyclovir required for a child with a BSA of 1 m² if the recommended dosage is 250 mg/m²? _____ mg

6. Child is 30 inches tall and weighs 25 pounds.

   Order: **Zovirax 122.5 mg IV q.8h**

   Supply: Zovirax 500 mg with directions to reconstitute with 10 mL sterile water for injection for a final concentration of 50 mg/mL.

   Recommended dosage from drug insert: 250 mg/m²

   BSA = _____ m²

   Recommended dosage for this child: _____ mg

   Is the ordered dosage safe? _____

   If safe, give _____ mL

   If not safe, what should you do? _____

7. Child is 45 inches tall and weighs 55 pounds.

   Order: **methotrexate 2.9 mg IV daily**

Supply: methotrexate 2.5 mg/mL

Recommended dosage from drug insert: 3.3 mg/m²

BSA = _____ m²

Recommended dosage for this child: _____ mg

Is the ordered dosage safe? _____

If safe, give _____ mL

If not safe, what should you do? _____

8. Order: **Benoject 22 mg IV q.8h.** Child has BSA of 0.44 m². Recommended safe dosage of Benoject is 150 mg/m²/day in divided dosages every 6 to 8 hours.

   Recommended daily dosage for this child: _____ mg/day

   Recommended single dosage for this child: _____ mg/dose

   Is the ordered dosage safe? _____

   If not safe, what should you do? _____

9. Order: **quinidine 198 mg p.o. daily for 5 days.** Child has BSA of 0.22 m². Recommended safe dosage of quinidine is 900 mg/m²/day given in 5 daily doses.

   Recommended dosage for this child: _____ mg/dose

   Is the dosage ordered safe? _____

   If not safe, what should you do? _____

   How much quinidine would this child receive over 5 days of therapy? _____ mg

10. Order: **deferoxamine mesylate IV per protocol.** Child has BSA of 1.02 m².

    Protocol: 600 mg/m² initially followed by 300 mg/m² at 4-hour intervals for 2 doses; then give 300 mg/m² q.12 h for 2 days. Calculate the total dosage received.

    Initial dosage: _____ mg

    Total for two q.4h dosages: _____ mg

    Total for 2 days of q.12h dosages: _____ mg

    Total dosage child would receive: _____ mg

11. Protocol: **Fludara 10 mg/m² bolus over 15 minutes followed by a continuous IV infusion of 30.5 mg/m²/day.** Child has BSA of 0.81 m². The bolus dosage is _____ mg, and the continuous 24-hour IV infusion will contain _____ mg of Fludara.

12. Order: **isotretinoin 83.75 mg IV q.12h** for a child with a BSA of 0.67 m². The recommended dosage range is 100 to 250 mg/m²/day in 2 divided doses.

    Recommended daily dosage range for this child: _____ mg/day to _____ mg/day

    Recommended single dosage range for this child: _____ mg/dose to _____ mg/dose

    Is the ordered dosage safe? _____

    If not, what should you do? _____

13. Order: **Cerubidine 9.6 mg IV on day 1 and day 8 of cycle.**

    Protocol: 25 to 45 mg/m² on days 1 and 8 of cycle. Child has BSA of 0.32 m².

    Recommended dosage range for this child: _____ mg/dose to _____ mg/dose

    Is the ordered dosage safe? _____

If not safe, what should you do? _____

Answer questions 14 and 15 based on the following information.

The recommended dosage of Oncaspar is 2,500 units/m²/dose IV daily × 14 days for adults and children with a BSA > 0.6 m².

Supply: Oncaspar 750 units/mL with directions to dilute in 100 mL D_5W and give over 2 hours. You will administer the drug via infusion pump.

14. Order: **Give Oncaspar 2,050 units IV today at 1600.** Child is 100 cm tall and weighs 24 kg. The child's BSA is _____ m².

    The recommended dosage for this child is _____ units. Is the ordered dosage of Oncaspar safe? _____

    If yes, add _____ mL of Oncaspar for a total IV fluid volume of _____ mL. Set the IV infusion pump at _____ mL/h.

    If the order is not safe, what should you do? _____

15. Order: **Oncaspar 4,050 units IV stat** for an adult patient who is 162 cm tall and weighs 58.2 kg. The patient's BSA is _____ m². The recommended dosage of Oncaspar for this adult is _____ units.

    Is the ordered dosage of Oncaspar safe? _____

    If safe, you would add _____ mL of Oncaspar for a total IV fluid volume of _____ mL. Set the infusion pump at _____ mL/h.

    If the order is not safe, what should you do? _____

After completing these problems, see page 565 to check your answers.

PEDIATRIC VOLUME CONTROL SETS

Volume control sets (Figure 16-3) are most frequently used to administer hourly fluids and intermittent IV medications to children. The fluid chamber will hold 100 to 150 milliliters of fluid to be infused in a specified time period as ordered, usually 60 minutes or less. The medication is added to the IV fluid in the chamber for a prescribed dilution volume.

The volume of fluid in the chamber is filled by the nurse every 1 to 2 hours or as needed. Only small, prescribed quantities of fluid are added, and the clamp above the chamber is fully closed. The IV bag acts only as a reservoir to hold future fluid infusions. The patient is protected from receiving more volume than intended. This is especially important for children because they can tolerate only a narrow range of fluid volume. This differs from standard IV infusions that run directly from the IV bag through the drip chamber and IV tubing into the patient's vein.

Volume control sets may also be used to administer intermittent IV medications to adults with fluid restrictions, such as for heart or kidney disease. An electronic controller or pump may also be used to regulate the flow rate. When used, the electronic device will alarm when the chamber empties.

Intermittent IV Medication Infusion via Volume Control Set

Children receiving IV medications may have a saline or heparin lock in place of a continuous IV infusion. The nurse will inject the medication into the volume control set chamber, add an appropriate volume of IV fluid to dilute the drug, and attach the IV tubing to the child's IV lock to infuse over a specified period of time. Realize that when the chamber empties, some medication still remains in the drip chamber, IV tubing, and the IV lock above the child's vein. After the chamber has emptied and the medication has infused, a flush of IV fluid is given to be sure all the medication has cleared the tubing. There is no standard amount of fluid used to flush peripheral or central IV lines. Because tubing varies

FIGURE 16-3 Volume control set

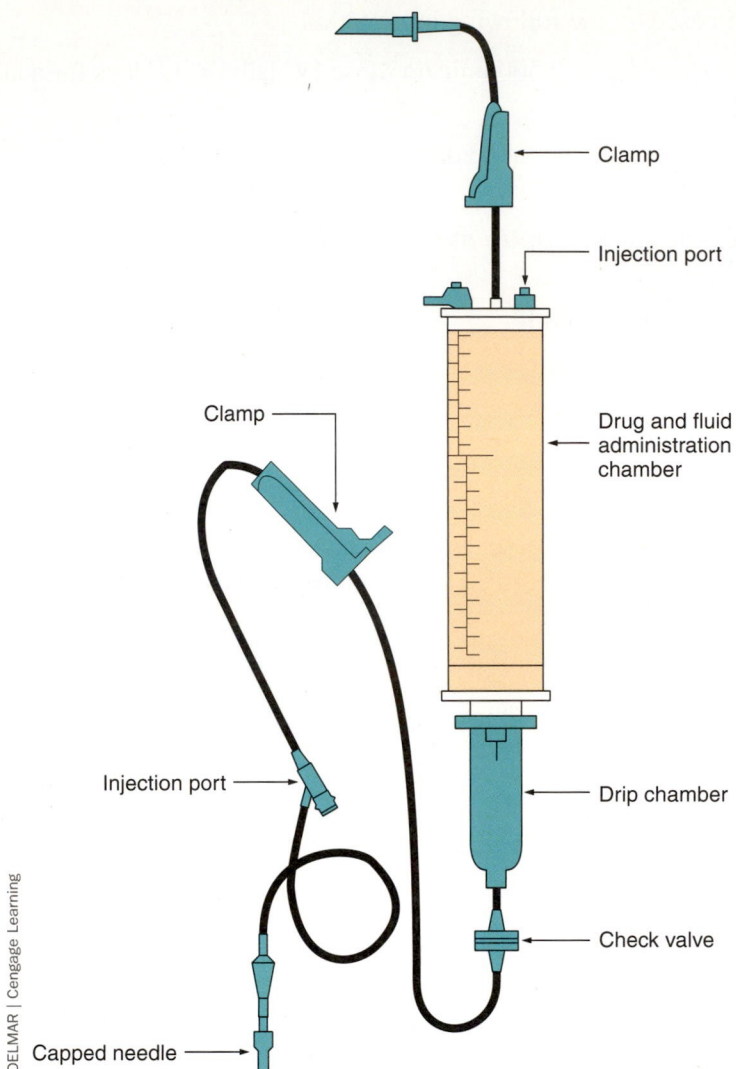

Clamp

Injection port

Clamp

Drug and fluid administration chamber

Injection port

Drip chamber

Check valve

Capped needle

DELMAR | Cengage Learning

by manufacturer, the flush can vary from 15 mL to as much as 50 mL, according to the overall length of the tubing and extra extensions added. Verify your hospital policy on the correct volume to flush peripheral and central IV lines in children. For the purpose of sample calculations, this text uses a 15 mL volume to flush a peripheral IV line, unless specified otherwise.

To calculate the IV flow rate for the volume control set, you must consider the total fluid volume of the medication, the IV fluid used for dilution, and the volume of IV flush fluid. Volume control sets are microdrip sets with a drop factor of 60 gtt/mL.

EXAMPLE ■

Order: *Claforan 250 mg IV q.6h in 50 mL $D_5\frac{1}{4}NS$ to infuse in 30 min followed by a 15 mL flush.* Child has a saline lock.

Supply: See label (Figure 16-4)

Instructions from package insert for IV use: Add 10 mL diluent for a total volume of 11 mL with a concentration of 180 mg/mL.

FIGURE 16-4 Claforan 2 g label

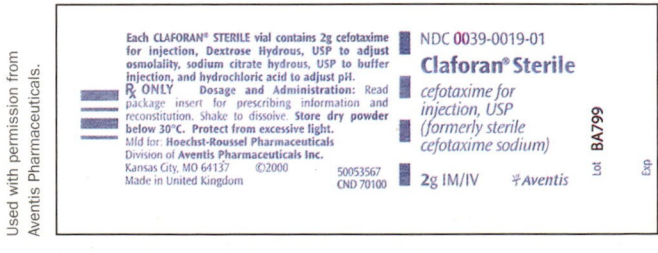

Each CLAFORAN® STERILE vial contains 2g cefotaxime for injection, Dextrose Hydrous, USP to adjust osmolality, sodium citrate hydrous, USP to buffer injection, and hydrochloric acid to adjust pH.
℞ ONLY Dosage and Administration: Read package insert for prescribing information and reconstitution. Shake to dissolve. **Store dry powder below 30°C. Protect from excessive light.**
Mfd for: Hoechst-Roussel Pharmaceuticals
Division of Aventis Pharmaceuticals Inc.
Kansas City, MO 64137   ©2000
Made in United Kingdom

50053567
CND 70100

NDC 0039-0019-01
Claforan® Sterile
cefotaxime for injection, USP (formerly sterile cefotaxime sodium)

2g IM/IV   ⚡Aventis

Lot BA799

Exp

Step 1 Calculate the total volume of the intermittent IV medication and the IV flush.
50 mL + 15 mL = 65 mL

Step 2 Calculate the flow rate of the IV medication and the IV flush. Remember: The drop factor is 60 gtt/mL.

$$\frac{V}{T} \times C = \frac{65\ \cancel{mL}}{\underset{1}{\cancel{30}\ min}} \times \overset{2}{\cancel{60}}\ gtt/\cancel{mL} = 130\ gtt/min$$

Step 3 Calculate the volume of the medication to be administered.

$$\frac{Dosage\ on\ hand}{Amount\ on\ hand} = \frac{Dosage\ desired}{X\ Amount\ desired}$$

$$\frac{180\ mg}{1\ mL} \diagdown \frac{250\ mg}{X\ mL}$$

$$180X = 250$$

$$\frac{180X}{180} = \frac{250}{180}$$

$$X = 1.38 = 1.4\ mL$$

Step 4 Add 1.4 mL Claforan 2 g to the chamber and fill with IV fluid to a volume of 50 mL. This provides the prescribed total volume of 50 mL in the chamber.

Step 5 Set the flow rate of the 50 mL of intermittent IV medication for 130 gtt/min. Follow with the 15 mL flush also set at 130 gtt/min. When complete, detach IV tubing, and follow saline lock policy.

The patient may also have an intermittent medication ordered as part of a continuous infusion at a prescribed IV volume per hour. In such cases the patient is to receive the same fluid volume each hour, regardless of the addition of intermittent medications. This means that the total prescribed fluid volume must include the intermittent IV medication volume.

EXAMPLE ■

Order: D_5NS IV at 30 mL/h for
continuous infusion and gentamicin
30 mg IV q.8h over 30 min

Supply: See label (Figure 16-5)

An electronic infusion pump is in use with the volume control set.

FIGURE 16-5 Gentamicin 40 mg/mL label

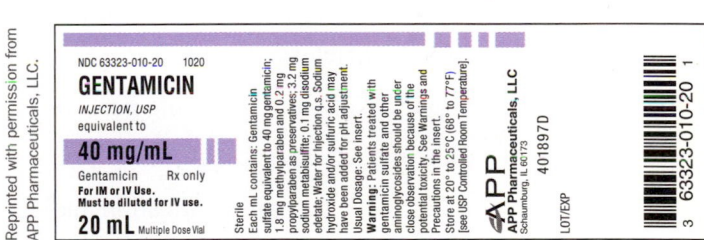

Step 1 Calculate the dilution volume required to administer the gentamicin at the prescribed continuous flow rate of 30 mL/h.

Think If 30 mL infuses in 1 h, then $\frac{1}{2}$ of 30, or 15 mL, will infuse in $\frac{1}{2}$ h or 30 min.

Calculate Use ratio-proportion to verify your estimate.

$$\frac{30\ mL}{60\ min} \diagdown \frac{X\ mL}{30\ min}$$

$$60X = 900$$

$$\frac{60X}{60} = \frac{900}{60}$$

$$X = 15\ mL\ (in\ 30\ min)$$

Therefore, the IV fluid dilution volume required to administer 30 mg of gentamicin in 30 minutes is 15 mL to maintain the prescribed, continuous infusion rate of 30 mL/h.

Step 2   Determine the volume of gentamicin and IV fluid to add to the volume control chamber.

$$\frac{\text{Dosage on hand}}{\text{Amount on hand}} = \frac{\text{Dosage desired}}{\text{X Amount desired}}$$

$$\frac{40\ \text{mg}}{1\ \text{mL}} \diagup\!\!\!\!\diagdown \frac{30\ \text{mg}}{\text{X mL}}$$

$$40\text{X} = 30$$

$$\frac{40\text{X}}{40} = \frac{30}{40}$$

$$\text{X} = 0.75\ \text{mL}$$

Add 0.75 mL gentamicin and fill the chamber with D_5NS to the total volume of 15 mL.

Step 3   Set the infusion pump to 30 mL/h to deliver 15 mL of intermittent IV gentamicin solution in 30 minutes. Resume the regular IV, which will also flush out the tubing. The continuous flow rate will remain at 30 mL/h.

QUICK REVIEW

- Volume control sets have a drop factor of 60 gtt/mL.

- The total volume of the medication, IV dilution fluid, and the IV flush fluid must be considered to calculate flow rates when using volume control sets.

- Use ratio-proportion to calculate flow rates for intermittent medications when a continuous IV rate in mL/h is prescribed.

Review Set 44

Calculate the IV flow rate to administer the following IV medications by using a volume control set, and determine the amount of IV fluid and medication to be added to the chamber. The ordered time includes the flush volume.

1. Order: Antibiotic X 60 mg IV q.8h in 50 mL D_5NS over 45 min. Flush with 15 mL.

   Supply: Antibiotic X 60 mg per 2 mL

   Flow rate: _____ gtt/min

   Add _____ mL medication and _____ mL IV fluid to the chamber.

2. Order: Medication Y 75 mg IV q.6h in 60 mL $D_5\frac{1}{4}NS$ over 60 min. Flush with 15 mL.

   Supply: Medication Y 75 mg per 3 mL

   Flow rate: _____ gtt/min

   Add _____ mL medication and _____ mL IV fluid to the chamber.

3. Order: Antibiotic Z 15 mg IV b.i.d. in 25 mL 0.9% NaCl over 20 min. Flush with 15 mL.

   Supply: Antibiotic Z 15 mg per 3 mL

   Flow rate: _____ gtt/min

   Add _____ mL medication and _____ mL IV fluid to the chamber.

4. Order: Ancef 0.6 g IV q.12h in 50 mL D_5NS over 60 min on an infusion pump. Flush with 30 mL.

   Supply: Ancef 1 g per 10 mL

   Flow rate: _____ mL/h

   Add _____ mL medication and _____ mL IV fluid to the chamber.

5. Order: **Cleocin 150 mg IV q.8h in 32 mL D₅NS over 60 min on an infusion pump. Flush with 28 mL.**

   Supply: Cleocin 150 mg/mL

   Flow rate: _____ mL/h

   Add _____ mL medication and _____ mL IV fluid to the chamber.

   Total IV volume after 3 doses are given is _____ mL.

Calculate the amount of IV fluid to be added to the volume control chamber.

6. Order: **0.9% NaCl at 50 mL/h for continuous infusion with Ancef 250 mg IV q.8h to be infused over 30 min by volume control set.**

   Supply: Ancef 125 mg/mL

   Add _____ mL medication and _____ mL IV fluid to the chamber.

7. Order: **D₅W at 30 mL/h for continuous infusion with Medication X 60 mg q.6h to be infused over 20 min by volume control set.**

   Supply: Medication X 60 mg per 2 mL

   Add _____ mL medication and _____ mL IV fluid to the chamber.

8. Order: **D₅ 0.225% NaCl IV at 85 mL/h with erythromycin 600 mg IV q.6h to be infused over 40 min by volume control set.**

   Supply: erythromycin 50 mg/mL

   Add _____ mL medication and _____ mL IV fluid to the chamber.

9. Order: **D₅NS IV at 66 mL/h with Fortaz 720 mg IV q.8h to be infused over 40 min by volume control set.**

   Supply: Fortaz 1 g per 10 mL

   Add _____ mL medication and _____ mL IV fluid to the chamber.

10. Order: **D₅ 0.45% NaCl IV at 48 mL/h with doxycycline 75 mg IV q.12h to be infused over 2 h by volume control set.**

    Supply: doxycycline 100 mg per 10 mL

    Add _____ mL medication and _____ mL IV fluid to the chamber.

After completing these problems, see page 566 to check your answers.

MINIMAL DILUTIONS FOR IV MEDICATIONS

IV medications in infants and young children (or adults on limited fluids) are often prescribed to be given in the smallest volume or *maximal safe concentration* to prevent fluid overload. Consult a pediatric reference, *Hospital Formulary,* or drug insert to assist you in problem solving. These types of medications are usually given via an electronic infusion pump.

Many pediatric IV medications allow a dilution *range* or a minimum and maximum allowable concentration. A solution of *lower* concentration may be given if the patient can tolerate the added volume (called *minimal safe concentration, maximal dilution,* or *largest volume*). A solution of *higher* concentration (called *maximal safe concentration, minimal dilution,* or *smallest volume*) must not exceed the recommended dilution instructions. Recall that the greater the volume of diluent or solvent, the less concentrated the resulting solution. Likewise, less volume of diluent or solvent results in a more concentrated solution.

CAUTION

An excessively high concentration of an IV drug can cause vein irritation and potentially life-threatening toxic effects. Dilution calculations are critical skills.

Let's examine how to follow the drug reference recommendations for a minimal IV drug dilution, when a minimal and maximal range is given for an IV drug dilution.

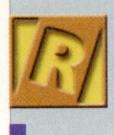

RULE

Ratio for recommended drug dilution equals ratio for desired drug dilution.

FIGURE 16-6   Portion of simulated vancomycin package insert

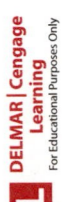 

> ### STERILE VANCOMYCIN HYDROCHLORIDE, USP
> #### INTRAVENOUS
>
> #### DOSAGE AND ADMINISTRATION
>
> Infusion-related events are related to both the concentration and the rate of administration of vancomycin. Concentrations of no more than 5 mg/mL and rates of no more than 10 mg/min are recommended in adults (see also age-specific recommendations). In selected patients in need of fluid restriction, <u>a concentration up to 10 mg/mL may be used;</u> use of such higher concentrations may increase the risk of infusion-related events. An infusion rate of 10 mg/min or less is associated with fewer infusion-related events. Infusion-related events may occur, however, at any rate or concentration.

EXAMPLE 1 ■

The physician orders *vancomycin 40 mg IV q.12h* for an infant who weighs 4,000 g. What is the minimal amount of IV fluid in which the vancomycin can be safely diluted? Look at the package insert provided for your reference (Figure 16-6) and find the *recommended maximal safe concentration* (10 mg/mL).

$$\frac{10 \text{ mg}}{1 \text{ mL}} \diagdown\!\!\!\!\diagup \frac{40 \text{ mg}}{X \text{ mL}}$$

$$10X = 40$$

$$\frac{10X}{10} = \frac{40}{10}$$

$$X = 4 \text{ mL (This is the minimal amount of IV fluid.)}$$

EXAMPLE 2 ■

The physician orders *Claforan 1.2 g IV q.8h* for a child who weighs 36 kg. The recommended safe administration of Claforan for intermittent IV administration is a final concentration of 20 to 60 mg/mL to infuse over 15 to 30 minutes. What is the minimal amount of IV fluid to safely dilute this dosage? (Remember this represents the **maximal safe concentration.**)

Step 1	**Convert**	$1.2 \text{ g} = 1.200. = 1,200 \text{ mg}$
Step 2	**Think**	1,200 is more than 10 times 60; in fact, it is 20 times 60. So you need at least 20 mL to dilute the drug.
Step 3	**Calculate**	$\dfrac{60 \text{ mg}}{1 \text{ mL}} \diagdown\!\!\!\!\diagup \dfrac{1,200 \text{ mg}}{X \text{ mL}}$

$$60X = 1,200$$

$$\frac{60X}{60} = \frac{1,200}{60}$$

$$X = 20 \text{ mL (minimal dilution for maximal safe concentration)}$$

What is the maximal amount of IV fluid recommended to safely dilute this drug to the minimal safe concentration?

Step 1 **Convert**   1.2 g $= 1,200$ mg

Step 2 **Think**   1,200 is more than 50 times 20; in fact, it is 60 times 20. So you can use up to 60 mL to dilute the drug.

Step 3 **Calculate**

$$\frac{20 \text{ mg}}{1 \text{ mL}} \diagup\!\!\!\!\diagdown \frac{1,200 \text{ mg}}{X \text{ mL}}$$

$$20X = 1,200$$

$$\frac{20X}{20} = \frac{1,200}{20}$$

$$X = 60 \text{ mL (maximal dilution for minimal safe concentration)}$$

CALCULATION OF DAILY VOLUME FOR MAINTENANCE FLUIDS

Another common pediatric IV calculation is to calculate 24-hour maintenance IV fluids for children.

RULE

Use this formula to calculate the daily rate of pediatric maintenance IV fluids:

- 100 mL/kg/day for first 10 kg of body weight
- 50 mL/kg/day for next 10 kg of body weight
- 20 mL/kg/day for each kg above 20 kg of body weight

This formula uses the child's weight in kilograms to estimate the 24-hour total fluid need, including oral intake. It does not include replacement for losses, such as diarrhea, vomiting, or fever. This accounts only for fluid needed to maintain normal cellular metabolism and fluid turnover.

Pediatric IV solutions that run over 24 hours usually include a combination of glucose, saline, and potassium chloride and are *hypertonic* solutions (see Figure 15-5, page 366). Dextrose (glucose) for energy is usually concentrated between 5% and 12% for peripheral infusions. Sodium chloride is usually concentrated between 0.225% and 0.9% ($\frac{1}{4}$ NS up to NS). Further, 20 mEq per liter of potassium chloride (20 mEq KCl/L) are usually added to continuous pediatric infusions. Any dextrose and saline combination without potassium should be used only as an intermittent or short-term IV fluid in children. Be wary of isotonic solutions such as 5% dextrose in water and 0.9% sodium chloride. They do not contribute enough electrolytes and can quickly lead to water intoxication.

CAUTION

A red flag should go up in your mind if either plain 5% dextrose in water or 0.9% sodium chloride (normal saline) are running continuously on an infant or child. Consult the ordering practitioner immediately!

Let's examine the daily rate of maintenance fluids and the hourly flow rate for the children in the following examples.

EXAMPLE 1 ■

Child who weighs 6 kg

100 mL/kg/day $\times$ 6 kg $= 600$ mL/day or per 24 h

$$\frac{600 \text{ mL}}{24 \text{ h}} = 25 \text{ mL/h}$$

EXAMPLE 2 ■

Child who weighs 12 kg

100 mL/kg/day × 10 kg = 1,000 mL/day (for first 10 kg)

50 mL/kg/day × 2 kg = 100 mL/day (for the remaining 2 kg)

Total: 1,000 mL/day + 100 mL/day = 1,100 mL/day or per 24 h

$\dfrac{1,100 \text{ mL}}{24 \text{ h}}$ = 45.8 mL/h = 46 mL/h

EXAMPLE 3 ■

Child who weighs 24 kg

100 mL/kg/day × 10 kg = 1,000 mL/day (for first 10 kg)

50 mL/kg/day × 10 kg = 500 mL/day (for next 10 kg)

20 mL/kg/day × 4 kg = 80 mL/day (for the remaining 4 kg)

Total: 1,000 mL/day + 500 mL/day + 80 mL/day = 1,580 mL/day or per 24 h

$\dfrac{1,580 \text{ mL}}{24 \text{ h}}$ = 65.8 mL/h = 66 mL/h

QUICK REVIEW

- Minimal and maximal dilution volumes for some IV drugs are recommended to prevent fluid overload and to minimize vein irritation and toxic effects.

- The ratio for recommended dilution equals the ratio for desired drug dilution.

- When mixing IV drug solutions,

   - the *smaller* the added volume, the *stronger* or *higher* the resulting *concentration* (minimal dilution).

   - the *larger* the added volume, the *weaker (more dilute)* or *lower* the resulting *concentration* (maximal dilution).

- Daily volume of pediatric maintenance IV fluids based on body weight is:

   - 100 mL/kg/day for first 10 kg

   - 50 mL/kg/day for next 10 kg

   - 20 mL/kg/day for each kg above 20

Review Set 45

1. If a child is receiving **chloramphenicol 400 mg IV q.6h** and the maximum concentration is 100 mg/mL, what is the minimum volume of fluid in which the medication can be safely diluted? _____ mL

2. If a child is receiving **gentamicin 25 mg IV q.8h** and the minimal concentration is 1 mg/mL, what is the maximum volume of fluid in which the medication can be safely diluted? _____ mL

3. Calculate the total volume and hourly IV flow rate for a 25 kg child receiving maintenance IV fluids. Infuse _____ mL at _____ mL/h

4. Calculate the total volume and hourly IV flow rate for a 13 kg child receiving maintenance IV fluids. Infuse _____ mL at _____ mL/h

5. Calculate the total volume and hourly IV flow rate for a 77 lb child receiving maintenance fluids. Infuse _____ mL at _____ mL/h

6. Calculate the total volume and hourly IV flow rate for a 3,500 g infant receiving maintenance fluids. Infuse _____ mL at _____ mL/h

7. A child is receiving 350 mg of a certain medication IV, and the minimal and maximal dilution range is 30 to 100 mg/mL. What is the minimum volume (maximal concentration) and the maximum volume (minimal concentration) for safe dilution? _____ mL (minimum volume); _____ mL (maximum volume). Hint: The equipment measures whole mL; round up to the next whole mL.

8. A child is receiving 52 mg of a certain medication IV, and the minimal and maximal dilution range is 0.8 to 20 mg/mL. What is the minimum volume and the maximum volume of fluid for safe dilution? _____ mL (minimum volume); _____ mL (maximum volume).

9. A child is receiving 175 mg of a certain medication IV, and the minimal and maximal dilution range is 5 to 75 mg/mL. What is the minimum volume and the maximum volume of fluid for safe dilution? _____ mL (minimum volume); _____ mL (maximum volume).

10. You are making rounds on your pediatric patients and notice that a 2-year-old child who weighs 14 kg has 1,000 mL of normal saline infusing at the rate of 50 mL/h. You decide to question this order. What is your rationale? _____

_____

After completing these problems, see page 567 to check your answers.

CRITICAL THINKING SKILLS

Let's look at an example in which the nurse *prevents* a medication error by calculating the safe dosage of a medication before administering the drug to an infant.

ERROR

Dosage that is too high for an infant.

Possible Scenario

Suppose a physician ordered KCl 25 mEq IV per 500 mL of $D_5\frac{1}{2}$ NS to infuse at the rate of 20 mL/h. The infant weighs $10\frac{1}{2}$ lb and is 24 in long. KCl for IV injection is supplied as 2 mEq/mL. The nurse looked up potassium chloride in a drug reference and noted that the safe dosage of potassium chloride is up to 3 mEq/kg or 40 mEq/m^2/day. The nurse calculated the infant's dosage as 14.4 mEq/day based on body weight and 11.2 mEq/day based on BSA.

First convert lb to kg.

$10\frac{1}{2}$ lb = 10.5 lb

$$\frac{1 \text{ kg}}{2.2 \text{ lb}} \diagdown\!\!\!\!\diagup \frac{X \text{ kg}}{10.5 \text{ lb}}$$

$$\frac{2.2X}{2.2} = \frac{10.5}{2.2}$$

$$X = 4.8 \text{ kg}$$

3 mEq/kg/day × 4.8 kg = 14.4 mEq/day

$$\text{BSA (m}^2) = \sqrt{\frac{\text{ht (in)} \times \text{wt (lb)}}{3,131}} = \sqrt{\frac{10.5 \times 24}{3,131}} = \sqrt{\frac{252}{3,131}} = \sqrt{0.080...} = 0.283 \text{ m}^2 = 0.28 \text{ m}^2$$

40 mEq/m^2/day × 0.28 m^2 = 11.2 mEq/day

The nurse further calculated that at the rate ordered, the infant would receive 480 mL of IV fluid per day, which is a reasonable daily rate of pediatric maintenance IV fluids.

20 mL/h̶ × 24 h̶/day = 480 mL/day

Maintenance pediatric IV fluids:
100 mL/kg/day for first 10 kg: 100 mL/k̶g̶/day × 4.8 k̶g̶ = 480 mL/day

But then the nurse calculated that the infant would receive 1 mEq KCl per hour.

$$\frac{25\ mEq}{500\ mL} \diagdown \frac{X\ mEq}{20\ mL}$$

$$500X = 500$$

$$X = 1\ mEq$$

Finally, the nurse calculated that at this rate the infant would receive 24 mEq/day, which is approximately twice the safe dosage. Therefore, the order is unsafe.

1 mEq/h̶ × 24 h̶/day = 24 mEq/day

The nurse notified the physician and questioned the order. The physician responded, "Thank you, you are correct. I intended to order one-half that amount of KCl or 25 mEq per L, which should have been 12.5 mEq per 500 mL. This was my error and I am glad you caught it."

Potential Outcome

If the nurse had not questioned the order, the infant would have received twice the safe dosage. The infant likely would have developed signs of hyperkalemia that could lead to ventricular fibrillation, muscle weakness progressing to flaccid quadriplegia, respiratory failure, and death.

Prevention

In this instance, the nurse prevented a medication error by checking the safe dosage and notifying the physician before administering the infusion. Let this be you!

PRACTICE PROBLEMS—CHAPTER 16

Calculate the volume for 1 dose of safe dosages. Refer to the BSA formulas or the West Nomogram on the next page (Figure 16-7) as needed to answer questions 1 through 20.

1. Order: **vincristine 2 mg direct IV stat** for a child who weighs 85 pounds and is 50 inches tall.

   Recommended dosage of vincristine for children: 1.5 to 2 mg/m² 1 time/week; inject slowly over a period of 1 minute.

   Supply: vincristine 1 mg/mL

   BSA (per formula) of this child: _____ m²

   Recommended dosage range for this child: _____ mg to _____ mg

   Is the ordered dosage safe? _____

   If safe, give _____ mL/min or _____ mL per 15 sec.

   If not, what should you do? _____

2. Use the BSA nomogram to calculate the safe oral dosage and amount to give of mercaptopurine for a child of normal proportions who weighs 25 pounds.

Recommended dosage: 80 mg/m²/day once daily p.o.

Supply: mercaptopurine 50 mg/mL

BSA: _____ m²

Safe dosage: _____ mg. Give _____ mL.

3. Use the BSA nomogram to calculate the safe IV dosage of sargramostim for a 1-year-old child who is 25 inches tall and weighs 20 pounds.

Recommended dosage: 250 mcg/m²/day once daily IV

BSA: _____ m²

Safe dosage: _____ mcg

FIGURE 16-7 West Nomogram for estimation of body surface area

Metric:

$$BSA\ (m^2) = \sqrt{\frac{ht\ (cm) \times wt\ (kg)}{3,600}}$$

Household:

$$BSA\ (m^2) = \sqrt{\frac{ht\ (in) \times wt\ (lb)}{3,131}}$$

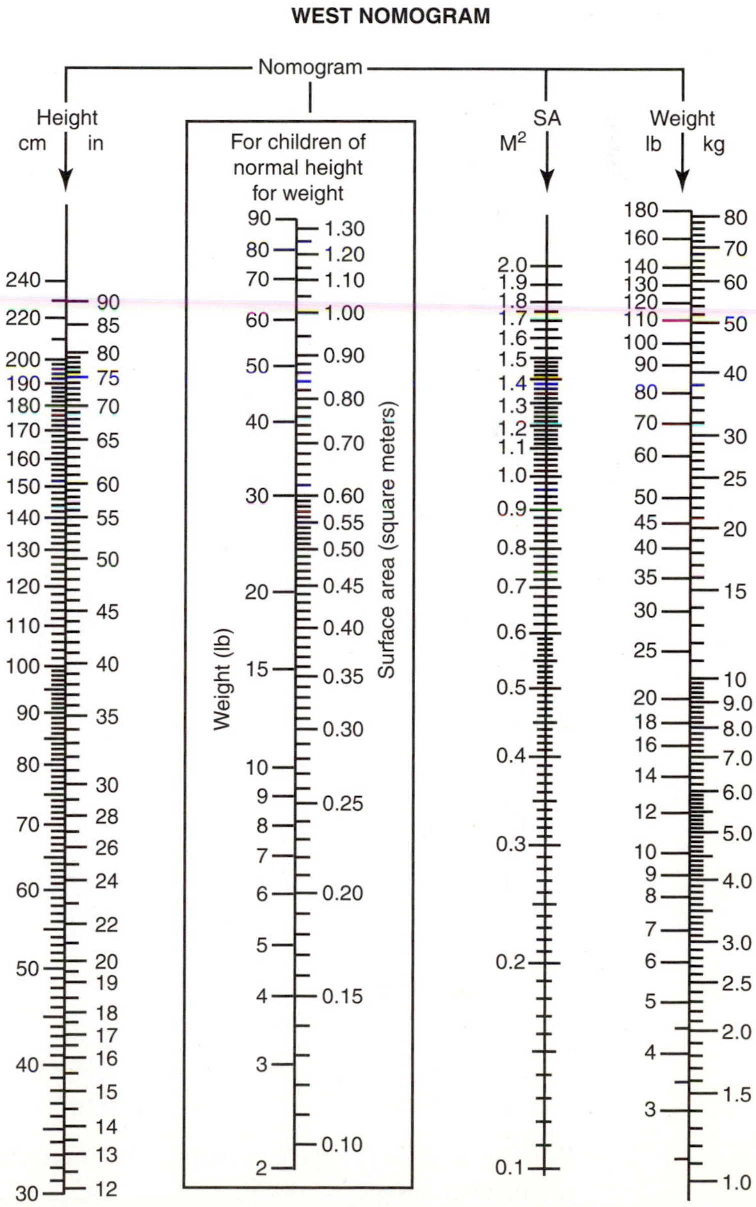

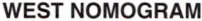

From Kliegman, R.M., Behrman, R.E., Jenson, H.B., and Stanton, B.F. (2007). *Nelson textbook of pediatrics* (18th ed.) Philadelphia: Saunders. Reprinted with permission.

4. Sargramostim is available in a solution strength of 500 mcg per 10 mL. Calculate 1 dose for the child in question 3.

   Give: _____ mL

5. Use the BSA nomogram to determine the BSA for a child who is 35 inches tall and weighs 40 pounds.

   BSA: _____ m^2

6. The child in question 5 will receive levodopa. The recommended oral dosage of levodopa is 0.5 g/m^2. What is the safe dosage for this child?

   Safe dosage: _____ mg

7. Levodopa is supplied in 100 mg and 250 mg capsules. Calculate 1 dose for the child in question 6.

   Give: _____ of the _____ mg capsule(s)

8. Use the BSA nomogram to determine the safe IM dosage of Oncaspar for a child who is 42 inches tall and weighs 45 pounds. The recommended IM dosage is 2,500 $units/m^2$/dose.

   BSA: _____ m^2

   Safe dosage: _____ units

9. Oncaspar is reconstituted to 750 units/mL. Calculate 1 dose for the child in question 8.

   Give: _____ mL

10. Should the Oncaspar in question 9 be given in one injection? _____

11. A child is 140 cm tall and weighs 43.5 kg. The recommended IV dosage of Adriamycin is 20 mg/m^2. Use the BSA formula to calculate the safe IV dosage of Adriamycin for this child.

    BSA: _____ m^2

    Safe dosage: _____ mg

12. Calculate the dose amount of Adriamycin for the child in question 11.

    Supply: Adriamycin 2 mg/mL

    Give: _____ mL

For questions 13 through 20, use the BSA formulas to calculate the BSA value.

13. Height: 5 ft 6 in   Weight: 136 lb   BSA: _____ m^2

14. Height: 4 ft   Weight: 80 lb   BSA: _____ m^2

15. Height: 60 cm   Weight: 6 kg   BSA: _____ m^2

16. Height: 68 in   Weight: 170 lb   BSA: _____ m^2

17. Height: 164 cm   Weight: 58 kg   BSA: _____ m^2

18. Height: 100 cm   Weight: 17 kg   BSA: _____ m^2

19. Height: 64 in   Weight: 63 kg   BSA: _____ m^2

20. Height: 85 cm   Weight: 11.5 kg   BSA: _____ m^2

21. What is the safe dosage of 1 dose of interferon alpha-2b required for a child with a BSA of 0.28 m^2 if the recommended dosage is 2 million $units/m^2$? _____ units

22. What is the safe dosage of calcium EDTA required for an adult with a BSA of 2.17 m^2 if the recommended dosage is 500 mg/m^2? _____ mg or _____ g

23. What is the total daily dosage range of mitomycin required for a child with a BSA of 0.19 m² if the recommended dosage range is 10 to 20 mg/m²/day? _____ mg/day to _____ mg/day

24. What is the total safe daily dosage of thiotepa required for an adult with a BSA of 1.34 m² if the recommended dosage is 6 mg/m²/day? _____ mg/day

25. After 5 full days of therapy receiving the recommended dosage, the patient in question 24 will have received a total of _____ mg of thiotepa.

26. Order: **Ancef 0.42 g IV q.12 h in 30 mL D₅NS over 30 min by volume control set on an electronic infusion pump. Flush with 15 mL.**

    Supply: Ancef 500 mg per 5 mL

    Total IV fluid volume: _____ mL

    Flow rate: _____ mL/h

    Add _____ mL Ancef and _____ mL D₅NS to the chamber.

27. After 7 days of IV therapy, the patient referred to in question 26 will have received a total of _____ mL of Ancef.

28. Order: **clindamycin 285 mg IV q.8h in 45 mL D₅NS over 60 min by volume control set on an electronic infusion pump. Flush with 15 mL.**

    Supply: clindamycin 75 mg per 0.5 mL

    Total IV fluid volume: _____ mL

    Flow rate: _____ mL/h

    Add _____ mL clindamycin and _____ mL D₅NS to the chamber.

29. When the patient in item 28 has received 4 days therapy of clindamycin, he will have received a total IV medication volume of _____ mL.

30. Order: **D₅ 0.225% NaCl IV at 65 mL/h c̄ erythromycin 500 mg IV q.6h to be infused over 40 min**

    You will use a volume control set and flush with 15 mL.

    Supply: erythromycin 50 mg/mL

    Add _____ mL of erythromycin and _____ mL D₅ NS to the chamber.

31. When the patient in question 30 has received 5 days of therapy of erythromycin, he will have received a total IV medication volume of _____ mL.

32. Order: **D₅ 0.45% NaCl IV at 66 mL/h with Fortaz 620 mg IV q.8h to be infused over 40 min**

    You will use a volume control set and flush with 15 mL.

    Supply: Fortaz 0.5 g per 5 mL

    Add _____ mL Fortaz and _____ mL D₅ 0.45% NaCl to the chamber.

33. When the patient in question 32 has received 7 days of therapy of Fortaz, he will have received a total IV medication volume of _____ mL.

For questions 34 through 38, calculate the daily volume of pediatric maintenance IV fluids using:

    100 mL/kg/day for first 10 kg of body weight

    50 mL/kg/day for next 10 kg of body weight

    20 mL/kg/day for each kg of body weight above 20 kg

34. Calculate the total volume and hourly IV flow rate for a child who weighs 10 kg and who is receiving maintenance fluids.

    Infuse _____ mL at _____ mL/h

35. Calculate the total volume and hourly IV flow rate for a 21 kg child receiving maintenance fluids.

   Infuse _____ mL at _____ mL/h

36. Calculate the total volume and hourly IV flow rate for a 78 lb child receiving maintenance fluids.

   Infuse _____ mL at _____ mL/h

37. Calculate the total volume and hourly IV flow rate for a 33 lb child receiving maintenance fluids.

   Infuse _____ mL at _____ mL/h

38. Calculate the total volume and hourly IV flow rate for a 2,400 g infant receiving maintenance fluids.

   Infuse _____ mL at _____ mL/h

For questions 39 through 49, verify the safety of the following pediatric dosages ordered. If the dosage is safe, calculate 1 dose and the IV volume to infuse 1 dose.

Order for a child weighing 15 kg:

D_5 0.45% NaCl IV at 53 mL/h c̄ ampicillin 275 mg IV q.4h infused over 40 min by volume control set

Recommended dosage: ampicillin 100 to 125 mg/kg/day in 6 divided doses

Supply: ampicillin 1 g per 10 mL

39. Safe daily dosage range for this child: _____ mg/day to _____ mg/day

   Safe single dosage range for this child: _____ mg/dose to _____ mg/dose

   Is the ordered dosage safe? _____ If safe, give _____ mL/dose.

   If not safe, describe your action. _____

40. IV fluid volume to be infused in 40 min: _____ mL

   Add _____ mL ampicillin and _____ mL D_5 0.45% NaCl to the chamber.

For questions 41 and 42, order for a child who weighs 27 lb:

D_5 NS IV at 46 mL/h c̄ oxacillin 308 mg IV q.6h to be infused over 30 min by volume control set

Recommended dosage: oxacillin 100 mg/kg/day in 4 divided doses

Supply: oxacillin 500 mg per 10 mL

41. Child's weight: _____ kg

   Safe daily dosage for this child: _____ mg/day

   Safe single dosage for this child: _____ mg/dose

   Is the ordered dosage safe? _____ If safe, give _____ mL/dose.

   If not safe, describe your action. _____

42. IV fluid volume to be infused in 30 min: _____ mL

   Add _____ mL oxacillin and _____ mL D_5 NS to the chamber.

For questions 43 and 44, order for a child who weighs 22 kg:

D_5 0.225% NaCl IV at 50 mL/h c̄ Amikin 165 mg IV q.8h to be infused over 30 min by volume control set

Recommended dosage: Amikin 15 to 22.5 mg/kg/day in 3 divided doses q.8h

Supply: Amikin 100 mg per 2 mL

43. Safe daily dosage range for this child: _____ mg/day to _____ mg/day

    Safe single dosage range for this child: _____ mg/dose to _____ mg/dose

    Is the ordered dosage safe? _____ If safe, give _____ mL/dose.

    If not safe, describe your action. _____

44. IV fluid volume to be infused in 30 min: _____ mL

    Add _____ mL Amikin and _____ mL D_5 0.225% NaCl to the chamber.

For questions 45 and 46, order for a child who weighs 9 kg:

D_5 NS IV at 38 mL/h $\bar{c}$ Timentin 800 mg IV q.4h to be infused over 40 min by volume control set

Recommended dosage: Timentin 200 to 300 mg/kg/day in 6 divided doses every 4 hours

Supply: Timentin 200 mg/mL

45. Safe daily dosage range for this child: _____ mg/day to _____ mg/day

    Safe single dosage range for this child: _____ mg/dose to _____ mg/dose

    Is the ordered dosage safe? _____ If safe, give _____ mL/dose.

    If not safe, describe your action. _____

46. IV fluid volume to be infused in 40 min: _____ mL

    Add _____ mL Timentin and _____ mL D_5 NS to the chamber.

For questions 47 through 49, order for a child who weighs 55 lbs:

D_5NS IV at 60 mL/h $\bar{c}$ penicillin G potassium 525,000 units q.4h to be infused over 20 min by volume control set

Recommended dosage: penicillin G potassium 100,000 to 250,000 units/kg/day in 6 divided doses q.4h

Supply: penicillin G potassium 200,000 units/mL

47. Child's weight: _____ kg

    Safe daily dosage for this child: _____ units/day to _____ units/day

    Safe single dosage for this child: _____ units/dose to _____ units/dose

48. Is the ordered dosage safe? _____ If safe, give _____ mL/dose.

    If not safe, describe your action. _____

49. IV fluid volume to be infused in 20 min: _____ mL

    Add _____ mL penicillin G potassium and _____ mL D_5 NS to the chamber.

50. Describe the strategy you would implement to prevent this medication error.

    Possible Scenario
    Suppose the physician came to the pediatric oncology unit to administer chemotherapy to a critically ill child whose cancer symptoms had recurred suddenly. The nurse assigned to care for the child was floated from the adult oncology unit and was experienced in administering chemotherapy to adults. The physician, recognizing the nurse, said, "Oh good, you know how to calculate and prepare chemo. Go draw up 2 mg/m² of vincristine for this child so I can get his chemotherapy started quickly." The nurse consulted the child's chart and saw the following weights written on his assessment sheet: 20/.45. No height was recorded.

    On the adult unit, that designation means __X__ kg or __Y__ lb. The nurse took the West Nomogram and estimated the child's BSA based on his weight of 45 lb to be 0.82 m². The nurse calculated $2 \text{ mg/m}^2 \times 0.82 \text{ m}^2 = 1.64$ mg. Vincristine is supplied as 1 mg/1 mL, so the nurse further calculated 1.6 mL was the dose and drew it up in a 3 mL syringe. As the nurse handed the syringe to the physician, the amount looked wrong. The physician asked the nurse how that amount was obtained. When the nurse told the physician the estimated BSA from the child's weight (45 pounds) is 0.82 m², and the dosage is 2 mg/m² × 0.82 m² = 1.64 mg or 1.6 mL, the physician said, "No! This child's *BSA is 0.45 m²*. I wrote it myself next to his weight—20 pounds." The physician, despite the need to give the medication as soon as possible, took the necessary extra step and examined the amount of medication in the syringe. Though the physician knew and trusted the nurse, the amount of medication in the syringe did not seem right. Perhaps the physician had figured a ball-park amount of about 1 mL, and the volume the nurse brought in made the physician question what was calculated. The correct dosage calculations are:

$$2 \text{ mg/m}^2 \times 0.45 \text{ m}^2 = 0.9 \text{ mg}$$

$$\frac{\text{Dosage on hand}}{\text{Amount on hand}} = \frac{\text{Dosage desired}}{\text{X Amount desired}}$$

$$\frac{1 \text{ mg}}{1 \text{ mL}} \diagup\hspace{-1.2em}\diagdown \frac{0.9 \text{ mg}}{\text{X mL}}$$

$$X = 0.9 \text{ mL}$$

Potential Outcome

The child, already critically ill, could have received almost double the amount of medication had the physician rushed to give the dose calculated and prepared by someone else. This excessive amount of medication probably could have caused a fatal overdose. What should have been done to prevent this error?

Prevention

_____

_____

After completing these problems, see pages 567–570 to check your answers.

REFERENCE

Kliegman, R. M., Behrman, R. E., Jenson, H. B., & Stanton, B. F. (2007). *Nelson textbook of pediatrics* (18th ed.). Philadelphia: Saunders.

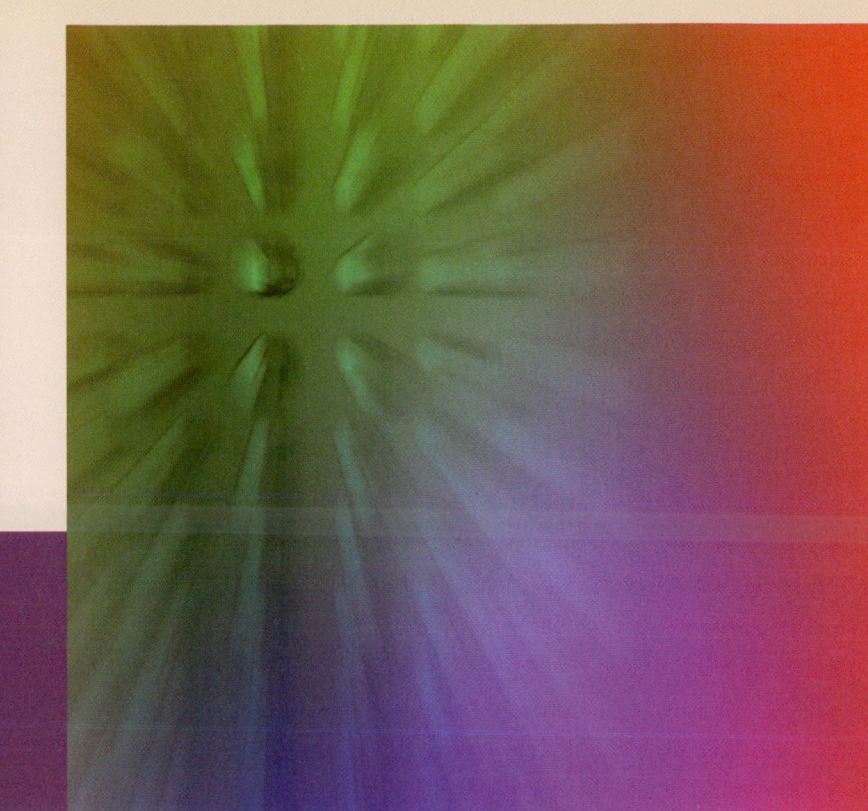

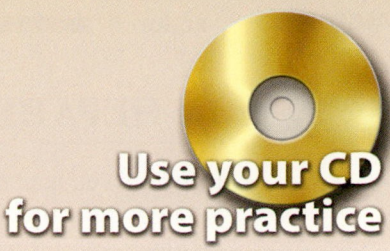

Use your CD for more practice

17

Advanced Adult Intravenous Calculations

OBJECTIVES

Upon mastery of Chapter 17, you will be able to perform advanced adult intravenous (IV) calculations and apply these skills to patients across the life span. To accomplish this you will also be able to:

- Calculate and assess safe hourly heparin dosage.
- Calculate heparin IV flow rate.
- Calculate the flow rate and assess safe dosages for critical care IV medications administered over a specified time period.
- Calculate the flow rate for primary IV and IV piggyback (IV PB) solutions for patients with restricted fluid intake requirements.

Nurses are becoming increasingly more responsible for the administration of IV medications in the critical care areas as well as on general nursing units. Patients in life-threatening situations require thorough and timely interventions that frequently involve specialized, potent drugs. This chapter focuses on advanced adult IV calculations with special requirements that can be applied to patients across the life span.

IV HEPARIN

Heparin is an anticoagulant for the prevention of clot formation. It is measured in USP units (Figure 17-1). IV heparin is frequently ordered in *units per hour (units/h)* and as such should be administered by an electronic infusion device. Because of the potential for hemorrhage or clots with incorrect dosage, careful monitoring of patients receiving heparin is a critical nursing skill. The nurse is responsible for administering the correct dosage and for ensuring that the dosage is safe.

FIGURE 17-1 Various heparin dosage strengths and container volumes

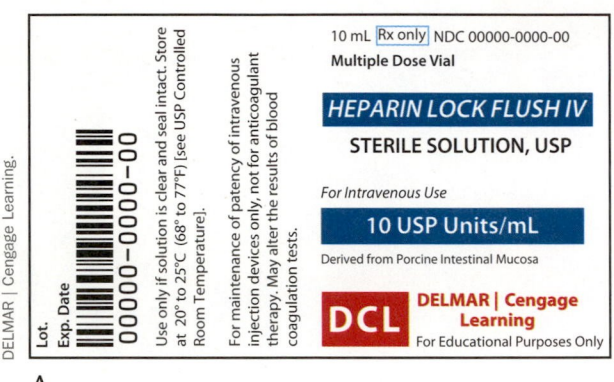

A

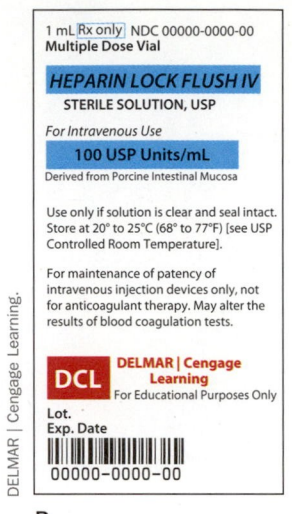

B

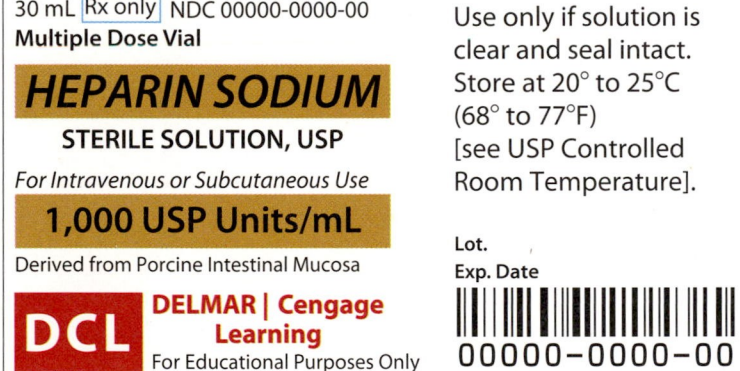

C

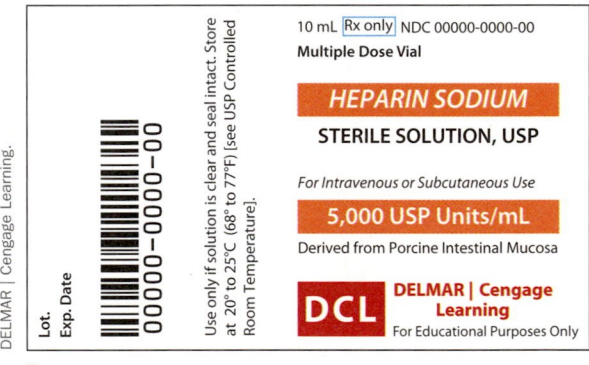

D

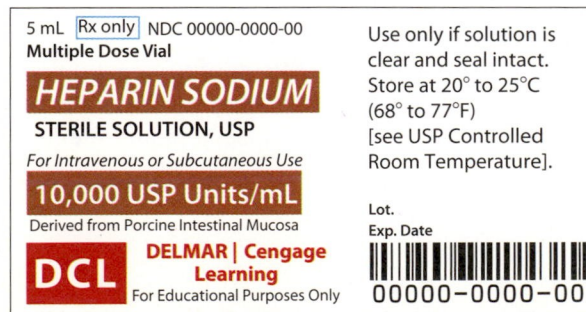

E

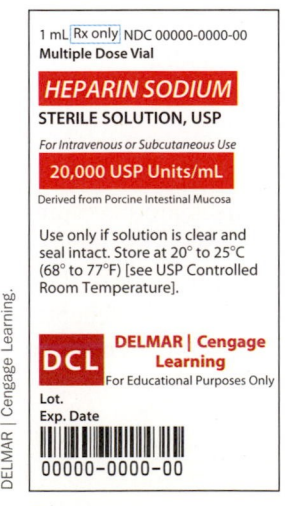

F

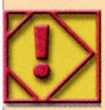

CAUTION

Heparin order, dosage, vial, and amount to give should be checked by another nurse before administering the dose.

Calculating Safe IV Heparin Flow Rate

When IV heparin is ordered in units/h, use ratio-proportion to calculate the flow rate in mL/h.

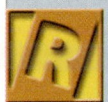

RULE

To calculate IV heparin flow rate in mL/h:

Ratio of supply dosage on hand is equivalent to ratio of desired dosage rate

$$\frac{\text{Dosage on hand}}{\text{Amount on hand}} = \frac{\text{Dosage desired/h}}{\text{X Amount desired/h}}$$

Note: This rule applies to drugs ordered in units/h, milliunits/h, mg/h, mcg/h, g/h, or mEq/h.

Let's apply the rule to some examples.

EXAMPLE 1 ■

Order: D₅W 500 mL c̄ heparin 25,000 units IV at 1,000 units/h

What is the flow rate in mL/h?

Calculate the flow rate in mL/h, which will administer 1,000 units/h.

$$\frac{\text{Dosage on hand}}{\text{Amount on hand}} = \frac{\text{Dosage desired/h}}{\text{X Amount desired/h}}$$

$$\frac{25,000 \text{ units}}{500 \text{ mL}} \diagtimes \frac{1,000 \text{ units/h}}{\text{X mL/h}}$$

$$25,000X = 500,000$$

$$\frac{25,000X}{25,000} = \frac{500,000}{25,000}$$

$$X = 20 \text{ mL/h}$$

Look at the labels in Figure 17-1, representing the various supply dosages of heparin you have available. Often, IV solutions with heparin additive come premixed. But, if you have to mix the solution, what label would you select to prepare the heparin infusion as ordered? The best answer is label E: 5 mL vial of heparin 10,000 units/mL. To add 25,000 units of heparin to 500 mL of IV solution, you would need 2.5 mL of heparin. Let's do the calculations.

$$\frac{\text{Dosage on hand}}{\text{Amount on hand}} = \frac{\text{Dosage desired}}{\text{X Amount desired}}$$

$$\frac{10,000 \text{ units}}{1 \text{ mL}} \diagtimes \frac{25,000 \text{ units}}{\text{X mL}}$$

$$10,000X = 25,000$$

$$\frac{10,000X}{10,000} = \frac{25,000}{10,000}$$

$$X = 2.5 \text{ mL}$$

However, notice that you could also select Label D and prepare 5 mL of heparin 5,000 units/mL. Label C (1,000 units/mL) is not a good choice, because drawing up 25 mL of heparin is impractical. Label F does not have sufficient volume per vial to fill the dosage required. Labels A and B are for maintenance of patency of IV injection devices and are not intended for anticoagulant therapy.

EXAMPLE 2 ■

Order: D₅W 500 mL c̄ heparin 25,000 units IV at 850 units/h

Calculate the flow rate in mL/h.

$$\frac{\text{Dosage on hand}}{\text{Amount on hand}} = \frac{\text{Dosage desired/h}}{\text{X Amount desired/h}}$$

$$\frac{25,000 \text{ units}}{500 \text{ mL}} \diagdown \frac{850 \text{ units/h}}{\text{X mL/h}}$$

$$25,000X = 425,000$$

$$\frac{25,000X}{25,000} = \frac{425,000}{25,000}$$

$$X = 17 \text{ mL/h}$$

EXAMPLE 3 ■

D₅W 500 mL with heparin 25,000 units IV is currently infusing at 850 units/h, or 17 mL/h. Based on laboratory results, it is determined that the patient's infusion must be increased by 120 units/h, so that it should now be infusing at 970 units/h.

Calculate the flow rate in mL/h.

$$\frac{\text{Dosage on hand}}{\text{Amount on hand}} = \frac{\text{Dosage desired/h}}{\text{X Amount desired/h}}$$

$$\frac{25,000 \text{ units}}{500 \text{ mL}} \diagdown \frac{970 \text{ units/h}}{\text{X mL/h}}$$

$$25,000X = 485,000$$

$$\frac{25,000X}{25,000} = \frac{485,000}{25,000}$$

$$X = 19.4 = 19 \text{ mL/h}$$

You would need to increase the infusion from 17 mL/h (850 units/h) to 19 mL/h (970 units/h).

IV Heparin Protocol

Because patients vary significantly in weight, the intravenous heparin dosage is individualized based on patient weight. Many hospitals have standard protocols related to intravenous heparin administration. Figure 17-2 shows a sample protocol. Note that the bolus or loading dosage and the initial infusion dosage of heparin are based on the patient's weight. Line 10 indicates that for this protocol, the standard heparin bolus dosage is 80 units/kg and the infusion rate is 18 units/kg/h. When the patient's response to heparin therapy changes, as measured by the APTT blood clotting value (activated partial thromboplastin time measured in seconds), the heparin dosage is adjusted as indicated in lines 11–15. These orders in Figure 17-2 are based on patient weight rounded to the nearest 10 kg. Some facilities use the patient's exact weight in kilograms. It is important to know the protocol for your clinical setting. Let's work through some examples of calculation of heparin dosage based on patient weight and a standardized heparin dosage protocol.

FIGURE 17-2 Sample orders for patient receiving heparin therapy

> ## Standard Weight-Based Heparin Protocol
>
> For all patients on heparin drips:
> 1. Weight in kilograms (rounded to nearest 10 kg). Required for order to be processed: _____ kg
> 2. Heparin 25,000 units in 250 mL of $\frac{1}{2}$NS. Boluses to be given as 1,000 units/mL.
> 3. APTT q.6h or 6 hours after rate change; daily after two consecutive therapeutic APTTs.
> 4. CBC initially and repeat every _____ days(s).
> 5. Obtain APTT and PT/INR on day 1 prior to initiation of therapy.
> 6. Guaiac stool initially then every _____ day(s) until heparin discontinued. Notify if positive.
> 7. Neuro checks every _____ hours while on heparin. Notify physician of any changes.
> 8. Discontinue APTT and CBC once heparin drip is discontinued, unless otherwise ordered.
> 9. Notify physician of any bleeding problems.
> 10. Bolus with 80 units/kg. Start drip at 18 units/kg/h.
> 11. If APTT is less than 35 secs: Rebolus with 80 units/kg and increase rate by 4 units/kg/h
> 12. If APTT is 36 to 44 secs: Rebolus with 40 units/kg and increase rate by 2 units/kg/h
> 13. If APTT is 45 to 75 secs: Continue current rate
> 14. If APTT is 76 to 90 secs: Decrease rate by 2 units/kg/h
> 15. If APTT is greater than 90 secs: Hold heparin for 1 hour and decrease rate by 3 units/kg/h

EXAMPLE 1 ■

Protocol: **Bolus patient with heparin 80 units/kg body weight and start drip at 18 units/kg/h**

Patient's weight: 110 lb

How many units of heparin should the patient receive?

Step 1 Calculate patient's weight in kilograms. Conversion: 1 kg = 2.2 lb

$$\frac{1 \text{ kg}}{2.2 \text{ lb}} \diagdown \frac{X \text{ kg}}{110 \text{ lb}}$$

$$2.2X = 110$$

$$\frac{2.2X}{2.2} = \frac{110}{2.2}$$

$$X = 50 \text{ kg}$$

Step 2 Calculate the heparin bolus dosage.

80 units/kg × 50 kg = 4,000 units

This patient should receive 4,000 units IV heparin as a bolus.

Step 3 Calculate the number of milliliters to administer for the bolus.

Supply: heparin 1,000 units/mL, as recommended by the protocol (see #2, Figure 17-2)

Think: You want to give 4,000 units, which is four times 1,000 units/mL, so you want to give four times 1 mL or 4 mL.

$$\frac{\text{Dosage on hand}}{\text{Amount on hand}} = \frac{\text{Dosage desired}}{\text{X Amount desired}}$$

$$\frac{1,000 \text{ units}}{1 \text{ mL}} \diagdown \frac{4,000 \text{ units}}{X \text{ mL}}$$

$$\frac{1,000X}{1,000} = \frac{4,000}{1,000}$$

$$1{,}000X = 4{,}000$$

$$X = 4 \text{ mL}$$

Administer 4 mL of heparin for the bolus.

Step 4 Calculate the infusion rate for the heparin IV drip.

Protocol: **Start drip at 18 units/kg/h** (see #10, Figure 17-2)

Supply: heparin 25,000 units per 250 mL (see #2, Figure 17-2) or 100 units/mL

18 units/kg/h × 50 kg = 900 units/h

Think: You want to administer 9 times 1 mL or 9 mL for the IV heparin infusion.

$$\frac{\text{Dosage on hand}}{\text{Amount on hand}} = \frac{\text{Dosage desired/h}}{\text{X Amount desired/h}}$$

$$\frac{100 \text{ units}}{1 \text{ mL}} \quad \times \quad \frac{900 \text{ units/h}}{\text{X mL/h}}$$

$$100X = 900$$

$$\frac{100X}{100} = \frac{900}{100}$$

$$X = 9 \text{ mL/h}$$

Set the flow rate at 9 mL/h.

EXAMPLE 2 ■

After 6 hours, the patient in Example 1 has an APTT of 43 secs. According to the protocol, you will **rebolus with 40 units/kg and increase the amount of IV heparin by 2 units/kg/h** (see #12, Figure 17-2).

Step 1 You already know the patient's weight: 50 kg

Step 2 Calculate the heparin rebolus dosage.

40 units/kg × 50 kg = 2,000 units

Step 3 Calculate the number of milliliters to prepare.

Supply: heparin 1,000 units/mL, as recommended by the protocol

Think: You want to give 2 times 1 mL or 2 mL.

$$\frac{\text{Dosage on hand}}{\text{Amount on hand}} = \frac{\text{Dosage desired}}{\text{X Amount desired}}$$

$$\frac{1{,}000 \text{ units}}{1 \text{ mL}} \quad \times \quad \frac{2{,}000 \text{ units}}{\text{X mL}}$$

$$1{,}000X = 2{,}000$$

$$\frac{1{,}000X}{1{,}000} = \frac{2{,}000}{1{,}000}$$

$$X = 2 \text{ mL}$$

Administer 2 mL of heparin for the rebolus.

Step 4 Calculate the number of units the patient's IV heparin will be increased.

2 units/kg/h × 50 kg = 100 units/h

Step 5 Calculate the new infusion rate.

Supply: heparin 25,000 units per 250 mL (see #2, Figure 17-2) or 100 units/mL

Think: You want to administer an additional 100 units/h and you have 100 units/mL, so you want to increase the infusion by 1 mL/h.

$$\frac{\text{Dosage on hand}}{\text{Amount on hand}} = \frac{\text{Dosage desired/h}}{\text{X Amount desired/h}}$$

$$\frac{100 \text{ units}}{1 \text{ mL}} \times \frac{100 \text{ units/h}}{\text{X mL/h}}$$

$$100X = 100$$

$$\frac{100X}{100} = \frac{100}{100}$$

$$X = 1 \text{ mL/h}$$

9 mL/h + 1 mL/h = 10 mL/h

Reset the infusion rate to 10 mL/h.

QUICK REVIEW

■ Use ratio-proportion to calculate mL/h when you know units/h and units/mL.

■ Many hospitals use standard protocols to initiate and maintain heparin therapy.

■ The protocols are based on patient weight in kilograms, and adjustments are made based on laboratory results (usually APTT).

Review Set 46

Calculate the flow rate.

1. Order: **0.45% NS 1,000 mL IV c̄ heparin 25,000 units to infuse at 1,000 units/h**

   Flow rate: _____ mL/h

2. Order: **D₅W 500 mL IV c̄ heparin 40,000 units to infuse at 1,100 units/h**

   Flow rate: _____ mL/h

3. Order: **0.45% NS 500 mL IV c̄ heparin 25,000 units to infuse at 500 units/h**

   Flow rate: _____ mL/h

4. Order: **D₅W 500 mL IV c̄ heparin 40,000 units to infuse at 1,500 units/h**

   Flow rate: _____ mL/h

5. Order: **D₅W 1 L IV c̄ heparin 25,000 units to infuse at 1,200 units/h.** On rounds, you assess the patient and observe that the infusion pump is set at 120 mL/h.

   At what rate should the pump be set? _____ mL/h

   What should your action be? _____

6. Order: **D₅W 500 mL IV with heparin 25,000 units to infuse at 800 units/h**

   Flow rate: _____ mL/h

Questions 7 through 10 refer to a patient who weighs 165 lb and has IV heparin ordered per the following Weight-Based Heparin Protocol. With this variation of the heparin protocol you will not round the patient's weight, and instead you will use the patient's actual weight.

Weight-Based Heparin Protocol:

Heparin IV infusion: Heparin 25,000 units in 250 mL of $\frac{1}{2}$ NS

IV boluses: Use heparin 1,000 units/mL

Calculate the patient's weight in kg. Weight: _____ kg

Bolus with heparin 80 units/kg. Then initiate heparin drip at 18 units/kg/h. Obtain APTT every 6 hours and adjust dosage and rate as follows:

If APTT is less than 35 seconds: Rebolus with 80 units/kg and increase rate by 4 units/kg/h.

If APTT is 36 to 44 seconds: Rebolus with 40 units/kg and increase rate by 2 units/kg/h.

If APTT is 45 to 75 seconds: Continue current rate.

If APTT is 76 to 90 seconds: Decrease rate by 2 units/kg/h.

If APTT is greater than 90 seconds: Hold heparin for 1 hour and then decrease rate by 3 units/kg/h.

---

7. Convert the patient's weight to kg: _____ kg

   Calculate the initial heparin bolus dosage: _____ units

   Calculate the bolus dose: _____ mL

   Calculate the initial heparin infusion rate: _____ units/h or _____ mL/h

8. At 0900, the patient's APTT is 33 seconds. According to the protocol, what will your action be?

   Rebolus with _____ units or _____ mL

   Increase infusion rate by _____ units/h or _____ mL/h for a new rate of _____ mL/h

9. At 1500, the patient's APTT is 40 seconds. According to the protocol, what will your action be?

   Rebolus with _____ units or _____ mL

   Increase infusion rate by _____ units/h or _____ mL/h for a new rate of _____ mL/h

10. At 2100, the patient's APTT is 60 seconds. What will your action be according to the protocol?

   _____

The same method can be used to calculate flow rates for other medications ordered at a specified dosage unit per hour. Calculate flow rate for questions 11 through 15.

11. Order: **0.9% NaCl 500 mL IV c̄ Humulin R Regular U-100 insulin 500 units to infuse at 10 units/h**

   Flow rate: _____ mL/h

12. Order: **D₅W 1 L IV c̄ KCl 40 mEq to infuse at 2 mEq/h**

   Flow rate: _____ mL/h

13. Order: **D₅W 100 mL IV c̄ Cardizem 125 mg to infuse at 5 mg/h**

   Flow rate: _____ mL/h

14. Order: **NS 250 mL IV c̄ Cardizem 125 mg to infuse at 10 mg/h**

   Flow rate: _____ mL/h

15. Order: **0.9% NaCl 500 mL IV c̄ Humulin R Regular U-100 insulin 300 units to infuse at 5 units/h**

   Flow rate: _____ mL/h

After completing these problems, see pages 571–572 to check your answers.

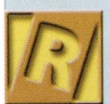

CRITICAL CARE IV CALCULATIONS: CALCULATING FLOW RATE OF AN IV MEDICATION TO BE GIVEN OVER A SPECIFIED TIME PERIOD

With increasing frequency, medications are ordered for patients in critical care situations as a prescribed amount to be administered in a specified time period, such as *X mg per minute*. Such medications are usually administered by electronic infusion devices, programmed in mL/h. Careful monitoring of patients receiving life-threatening therapies is a critical nursing skill.

IV Medication Ordered per Minute

> **RULE**
>
> To determine the flow rate (mL/h) for IV medications ordered per minute (such as mg/min):
>
> **Step 1** Calculate the dosage flow rate in mL/min
>
> Ratio for supply dosage on hand is equivalent to the desired dosage flow rate. In this case it is *per minute*.
>
> $$\frac{\text{Dosage on hand}}{\text{Amount of solution on hand}} = \frac{\text{Dosage desired/min}}{\text{X Amount desired/min}}$$
>
> **Step 2** Calculate the flow rate in mL/h of the volume to administer per minute:
>
> $$\frac{\text{Volume on hand}}{\text{Min to be infused}} = \frac{\text{X volume to be infused/h}}{60 \text{ min/h}}$$
>
> Or,
>
> mL/min × 60 min/h = mL/h
>
> Note: The order may specify mg/min, mcg/min, g/min, units/min, milliunits/min, or mEq/min.

EXAMPLE 1 ■

Order: **lidocaine 2 g IV in 500 mL D₅W at 2 mg/min via infusion pump.** You must prepare and hang 500 mL of D₅W IV solution that has 2 g of lidocaine added to it. Then, you must regulate the flow rate so the patient receives 2 mg of the lidocaine every minute. Determine the flow rate in mL/h.

Step 1 Calculate mL/min (change mg/min to mL/min)

$$\frac{\text{Dosage on hand}}{\text{Amount of solution on hand}} = \frac{\text{Dosage desired/min}}{\text{X Amount desired/min}}$$

Dosage on hand: 2 g = 2,000 mg

Amount of solution on hand: 500 mL

Dosage desired/min: 2 mg/min

Amount desired/min: X mL/min

$$\frac{2{,}000 \text{ mg}}{500 \text{ mL}} \diagdown\diagup \frac{2 \text{ mg/min}}{\text{X mL/min}}$$

$$2{,}000\text{X} = 1{,}000$$

$$\frac{2{,}000\text{X}}{2{,}000} = \frac{1{,}000}{2{,}000}$$

$$\text{X} = 0.5 \text{ mL/min}$$

Step 2 Determine the flow rate in mL/h (change mL/min to mL/h)

$$\frac{\text{Volume on hand}}{\text{Min to be infused}} = \frac{\text{X volume to be infused/h}}{60 \text{ min/h}}$$

Now you know the following information:

Volume on hand: 0.5 mL

Minutes to infuse 0.5 mL: 1 min

Minutes per hour: 60 min/h

Flow rate: X mL/h

$$\frac{0.5\ mL}{1\ min} \quad\nwarrow\!\!\swarrow\quad \frac{X\ mL/h}{60\ min/h}$$

$$X \quad = \quad 30\ mL/h$$

Or, you know that there are 60 minutes per hour, so you can just multiply mL/min by 60 min/h. Notice that *min* cancel out so you have *mL/h* remaining.

mL/min × 60 min/h = mL/h

0.5 mL/m̶i̶n̶ × 60 m̶i̶n̶/h = 30 mL/h

Regulate the flow rate to 30 mL/h to deliver 2 mg/min of lidocaine that is prepared at the concentration of 2 g per 500 mL of D_5W IV solution.

EXAMPLE 2 ■

Order: **nitroglycerin 125 mg IV in 500 mL D_5W to infuse at 42 mcg/min**

Calculate the flow rate in mL/h to program the infusion pump.

Step 1   Calculate mL/min (change mcg/min to mL/min)

First, convert mg to mcg: 1 mg = 1,000 mcg

$$\frac{1\ mg}{1,000\ mcg} \quad\nwarrow\!\!\swarrow\quad \frac{125\ mg}{X\ mcg}$$

$$X \quad = \quad 125,000\ mcg$$

Then, calculate mL/min:

$$\frac{\text{Dosage on hand}}{\text{Amount of solution on hand}} \quad = \quad \frac{\text{Dosage desired/min}}{\text{X Amount desired/min}}$$

$$\frac{125,000\ mcg}{500\ mL} \quad\nwarrow\!\!\swarrow\quad \frac{42\ mcg/min}{X\ mL/min}$$

$$125,000X \quad = \quad 21,000$$

$$\frac{125,000X}{125,000} \quad = \quad \frac{21,000}{125,000}$$

$$X \quad = \quad 0.168\ mL/min = 0.17\ mL/min$$

Step 2   Determine the flow rate in mL/h (change mL/min to mL/h)

$$\frac{\text{Volume on hand}}{\text{Min to be infused}} \quad = \quad \frac{\text{X volume to be infused/h}}{60\ min/h}$$

$$\frac{0.17\ mL}{1\ min} \quad\nwarrow\!\!\swarrow\quad \frac{X\ mL/h}{60\ min/h}$$

$$X \quad = \quad 10.2\ mL/h = 10\ mL/h$$

Or, you can just multiply mL/min by 60 min/h.

mL/min × 60 min/h = mL/h

0.17 mL/m̶i̶n̶ × 60 m̶i̶n̶/h = 10.2 mL/h = 10 mL/h

Regulate the flow rate to 10 mL/h to deliver 42 mcg/min of nitroglycerin that is prepared at the concentration of 125 mg per 500 mL of D_5W IV solution.

IV Medication Ordered Per Kilogram Per Minute

The physician may also order the amount of medication in an IV solution that a patient should receive in a specified time period per kilogram of body weight. An electronic infusion device is usually used to administer these orders.

RULE

To determine the flow rate (mL/h) for IV medications ordered per minute (such as mg/min):

Step 1 Convert to like units, such as mg to mcg or lb to kg

Step 2 Calculate desired dosage per minute: mg/kg/min × kg = mg/min

Step 3 Calculate the dosage flow rate in mL/min:

$$\frac{\text{Dosage on hand}}{\text{Amount of solution on hand}} = \frac{\text{Dosage desired/min}}{\text{X Amount desired/min}}$$

Step 4 Calculate the flow rate in mL/h of the volume to administer per minute:

$$\frac{\text{Volume on hand}}{\text{Min to be infused}} = \frac{\text{X volume to be infused/h}}{\text{60 min/h}}$$

Or,

mL/min × 60 min/h = mL/h

Note: The order may specify mg/min, mcg/min, g/min, units/min, milliunits/min, or mEq/min; or mg/h, mcg/h, g/h, units/h, milliunits/h, or mEq/h

EXAMPLE 1 ■

Order: **250 mL of IV solution with 225 mg of a medication to infuse at 3 mcg/kg/min via infusion pump** for a person who weighs 110 lb.

Determine the flow rate in mL/h.

Step 1 Convert mg to mcg: 1 mg = 1,000 mcg

$$\frac{1 \text{ mg}}{1,000 \text{ mcg}} \times \frac{225 \text{ mg}}{\text{X mcg}}$$

$$X = 225,000 \text{ mcg}$$

Convert lb to kg: 1 kg = 2.2 lb

$$\frac{1 \text{ kg}}{2.2 \text{ lb}} \times \frac{\text{X kg}}{110 \text{ lb}}$$

$$2.2X = 110$$

$$\frac{2.2X}{2.2} = \frac{110}{2.2}$$

$$X = 50 \text{ kg}$$

Step 2 Calculate desired mcg/min

3 mcg/k̶g̶/min × 50 k̶g̶ = 150 mcg/min

Step 3 Calculate mL/min

$$\frac{\text{Dosage on hand}}{\text{Amount of solution on hand}} = \frac{\text{Dosage desired/min}}{\text{X Amount desired/min}}$$

$$\frac{225,000 \text{ mcg}}{250 \text{ mL}} \times \frac{150 \text{ mcg/min}}{\text{X mL/min}}$$

$$225,000X = 37,500$$

$$\frac{225,000X}{225,000} = \frac{37,500}{225,000}$$

$$X = 0.166 \text{ mL/min} = 0.17 \text{ mL/min}$$

Step 4   Calculate mL/h

$$\frac{\text{Volume on hand}}{\text{Min to be infused}} = \frac{\text{X volume to be infused/h}}{60 \text{ min/h}}$$

$$\frac{0.17 \text{ mL}}{1 \text{ min}} \diagdown \frac{\text{X mL/h}}{60 \text{ min/h}}$$

$$\text{X} = 10.2 \text{ mL/h} = 10 \text{ mL/h}$$

Or, you can just multiply mL/min by 60 min/h.

mL/min × 60 min/h = mL/h

0.17 mL/min × 60 min/h = 10.2 mL/h = 10 mL/h

Regulate the flow rate to 10 mL/h to deliver 150 mcg/min (3 mcg/kg/min) of the drug that is prepared at the concentration of 225 mg per 250 mL of IV solution for a person who weighs 110 lb or 50 kg.

Titrating IV Drugs

Sometimes IV medications may be prescribed to be administered at an initial dosage over a specified time period and then continued at a different dosage and time period. These situations are common in obstetrics and critical care. Medications, such as magnesium sulfate, dopamine, Isuprel, and Pitocin, are ordered to be *titrated* or *regulated* to obtain measurable physiologic responses. Dosages will be adjusted until the desired effect is achieved. In some cases, a loading or bolus dose is infused and monitored closely. Most IV medications that require titration usually start at the lowest dosage and are increased or decreased as needed. An upper titration limit is usually set and is not exceeded unless the desired response is not obtained. A new drug order is then required.

Let's look at some of these situations.

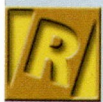

RULE

To calculate flow rate (mL/h) for IV medications ordered over a specific time period (such as mg/min):

Step 1   Calculate mg/mL

Step 2   Calculate mL/h

Note: The order may specify mg/min, mcg/min, g/min, units/min, milliunits/min, or mEq/min; or it may specify mg/h, mcg/h, g/h, units/h, milliunits/h, or mEq/h.

EXAMPLE 1 ▪

Order: RL 1,000 mL IV c̄ magnesium sulfate 20 g. Start with bolus of 4 g for 30 min, then maintain a continuous infusion at 2 g/h.

1. What is the flow rate in mL/h for the bolus order?

Step 1   Calculate the bolus dosage in g/mL

There are 20 g in 1,000 mL. How many mL are necessary to infuse 4 g?

$$\frac{\text{Dosage on hand}}{\text{Amount of solution on hand}} = \frac{\text{Dosage desired}}{\text{X Amount desired}}$$

$$\frac{20 \text{ g}}{1,000 \text{ mL}} \diagdown \frac{4 \text{ g}}{\text{X mL}}$$

$$20\text{X} = 4,000$$

$$\frac{20X}{20} = \frac{4{,}000}{20}$$

$$X = 200 \text{ mL}$$

Therefore, 200 mL contain 4 g, to be administered over 30 min.

Step 2 Calculate the bolus rate in mL/h

What is the flow rate in mL/h to infuse 200 mL (which contain 4 g of magnesium sulfate)? Remember 1 h = 60 min.

$$\frac{\text{Volume on hand}}{\text{Min to be infused}} = \frac{X \text{ volume to be infused/h}}{60 \text{ min/h}}$$

$$\frac{200 \text{ mL}}{30 \text{ min}} \diagdown \frac{X \text{ mL/h}}{60 \text{ min/h}}$$

$$30X = 12{,}000$$

$$\frac{30X}{30} = \frac{12{,}000}{30}$$

$$X = 400 \text{ mL/h}$$

Set the infusion pump at 400 mL/h to deliver the bolus of 4 g for 30 min as ordered.

Now calculate the continuous IV rate in mL/h.

2. What is the flow rate in mL/h for the continuous infusion of magnesium sulfate of 2 g/h? You know from the bolus dosage calculation that 200 mL contain 4 g.

$$\frac{\text{Dosage on hand}}{\text{Amount of solution on hand}} = \frac{\text{Dosage desired/h}}{X \text{ Amount desired/h}}$$

$$\frac{4 \text{ g}}{200 \text{ mL}} \diagdown \frac{2 \text{ g/h}}{X \text{ mL/h}}$$

$$4X = 400$$

$$\frac{4X}{4} = \frac{400}{4}$$

$$X = 100 \text{ mL/h}$$

After the bolus has infused in the first 30 min, reset the infusion pump to 100 mL/h to deliver the continuous infusion of 2 g/h.

Let's look at an example using Pitocin (a drug used to induce or augment labor), measured in units and milliunits.

EXAMPLE 2 ■

A drug order is written to induce labor: LR 1,000 mL IV c̄ Pitocin 20 units. Begin a continuous infusion IV at 1 milliunit/min, increase by 1 milliunit/min q.15 min to a maximum of 20 milliunits/min.

1. What is the flow rate in mL/h to deliver 1 milliunit/min?

In this example, the medication is measured in units (instead of g or mg).

Step 1 Calculate milliunits/mL

Convert: 1 unit = 1,000 milliunits; 20 units = 20,000 milliunits

$$\frac{\text{Dosage on hand}}{\text{Amount of solution on hand}} = \frac{\text{Dosage desired}}{X \text{ Amount desired}}$$

Dosage on hand: 20,000 milliunits

Amount of solution on hand: 1,000 mL

Dosage desired: 1 milliunit

$$\frac{20{,}000 \text{ milliunits}}{1{,}000 \text{ mL}} \times \frac{1 \text{ milliunit}}{X \text{ mL}}$$

$$20{,}000X = 1{,}000$$

$$\frac{20{,}000X}{20{,}000} = \frac{1{,}000}{20{,}000}$$

$$X = 0.05 \text{ mL}$$

Therefore, 0.05 mL contains 1 milliunit of Pitocin, or there is 1 milliunit per 0.05 mL.

Step 2   Calculate mL/h

What is the flow rate in mL/h to infuse 0.05 mL/min (which is 1 milliunit Pitocin/min)?

$$\frac{\text{Volume on hand}}{\text{Min to be infused}} = \frac{X \text{ volume to be infused/h}}{60 \text{ min/h}}$$

$$\frac{0.05 \text{ mL}}{1 \text{ min}} \times \frac{X \text{ mL/h}}{60 \text{ min/h}}$$

$$X = 3 \text{ mL/h}$$

Set the infusion pump at 3 mL/h to infuse Pitocin 1 milliunit/min as ordered.

2. What is the maximum flow rate in mL/h that the Pitocin infusion can be set for the titration as ordered? Notice that the order allows a maximum of 20 milliunits/min. You know from the bolus dosage calculation that there is 1 milliunit per 0.05 mL.

$$\frac{\text{Dosage on hand}}{\text{Amount of solution on hand}} = \frac{\text{Dosage desired/min}}{X \text{ Amount desired/min}}$$

Dosage on hand: 1 milliunit

Amount of solution: 0.05 mL

Dosage desired: 20 milliunits/min

$$\frac{1 \text{ milliunit}}{0.05 \text{ mL}} \times \frac{20 \text{ milliunits/min}}{X \text{ mL/min}}$$

$$X = 0.05 \times 20$$

$$X = 1 \text{ mL/min}$$

Now convert mL/min to mL/h, so you can program the electronic infusion device.

$$\frac{\text{Volume on hand}}{\text{Min to be infused}} = \frac{X \text{ volume to be infused/h}}{60 \text{ min/h}}$$

$$\frac{1 \text{ mL}}{1 \text{ min}} \times \frac{X \text{ mL/h}}{60 \text{ min/h}}$$

$$X = 60 \text{ mL/h}$$

Or, you can just multiply mL/min by 60 min/h.

mL/min × 60 min/h = mL/h

1 mL/min × 60 min/h = 60 mL/h

You know that 1 milliunit/min is infused at 3 mL/h.

$$\frac{3 \text{ mL/h}}{1 \text{ milliunit/min}} \times \frac{X \text{ mL/h}}{20 \text{ milliunits/min}}$$

$$X = 60 \text{ mL/h}$$

Rate of 60 mL/h will deliver 20 milliunits/min.

Verifying Safe IV Medication Dosage Recommended Per Minute

It is also a critical nursing skill to be sure that patients are receiving safe dosages of medications. Therefore, you must also be able to convert critical care IVs with additive medications to **mg/h** or **mg/min** to check safe or normal dosage ranges.

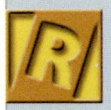

RULE

To check safe dosage of IV medications ordered in mL/h:

Step 1 Calculate mg/h

Step 2 Calculate mg/min

Step 3 Compare recommended dosage and ordered dosage to decide if the dosage is safe.

Note: The ordered and recommended dosages may specify mg/min, mcg/min, g/min, units/min, milliunits/min, or mEq/min.

EXAMPLE ■

The *Hospital Formulary* states that the recommended dosage of Lidocaine is 1 to 4 mg/min. The patient has an order for D₅W 500 mL IV c̄ lidocaine 1 g to infuse at 30 mL/h. Is the lidocaine dosage within the safe range?

Step 1 Calculate mg/h

Convert: 1 g = 1,000 mg

Remember, the unknown X is mg/h. Notice that X is in the numerator of the second ratio in this proportion.

$$\frac{\text{Dosage on hand}}{\text{Amount of solution on hand}} = \frac{\text{X Dosage desired/h}}{\text{Amount desired/h}}$$

$$\frac{1,000 \text{ mg}}{500 \text{ mL}} \diagdown \frac{\text{X mg/h}}{30 \text{ mL/h}}$$

$$500\text{X} = 30,000$$

$$\frac{500\text{X}}{500} = \frac{30,000}{500}$$

$$\text{X} = 60 \text{ mg/h} \quad \text{60 mg are administered in one hour when the flow rate is 30 mL/h.}$$

Step 2 Calculate mg/min. THINK: It is obvious that 60 mg/h is the same as 60 mg per 60 min or 1 mg/min.

$$\frac{60 \text{ mg}}{60 \text{ min}} \diagdown \frac{\text{X mg}}{1 \text{ min}}$$

$$60\text{X} = 60$$

$$\frac{60\text{X}}{60} = \frac{60}{60}$$

$$\text{X} = 1 \text{ mg}$$

Rate is 1 mg/min.

Step 3 Compare ordered and recommended dosages.

1 mg/min is within the safe range of 1 to 4 mg/min. The dosage is safe.

Likewise, IV medications ordered as mL/h and recommended in mg/kg/min require verification of their safety or normal dosage range.

> **RULE**
>
> To check safe dosage of IV medications recommended in mg/kg/min and ordered in mL/h:
>
> **Step 1** Convert to like units, such as mg to mcg or lb to kg
>
> **Step 2** Calculate recommended mg/min
>
> **Step 3** Calculate ordered mg/h
>
> **Step 4** Calculate ordered mg/min
>
> **Step 5** Compare ordered and recommended dosages. Decide if the dosage is safe
>
> Note: The ordered and recommended dosages may specify mg/kg/min, mcg/kg/min, g/kg/min, units/kg/min, milliunits/kg/min, or mEq/kg/min.

EXAMPLE ■

The recommended dosage range of Nitropress for adults is 0.3–10 mcg/kg/min. The patient has an order for **D₅W 100 mL IV with Nitropress 420 mg to infuse at 1 mL/h**. The patient weighs 154 lb. Is the Nitropress dosage within the normal range?

Step 1 Convert lb to kg

$$\frac{1\ kg}{2.2\ lb} \bowtie \frac{X\ kg}{154\ lb}$$

$$2.2X = 154$$

$$\frac{2.2X}{2.2} = \frac{154}{2.2}$$

$$X = 70\ kg$$

Convert mg to mcg: 420 mg = 420.000. = 420,000 mcg

Step 2 Calculate recommended mcg/min range.

minimum: 0.3 mcg/kg/min × 70 kg = 21 mcg/min

maximum: 10 mcg/kg/min × 70 kg = 700 mcg/min

Step 3 Calculate ordered mcg/h

$$\frac{Dosage\ on\ hand}{Amount\ on\ hand} = \frac{Dosage\ desired/h}{X\ Amount\ desired/h}$$

$$\frac{420,000\ mcg}{100\ mL} \bowtie \frac{X\ mcg/h}{1\ mL/h}$$

$$100X = 420,000$$

$$\frac{100X}{100} = \frac{420,000}{100}$$

$$X = 4,200\ mcg/h$$

Step 4 Calculate ordered mcg/min

You know 1 h = 60 min; therefore, 4,200 mcg/h = 4,200 mcg per 60 min. How many mcg can be infused in 1 min?

$$\frac{4,200\ mcg}{60\ min} \bowtie \frac{X\ mcg}{1\ min}$$

$$60X = 4,200$$

$$\frac{60X}{60} = \frac{4,200}{60}$$

$$X = 70\ mcg\ (per\ minute)$$

This is also a simple division problem.

$$\frac{4,200\ mcg}{60\ min} = 70\ mcg/min$$

Step 5 Compare ordered and recommended dosages. Decide if the dosage is safe. 70 mcg/min is within the allowable range of 21 to 700 mcg/min. The ordered dosage is safe.

QUICK REVIEW

- For IV medications ordered in mg/min:

  Step 1 Calculate mL/min

  Step 2 Calculate mL/h

- To check safe dosages of IV medications recommended in mg/min and ordered in mL/h:

  Step 1 Calculate mg/h

  Step 2 Calculate mg/min

  Step 3 Compare recommended and ordered dosages. Decide if the dosage is safe.

- To check safe dosage of IV medications recommended in mg/kg/min and ordered in mL/h:

  Step 1 Convert to like units, such as mg to mcg or lb to kg

  Step 2 Calculate recommended mg/min

  Step 3 Calculate ordered mg/h

  Step 4 Calculate ordered mg/min

  Step 5 Compare ordered and recommended dosages. Decide if the dosage is safe.

Review Set 47

Compute the flow rate for each of these medications administered by infusion pump.

1. Order: lidocaine 2 g IV per 1,000 mL D₅W at 4 mg/min

   Rate: _____ mL/min and _____ mL/h

2. Order: Pronestyl 0.5 g IV per 250 mL D₅W at 2 mg/min

   Rate: _____ mL/min and _____ mL/h

3. Order: Isuprel 2 mg IV per 500 mL D₅W at 6 mcg/min

   Rate: _____ mL/min and _____ mL/h

4. Order: Medication X 450 mg IV per 500 mL NS at 4 mcg/kg/min

   Weight: 198 lb

   Weight: _____ kg   Give: _____ mcg/min

   Rate: _____ mL/min and _____ mL/h

5. Order: dopamine 800 mg in 500 mL NS IV at 15 mcg/kg/min

   Weight: 70 kg

   Give: _____ mcg/min

   Rate: _____ mL/min and _____ mL/h

Refer to this order for questions 6 through 8.

Order: D₅W 500 mL IV c̄ dobutamine hydrochloride 500 mg to infuse at 15 mL/h. The patient weighs 125 lb. Recommended range: 2.5 to 10 mcg/kg/min

6. What mcg/min range of dobutamine should this patient receive?

   _____ to _____ mcg/min

7. What mg/min range of dobutamine should this patient receive?

_____ to _____ mg/min

8. Is the dobutamine as ordered within the safe range? _____

Refer to this order for questions 9 and 10.

Order: D$_5$W 500 mL IV $\bar{c}$ Pronestyl 2 g to infuse at 60 mL/h. Normal range: 2 to 6 mg/min

9. How many mg/min of Pronestyl is the patient receiving? _____ mg/min

10. Is the dosage of Pronestyl within the normal range? _____

11. Order: magnesium sulfate 20 g IV in LR 500 mL. Start with a bolus of 2 g to infuse over 30 min. Then maintain a continuous infusion at 1 g/h.

    Rate: _____ mL/h for bolus

    _____ mL/h for continuous infusion

12. A drug order is written to induce labor as follows:

    Pitocin 15 units IV in 250 mL LR. Begin a continuous infusion at the rate of 1 milliunit/min.

    Rate: _____ mL/h

Refer to this order for questions 13 through 15.

Order: D$_5$W 1,000 mL IV with terbutaline sulfate 10 mg to infuse at 150 mL/h

Normal dosage range: 10 to 80 mcg/min

13. How many mg/min of terbutaline is the patient receiving? _____ mg/min

14. How many mcg/min of terbutaline is the patient receiving? _____ mcg/min

15. Is the dosage of terbutaline within the normal range? _____

After completing these problems, see pages 572–574 to check your answers.

LIMITING INFUSION VOLUMES

Calculating IV rates to include the IV piggyback (PB) volume may be necessary to limit the total volume of IV fluid a patient receives. To do this, you must calculate the flow rate for both the regular IV and the piggyback IV. In such instances of restricted fluids, the piggyback IVs are to be included as part of the total prescribed IV volume and time.

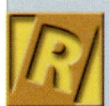

RULE

Follow these six steps to calculate the flow rate of an IV, which includes IV PB.

Step 1 *IV PB flow rate:* $\frac{V}{T} \times C = R$

or use $\dfrac{\text{mL/h}}{\text{Drop factor constant}} = R$

Step 2 *Total IV PB time:*   Time for 1 dose × # of doses in 24 h

Step 3 *Total IV PB volume:*   Volume of 1 dose × # of doses in 24 h

Step 4 *Total regular IV volume:*   Total volume − IV PB volume = Regular IV volume

Step 5 *Total regular IV time:*   Total time − IV PB time = Regular IV time

Step 6 *Regular IV flow rate:* $\frac{V}{T} \times C = R$

or use $\dfrac{\text{mL/h}}{\text{Drop factor constant}} = R$

EXAMPLE 1 ▪

Order: D₅LR 3,000 mL IV for 24 h with cefazolin 1 g IV PB per 100 mL D₅W q.6h to run 1 hour. Limit total fluids to 3,000 mL daily.

The drop factor is 10 gtt/mL.

Note: The order intends that the patient will receive a maximum of 3,000 mL in 24 hours. Remember, when fluids are restricted, the piggybacks are to be *included* in the total 24-hour intake, not added to it.

Step 1 Calculate the flow rate of the IV PB.

$$\frac{V}{T} \times C = \frac{100 \text{ mL}}{\underset{6}{60 \text{ min}}} \times \overset{1}{10} \text{ gtt/mL} = \frac{100 \text{ gtt}}{6 \text{ min}} = 16.6 \text{ gtt/min} = 17 \text{ gtt/min}$$

or $\dfrac{\text{mL/h}}{\text{Drop factor constant}}$ = gtt/min (Drop factor constant is 6)

$$\frac{100 \text{ mL/h}}{6} = 16.6 \text{ gtt/min} = 17 \text{ gtt/min}$$

Set the flow rate for the IV PB at 17 gtt/min to infuse 1 g cefazolin in 100 mL over 1 hour or 60 min.

Step 2 Calculate the total time the IV PB will be administered.

q.6h = 4 times per 24 h; 4 × 1 h = 4 h

Step 3 Calculate the total volume of the IV PB.

100 mL × 4 = 400 mL IV PB per 24 hours

Step 4 Calculate the volume of the regular IV fluids to be administered between IV PB. Total volume of regular IV minus total volume of IV PB: 3,000 mL − 400 mL = 2,600 mL

Step 5 Calculate the total regular IV fluid time or the time between IV PB. Total IV time minus total IV PB time: 24 h − 4 h = 20 h

Step 6 Calculate the flow rate of the regular IV.

$$\text{mL/h} = \frac{2,600 \text{ mL}}{20 \text{ h}} = 130 \text{ mL/h}$$

$$\frac{V}{T} \times C = \frac{130 \text{ mL}}{\underset{6}{60 \text{ min}}} \times \overset{1}{10} \text{ gtt/mL} = \frac{130 \text{ gtt}}{6 \text{ min}} = 21.6 \text{ gtt/min} = 22 \text{ gtt/min}$$

or $\dfrac{\text{mL/h}}{\text{Drop factor constant}}$ = gtt/min (Drop factor constant is 6)

$$\frac{130 \text{ mL/h}}{6} = 21.6 \text{ gtt/min} = 22 \text{ gtt/min}$$

Set the regular IV of D₅LR at the flow rate of 22 gtt/min. Then after 5 hours, switch to the cefazolin IV PB at the flow rate of 17 gtt/min for 1 hour. Repeat this process 4 times in 24 hours.

EXAMPLE 2 ▪

Order: NS 2,000 mL IV for 24 h with 80 mg gentamycin in 80 mL IV PB q.8h to run for 30 min. Limit fluid intake to 2,000 mL daily.

Drop factor: 15 gtt/mL

Calculate the flow rate for the regular IV and for the IV PB.

Step 1 IV PB flow rate:

$$\frac{V}{T} \times C = \frac{80 \text{ mL}}{\underset{2}{30 \text{ min}}} \times \overset{1}{15} \text{ gtt/mL} = \frac{80 \text{ gtt}}{2 \text{ min}} = 40 \text{ gtt/min}$$

Step 2 Total IV PB time: q.8h = 3 times per 24 h; 3 × 30 min = 90 min

$$90 \text{ min} \div 60 \text{ min/h} = \frac{90}{60} \text{ h} = 1\frac{1}{2} \text{ h}$$

Step 3   Total IV PB volume: 80 mL × 3 = 240 mL

Step 4   Total regular IV volume: 2,000 mL − 240 mL = 1,760 mL

Step 5   Total regular IV time: $24 \text{ h} - 1\frac{1}{2} \text{ h} = 22\frac{1}{2} \text{ h} = 22.5 \text{ h}$

Step 6   Regular IV flow rate:

$$\text{mL/h} = \frac{1,760 \text{ mL}}{22.5 \text{ h}} = 78.2 \text{ mL/h} = 78 \text{ mL/h}$$

$$\frac{V}{T} \times C = \frac{78 \text{ mL}}{\overset{60 \text{ min}}{4}} \times \overset{1}{15} \text{ gtt/mL} = \frac{78 \text{ gtt}}{4 \text{ min}} = 19.5 \text{ gtt/min} = 20 \text{ gtt/min}$$

or $\dfrac{\text{mL/h}}{\text{Drop factor constant}} = \text{R}$ (Drop factor constant is 4)

$$\frac{78 \text{ mL/h}}{4} = 19.5 \text{ gtt/min} = 20 \text{ gtt/min}$$

Set the regular IV of NS at the flow rate of 20 gtt/min. After $7\frac{1}{2}$ hours, switch to the genta-mycin IV PB at the flow rate of 40 gtt/min for 30 minutes. Repeat this process 3 times in 24 hours.

Patients receiving a primary IV at a specific rate via an electronic infusion pump may require that the infusion rate be altered when a secondary (piggyback) medication is being administered. To do this, calculate the flow rate of the secondary medication in mL/h as you would for the primary IV, and reset the infusion device.

Some infusion pumps allow you to set the flow rate for the secondary IV independent of the primary IV. Upon completion of the secondary infusion, the infusion device automatically returns to the original flow rate. If this is not the case, be sure to manually readjust the primary flow rate after the completion of the secondary set.

QUICK REVIEW

- To calculate the flow rate of a regular IV with an IV PB and restricted fluids, calculate:

  Step 1   IV PB flow rate

  Step 2   Total IV PB time

  Step 3   Total IV PB volume

  Step 4   Total regular IV volume

  Step 5   Total regular IV time

  Step 6   Regular IV flow rate

Review Set 48

Calculate the flow rates for the IV and IV PB orders. These patients are on limited fluid volume (restricted fluids).

1. Orders: NS 3,000 mL IV for 24 h

   Limit total IV fluids to 3,000 mL daily

   penicillin G potassium 1,000,000 units IV PB q.4h in 100 mL NS to run for 30 min

   Drop factor: 10 gtt/mL

   IV PB flow rate: _____ gtt/min

   IV flow rate: _____ gtt/min

2. Orders: D$_5$W 1,000 mL IV for 24 h

Limit total IV fluids to 1,000 mL daily

gentamicin 40 mg q.i.d. in 40 mL IV PB to run 1 h

Drop factor: 60 gtt/mL

IV PB flow rate: _____ gtt/min

IV flow rate: _____ gtt/min

3. Orders: D$_5$ LR 3,000 mL IV for 24 h

Limit total IV fluids to 3,000 mL daily

ampicillin 0.5 g q.6h IV PB in 50 mL D$_5$W to run 30 min

Drop factor: 15 gtt/mL

IV PB flow rate: _____ gtt/min

IV flow rate: _____ gtt/min

4. Orders: $\frac{1}{2}$ NS 2,000 mL IV for 24 h

Limit total IV fluids to 2,000 mL daily

Chloromycetin 500 mg per 50 mL NS IV PB q.6h to run 1 h

Drop factor: 60 gtt/mL

IV PB flow rate: _____ gtt/min

IV flow rate: _____ gtt/min

5. Orders: LR 1,000 mL IV for 24 h

Limit total IV fluids to 1,000 mL daily

cefazolin 250 mg IV PB per 50 mL D$_5$W q.8h to run 1 h

Drop factor: 60 gtt/mL

IV PB flow rate: _____ gtt/min

IV flow rate: _____ gtt/min

6. Orders: D$_5$ LR 2,400 mL IV for 24 h

Limit total IV fluids to 2,400 mL daily

Ancef 1 g IV PB q.6h in 50 mL D$_5$W to run 30 min

Drop factor: On electronic infusion pump

IV PB flow rate: _____ mL/h

IV flow rate: _____ mL/h

7. Orders: NS 2,000 mL IV for 24 h

Limit total IV fluids to 2,000 mL daily

gentamicin 100 mg IV PB q.8h in 100 mL D$_5$W to run in over 30 min

Drop factor: On electronic infusion pump

IV PB flow rate: _____ mL/h

IV flow rate: _____ mL/h

8. Orders: D$_5$ 0.45% NS 3,000 mL IV to run 24 h

Limit total IV fluids to 3,000 mL daily

Zantac 50 mg q.6h in 50 mL D$_5$W to infuse 15 min

Drop factor: On electronic infusion pump

IV PB flow rate: _____ mL/h

IV flow rate: _____ mL/h

9. Orders: D₅ NS 1,500 mL IV to run 24 h

Limit total IV fluids to 1,500 mL daily

cefazolin 500 mg IV PB per 50 mL D₅W q.8 h to run 1 h

Drop factor: 20 gtt/mL

IV PB flow rate: _____ gtt/min

IV flow rate: _____ gtt/min

10. Orders: NS 2,700 mL IV for 24 h

Limit total IV fluids to 2,700 mL per day

gentamicin 60 mg in 60 mL D₅W IV PB q.8h to run for 30 min

Drop factor: On electronic infusion pump

IV PB flow rate: _____ mL/h

IV flow rate: _____ mL/h

After completing these problems, see pages 574–575 to check your answers.

CRITICAL THINKING SKILLS

The importance of knowing the therapeutic dosage of a given medication is a critical nursing skill. Let's look at an example in which the order was unclear and the nurse did not verify the order with the appropriate person.

ERROR

Failing to clarify an order.

Possible Scenario

Suppose the physician ordered a heparin infusion for a patient with thrombophlebitis who weighs 100 kg. The facility uses the Standard Weight-Based Heparin Protocol as seen in Figure 17-2. The order was written this way:

heparin 25,000 units in 250 mL $\frac{1}{2}$ NS IV at 18000/h

The order was difficult to read, and the nurse asked a co-worker to help her decipher it. They both agreed that it read 18,000 units per hour. The nurse calculated mL/h to be:

$$\frac{\text{Dosage on hand}}{\text{Amount of solution on hand}} = \frac{\text{Dosage desired/h}}{\text{X Amount desired/h}}$$

$$\frac{25,000 \text{ units}}{250 \text{ mL}} \quad\times\quad \frac{18,000 \text{ units/h}}{\text{X mL/h}} \qquad \textbf{INCORRECT}$$

$$25,000\text{X} = 4,500,000$$

$$\frac{25,000\text{X}}{25,000} = \frac{4,500,000}{25,000}$$

$$\text{X} = 180 \text{ mL/h}$$

The nurse proceeded to start the heparin drip at 180 mL/h. The patient's APTT prior to initiation of the infusion was 37 seconds. Six hours into the infusion, an APTT was drawn according to protocol. The nurse was shocked when the results returned and were 95 seconds, which is abnormally high. The nurse called the physician, who asked, "What is the rate of the heparin drip?" The nurse replied, "I have the infusion set at 180 mL/h so that the patient receives the prescribed amount of 18,000 units per hour." The physician was astonished and replied, "I ordered the drip at 1,800 units per hour, not 18,000 units per hour."

Potential Outcome

The physician would likely have discontinued the heparin; ordered protamine sulfate, the antidote for heparin overdosage; and obtained another APTT. The patient may have started to show signs of abnormal bleeding, such as blood in the urine, bloody nose, and increased tendency to bruise.

Prevention

When the physician wrote the order for 1800 U/h, the U for "units" looked like an 0 and the nurse misinterpreted the order as 18,000 units. The nurse missed three opportunities to prevent this error. The order as written is unclear, unsafe, and incomplete. Contacting the physician and requesting a clarification of the order are appropriate actions for several reasons. First, the writing is unclear and does not follow The Joint Commission guidelines, which are automatic cautions to contact the prescribing practitioner for clarification. The prescriber should have used commas to write amounts of 1,000 and greater, and the prescriber should have spelled out *units* rather than use the *U* abbreviation. Guessing about the exact meaning of an order is dangerous, as this scenario demonstrates.

Second, the Standard Weight-Based Heparin Protocol recommends a safe heparin infusion rate of 1,800 units/h or 18 mL/h (with a supply dosage of 25,000 units per 250 mL or 100 units/mL) for an individual weighing 100 kg. It is the responsibility of the individual administering a medication to be sure the Six Rights of medication administration are observed. The first three rights state that the *"**right** patient must receive the **right** drug in the **right** amount."* The order of 18,000 units as understood by the nurse was unsafe. The patient was overdosed by 10 times the recommended amount of heparin.

Third, if the nurse clearly interpreted the order as 18,000, then no unit of measure was specified, which is a medication error that requires contact with the physician for correction. An incomplete order must not be filled.

PRACTICE PROBLEMS—CHAPTER 17

You are working on the day shift 0700–1500 hours. You observe that one of the patients assigned to you has an IV infusion with a volume control set (as shown in Figure 16-3). His orders include:

D₅W IV at 50 mL/h for continuous infusion

piperacillin 1 g IV q.6h

The pharmacy supplies the piperacillin in a prefilled syringe labeled *1 g per 5 mL* with instructions to *add piperacillin to volume control set, and infuse over 30 minutes.* Answer questions 1 through 5.

1. What is the drop factor of the volume control set? _____ gtt/mL

2. What amount of piperacillin will you add to the chamber? _____ mL

3. How much D₅W IV fluid will you add to the chamber with the piperacillin? _____ mL

4. To maintain the flow rate at 50 mL/h, you will time the IV piperacillin to infuse at _____ gtt/min.

5. The medication administration record indicates that the patient received his last dose of IV piperacillin at 0600. How many doses of piperacillin will you administer during your shift? _____

6. Order: **heparin 25,000 units in 250 mL 0.45% NS to infuse at 1,200 units/h**

   Drop factor: On electronic infusion pump

   Flow rate: _____ mL/h.

7. Order: **thiamine 100 mg per L D₅W IV to infuse at 5 mg/h**

   Drop factor: On electronic infusion pump

   Flow rate: _____ mL/h

8. Order: **magnesium sulfate 4 g in 500 mL D₅W at 500 mg/h**

   Drop factor: On electronic infusion pump

   Flow rate: _____ mL/h

9. A patient is to receive **D₅W 500 mL c̄ heparin 20,000 units at 1,400 units/h.**

   Set the infusion pump at _____ mL/h.

10. At the rate of 4 mL/min, how long will it take to administer 1.5 L of IV fluid? _____ h and _____ min

11. Order: **lidocaine 2 g in 500 mL D₅W IV to run at 4 mg/min**

    Drop factor: On electronic infusion pump

    Flow rate: _____ mL/h

12. Order: **Xylocaine 1 g IV in 250 mL D₅W at 3 mg/min**

    Drop factor: On electronic infusion pump

    Flow rate: _____ mL/h

13. Order: **procainamide 1 g IV in 500 mL D₅W to infuse at 2 mg/min**

    Drop factor: On electronic infusion pump

    Flow rate: _____ mL/h

14. Order: **dobutamine 250 mg IV in 250 mL D₅W to infuse at 5 mcg/kg/min**

    Weight: 80 kg

    Drop factor: On electronic infusion pump

    Flow rate: _____ mL/h

15. Your patient has **D₅W 1 L IV with 2 g lidocaine added infusing at 75 mL/h.** The recommended continuous IV dosage of lidocaine is 1 to 4 mg/min. Is this dosage safe? _____

16. Order: **Restricted fluids: 3,000 mL D₅ NS IV for 24 h**

    Chloromycetin 1 g IV PB in 100 mL NS q.6h to run 1 h

    Drop factor: 10 gtt/mL

    Flow rate: _____ gtt/min IV PB and _____ gtt/min primary IV

17. Order: **Restricted fluids: 3,000 mL D₅W IV for 24 h**

    ampicillin 500 mg in 50 mL D₅W IV PB q.i.d. for 30 min

    Drop factor: On electronic infusion pump

    Flow rate: _____ mL/h IV PB and _____ mL/h primary IV

18. Order: **50 mg Nitropress IV in 500 mL D₅W to infuse at 3 mcg/kg/min**

    Weight: 125 lb

    Drop factor: On electronic infusion pump

    Flow rate: _____ mL/h

19. Order: **KCl 40 mEq to each liter IV fluid**

    Situation: IV discontinued with 800 mL remaining

    How much KCl infused? _____

20. A patient's infusion rate is 125 mL/h. The rate is equivalent to _____ mL/min

21. Order: $\frac{1}{2}$ **NS 1,500 mL IV to run at 100 mL/h.** Calculate the infusion time. _____ h

22. Order: **KCl 40 mEq/L D₅W IV to infuse at 2 mEq/h**

    Rate: _____ mL/h

23. Order: **heparin 50,000 units/L D₅W IV to infuse at 1,250 units/h**

    Rate: _____ mL/h

24. If the minimal dilution for tobramycin is 5 mg/mL and you are giving 37 mg, what is the least amount of fluid in which you could safely dilute the dosage? _____ mL

25. Order: **oxytocin 10 units IV in 500 mL NS. Infuse 4 milliunits/min for 20 min, followed by 6 milliunits/min for 20 min. Use electronic infusion pump.**

    Rate: _____ mL/h for first 20 min

    Rate: _____ mL/h for next 20 min

26. Order: **magnesium sulfate 20 g IV in 500 mL of LR solution. Start with a bolus of 3 g to infuse over 30 min. Then maintain a continuous infusion at 2 g/h.**

    You will use an electronic infusion pump.

    Rate: _____ mL/h for bolus

    Rate: _____ mL/h for continuous infusion

27. Order: **Pitocin 15 units IV in 500 mL of LR solution. Infuse at 1 milliunit/min**

    You will use an electronic infusion pump.

    Rate: _____ mL/h

28. Order: **heparin drip 40,000 units/L D₅W IV to infuse at 1,400 units/h**

    Drop factor: On infusion pump

    Flow rate: _____ mL/h

Refer to this order for questions 29 and 30.

Order: **magnesium sulfate 4 g IV in 500 mL D₅W at 500 mg/h on an infusion pump**

29. What is the solution concentration? _____ mg/mL

30. What is the hourly flow rate? _____ mL/h

Calculate the drug concentration of the following IV solutions as requested.

31. A solution containing 80 units of oxytocin in 1,000 mL of D₅W: _____ milliunits/mL

32. A solution containing 200 mg of nitroglycerin in 500 mL of D₅W: _____ mg/mL

33. A solution containing 4 mg of Isuprel in 1,000 mL of D₅W: _____ mcg/mL

34. A solution containing 2 g of lidocaine in 500 mL of D₅W: _____ mg/mL

Refer to this order for questions 35 through 37.

Order: **venuronium bromide IV I mg/kg/min** to control respirations for a patient who is ventilated.

35. The patient weighs 220 pounds, which is equal to _____ kg.

36. The available venuronium bromide 20 mg is dissolved in 100 mL NS. This available solution concentration is _____ mg/mL, which is equivalent to _____ mcg/mL.

37. The IV is infusing at the rate of 1 mcg/kg/min on an infusion pump. The hourly rate is _____ mL/h.

Refer to this order for questions 38 through 43.

Order: **Restricted fluids: 3,000 mL per 24 h. Primary IV of D_5LR running via infusion pump**
       ampicillin 3 g IV PB q.6h in 100 mL of D_5W over 30 min
       gentamicin 170 mg IV PB q.8h in 50 mL of D_5W to infuse in 1 h

38. Calculate the IV PB flow rates. ampicillin: _____ mL/h; gentamicin: _____ mL/h

39. Calculate the total IV PB time. _____ h

40. Calculate the total IV PB volume. _____ mL

41. Calculate the total regular IV volume. _____ mL

42. Calculate the total regular IV time. _____ h

43. Calculate the regular IV flow rate. _____ mL/h

44. A patient who weighs 190 lb receives **dopamine 800 mg in 500 mL of D_5W IV at 4 mcg/kg/min.** As the patient's blood pressure drops, the nurse titrates the drip to **12 mcg/kg/min** as ordered.

    What is the initial flow rate? _____ mL/h

    After titration, what is the flow rate? _____ mL/h

Questions 45 through 49 refer to your patient who has left-leg deep vein thrombosis. He has orders for IV heparin therapy. He weighs 225 lb. On admission his APTT is 25 seconds. You initiate therapy at 1130 on 5/10/xx. Follow the Standard Weight-Based Heparin Protocol (Figure 17-3) and record your answers on the Standard Weight-Based Heparin Protocol Worksheet (Figure 17-4).

FIGURE 17-3

Standard Weight-Based Heparin Protocol

For all patients on heparin drips:
1. Weight in kilograms (round to nearest 10 kg). Required for order to be processed: _____ kg
2. Heparin 25,000 units in 250 mL of $\frac{1}{2}$NS. Boluses to be given as 1,000 units/mL.
3. APTT q.6h or 6 hours after rate change; daily after two consecutive therapeutic APTTs.
4. CBC initially and repeat every _____ days(s).
5. Obtain APTT and PT/INR on day 1 prior to initiation of therapy.
6. Guaiac stool initially then every _____ day(s) until heparin discontinued. Notify if positive.
7. Neuro checks every _____ hours while on heparin. Notify physician of any changes.
8. Discontinue APTT and CBC once heparin drip is discontinued, unless otherwise ordered.
9. Notify physician of any bleeding problems.
10. Bolus with 80 units/kg. Start drip at 18 units/kg/h.

11. If APTT is less than 35 secs:	Rebolus with 80 units/kg and increase rate by 4 units/kg/h
12. If APTT is 36 to 44 secs:	Rebolus with 40 units/kg and increase rate by 2 units/kg/h
13. If APTT is 45 to 75 secs:	Continue current rate
14. If APTT is 76 to 90 secs:	Decrease rate by 2 units/kg/h
15. If APTT is greater than 90 secs:	Hold heparin for 1 hour and decrease rate by 3 units/kg/h

FIGURE 17-4

STANDARD WEIGHT-BASED HEPARIN PROTOCOL WORKSHEET

Round Patient's Total Body Weight to Nearest 10 kg: _____ kg
DO NOT Change the Weight Based on Daily Measurements

FOUND ON THE ORDER FORM
Initial Bolus (80 units/kg) _____ units   _____ mL
Initial Infusion Rate (18 units/kg/h) _____ units/h   _____ mL/h

Make adjustments to the heparin drip rate as directed by the order form.
ALL DOSES ARE ROUNDED TO THE NEAREST 100 UNITS

Date	Time	APTT	Bolus	Rate Change		New Rate	RN 1	RN 2
				units/h	mL/h			

If APTT is	Then
Less than 35 secs:	Rebolus with 80 units/kg and increase rate by 4 units/kg/h
36 to 44 secs:	Rebolus with 40 units/kg and increase rate by 2 units/kg/h
45 to 75 secs:	Continue current rate
76 to 90 secs:	Decrease rate by 2 units/kg/h
Greater than 90 secs:	Hold heparin for 1 hour and decrease rate by 3 units/kg/h

Signatures   Initials

_____

_____

_____

_____

45. What is the patient's weight in kilograms? Calculate the weight as instructed in the protocol and record weight on the worksheet. _____ kg. What does the protocol indicate for the standard bolus dosage of heparin? _____ units/kg

46. Calculate the dosage of heparin that should be administered for the bolus for this patient, and record your answer on the worksheet. _____ units

    What does the protocol indicate as the required solution concentration (supply dosage) of heparin to use for the bolus? _____ units/mL

    Calculate the dose volume of heparin that should be administered for the bolus for this patient, and record your answer on the worksheet. _____ mL

47. What does the protocol indicate for the initial infusion rate? _____ units/kg/h

    Calculate the dosage of heparin this patient should receive each hour, and record your answer on the worksheet. _____ units/h

    What does the protocol indicate as the required solution concentration (supply dosage) of heparin to use for the initial infusion? _____ units/mL

    Calculate the heparin solution volume this patient should receive each hour to provide the correct infusion for his weight, and record your answer on the worksheet. _____ mL/h

48. According to the protocol, how often should the patient's APTT be checked? q._____ h

    At 1730, the patient's APTT is 37 seconds. Calculate the new heparin bolus and record your answer on the worksheet. Give _____ units/kg or _____ units measured as _____ mL

    Calculate the change in heparin infusion rate (increase or decrease) and record on worksheet. How much should you change the infusion rate? _____ by _____ units/kg/h or _____ units/h for a rate of _____ mL/h

    Calculate the new infusion rate and record on worksheet. _____ mL/h

49. At 2330, the patient's APPT is 77 seconds. What should you do now?

    _____

    Calculate the new infusion rate and record your answer on the worksheet. _____ mL/h

50. Describe the strategy you would implement to prevent this medication error.

    Possible Scenario
    Suppose the physician writes an order to induce labor, as follows: **Pitocin 20 U IV added to 1 liter of LR beginning at 1 mU/min, then increase by 1 mU/min q 15 min to a maximum of 20 mU/min until adequate labor is reached.** The labor and delivery unit stocks Pitocin ampules 10 units per mL in boxes of 50 ampules. The nurse preparing the IV solution misread the order as "20 mL of Pitocin added to 1 liter of lactated Ringer's . . ." and pulled 20 ampules of Pitocin from the supply shelf. Another nurse, seeing this nurse drawing up medication from several ampules, asked what the nurse was preparing. When the nurse described the IV solution being prepared, he suddenly realized he had misinterpreted the order.

    Potential Outcome
    The amount of Pitocin that was being drawn up (20 mL) to be added to the IV solution would have been 10 units/mL × 20 mL = 200 units of Pitocin, 10 times the ordered amount of 20 units. Starting this Pitocin solution, even at the usual slow rate, would have delivered an excessively high amount of Pitocin that could have led to fatal consequences for both the fetus and laboring mother. What should the nurse have done to avoid this type of error?

    Prevention

    _____

    _____

After completing these problems, see pages 576–580 to check your answers.

SECTION 4 SELF-EVALUATION

Chapter 15—Intravenous Solutions, Equipment, and Calculations

1. Which of the following IV solutions is normal saline? _____ 0.45% NaCl

   _____ 0.9% NaCl   _____ D_5W

2. What is the solute and concentration of 0.9% NaCl? _____

3. What is the solute and concentration of 0.45% NaCl? _____

Use the following information to answer questions 4 and 5.

Order: D_5 0.45% NaCl 1,000 mL IV q.8h

4. The IV solution contains _____ g dextrose.

5. The IV solution contains _____ g sodium chloride.

6. Order: **0.45% NaCl 500 mL IV q.6h.** The IV solution contains _____ g sodium chloride.

Refer to this order for questions 7 and 8.

Order: D_{10} 0.9% NaCl 750 mL IV q.8h

7. The IV solution contains _____ g dextrose.

8. The IV solution contains _____ g sodium chloride.

9. Are most electronic infusion devices calibrated in gtt/min, mL/h, mL/min, or gtt/mL? _____

Use the following information to answer questions 10 and 11.

Mrs. Wilson has an order to receive **2,000 mL of D_5NS IV fluids over 24 h.** The IV tubing is calibrated for a drop factor of 15 gtt/mL.

10. Calculate the watch count flow rate for Mrs. Wilson's IV. _____ gtt/min

11. An electronic infusion pump becomes available, and you decide to use it to regulate Mrs. Wilson's IV. Set the pump at _____ mL/h.

12. Mrs. Hawkins returns from the delivery room at 1530 with 400 mL D_5LR infusing at 24 gtt/min with your hospital's standard macrodrop infusion control set calibrated at 15 gtt/mL. You anticipate that Mrs. Hawkins's IV will be complete at _____ (hours).

13. You start your shift at 3:00 PM. On your nursing assessment rounds, you find that Mr. Johnson has an IV of $D_5 \frac{1}{2}$ NS infusing at 32 gtt/min. The tubing is calibrated for 10 gtt/mL. Mr. Johnson will receive _____ mL during your 8-hour shift.

Use the following information to answer questions 14 through 16.

As you continue on your rounds, you find Mr. Boyd with an infiltrated IV and decide to restart it and regulate it on an electronic infusion pump. The orders specify:
NS 1,000 mL IV c̄ 20 mEq KCl q.8h
cefazolin 250 mg IV PB per 100 mL NS q.8h over 30 min
Limit IV total fluids to 3,000 mL daily

14. Interpret Mr. Boyd's IV and medication orders. _____

   _____

15. Regulate the electronic infusion pump for Mr. Boyd's standard IV at _____ mL/h.

16. Regulate the electronic infusion pump for Mr. Boyd's IV PB at _____ mL/h.

17. Order: **D₅LR 1,200 mL IV at 100 mL/h.** You start this IV at 1530 and during your nursing assessment at 2200, you find 650 mL remaining. The flow rate is 100 gtt/min using a microdrip infusion set. Describe your action now. _____

_____

Chapter 16—Body Surface Area and Advanced Pediatric Calculations

Calculate the hourly maintenance IV rate for the children described in questions 18 through 21. Use the following recommendations:

First 10 kg of body weight: 100 mL/kg/day

Next 10 kg of body weight: 50 mL/kg/day

Each additional kg over 20 kg of body weight: 20 mL/kg/day

18. A child who weighs 40 lb requires _____ mL/day for maintenance IV fluids.

19. The infusion rate for the same child who weighs 40 lb is _____ mL/h.

20. An infant who weighs 1,185 g requires _____ mL/day for maintenance IV fluids.

21. The infusion rate for the same infant who weighs 1,185 g is _____ mL/h.

Use the BSA formula method on the following page to answer questions 22 through 24.

22. Height: 30 in   Weight: 24 lb   BSA: _____ m²

23. Height: 155 cm   Weight: 39 kg   BSA: _____ m²

24. Height: 52 in   Weight: 65 lb   BSA: _____ m²

Questions 25 through 31 refer to the following situation.

A child who is 28 in tall and weighs 25 lb will receive 1 dosage of cisplatin IV. The recommended dosage is 37 to 75 mg/m² once every 2 to 3 weeks. The order reads **cisplatin 18.5 mg IV at 1 mg/min today at 1500 hours.** You have available a 50 mg vial of cisplatin. Reconstitution directions state to *add 50 mL of sterile water to yield 1 mg/mL.* Minimal dilution instructions require 2 mL of IV solution for every 1 mg of cisplatin.

25. According to the nomogram on the following page, the child's BSA is _____ m².

26. The safe dosage range for this child is _____ mg to _____ mg.

27. Is this dosage safe? _____.

28. If safe, you will prepare _____ mL. If not, describe your action. _____

_____

29. How many mL of IV fluid are required for safe dilution of the cisplatin? _____ mL

30. Given the ordered rate of 1 mg/min, set the infusion pump at _____ mL/h.

31. How long will this infusion take? _____ min

WEST NOMOGRAM

Metric:

$$\text{BSA (m}^2) = \sqrt{\frac{\text{ht (cm)} \times \text{wt (kg)}}{3,600}}$$

Household:

$$\text{BSA (m}^2) = \sqrt{\frac{\text{ht (in)} \times \text{wt (lb)}}{3,131}}$$

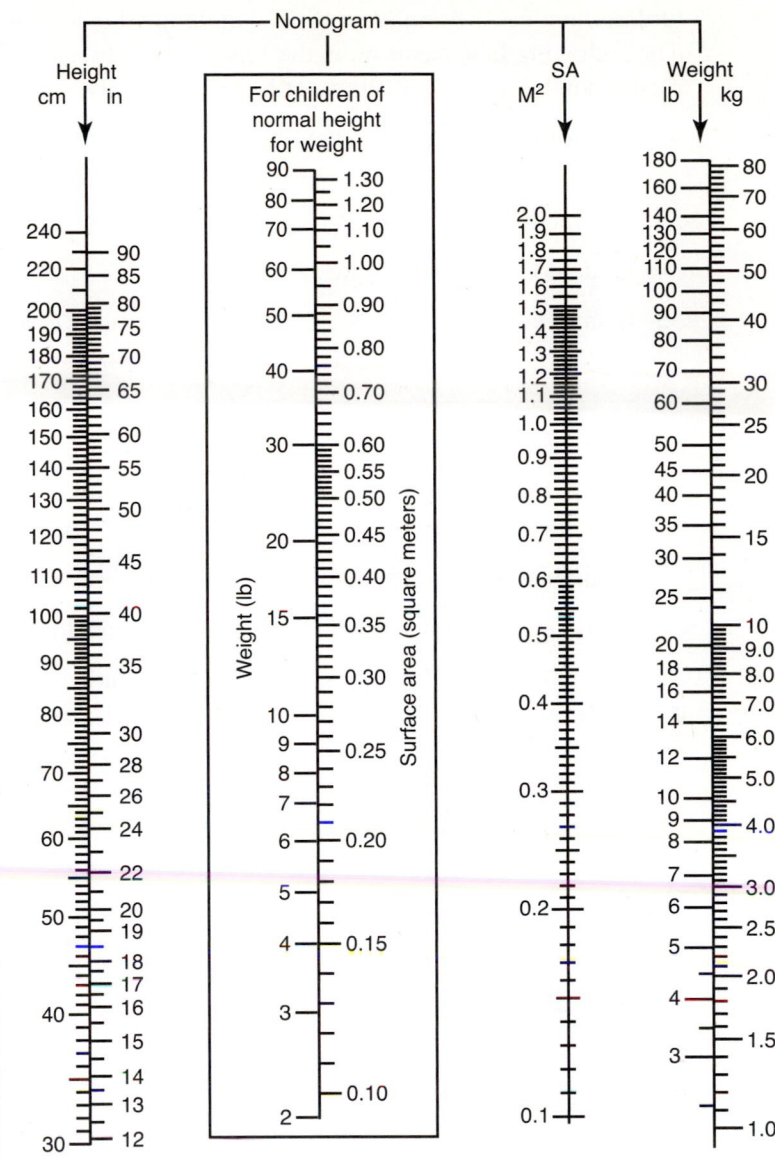

West Nomogram for estimation of body surface area. (From Kliegman, R.M., Behrman, R.E., Jenson, H.B., & Stanton, B.F. [2007]. Nelson textbook of pediatrics [18th ed.]. Philadelphia: Saunders. Reprinted with permission.)

Questions 32 through 35 refer to the following situation.

Order: **Vincasar 1.6 mg IV stat.** The child is 50 inches tall and weighs 40 lb. The following label represents the Vincasar solution you have available. The recommended dosage of Vincasar is 2 mg/m² daily.

32. According to the nomogram on the previous page, the child's BSA is _____ m².

33. The recommended safe dosage for this child is _____ mg.

34. Is the dosage ordered safe? _____

35. If safe, you will prepare _____ mL Vincasar to add to the IV. If not safe, describe your action.

_____

_____

36. Order: **NS IV for continuous infusion at 40 mL/h c̄ Ancef 250 mg IV q.8h over 30 min by volume control set**

    Available: Ancef 125 mg/mL

    Add _____ mL NS and _____ mL Ancef to the chamber to infuse at 40 mL/h.

37. Order: **Timentin 750 mg IV q.6h.** Recommended minimal dilution (maximal concentration) is 100 mg/mL. Calculate the number of mL to be used for minimal dilution of the Timentin as ordered. _____ mL

Chapter 17—Advanced Adult Intravenous Calculations

Use the following information to answer questions 38 through 41.

Mr. Smith is on restricted fluids. His IV order is: **NS 1,500 mL IV q.24h c̄ 300,000 units penicillin G potassium IV PB in 100 mL NS q.4h over 30 min.** The infusion set is calibrated at 60 gtt/mL.

38. Set Mr. Smith's regular IV at _____ gtt/min.

39. Set Mr. Smith's IV PB at _____ gtt/min.

40. Later during your shift, an electronic infusion pump becomes available. You decide to use it to regulate Mr. Smith's IVs. Regulate Mr. Smith's regular IV at _____ mL/h.

41. Regulate Mr. Smith's IV PB at _____ mL/h.

42. Order: **KCl 40 mEq/L D₅W IV at 2 mEq/h**

    Regulate the infusion pump at _____ mL/h.

43. Order: **nitroglycerin 25 mg/L D₅W IV at 5 mcg/min**

    Regulate the infusion pump at _____ mL/h.

Refer to this order for questions 44 through 47.

Order: **Induce labor c̄ Pitocin 15 units/L LR IV continuous infusion at 2 milliunits/min; increase by 1 milliunit/min q.30 min to a maximum of 20 milliunits/min**

44. The initial concentration of Pitocin is _____ milliunits/mL.

45. The initial Pitocin order will infuse at the rate of _____ mL/min.

46. Regulate the electronic infusion pump at _____ mL/h to initiate the order.

NDC 0703-4402-11

VINCASAR PFS®
(vincristine sulfate injection, USP)

PRESERVATIVE FREE SOLUTION
1 mg/mL

FATAL IF GIVEN INTRATHECALLY
FOR INTRAVENOUS USE ONLY
Single Dose Vial
REFRIGERATE
Protect From Light

sicor™
SICOR Pharmaceuticals, Inc.,
Irvine, CA 92618

(01)00307034402115

440202

47. The infusion pump will be regulated at a maximum of _____ mL/h to infuse the maximum of 20 milliunits/min.

Use the following information to answer questions 48 and 49.

Order for Ms. Hill, who weighs 150 lb, to stabilize her blood pressure: **dopamine 400 mg per 0.5 L D₅W at 4 mcg/kg/min titrated to 12 mcg/kg/min**

48. Regulate the electronic infusion pump for Ms. Hill's IV at _____ mL/h to initiate the order.

49. Anticipate that the maximum flow rate for Ms. Hill's IV to achieve the maximum safe titration would be _____ mL/h.

50. Mr. Black has a new order for **heparin 10,000 units in 500 mL NS IV at 750 units/h.** Regulate the infusion pump at _____ mL/h.

After completing these problems, refer to pages 581–583 to check your answers. Give yourself 2 points for each correct answer.

Perfect score = 100   My score = _____

Minimum mastery score = 86 (43 correct)

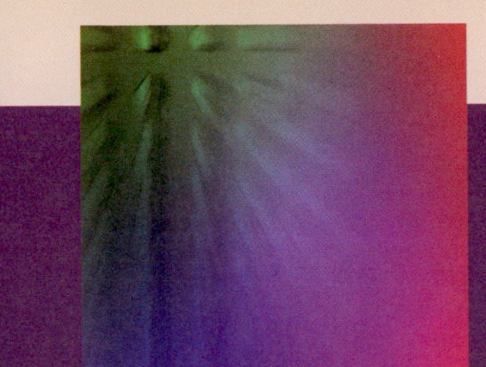

Essential Skills Evaluation

This evaluation is designed to assess your mastery of essential dosage calculation skills. It is similar to the type of entry-level test given by hospitals and health care agencies during orientation for new graduates and new employees. It excludes the advanced calculation skills presented in Chapters 16 and 17.

You are assigned to give Team Medications on a busy Adult Medical Unit. The following labels represent the medications available in your medication cart to fill the orders given in questions 1 through 17. Calculate the amount you will administer for 1 dose. Assume that all tablets are scored. Draw an arrow on the appropriate syringe to indicate how much you will prepare for parenteral medications.

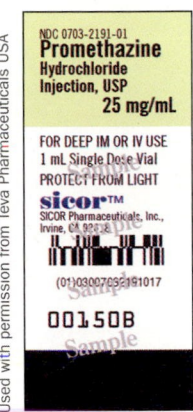

1. Order: **promethazine 12.5 mg IV q.4h p.r.n., nausea**

   Give: _____ mL

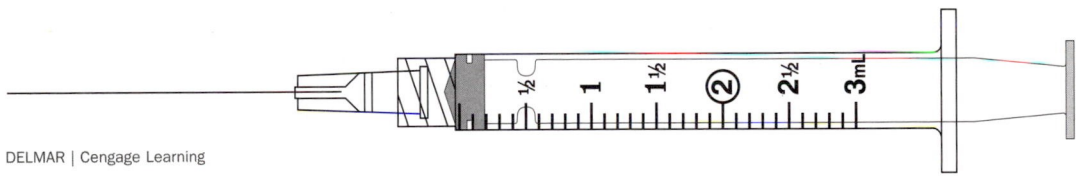

DELMAR | Cengage Learning

2. Order: **gentamicin 35 mg IM stat**

   Give: _____ mL

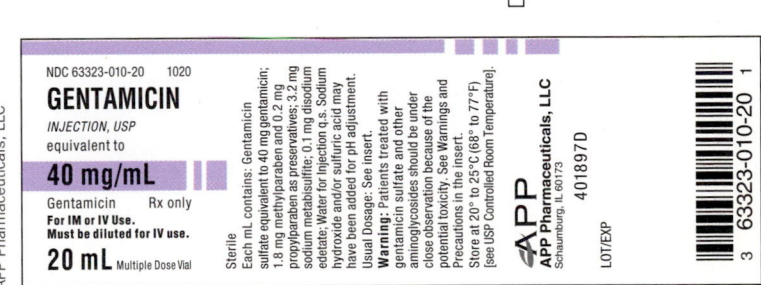

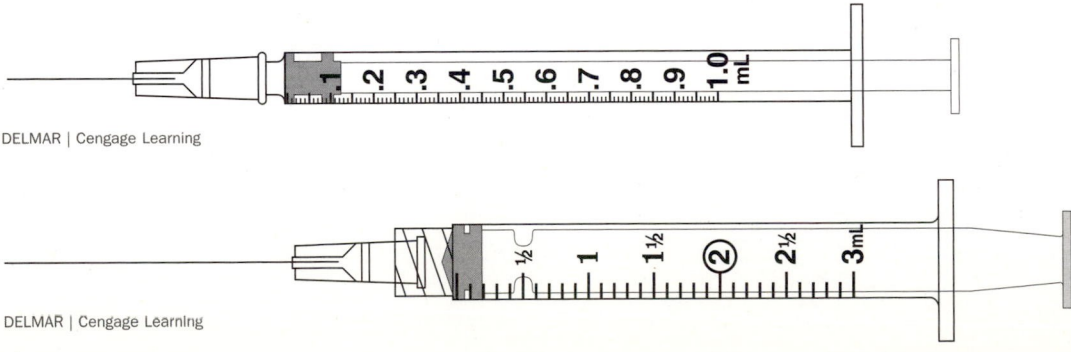

DELMAR | Cengage Learning

3. Order: **phenytoin 50 mg IV push q.8h**
(administer at the rate recommended
on the label)

Give: _____ mL at _____ mL/min
or _____ mL per 15 sec

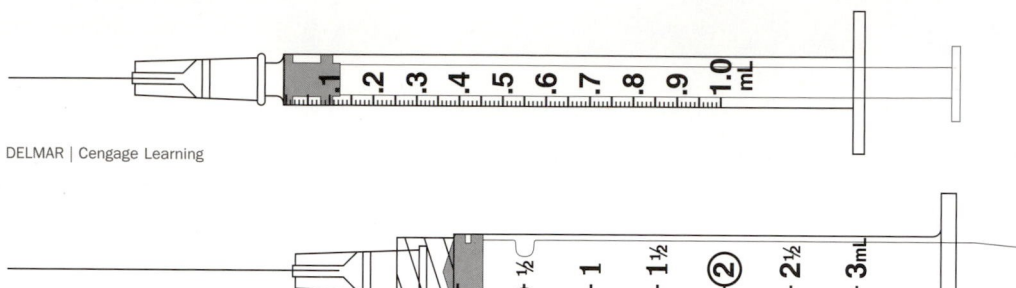

Dosage—See package insert.

℞ only

STERI-VIAL®
Dilantin®
(Phenytoin Sodium
Injection, USP)
ready/mixed

N 0071-4475-45

Manufactured by:
Parkedale Pharmaceuticals, Inc.
Rochester, MI 48307
For:
PARKE-DAVIS
Div of Warner-Lambert Co
Morris Plains, NJ 07950 USA

250 mg in 5 mL
5 mL

Do not exceed
50 mg/minute IV
IM/IV (no infusion)

© 1997-'98, Warner-Lambert Co.

4475G233

DELMAR | Cengage Learning

DELMAR | Cengage Learning

4. Order: **Robinul 200 mcg IV stat**

Give: _____ mL

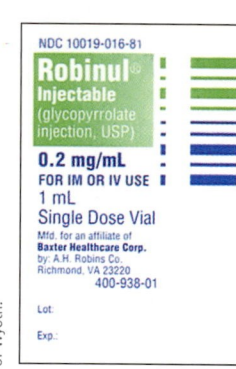

NDC 10019-016-81
Robinul®
Injectable
(glycopyrrolate
injection, USP)
0.2 mg/mL
FOR IM OR IV USE
1 mL
Single Dose Vial
Mfd. for an affiliate of
Baxter Healthcare Corp.
by: A.H. Robins Co.
Richmond, VA 23220
400-938-01
Lot:
Exp.:

DELMAR | Cengage Learning

5. Order: **Lortab 7.5 mg p.o.
q.3h p.r.n., pain**

Dosage is based on
hydrocodone.

Give: _____ tablet(s)

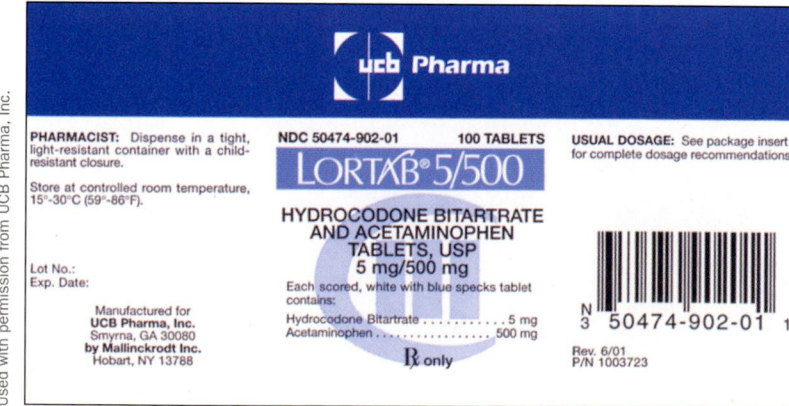

ucb Pharma

PHARMACIST: Dispense in a tight,
light-resistant container with a child-
resistant closure.

Store at controlled room temperature,
15°–30°C (59°–86°F).

Lot No.:
Exp. Date:

Manufactured for
UCB Pharma, Inc.
Smyrna, GA 30080
by Mallinckrodt Inc.
Hobart, NY 13788

NDC 50474-902-01   100 TABLETS

LORTAB® 5/500

HYDROCODONE BITARTRATE
AND ACETAMINOPHEN
TABLETS, USP
5 mg/500 mg

Each scored, white with blue specks tablet
contains:

Hydrocodone Bitartrate . . . . .5 mg
Acetaminophen . . . . .500 mg

℞ only

USUAL DOSAGE: See package insert
for complete dosage recommendations.

3 50474-902-01 1

Rev. 6/01
P/N 1003723

6. Order: **Lanoxin 0.125 mg IV q.** AM

   Give: _____ mL

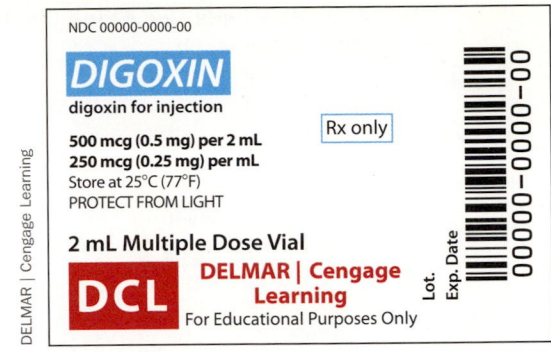

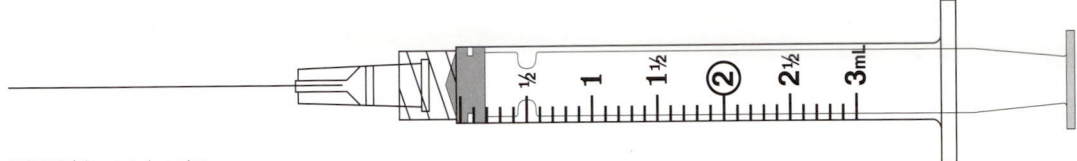

DELMAR | Cengage Learning

7. Order: **morphine sulfate gr $\frac{1}{15}$ slow IV push q.4h p.r.n., severe pain**

   Give: _____ mL (will then be further diluted for safe administration)

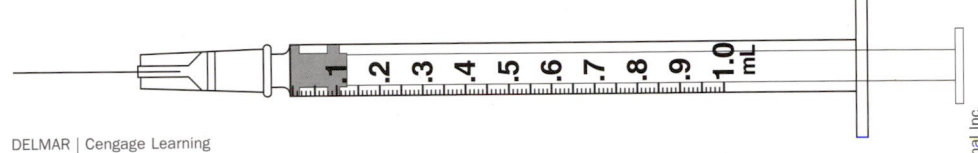

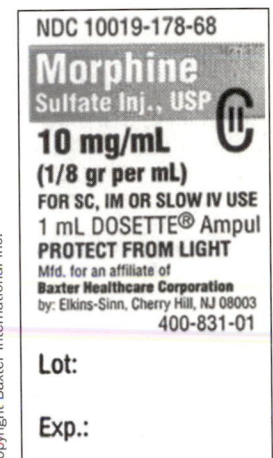

DELMAR | Cengage Learning

8. Order: **Kantrex 350 mg IV q.8h**

   Give: _____ mL

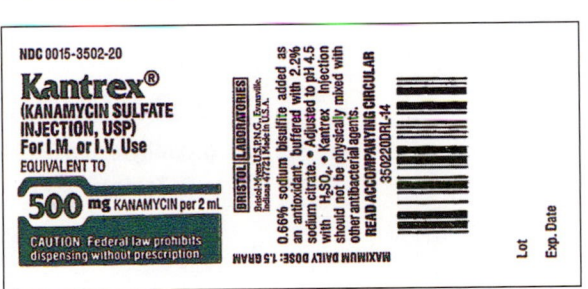

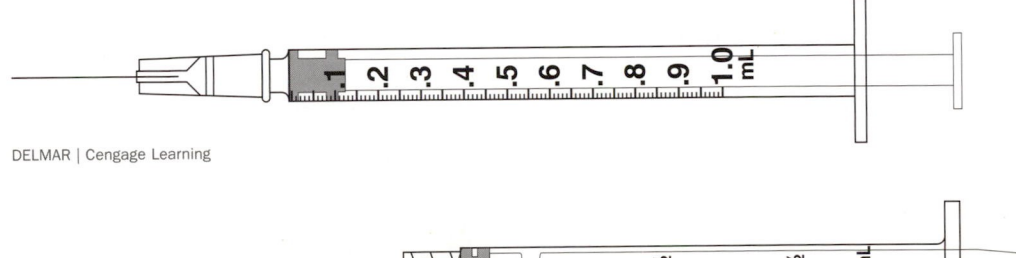

DELMAR | Cengage Learning

DELMAR | Cengage Learning

9. Order: Novolin N U-100 insulin 46 units c̄ Novolin R Regular U-100 insulin 22 units subcut stat

You will give _____ units total.

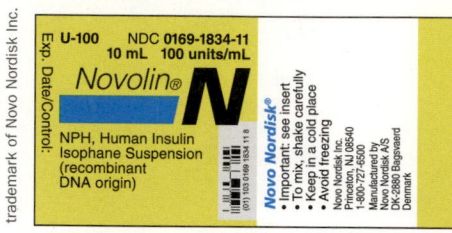
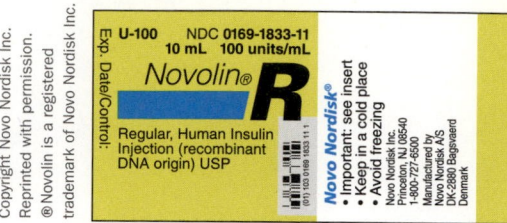

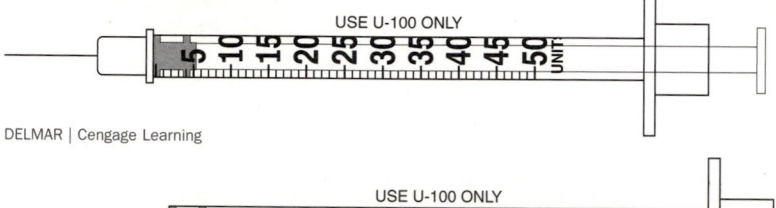

DELMAR | Cengage Learning

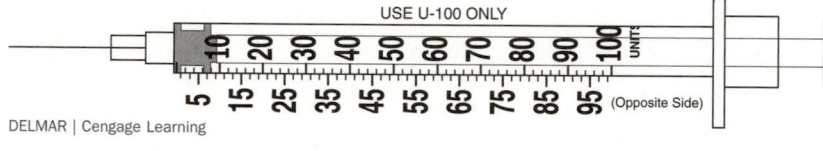

DELMAR | Cengage Learning

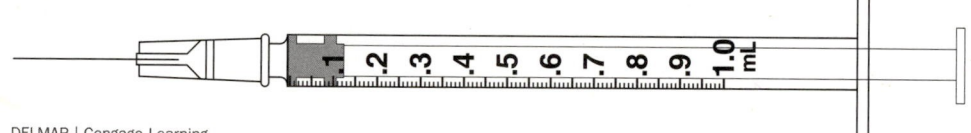

DELMAR | Cengage Learning

10. Order: **Synthroid 0.3 mg p.o. q.** AM

Give: _____ tablet(s)

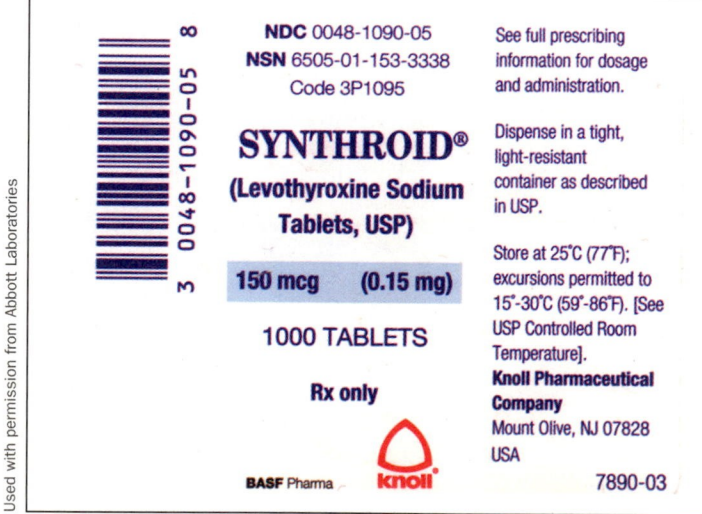

11. Order: **Calan 40 mg p.o. t.i.d.**

    Give: _____ tablet(s)

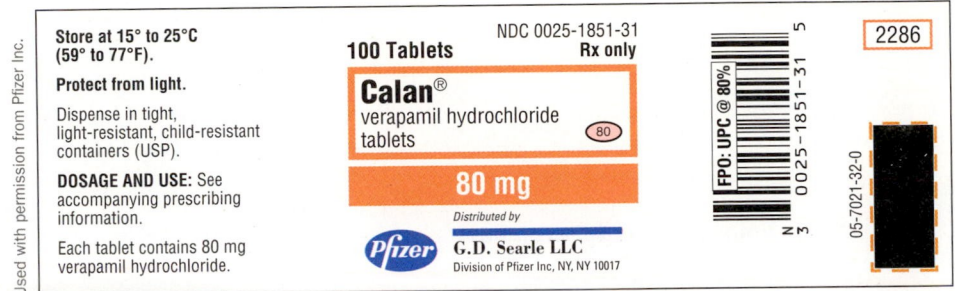

12. Order: **Naprosyn 375 mg p.o. b.i.d.**

    Give: _____ tablet(s)

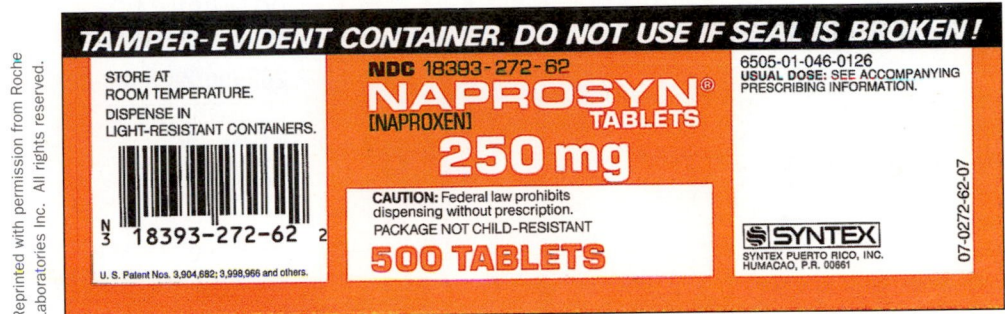

13. Order: **promethazine 40 mg IM stat**

    Give: _____ mL

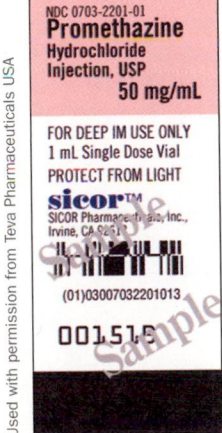

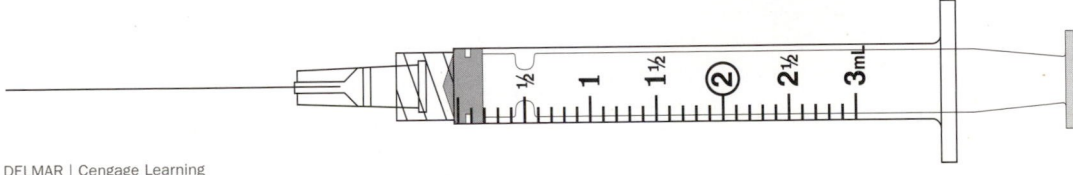

14. Order: butorphanol 3 mg IM stat

Give: _____ mL

BUTORPHANOL
TARTRATE INJECTION, USP

2 mg/mL

SINGLE DOSE VIAL
FOR IM OR IV USE
Rx ONLY

Used with permission from Bedford Laboratories. A Division of Ben Venue Laboratories Inc. A Boehringer-Ingelheim Company.

NDC 5390-184-01
1 mL vial

USUAL DOSAGE: See package insert.
Store at room temperature, 15° to 30°C (59° to 86°F).
Manufactured for:
Bedford Laboratories™
Bedford, OH 44146

BTP-VB05

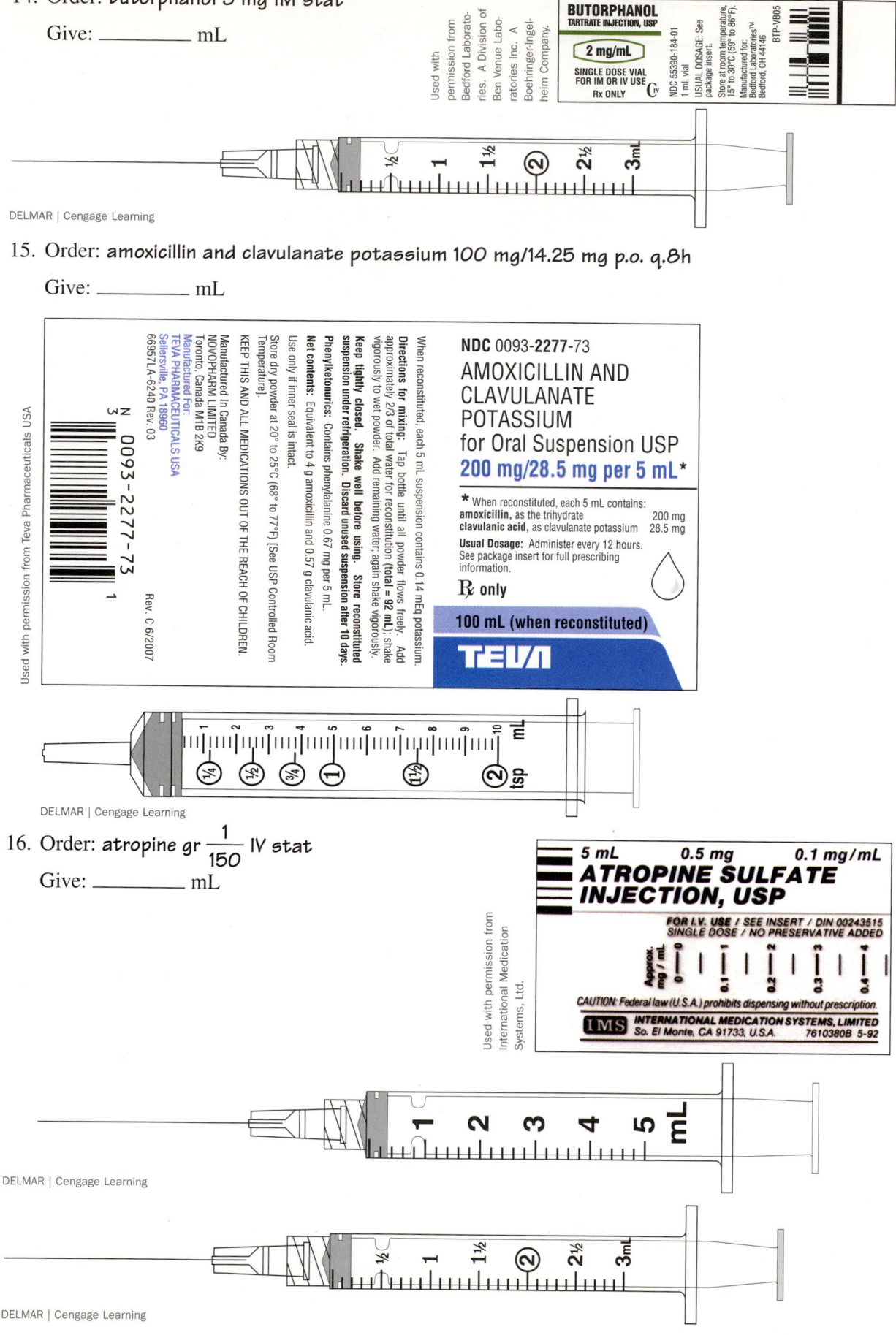

15. Order: amoxicillin and clavulanate potassium 100 mg/14.25 mg p.o. q.8h

Give: _____ mL

NDC 0093-2277-73

AMOXICILLIN AND CLAVULANATE POTASSIUM
for Oral Suspension USP
200 mg/28.5 mg per 5 mL*

* When reconstituted, each 5 mL contains:
amoxicillin, as the trihydrate   200 mg
clavulanic acid, as clavulanate potassium   28.5 mg

Usual Dosage: Administer every 12 hours. See package insert for full prescribing information.

Rx only

100 mL (when reconstituted)

TEVA

When reconstituted, each 5 mL suspension contains 0.14 mEq potassium.
Directions for mixing: Tap bottle until all powder flows freely. Add approximately 2/3 of total water for reconstitution (**total = 92 mL**); shake vigorously to wet powder. Add remaining water, again shake vigorously.
Keep tightly closed. Shake well before using. Store reconstituted suspension under refrigeration. Discard unused suspension after 10 days.
Phenylketonurics: Contains phenylalanine 0.67 mg per 5 mL.
Net contents: Equivalent to 4 g amoxicillin and 0.57 g clavulanic acid.
Use only if inner seal is intact.
Store dry powder at 20° to 25°C (68° to 77°F) [See USP Controlled Room Temperature].
KEEP THIS AND ALL MEDICATIONS OUT OF THE REACH OF CHILDREN.

Manufactured in Canada By:
NOVOPHARM LIMITED
Toronto, Canada M1B 2K9
Manufactured For:
TEVA PHARMACEUTICALS USA
Sellersville, PA 18960
66957LA-6240 Rev. 03

Rev. C 6/2007

N 0093-2277-73

Used with permission from Teva Pharmaceuticals USA

16. Order: atropine gr $\frac{1}{150}$ IV stat

Give: _____ mL

5 mL   0.5 mg   0.1 mg/mL

ATROPINE SULFATE INJECTION, USP

FOR I.V. USE / SEE INSERT / DIN 00243515
SINGLE DOSE / NO PRESERVATIVE ADDED

Approx. mg / mL
0 0.1 0.2 0.3 0.4

CAUTION: Federal law (U.S.A.) prohibits dispensing without prescription.

IMS INTERNATIONAL MEDICATION SYSTEMS, LIMITED
So. El Monte, CA 91733, U.S.A.   7610380B 5-92

Used with permission from International Medication Systems, Ltd.

DELMAR | Cengage Learning

17. Order: **ranitidine 35 mg in 100 mL D$_5$W IV PB over 20 min**

Add _____ mL ranitidine to the IV fluid, and set the flow rate to _____ gtt/min.

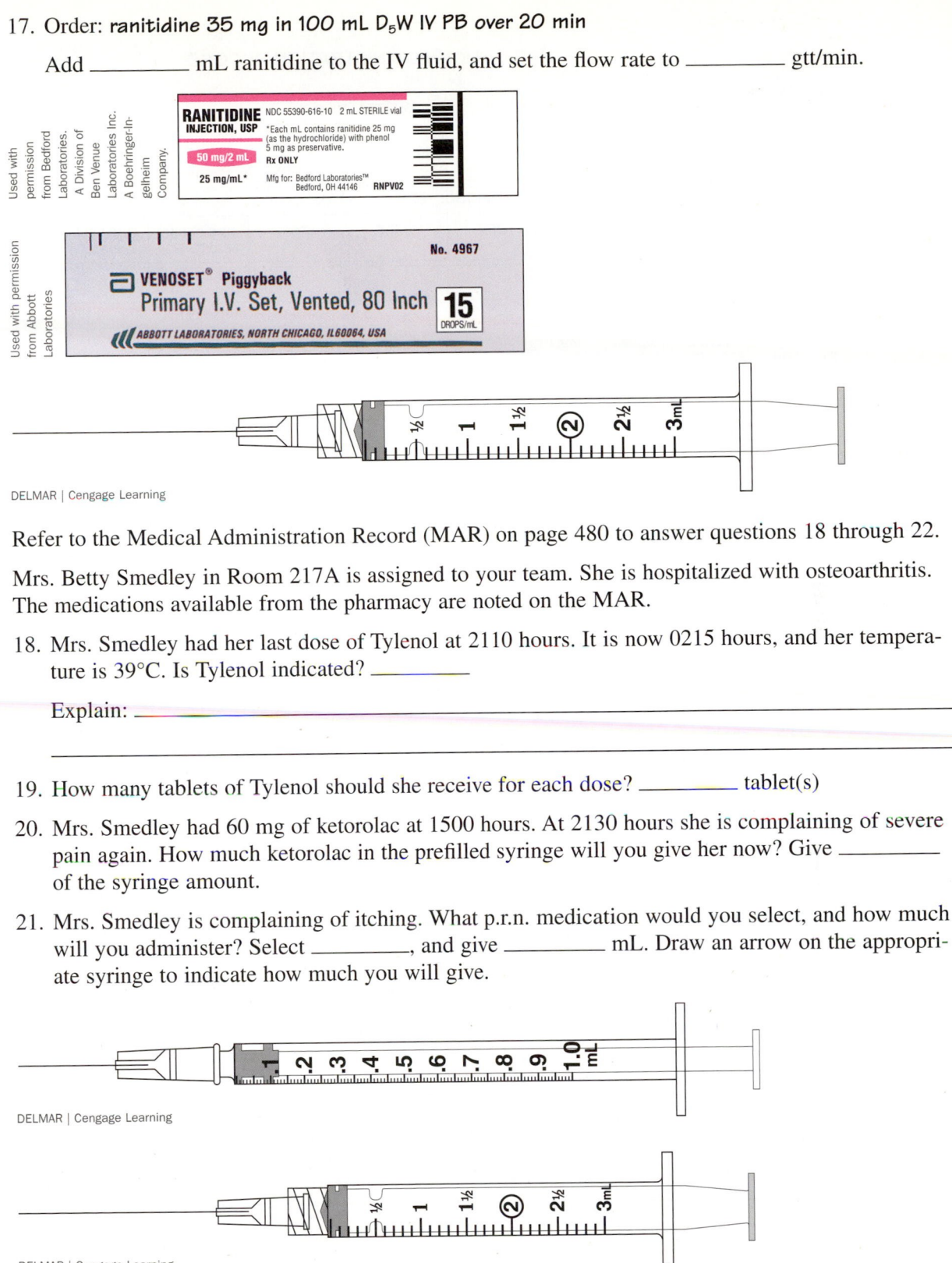

DELMAR | Cengage Learning

Refer to the Medical Administration Record (MAR) on page 480 to answer questions 18 through 22.

Mrs. Betty Smedley in Room 217A is assigned to your team. She is hospitalized with osteoarthritis. The medications available from the pharmacy are noted on the MAR.

18. Mrs. Smedley had her last dose of Tylenol at 2110 hours. It is now 0215 hours, and her temperature is 39°C. Is Tylenol indicated? _____

    Explain: _____

    _____

19. How many tablets of Tylenol should she receive for each dose? _____ tablet(s)

20. Mrs. Smedley had 60 mg of ketorolac at 1500 hours. At 2130 hours she is complaining of severe pain again. How much ketorolac in the prefilled syringe will you give her now? Give _____ of the syringe amount.

21. Mrs. Smedley is complaining of itching. What p.r.n. medication would you select, and how much will you administer? Select _____, and give _____ mL. Draw an arrow on the appropriate syringe to indicate how much you will give.

DELMAR | Cengage Learning

DELMAR | Cengage Learning

DELMAR | Cengage Learning

09/15/xx
0826
CHECKED BY: – – – – – – – – – – – – – – – – –

MEDICATION ADMINISTRATION RECORD

PAGE: 1
REPT: PHR20B

2ND   241
  217A   532729
       Smedley, Betty

DIAGNOSIS: 71590
ALLERGIES: NKA
NOTES:

DIET: Regular

ADMIT: 09/15/xx
WT: 154 lb

DX: OSTEOARTHRITIS-UNSPEC

ADMINISTRATION PERIOD:	0730	09/15/xx	TO	0729	09/16/xx

ORDER # DRUG NAME, STRENGTH, DOSAGE FORM DOSE RATE ROUTE SCHEDULE	START	STOP	TIME PERIOD 0730 TO 1529	TIME PERIOD 1530 TO 2329	TIME PERIOD 2330 TO 0729
NURSE:					
• • • PRN's FOLLOW • • •		• • • PRN's FOLLOW • • •			
264077 TYLENOL 325 MG TABLET PRN **650 MG** ORAL Q4H/PRN FOR TEMP GREATER THAN 101 F	0930 09/15/xx			2110 GP	

264147   KETOROLAC 60 MG   SYRINGE
PRN   **60 MG**   IM   PRN
    GIVE 60 MG FOR BREAKTHROUGH PAIN X1 DOSE
    THEN 30 MG Q6H/PRN
	0930
	
	09/15/xx
			1500
			MS		

264148   KETOROLAC 60 MG   SYRINGE
PRN   **30 MG**   IM   Q6H/PRN
    GIVE 6 HOURS AFTER 60 MG DOSE FOR BREAK-
    THROUGH PAIN.
	0930
	
	09/15/xx				

264151   INAPSINE   2.5 MG/ML AMPULE
PRN   **SEE NOTE**   IV   Q6H/PRN
    SAME AS DROPERIDOL; DOSE IS 0.625 MG TO
    1.25 MG (0.5-1.0 ML) FOR NAUSEA
	0930
	
	09/15/xx				

264152 BENADRYL 50 MG/ML AMPULE PRN **35 MG** IV Q4H/PRN FOR ITCHING	0930 09/15/xx				
264153 NARCAN 0.4 MG/ML AMPULE PRN **0.4 MG** IV PRN FOR RR LESS THAN 8 AND IF PT. IS UNAROUSABLE	0930 09/15/xx				
264154 MORPHINE SULFATE AMPULE PRN **4 MG** IV Q2H/PRN SEVERE PAIN NOT RESPONSIVE TO KETOROLAC	0930 09/15/xx			2330 GP	

INITIALS	SIGNATURE	INITIALS	SIGNATURE	NOTES
GP	G. Pickar, R.N.			
MS	M. Smith, R.N.			

217A   Betty Smedley
          ID# 532729

AGE: 73   SEX: F   PHYSICIAN: J. Physician, MD

22. At 2400 Mrs. Smedley's respiratory rate (RR) is 7, and she is difficult to arouse. What medication is indicated? _____ Give _____ mL. Draw an arrow on the syringe to indicate how much of this medication you will give.

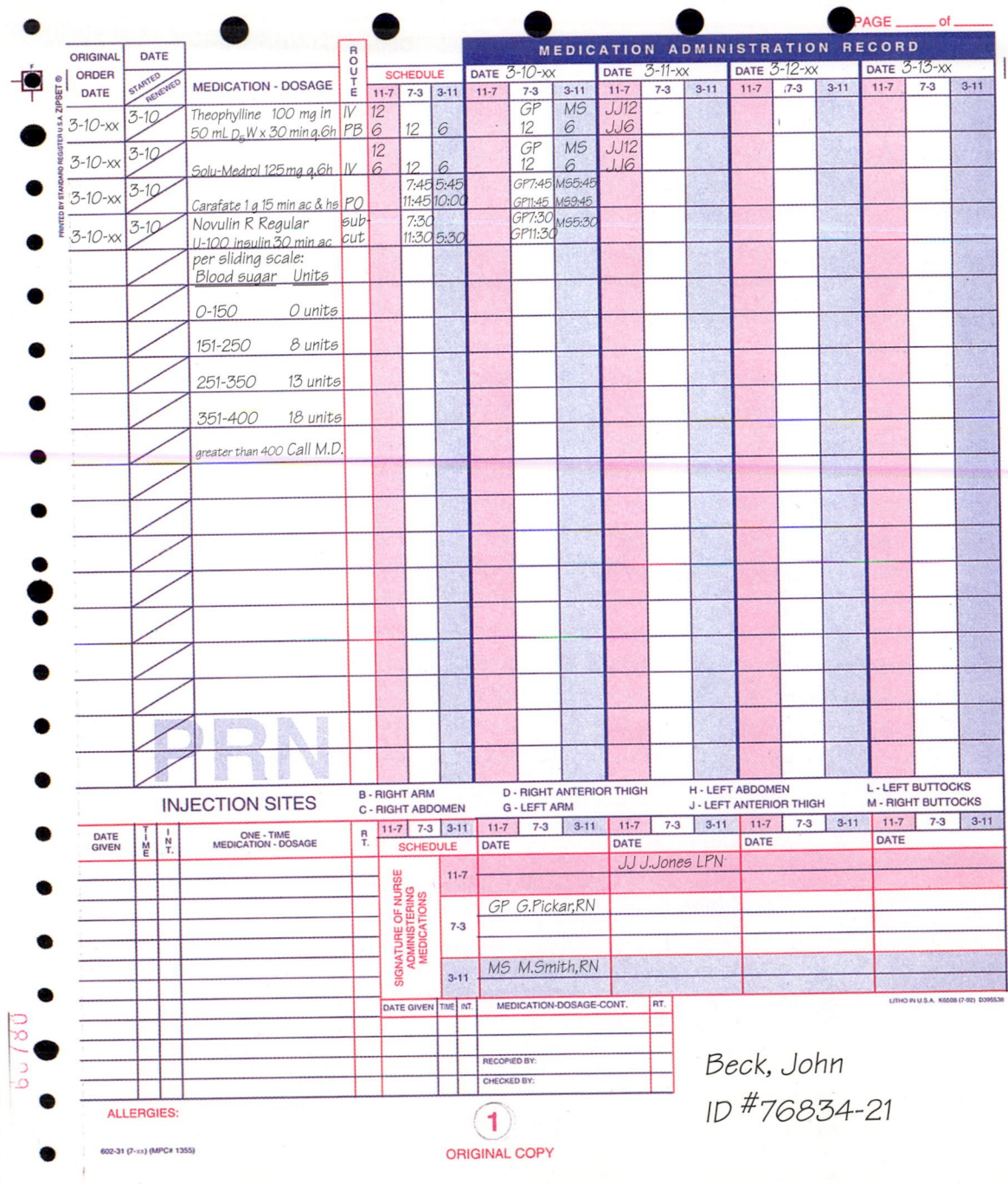

DELMAR | Cengage Learning

Refer to the following MAR to answer questions 23 through 27.

ORIGINAL ORDER DATE	DATE STARTED/RENEWED	MEDICATION - DOSAGE	ROUTE	SCHEDULE 11-7	7-3	3-11	DATE 3-10-xx 11-7	7-3	3-11	DATE 3-11-xx 11-7	7-3	3-11	DATE 3-12-xx 11-7	7-3	3-11	DATE 3-13-xx 11-7	7-3	3-11
3-10-xx	3-10	Theophylline 100 mg in 50 mL D₅W x 30 min q.6h	IV PB	12 6	12	6		GP 12	MS 6	JJ12 JJ6								
3-10-xx	3-10	Solu-Medrol 125 mg q.6h	IV	12 6	12	6		GP 12	MS 6	JJ12 JJ6								
3-10-xx	3-10	Carafate 1 g 15 min ac & hs	PO		7:45 11:45	5:45 10:00	GP7:45 GP11:45	MS5:45 MS9:45										
3-10-xx	3-10	Novulin R Regular U-100 insulin 30 min ac per sliding scale: Blood sugar Units	sub-cut		7:30 11:30	5:30	GP7:30 GP11:30	MS5:30										
		0-150 0 units																
		151-250 8 units																
		251-350 13 units																
		351-400 18 units																
		greater than 400 Call M.D.																

MEDICATION ADMINISTRATION RECORD

PRN

INJECTION SITES

B - RIGHT ARM
C - RIGHT ABDOMEN
D - RIGHT ANTERIOR THIGH
G - LEFT ARM
H - LEFT ABDOMEN
J - LEFT ANTERIOR THIGH
L - LEFT BUTTOCKS
M - RIGHT BUTTOCKS

DATE GIVEN	TIME	INT.	ONE - TIME MEDICATION - DOSAGE	R.T.	SCHEDULE 11-7	7-3	3-11	DATE 11-7	7-3	3-11	DATE 11-7	7-3	3-11	DATE 11-7	7-3	3-11

SIGNATURE OF NURSE ADMINISTERING MEDICATIONS

11-7	JJ J.Jones LPN
7-3	GP G.Pickar,RN
3-11	MS M.Smith,RN

DATE GIVEN	TIME	INT.	MEDICATION-DOSAGE-CONT.	RT.

RECOPIED BY:

CHECKED BY:

LITHO IN U.S.A. K6508 (7-92) D095538

ALLERGIES:

602-31 (7-xx) (MPC# 1355)

① ORIGINAL COPY

Beck, John
ID #76834-21

DELMAR | Cengage Learning

John Beck, 19 years old, is diabetic. He is admitted to the medical unit with asthma. You are administering his medications. The MAR on page 480 is in the medication notebook on your medication cart. The labels represent the infusion set available and the medications in his medication cart drawer. Questions 23 through 27 refer to Mr. Beck.

23. Theophylline is available in a solution strength of 80 mg per 15 mL. There will be _____ mL theophylline in the IV PB. Set the flow rate at _____ gtt/min.

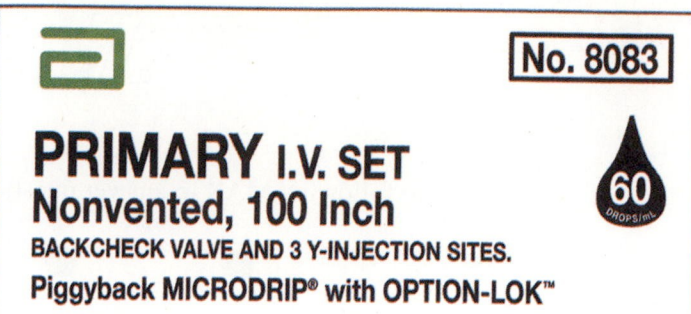

24. An infusion pump becomes available, and you decide to use it for Mr. Beck's IV. It is calibrated in mL/h. To administer the theophylline by infusion pump, set the pump at _____ mL/h.

25. Reconstitute the Solu-Medrol with _____ mL diluent, and give _____ mL.

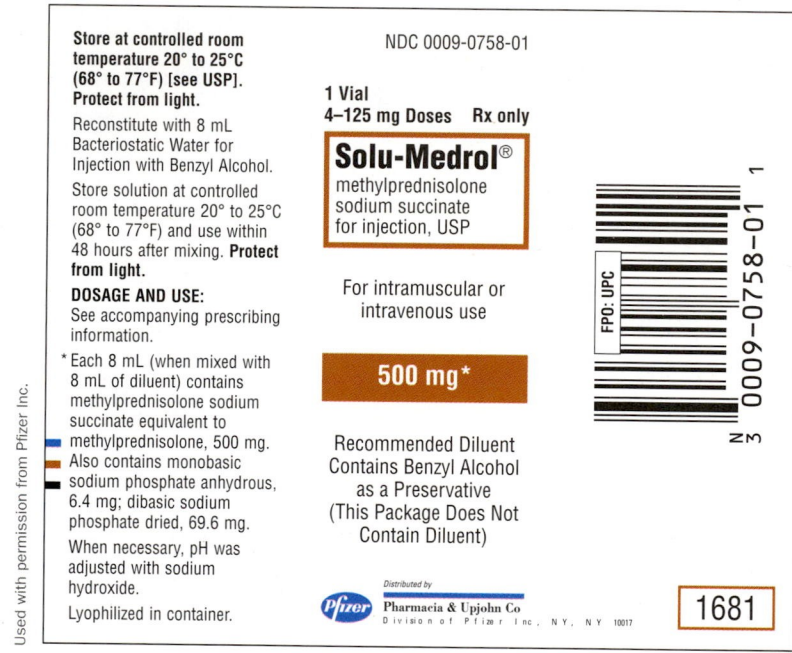

26. Mealtimes and bedtime are 8 AM, 12 NOON, 6 PM, and 10 PM. Using international time, give _____ tablet(s) of Carafate per dose each day at _____, _____, _____, and _____ hours.

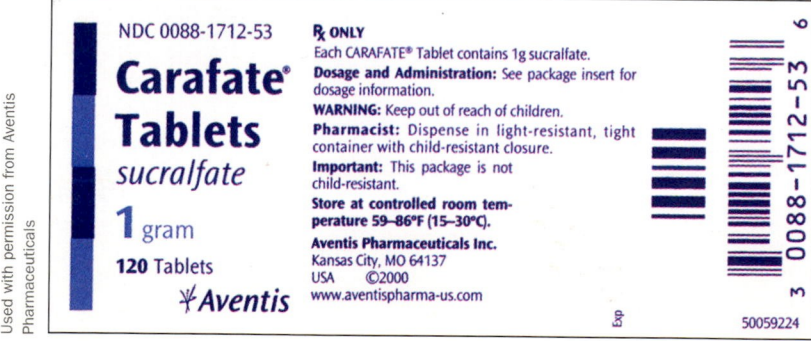

27. At 0730 Mr. Beck's blood sugar is 360. You will give him _____ units of insulin by the _____ route. Draw an arrow on the appropriate syringe to indicate the correct dosage.

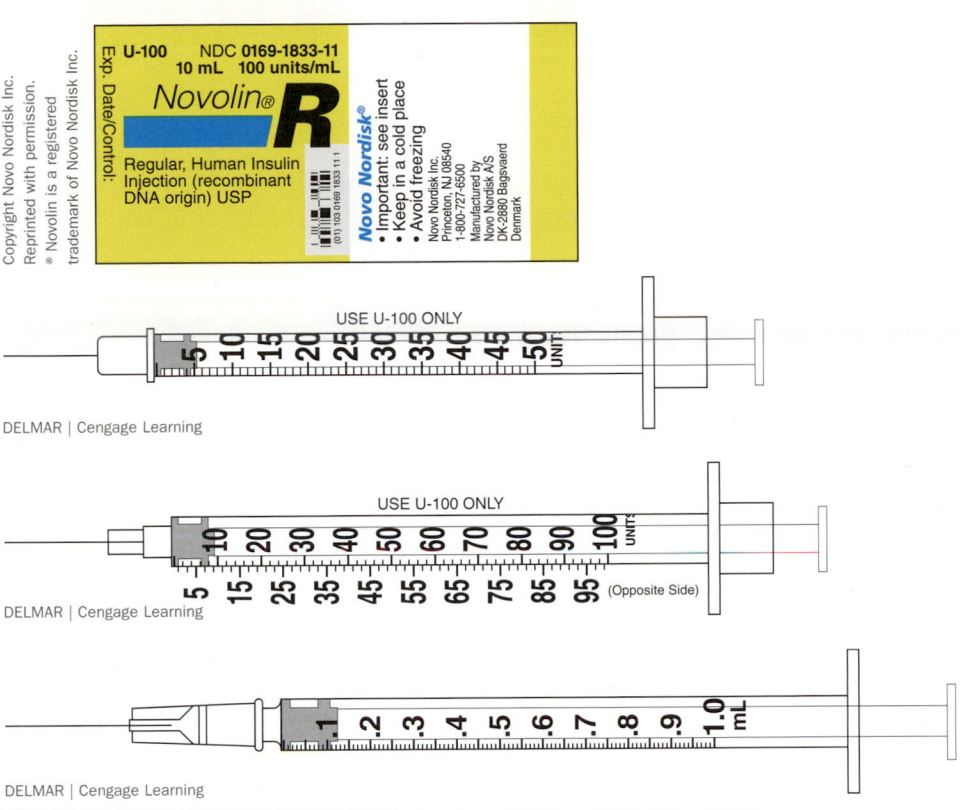

Jimmy Bryan is brought to the pediatric clinic by his mother. He is a 22 lb baby with an ear infection. Questions 28 through 31 refer to Jimmy.

28. The physician orders **amoxicillin 100 mg p.o. q.8h** for Jimmy. To reconstitute the amoxicillin, add _____ mL water.

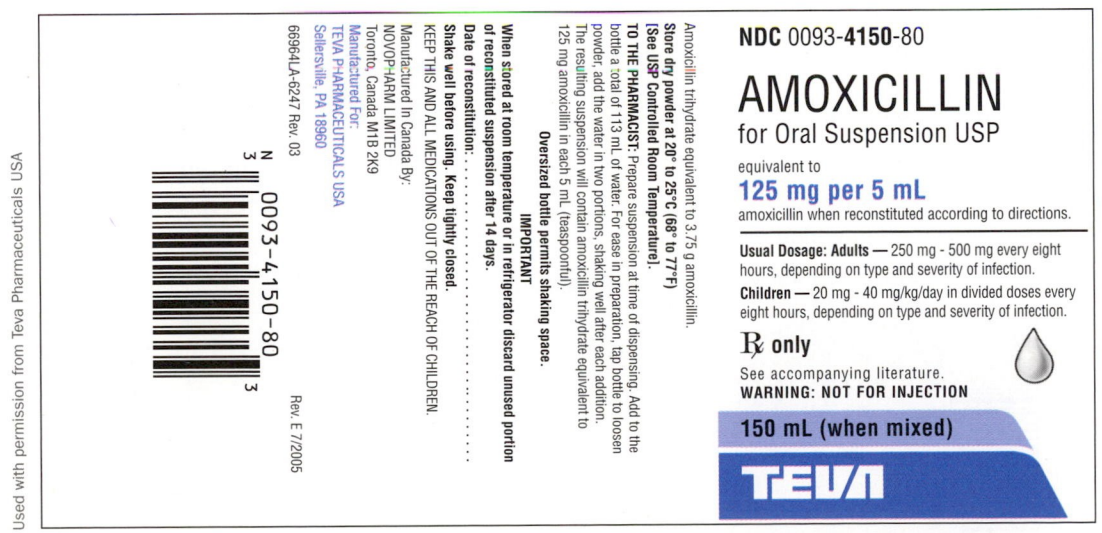

29. Is Jimmy's amoxicillin order safe and reasonable? _____ Explain: _____

30. The physician asks you to give Jimmy 1 dose of the amoxicillin stat. You will give Jimmy _____ mL.

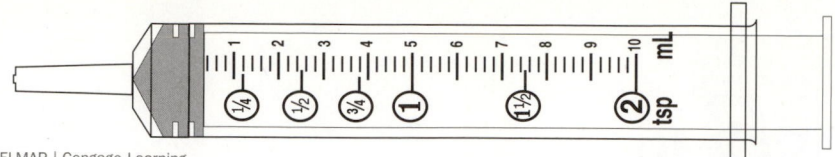

31. The physician also asks you to instruct Jimmy's mother about administering the medication at home. Tell Jimmy's mother to fill the oral syringe to the _____ mL line for each dose. How often? _____

32. Jill Jones is a 16-year-old, 110 lb teenager with a duodenal ulcer and abdominal pain. Order: **cimetidine 250 mg q.6h in 50 mL D$_5$W IV PB to be infused in 20 min**

    The recommended cimetidine dosage is 20 to 40 mg/kg/day in 4 divided doses. Available is cimetidine for injection, 300 mg per 2 mL. The label represents the infusion set available. What is the safe single dosage range for this child? _____ mg/dose to _____ mg/dose. Is this ordered dosage safe? _____

    If safe, add _____ mL cimetidine, and set the flow rate at _____ gtt/min.

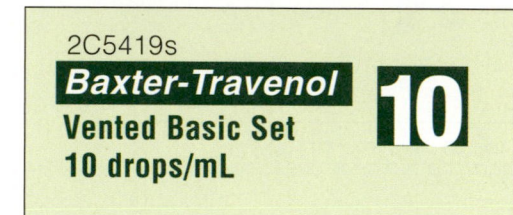

2C5419s
Baxter-Travenol **10**
Vented Basic Set
10 drops/mL

33. The doctor writes a new order for strict intake and output assessment for a child. During your 8 hour shift, in addition to his IV fluids of 200 mL D$_5$NS, he consumed the following oral fluids:

    gelatin—4 fl oz

    water—3 fl oz × 2

    apple juice—16 fl oz

    What is his total fluid intake during your shift? _____ mL

Use the following information to answer questions 34 and 35.

Order for a child with severe otitis media (inner ear infection) who weighs 40 lb: **amoxicillin clavulanate 240 mg/34.2 mg p.o. q.8h.** The following **amoxicillin clavulanate** label represents the dosage you have available. Recommended **amoxicillin clarularate** dosage is 40 mg/kg/day q.8h in divided doses.

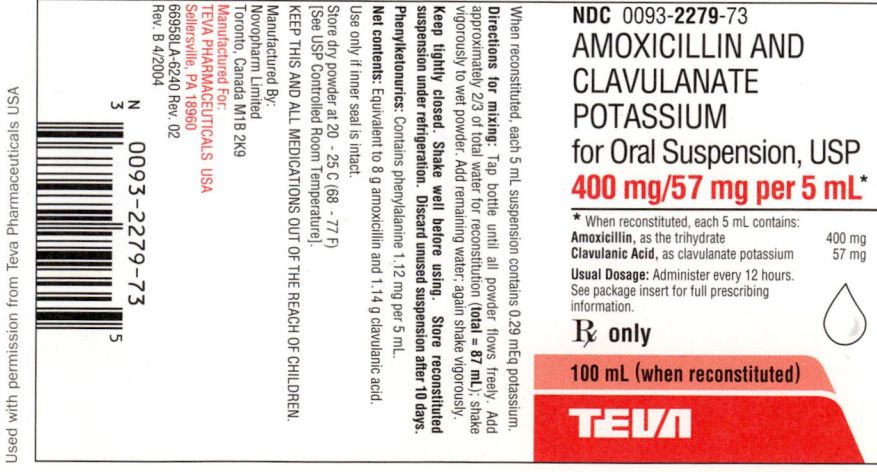

NDC 0093-2279-73
AMOXICILLIN AND CLAVULANATE POTASSIUM
for Oral Suspension, USP
400 mg/57 mg per 5 mL*

* When reconstituted, each 5 mL contains:
Amoxicillin, as the trihydrate .... 400 mg
Clavulanic Acid, as clavulanate potassium ..... 57 mg
Usual Dosage: Administer every 12 hours. See package insert for full prescribing information.

R only

100 mL (when reconstituted)

TEVA

34. Is the ordered dosage safe? _____

35. If it is safe, how much would you administer to the child? _____ mL per dose. If it is not safe, what would you do next? _____

36. The physician has ordered **washed, packed red blood cells 2 units (600 mL) IV to infuse in 4 h.** The IV tubing has a drop factor of 10 gtt/mL. You will regulate the IV flow rate at _____ gtt/min.

Use the following information to answer questions 37 and 38.

A child who weighs 61 lb 8 oz has an elevated temperature. For hyperthermia in children, the recommended dosage of acetaminophen is 10 to 15 mg/kg p.o. q.4h, not to exceed 5 doses per day.

37. What is the safe single dosage range of acetaminophen for this child? _____ mg/dose to _____ mg/dose

38. If the physician orders the maximum safe dosage and acetaminophen is available as a suspension of 80 mg per 2.5 mL, how many mL will you give per dose? _____ mL

Use the following information to answer questions 39 and 40 for a child who weighs 52 lb.

Order: **Benadryl 25 mg IV q.6h**

Supply: Benadryl 10 mg/mL

Recommended dosage: 5 mg/kg/day in 4 divided doses

39. A safe single dosage for this child is _____ mg/dose. Is the order safe? _____

40. If safe, administer _____ mL. If not safe, what should you do? _____

Use the following information to answer questions 41 through 44.

At 1430, a patient is started on **morphine sulfate PCA IV pump at 1 mg q.10 min.** The morphine sulfate syringe in the pump contains 50 mg per 50 mL.

41. The patient can receive _____ mL every 10 minutes.

42. If the patient attempts 5 doses this hour, he would receive _____ mg and _____ mL of morphine.

43. Based on the amount of morphine in the syringe in the PCA pump, how many total doses can the patient receive? _____ dose(s)

44. If the patient receives 5 doses every hour, the morphine will be empty at _____ hours. Convert this time to traditional AM/PM time. _____

45. Order: **methyldopa 250 mg stat in 100 mL D$_5$W IV PB, infuse over 30 min**

    Regulate the electronic infusion pump at _____ mL/h.

Use the following information to answer questions 46 through 49.

Order: **Rocephin 0.5 g IV q.8h**

The following label represents the drug you have available. You reconstitute the drug at 1400 on 1/30/xx.

EXP
Rocephin®
(Ceftriaxone for Injection USP)
1 gram
Single-Use Vial
Batch
R only (Roche)
For I.M. or I.V. Use
Equivalent to 1 gram ceftriaxone
For I.M. Administration:
Reconstitute with 2.1 mL
1% Lidocaine Hydrochloride
Injection (USP) or Sterile Water
for Injection (USP). Each 1 mL of
solution contains approximately
350 mg equivalent of ceftriaxone
as ceftriaxone sodium.
For I.V. Administration:
Reconstitute with 9.6 mL of an
I.V. diluent specified in the
accompanying package insert.
Each 1 mL of solution contains
approximately 100 mg equivalent
of ceftriaxone as ceftriaxone
sodium. Withdraw entire
contents and dilute to the desired
concentration with the appropriate
I.V. diluent. USUAL DOSAGE: See
package insert.
Storage Prior to Reconstitution:
Store at 20°–25°C (68°–77°F) [see
USP Controlled Room Temperature].
Protect From Light.
Storage After Reconstitution:
See package insert.
Made in Switzerland
Distributed by:
Roche Laboratories Inc.
Nutley, New Jersey 07110
10079638 USA 1111
(01) 103 0004 1964 04 8

According to the Rocephin package insert, "Reconstituted intravenous solution is stable at room temperature for 2 days and refrigerated for 10 days."

46. The total volume of Rocephin after reconstitution is _____ mL.

47. The resulting dosage strength of Rocephin is _____ mg per _____ mL or _____ mg/mL.

48. Give _____ mL of Rocephin.

49. Prepare a reconstitution label for Rocephin.

```
┌─────────────────────────────────────────────┐
│                                               │
│                                               │
│                                               │
│                                               │
│                                               │
└─────────────────────────────────────────────┘
```
Reconstitution label

50. Describe the strategy you would implement to prevent this medication error.

   Possible Scenario
   Order: **dexamethasone 4 mg IV q.6h**

   Day 1 Supply: dexamethasone 4 mg/mL

   Student nurse prepared and administered 1 mL.

   Day 2 Supply: dexamethasone 10 mg/mL

   Student nurse prepared 1 mL.

   Potential Outcome
   Day 2, the student's instructor asked the student to recheck the order, think about the action, check the calculation, and provide the rationale for the amount prepared. The student was alarmed at the possibility of administering two-and-a-half times the prescribed dosage. The student insisted that the pharmacy should consistently supply the same unit dosage. The instructor advised the student of the possibility that different pharmacy technicians could be involved or possibly the original supply dosage was not available.

   Prevention
   _____

   _____

After completing these problems, see pages 584–590 to check your answers. Give yourself 2 points for each correct answer.

Perfect score = 100   My score = _____

Minimum mastery score = 90 (45 correct)

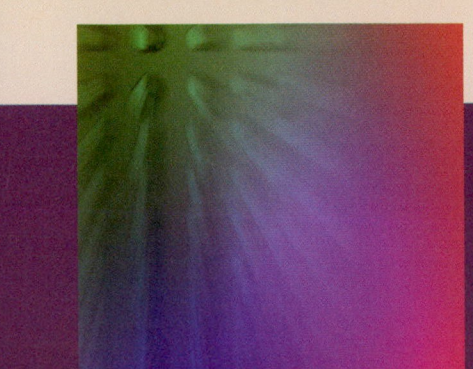

Comprehensive Skills Evaluation

This evaluation is a comprehensive assessment of your mastery of the concepts presented in all 17 chapters of *Dosage Calculations*.

Donna Smith, a 46-year-old patient of Dr. J. Physician, has been admitted to the Progressive Care Unit (PCU) with complaints of an irregular heartbeat, shortness of breath, and chest pain relieved by nitroglycerin. Questions 1 through 14 refer to the admitting orders on page 488 for Mrs. Smith. The labels shown represent available medications and infusion set.

1. How many capsules of nitroglycerin will you give Mrs. Smith?

   Give: _____ capsules

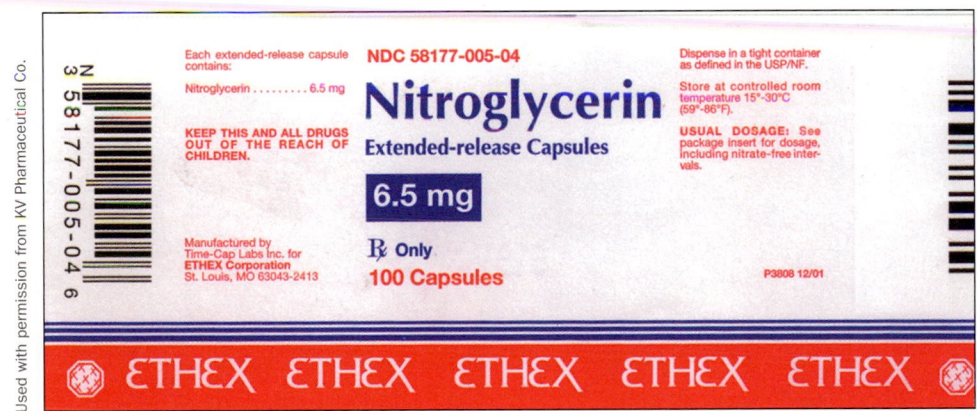

2. Frequently nitroglycerin is ordered by the SL route. SL is the medical abbreviation for _____

   Explain: _____

		ENTERED	FILLED	CHECKED	VERIFIED
					—

NOTE: A NON-PROPRIETARY DRUG OF EQUAL QUALITY MAY BE DISPENSED - IF THIS COLUMN IS NOT CHECKED!

DATE	TIME WRITTEN	PLEASE USE BALL POINT - PRESS FIRMLY	✓	TIME NOTED	NURSES SIGNATURE
9/3/xx	1600	Admit to PCU, monitored bed			
		Bedrest c̄ bathroom privileges			
		nitroglycerin ER 13 mg p.o. q.8h			
		furosemide 20 mg IV Push stat, then 20 mg p.o. b.i.d.			
		digoxin 0.25 mg IV Push stat, repeat in 4 hours,	✓	1610 GP	
		then 0.125 mg p.o. daily			
		KCl 10 mEq per L D₅ ½ NS IV at 80 mL/h			
		Tylenol 1 g p.o. q.4h p.r.n, headache	✓		
		Labwork: Electrolytes and CBC in am			
		Soft diet, advance as tolerated			
		J. Physician, MD			

AUTO STOP ORDERS: UNLESS REORDERED, FOLLOWING WILL BE D/C'D AT 0800 ON:

DATE	ORDER		PHYSICIAN SIGNATURE
		☐ CONT	
		☐ D/C	
		☐ CONT	PHYSICIAN SIGNATURE
		☐ D/C	
		☐ CONT	PHYSICIAN SIGNATURE
		☐ D/C	

CHECK WHEN ANTIBIOTICS ORDERED   ☐ Prophylactic   ☐ Empiric   ☐ Therapeutic

Allergies: None Known

Chest Pain

PATIENT DIAGNOSIS

Smith, Donna
ID #257-226-3

HEIGHT 5' 6"   WEIGHT 110 lb

FORM 959-708 (8xx)   **PHYSICIAN'S ORDER**   Reynolds + Reynolds LITHO IN U.S.A. K41814 (7-93) D330060

3. How much and at what rate will you administer Mrs. Smith's first dose of furosemide? Draw an arrow on the appropriate syringe to indicate how much you will prepare. The recommended direct IV administration rate for furosemide is 40 mg per 2 min.

Give: _____ mL at the rate of _____ mL/min or _____ mL per 15 sec

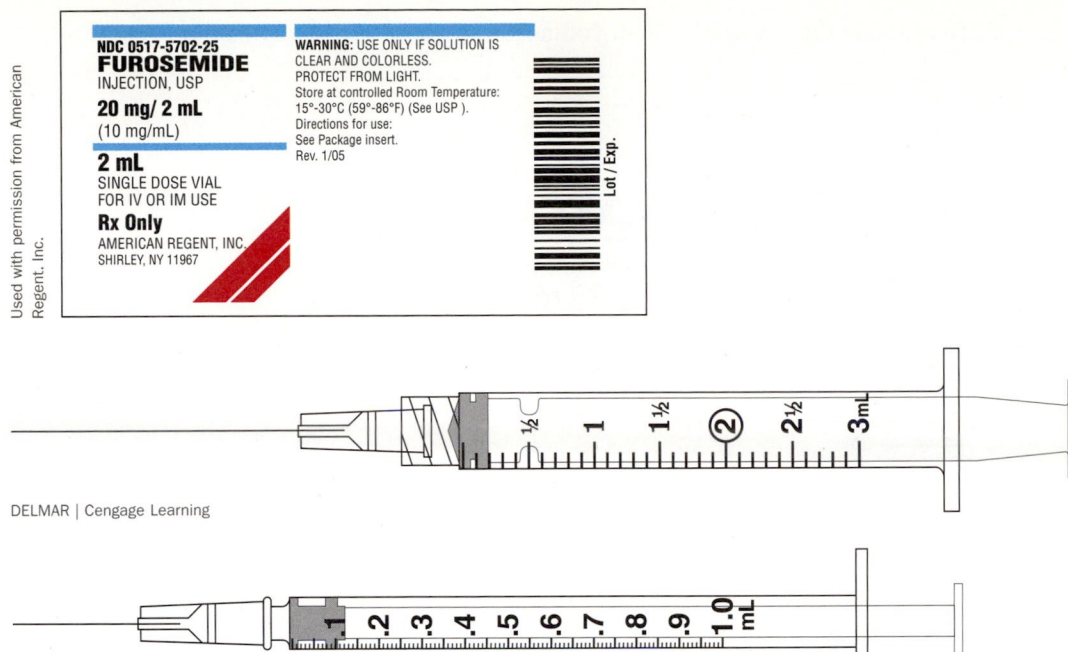

DELMAR | Cengage Learning

DELMAR | Cengage Learning

4. After the initial dose of furosemide, how much will you administer for each subsequent dose?

Give: _____ tablet(s)

5. How much and at what rate will you administer the IV digoxin on admission? Draw an arrow on the syringe to indicate how much you will prepare. The recommended direct IV rate for digoxin is 0.25 mg in 4 mL NS administered IV at the rate of 0.25 mg per 5 min.

Give: _____ mL at the rate of _____ mL/min or _____ mL per 15 sec

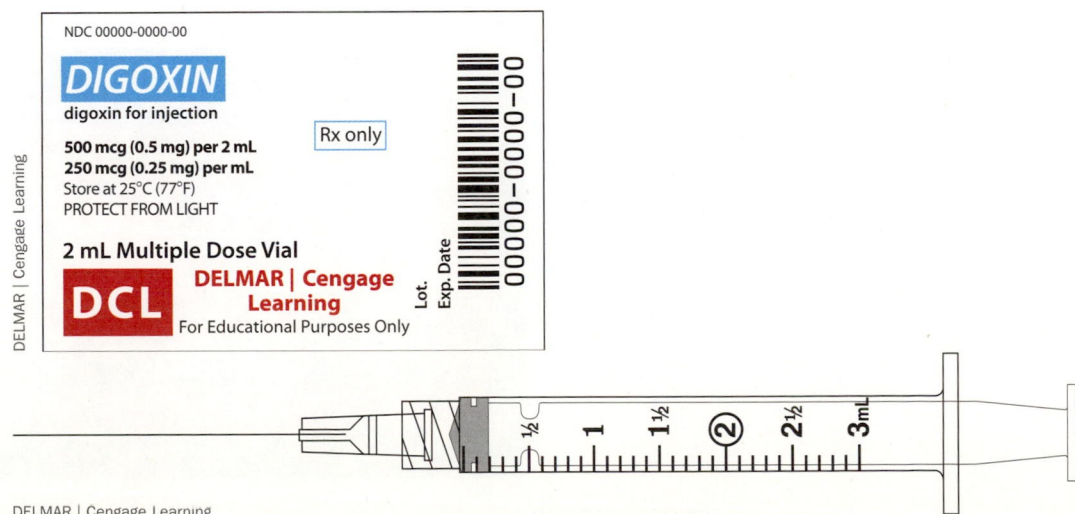

DELMAR | Cengage Learning

6. How many digoxin tablets will you need for a 24 hour supply of the p.o. order? _____ tablet(s)

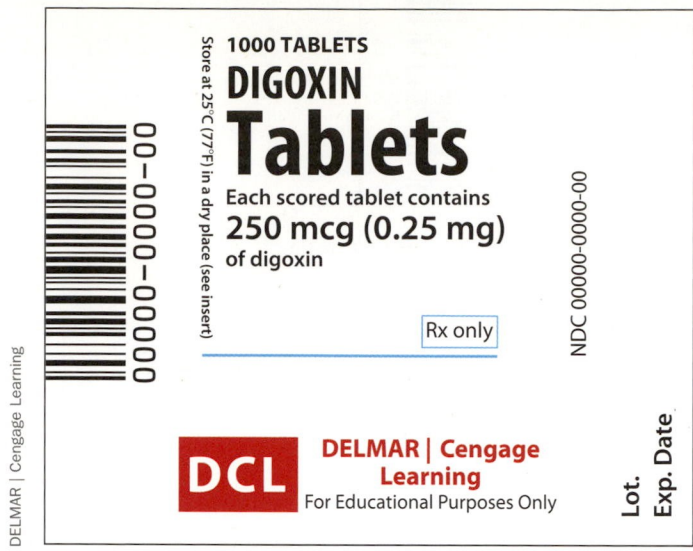

1000 TABLETS
DIGOXIN
Tablets
Each scored tablet contains
250 mcg (0.25 mg)
of digoxin

Store at 25°C (77°F) in a dry place (see insert)

Rx only

NDC 00000-0000-00

00000-0000-00

DCL **DELMAR | Cengage Learning** For Educational Purposes Only

Lot.
Exp. Date

7. Calculate the watch count flow rate for the IV fluid ordered. _____ gtt/min

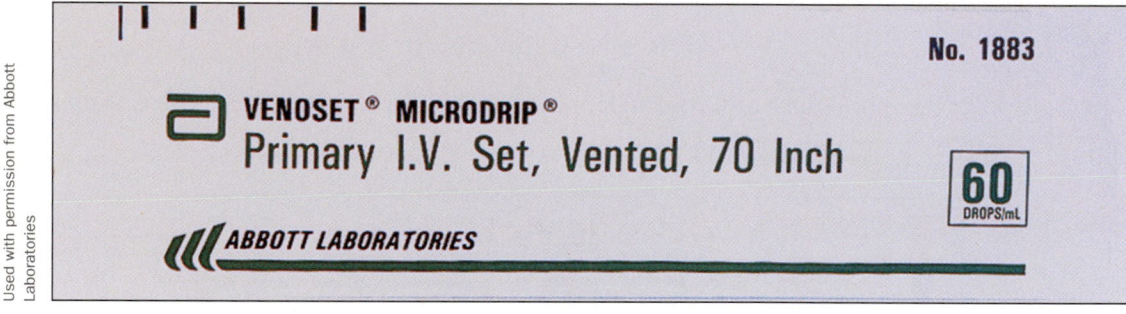

No. 1883

VENOSET® MICRODRIP®
Primary I.V. Set, Vented, 70 Inch

60 DROPS/mL

ABBOTT LABORATORIES

8. How many mEq KCl will Mrs. Smith receive per hour? _____ mEq/h

9. How many mEq KCl will Mrs. Smith receive in a 24-hour period? _____ mEq/day

10. At the present infusion rate, how much $D_5\frac{1}{2}$ NS will Mrs. Smith receive in a 24 hour period? _____ mL/day

11. The IV is started at 1630. Estimate the time and date that you should plan to hang the next liter of $D_5\frac{1}{2}$ NS. _____ hours _____ date

12. Mrs. Smith has a headache. Howmuch Tylenol will you give her?

    Give: _____ tablet(s)

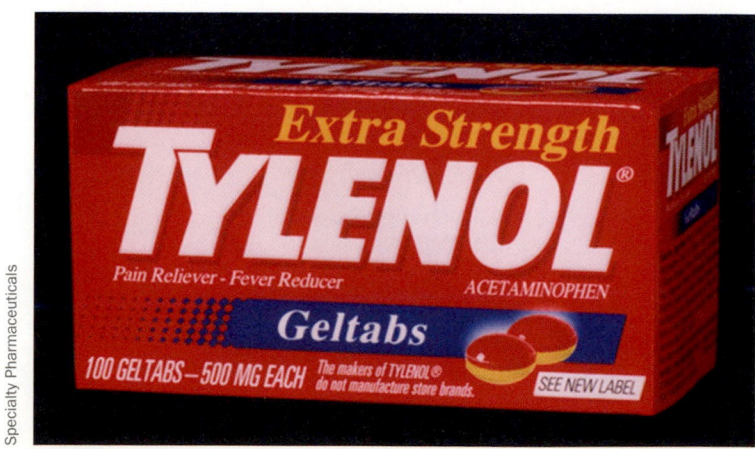

Extra Strength
TYLENOL®
Pain Reliever - Fever Reducer   ACETAMINOPHEN
Geltabs
100 GELTABS—500 MG EACH   The makers of TYLENOL® do not manufacture store brands.
SEE NEW LABEL

13. You have located an electronic infusion pump for Mrs. Smith's IV. At what rate will you set the pump? _____ mL/h

14. Compare the drug order and the labels to determine which of Mrs. Smith's medications are ordered by their generic or chemical names. _____

_____

Despite your excellent care, Mrs. Smith's condition worsens. She is transferred into the coronary care unit (CCU) with the medical orders on page 492. Questions 15 through 20 refer to those orders. She weighs 110 lb.

15. You have lidocaine 10 mg/mL available. How much lidocaine will you give for the bolus? Draw an arrow on the appropriate syringe to indicate the amount you will give.

    Give: _____ mL

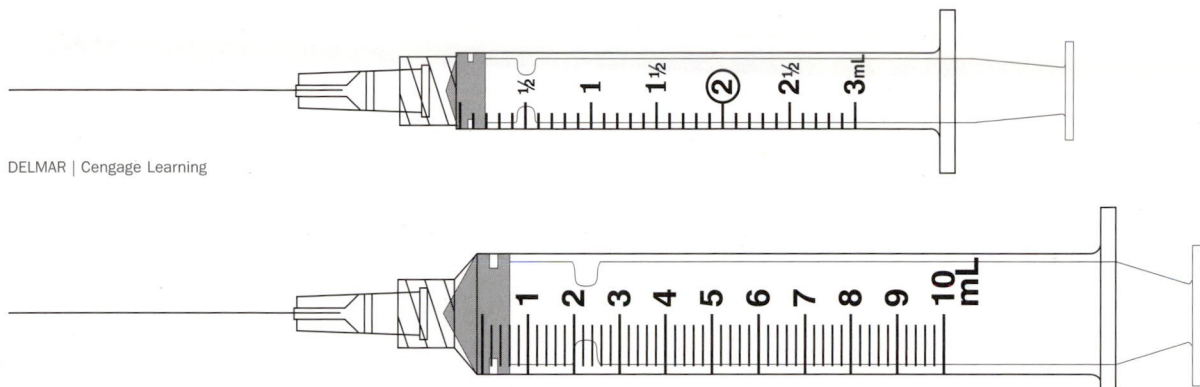

DELMAR | Cengage Learning

DELMAR | Cengage Learning

16. The electronic infusion pump is calibrated to administer mL/h. At what rate will you initially set the infusion pump for the lidocaine drip? _____ mL/h

17. The recommended dosage of dopamine is 5 to 10 mcg/kg/min. Is the dosage ordered for Mrs. Smith safe? _____ If safe, how much dopamine will you add to mix the dopamine drip? You have dopamine 80 mg/mL available. Draw an arrow on the appropriate syringe to indicate the amount you will add. Add: _____ mL

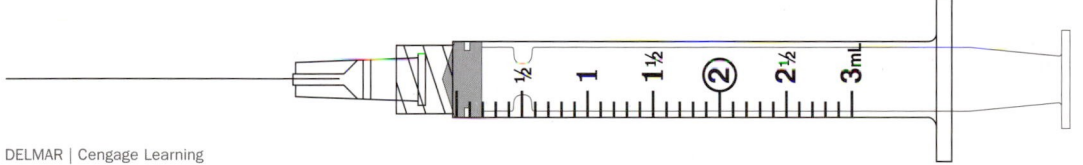

DELMAR | Cengage Learning

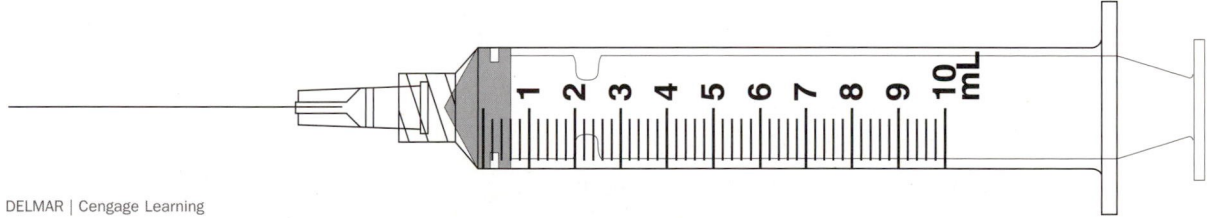

DELMAR | Cengage Learning

18. Calculate the rate for the infusion pump for the dopamine drip. _____ mL/h

19. How much dopamine will Mrs. Smith receive per hour? _____ mcg/h or _____ mg/h

20. Mrs. Smith is having increasing amounts of PVCs. To increase her lidocaine drip to 4 mg/min, you will now change the IV infusion pump setting to _____ mL/h.

		ENTERED	FILLED	CHECKED	VERIFIED

NOTE: A NON-PROPRIETARY DRUG OF EQUAL QUALITY MAY BE DISPENSED - IF THIS COLUMN IS NOT CHECKED!

DATE	TIME WRITTEN	PLEASE USE BALL POINT - PRESS FIRMLY	✓	TIME NOTED	NURSES SIGNATURE
9/4/xx	2230	Transfer to CCU			
		NPO			
		Discontinue nitroglycerin			
		lidocaine bolus 50 mg IV stat, then begin			
		lidocaine drip 2 g IV in 500 mL D_5W			
		at 2 mg/min by infusion pump			
		Increase lidocaine to 4 mg/min IV if PVCs			
		(premature ventricular contractions)			
		persist		2235 MS	
		dopamine 400 mg IV PB in 250 mL D_5W			
		at 500 mcg/min by infusion pump			
		Increase KCl to 20 mEq per L D_5W			
		$^1/_2$ NS IV at 50 mL/h			
		Increase furosemide to 40 mg IV q.12h			
		O_2 at 30% p̄ ABGs (arterial blood gases)			
		Labwork: Electrolytes stat and in am and			
		ABGs stat and p.r.n.			
		J. Physician, MD			

AUTO STOP ORDERS: UNLESS REORDERED, FOLLOWING WILL BE D/C'D AT 0800 ON:

DATE	ORDER		PHYSICIAN SIGNATURE
		☐ CONT ☐ D/C	
		☐ CONT ☐ D/C	PHYSICIAN SIGNATURE
		☐ CONT ☐ D/C	PHYSICIAN SIGNATURE

CHECK WHEN ANTIBIOTICS ORDERED   ☐ Prophylactic   ☐ Empiric   ☐ Therapeutic

Allergies:
None Known

Chest Pain
PATIENT DIAGNOSIS

Smith, Donna
ID #257-226-3

HEIGHT 5' 6"   WEIGHT 110 lb

PHYSICIAN'S ORDER

FORM 959-708 (8xx)   Reynolds + Reynolds LITHO IN U.S.A. K41814 (7-90) D339380

①

21. Julie Thomas is a 6-year-old pediatric patient who weighs 33 lb. She is in the hospital for fever of unknown origin. Julie complains of burning on urination and her urinalysis shows *E. coli* bacterial infection. The doctor prescribes **Kantrex 75 mg IV q.8h to be administered by volume control set on an infusion pump in 25 mL D$_5\frac{1}{2}$ NS followed by 15 mL flush over 1 hour.** The maximum recommended dosage of Kantrex is 15 mg/kg/day IV in 3 doses.

    Is the order safe? _____

    NDC 0015-3512-20
    EQUIVALENT TO   NSN 6505-00-926-9202
    75 mg KANAMYCIN per 2 mL
    KANTREX®
    Kanamycin Sulfate Injection, USP
    Pediatric Injection
    FOR I.M. OR I.V. USE
    CAUTION: Federal law prohibits dispensing without prescription.
    MAXIMUM DOSE: 15 MG/KG/DAY
    Cont:
    Exp. Date:

    Explain: _____

    If safe, add _____ mL Kantrex and _____ mL D$_5\frac{1}{2}$ NS to the chamber, and set the flow rate for _____ mL/h.

22. Order: **Cardizem 125 mg in 100 mL D$_5$W IV at 15 mg/h**

    Set the IV pump at _____ mL/h.

23. Jamie Smith is hospitalized with a staphylococcal bone infection. He weighs 66 lb.

    Orders: **D$_5\frac{1}{2}$ NS IV at 50 mL/h for continuous infusion**

    vancomycin 300 mg IV q.6h

    Supply: vancomycin 500 mg per 10 mL with instructions to "add to volume control set and infuse over 60 min."

    Recommended dosage: vancomycin 40 mg/kg/day IV in 4 equally divided doses.

    Is this drug order safe? _____. Explain: _____

    If safe, how much vancomycin will you add to the chamber? _____ mL

    How much IV fluid will you add to the chamber with the vancomycin? _____ mL

    How much IV fluid will Jamie receive in 24 hours? _____ mL

24. Calculate the hourly maintenance IV rate for the child described in question 23. Use the following recommendations:

    First 10 kg of body weight: 100 mL/kg/day

    Second 10 kg of body weight: 50 mL/kg/day

    Each additional kg over 20 kg of body weight: 20 mL/kg/day

    The child requires _____ mL/day for maintenance IV fluids.

    The infusion rate should be _____ mL/h. Does the recommended rate match the ordered rate? _____

Use the related orders and labels to answer questions 25 through 29. Select and mark the dose volume on the appropriate syringe, as indicated.

25. Order: Unasyn 500 mg IV q.6h in 50 mL D₅W IV PB over 30 min

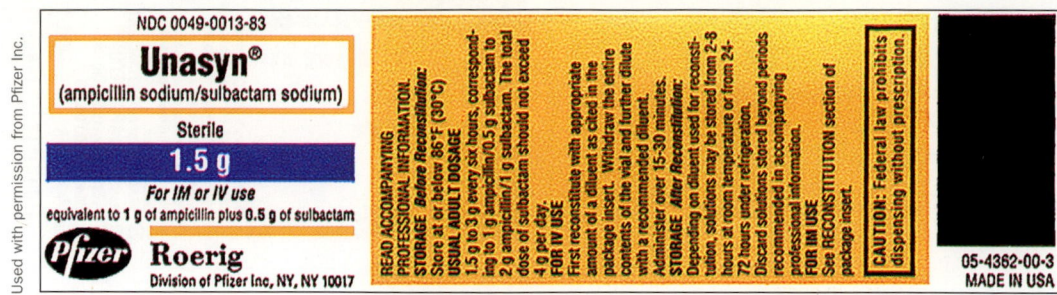

Package insert directions state:

Unasyn Vial Size	Volume Diluent to Be Added	Withdrawal Volume
1.5 g	3.2 mL	4.0 mL
3.0 g	6.4 mL	8.0 mL

Reconstitute with _____ mL diluent.

26. Prepare a reconstitution label for the Unasyn.

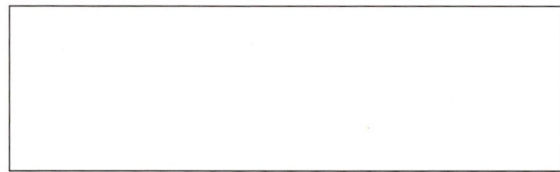

Reconstitution label

27. Add _____ mL Unasyn to the 50 mL IV PB.

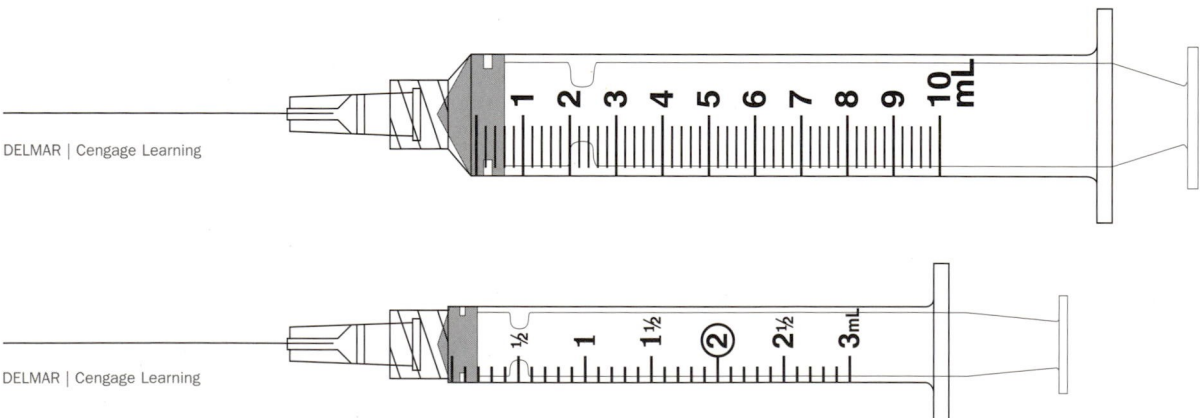

DELMAR | Cengage Learning

DELMAR | Cengage Learning

28. The IV Unasyn is regulated on an electronic infusion pump. Set the volume control set flow rate at _____ mL/h.

29. Order: heparin 10,000 units IV in 500 mL D₅W to infuse at 1,200 units/h

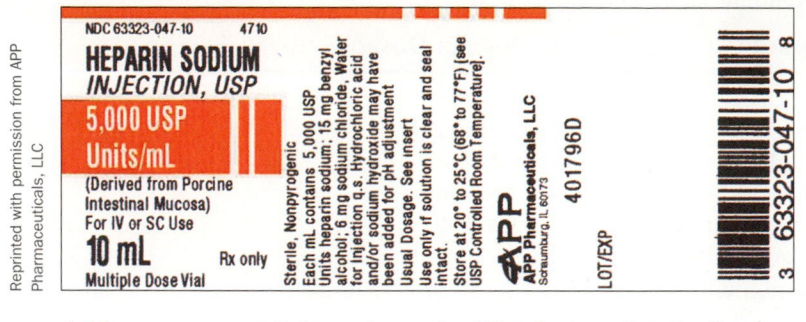

Add _____ mL heparin to the IV solution. Set the flow rate to _____ mL/h on an IV infusion pump.

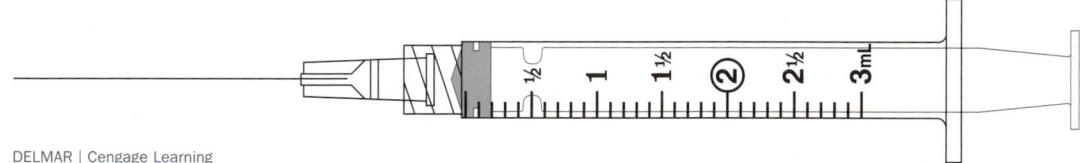

DELMAR | Cengage Learning

Questions 30 and 31 refer to a patient who weighs 125 lb and has IV heparin ordered per the following Weight-Based Heparin Protocol.

Weight-Based Heparin Protocol:

Heparin IV infusion: heparin 25,000 units IV in 250 mL of $\frac{1}{2}$ NS

IV boluses: Use heparin 1,000 units/mL

Bolus with heparin 80 units/kg. Then initiate heparin drip at 18 units/kg/h. Obtain APTT every 6 hours and adjust dosage and rate as follows:

If APTT is less than 35 seconds: Rebolus with 80 units/kg and increase rate by 4 units/kg/h.

If APTT is 36 to 44 seconds: Rebolus with 40 units/kg and increase rate by 2 units/kg/h.

If APTT is 45 to 75 seconds: Continue current rate.

If APTT is 76 to 90 seconds: Decrease rate by 2 units/kg/h.

If APTT is greater than 90 seconds: Hold heparin for 1 hour and then decrease rate by 3 units/kg/h.

---

30. Convert the patient's weight to kg (rounded to tenths): _____ kg

Calculate the initial heparin bolus dosage: _____ units

Calculate the bolus dose: _____ mL

Calculate the initial heparin infusion rate: _____ units/h or _____ mL/h

31. At 0930, the patient's APTT is 77 seconds. According to the protocol, what will your action be?

_____

_____

Decrease infusion rate by _____ units/h or _____ mL/h. Reset infusion rate to _____ mL/h.

32. Order: Novolin R Regular U-100 insulin subcut ac per sliding scale and blood sugar (BS) level
The patient's blood sugar at 1730 hours is 238

Sliding Scale	Insulin Dosage
BS: 0–150	0 units
BS: 151–250	8 units
BS: 251–350	13 units
BS: 351–400	18 units
BS: greater than 400	Call MD

Give: _____ units, which equals _____ mL (Mark dose on appropriate syringe.)

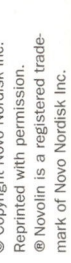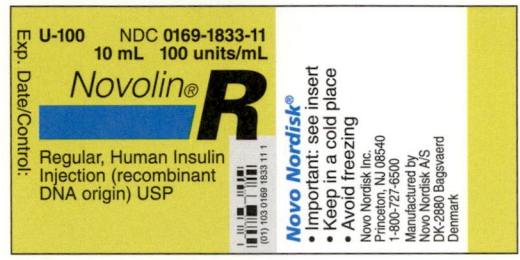

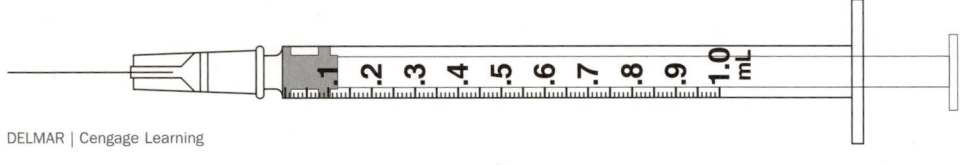

DELMAR | Cengage Learning

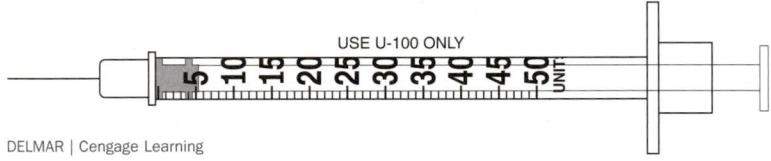

DELMAR | Cengage Learning

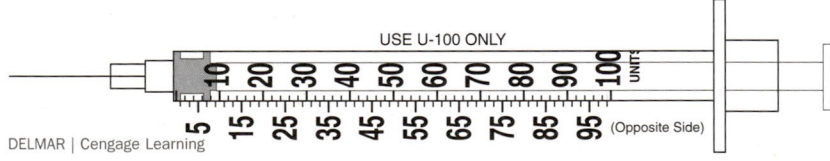

DELMAR | Cengage Learning

33. Order: Humulin R Regular U-100 insulin 15 units c̄ Humulin N NPH U-100 insulin 45 units sub-cut at 0730

    You will give a total of _____ units insulin. (Mark dose on appropriate syringe, designating Regular and NPH insulin.)

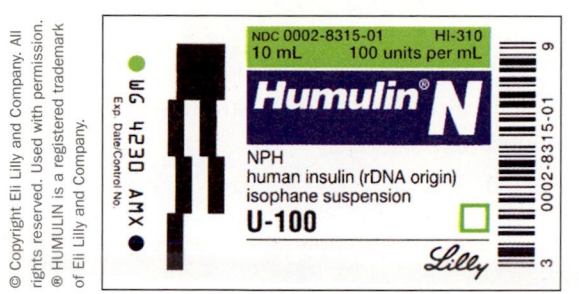
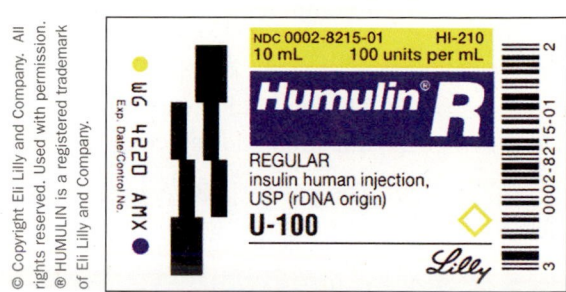

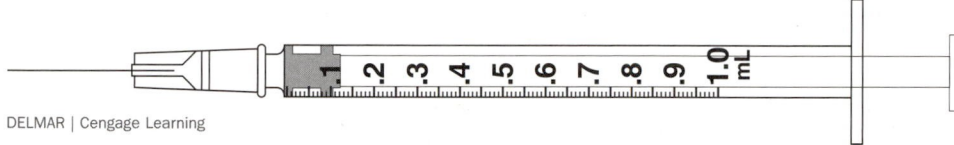

DELMAR | Cengage Learning

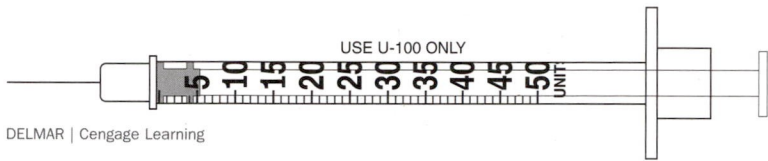

DELMAR | Cengage Learning

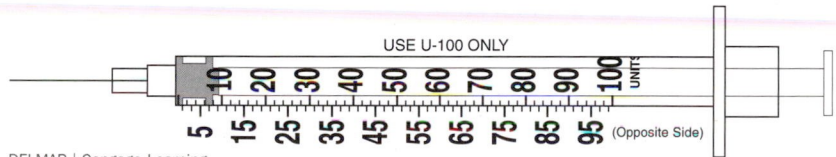

DELMAR | Cengage Learning

34. A patient with diabetes is receiving an insulin drip of Humulin R Regular U-100 insulin 300 units in 150 mL NS IV infusing at 10 mL/h. How many units/h of insulin is this patient receiving? _____ units/h

Questions 35 and 36 refer to an infant who weighs 16 lb and is admitted to the pediatric unit with vomiting and diarrhea for 3 days' duration.

Order: $\frac{1}{4}$ strength Isomil 80 mL q.3h for 4 feedings; if tolerated, increase Isomil to $\frac{1}{2}$ strength 80 mL q.3h for 4 feedings

Supply: Isomil Ready-to-Feed formula in 8 fluid ounce cans

35. To reconstitute a full 8 fluid ounce can of Isomil ready-to-feed to $\frac{1}{4}$ strength, you would add _____ mL water to mix a total of _____ mL of $\frac{1}{4}$ strength reconstituted Isomil.

36. The child is not tolerating the oral feedings. Calculate this child's allowable daily and hourly IV maintenance fluids using the following recommendation. _____ mL/day or _____ mL/h.

    Daily rate of pediatric maintenance IV fluids:

    100 mL/kg for first 10 kg of body weight

    50 mL/kg for next 10 kg of body weight

    20 mL/kg for each kg above 20 kg of body weight

Use the following information and order to answer questions 37 through 39.

Metric: BSA $(m^2) = \sqrt{\dfrac{ht\ (cm) \times wt\ (kg)}{3,600}}$ Household: BSA $(m^2) = \sqrt{\dfrac{ht\ (in) \times wt\ (lb)}{3,131}}$

Order: **mitomycin 28 mg IV push stat**

Recommended dosage is 10 to 20 mg/m²/single IV dose

Patient is 5 ft 2 in tall and weighs 103 lb

Mitomycin is available in a 40 mg vial with directions to reconstitute with 80 mL sterile water for injection and inject slowly over 10 minutes

37. The patient's BSA is _____ m²

38. What is the recommended dosage of mitomycin for this patient? _____ mg to _____ mg

    Is the ordered dosage safe? _____

39. What is the concentration of mitomycin after reconstitution? _____ mg/mL

    If the order is safe, administer _____ mL mitomycin at the rate of _____ mL/min or _____ mL per 15 sec.

40. A child's IV is **1 L D₅ 0.45% NaCl.** Calculate the amount of solute in this IV solution.
    _____ g dextrose and _____ g NaCl.

Use the following order and label for the available drug to answer questions 41 and 42.

Order: **Rocephin 600 mg IV q.12h for total volume of 50 mL to infuse over 1 h via volume control set**

41. Add _____ mL Rocephin and _____ mL IV fluid to the chamber.

42. The package insert states "...recommended dilution concentration is 10 mg/mL to 40 mg/mL..." Is the ordered amount of IV fluid sufficient to safely dilute the Rocephin? _____.
    Explain: _____

    _____

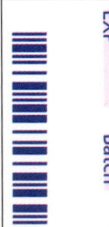

Use the following information to answer questions 43 and 44.

Order: **penicillin G potassium 400,000 units IV PB q.6h** for a child who weighs 10 kg. Recommended dosage for children: Give penicillin G potassium 150,000 to 250,000 units/kg/day in divided doses q.6h; dilute with 100 mL NS and infuse over 60 minutes.

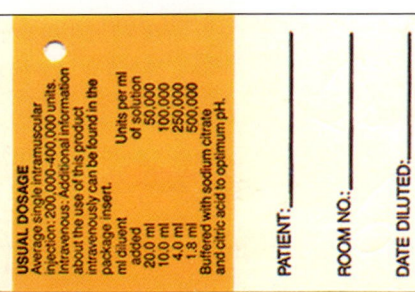

43. How many units per day of penicillin G potassium is this child ordered to receive? _____ units/day

Is the ordered dosage safe? _____ Explain: _____

If safe, reconstitute with _____ mL diluent for a concentration of _____ units/mL and prepare a reconstitution label.

```
┌─────────────────────────────────────┐
│                                     │
│                                     │
│                                     │
│                                     │
│                                     │
└─────────────────────────────────────┘
```

Reconstitution label

Prepare to give _____ mL

If not safe, what should you do? _____

44. The child's IV is infusing on an electronic infusion pump. If the dosage is safe, set the IV flow rate at _____ mL/h.

Use the following patient situation to answer questions 45 through 48.

A patient has been admitted to the hospital with fever and chills, productive cough with yellow-green sputum, shortness of breath, malaise, and anorexia. Laboratory tests and X-rays confirmed a diagnosis of pneumonia. The patient is complaining of nausea. The physician writes the following orders. The labels represent the drugs you have available.

NS 1,000 mL IV at 125 mL/h

ceftriaxone 1,500 mg IV PB q.8h in 100 mL NS over 30 min

promethazine 12.5 mg IV push q.4h p.r.n., nausea and vomiting

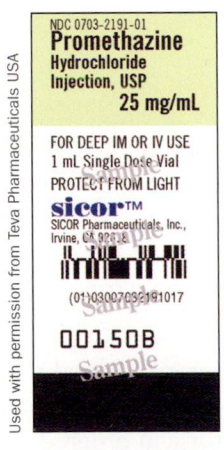

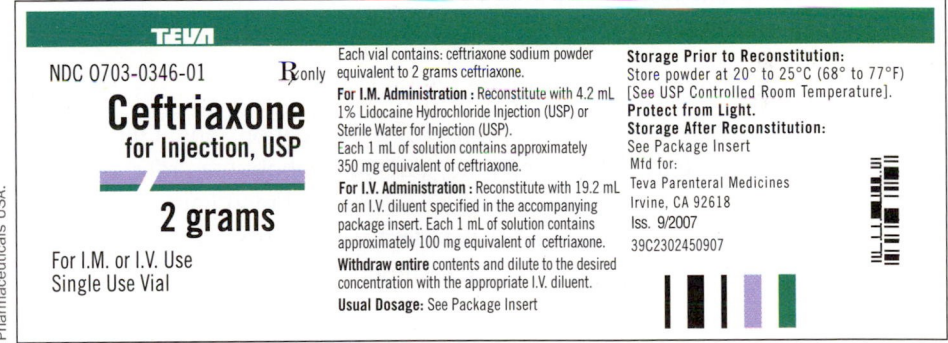

Intravenous Administration

Ceftriaxone for injection, USP should be administered intravenously by infusion over a period of 30 minutes. Concentrations between 10 mg/mL and 40 mg/mL are recommended; however, lower concentrations may be used if desired. Reconstitute vials with an appropriate IV diluent (see **COMPATIBILITY AND STABILITY**).

Vial Dosage Size	Amount of Diluent to be Added
250 mg	2.4 mL
500 mg	4.8 mL
1 g	9.6 mL
2 g	19.2 mL

After reconstitution, each 1 mL of solution contains approximately 100 mg equivalent of ceftriaxone. Withdraw entire contents and dilute to the desired concentration with the appropriate IV diluent.

45. You start the primary IV at 1:15 PM on an electronic infusion pump. When do you estimate (using international time) the primary IV and one IVPB administration will be completely infused and the primary IV will have to be replaced? _____ hours

46. Promethazine recommendation for direct IV administration is "not to exceed 25 mg/min." You will give _____ mL of promethazine per min or _____ mL per 15 sec.

47. You will give _____ mL ceftriaxone per dose.

48. Set the IV PB flow rate for each dose of ceftriaxone at _____ mL/h.

49. Describe the strategy you would implement to prevent this medication error.

Possible Scenario
A student nurse was preparing for medication administration. One of the orders on the Medical Administration Record (MAR) was written as **Lanoxin 0.125 mg od.** The student nurse crushed the Lanoxin tablet. Prior to giving the medication, the nursing instructor checked the medications that the student had prepared. The instructor asked the student to explain the rationale for crushing the Lanoxin tablet. The student explained to the instructor that the Lanoxin order was for the right eye ("O.D." is an outdated abbreviation for right eye) and the student planned to add a small amount of sterile water to the crushed tablet and put it in the patient's eye.

Potential Outcome
What is wrong with the Lanoxin order? _____

_____

What could be the result? _____

Prevention

_____

_____

50. Describe the strategy you would implement to prevent this medication error.

Possible Scenario
Order: **Quinapril 30 mg p.o. daily**

Supply: quinidine 300 mg tablets

A student nurse administering medications noted the difference between the order and the supply drug and questioned the staff nurse about the order and what had been administered. The staff nurse at first dismissed it as only the brand name versus the generic name of the drug. Later the nurse realized that the student was exactly right to question the order and the drug supplied; and the nurse admitted to the student that the patient had been receiving the wrong drug all week.

Potential Outcome
The student referred to a drug reference book and compared the therapeutic and side effects of both drugs. The quinapril was correctly ordered for hypertension. Quinidine is an anti-arrhythmic heart medication. The physician was notified of the medication error and ordered a stat electrocardiogram. Indeed, on the electrocardiogram the patient had a long QT interval, putting the patient at grave risk for a fatal arrythmia.

Prevention

_____

_____

After completing these problems, see pages 590–596 to check your answers. Give yourself 2 points for each correct answer.

Perfect score = 100   My score = _____

Minimum mastery score = 90 (45 correct)

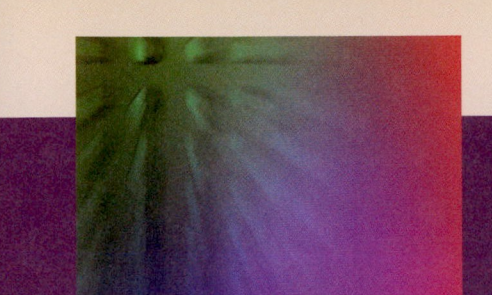

Answers

Mathematics Diagnostic Evaluation from pages 2–4

1) 1,517.63 **2)** 20.74 **3)** 100.66 **4)** $323.72 **5)** 46.11 **6)** 754.5 **7)** 16.91 **8)** 19,494.7 **9)** $173.04 **10)** 403.26 **11)** 36

12) 2,500 **13)** $\frac{2}{3}$ **14)** 6.25 **15)** $\frac{4}{5}$ **16)** 40% **17)** 0.4% **18)** 0.05 **19)** 1:3 **20)** 0.02 **21)** $1\frac{1}{4}$ **22)** $6\frac{13}{24}$ **23)** $1\frac{11}{18}$ **24)** $\frac{3}{5}$ **25)** $14\frac{7}{8}$

26) $\frac{1}{100}$ **27)** 0.009 **28)** 320 **29)** 3 **30)** 0.05 **31)** 4 **32)** 0.09 **33)** 0.22 **34)** 25 **35)** 4 **36)** 0.75 **37)** 3 **38)** 500 **39)** 18.24

40) 2.4 **41)** $\frac{1}{5}$ **42)** 1:50 **43)** 5 tablets **44)** 2 milligrams **45)** 30 kilograms **46)** 3.3 pounds **47)** $6\frac{2}{3}$ = 6.67 centimeters

48) 7.5 centimeters **49)** 90% **50)** 5:1

Solutions—Mathematics Diagnostic Evaluation

3)
```
    9.50
   17.06
   32.00
   41.11
 +  0.99
 -------
  100.66
```

6)
```
  1,005.0
 -  250.5
 --------
    754.5
```

10)
```
    17.16
 ×  23.5
 -------
   8580
  5148
 3432
 ------
 403.260 = 403.26
```

12)
$$0.001\overline{)2.500.} = 2,500$$

19) $33\frac{1}{3}\% = \dfrac{33\frac{1}{3}}{100} = \dfrac{\frac{100}{3}}{100} = \dfrac{100}{3} \div \dfrac{100}{1} = \dfrac{\cancel{100}}{3} \times \dfrac{1}{\cancel{100}} = \dfrac{1}{3} = 1:3$

23)
$$1\frac{5}{6} = 1\frac{15}{18}$$
$$-\frac{2}{9} = -\frac{4}{18}$$
$$\overline{\qquad 1\frac{11}{18}}$$

25) $4\frac{1}{4} \times 3\frac{1}{2} = \dfrac{17}{4} \times \dfrac{7}{2} = \dfrac{119}{8} = 14\frac{7}{8}$

29) $\dfrac{0.02 + 0.16}{0.4 - 0.34}$

```
   0.02      0.40
 + 0.16    - 0.34
 ------    ------
   0.18      0.06
```
$$\dfrac{0.18}{0.06} = 0.06\overline{)0.18.} = 3$$

32) $\dfrac{1}{2}\% = 0.5\% = 0.005$
```
       18
   × 0.005
  -------
   0.090 = 0.09
```

34) $\dfrac{1:1,000}{1:100} \times 250 =$
$$\dfrac{\frac{1}{1,000}}{\frac{1}{100}} \times 250 = \dfrac{1}{1,000} \times \dfrac{\cancel{100}}{1} \times \dfrac{250}{1} = \dfrac{250}{10} = 25$$

45) 66 pounds = $\dfrac{66}{2.2}$ = 30 kilograms or

2.2 pounds ⟍⟋ 66 pounds
1 kilogram ⟋⟍ X kilograms

$$2.2X = 66$$
$$\dfrac{2.2X}{2.2} = \dfrac{66}{2.2}$$
$$X = 30 \text{ kilograms}$$

49)
```
   50
 -  5
 ----
   45
```
$\dfrac{45}{50} = \dfrac{9}{10} = 90\%$

Review Set 1 from pages 10–12

1) $\frac{6}{6}, \frac{7}{5}$ **2)** $\dfrac{\frac{1}{100}}{\frac{1}{150}}$ **3)** $\frac{1}{4}, \frac{1}{14}$ **4)** $1\frac{2}{9}, 1\frac{1}{4}, 5\frac{7}{8}$ **5)** $\frac{3}{4} = \frac{6}{8}, \frac{1}{5} = \frac{2}{10}, \frac{3}{9} = \frac{1}{3}$ **6)** $\frac{13}{2}$ **7)** $\frac{6}{5}$ **8)** $\frac{32}{3}$ **9)** $\frac{47}{6}$ **10)** $\frac{411}{4}$ **11)** 2 **12)** 1

13) $3\frac{1}{3}$ **14)** $1\frac{1}{3}$ **15)** $2\frac{3}{4}$ **16)** $\frac{6}{8}$ **17)** $\frac{4}{16}$ **18)** $\frac{8}{12}$ **19)** $\frac{4}{10}$ **20)** $\frac{6}{9}$ **21)** $\frac{1}{100}$ **22)** $\frac{1}{10,000}$ **23)** $\frac{5}{9}$ **24)** $\frac{3}{10}$ **25)** $\frac{2}{5}$ bottle **26)** $1\frac{1}{2}$ bottles

27) $\frac{1}{20}$ of the students are men **28)** $\frac{9}{10}$ of the questions were answered correctly **29)** $\frac{1}{2}$ dose **30)** $\frac{1}{2}$ teaspoon

Solutions—Review Set 1

8) $10\frac{2}{3} = \frac{(3 \times 10) + 2}{3} = \frac{32}{3}$

14) $\frac{100}{75} = 1\frac{25}{75} = 1\frac{1}{3}$

18) $\frac{2}{3} \times \frac{4}{4} = \frac{8}{12}$

25) 10 ounces – 6 ounces = 4 ounces remaining

$\frac{\overset{2}{\cancel{4}}}{\underset{5}{\cancel{10}}} = \frac{2}{5}$ bottle remaining

27) $\begin{array}{r} 57 \\ + 3 \\ \hline 60 \end{array}$ people in class

The men represent $\frac{3}{60}$ or $\frac{1}{20}$ of the students in the class.

29) $\frac{80}{160} = \frac{1}{2}$ of a dose

30) $\frac{1}{2}$ of 1 teaspoon $= \frac{1}{2}$ teaspoon

Review Set 2 from page 14

1) $8\frac{7}{15}$ **2)** $1\frac{5}{12}$ **3)** $17\frac{5}{24}$ **4)** $1\frac{1}{24}$ **5)** $32\frac{5}{6}$ **6)** $5\frac{7}{12}$ **7)** $1\frac{1}{3}$ **8)** $5\frac{53}{72}$ **9)** 43 **10)** $5\frac{118}{119}$ **11)** $2\frac{8}{15}$ **12)** $\frac{53}{132}$ **13)** $\frac{1}{2}$ **14)** $4\frac{5}{6}$ **15)** $\frac{1}{24}$ **16)** $63\frac{2}{3}$ **17)** $299\frac{4}{5}$ **18)** $\frac{1}{6}$ **19)** $1\frac{2}{5}$ **20)** $7\frac{1}{16}$ **21)** $7\frac{2}{9}$ **22)** $1\frac{1}{4}$ **23)** $24\frac{6}{11}$ **24)** $\frac{7}{12}$ **25)** $\frac{1}{25}$ **26)** $\frac{7}{12}$ fluid ounce **27)** $1\frac{1}{8}$ inches **28)** 8 inches **29)** $21\frac{1}{2}$ pints **30)** $13\frac{1}{4}$ pounds

Solutions—Review Set 2

1) $\begin{array}{l} 7\frac{4}{5} + \frac{2}{3} : 7\frac{12}{15} \\ \qquad + \frac{10}{15} \\ \hline \qquad 7\frac{22}{15} = 8\frac{7}{15} \end{array}$

3) $\begin{array}{l} 4\frac{2}{3} + 5\frac{1}{24} + 7\frac{1}{2} : 4\frac{16}{24} \\ \qquad 5\frac{1}{24} \\ \qquad + 7\frac{12}{24} \\ \hline \qquad 16\frac{29}{24} = 17\frac{5}{24} \end{array}$

4) $\frac{3}{4} + \frac{1}{8} + \frac{1}{6} = \frac{18}{24} + \frac{3}{24} + \frac{4}{24} = \frac{18+3+4}{24} = \frac{25}{24} = 1\frac{1}{24}$

14) $\begin{array}{l} 8\frac{1}{12} - 3\frac{1}{4} = 8\frac{1}{12} - 3\frac{3}{12} : 7\frac{13}{12} \\ \qquad - 3\frac{3}{12} \\ \hline \qquad 4\frac{10}{12} = 4\frac{5}{6} \end{array}$

25) 50 pounds – 48 pounds = 2 pounds lost

$\frac{2}{50} = \frac{1}{25}$ of weight lost

26) $\frac{1}{4}$ fluid ounce $+ \frac{1}{3}$ fluid ounce $= \frac{3}{12} + \frac{4}{12} =$

$\frac{7}{12}$ fluid ounce

29) $\begin{array}{l} 56 - 34\frac{1}{2} : 55\frac{2}{2} \\ \qquad - 34\frac{1}{2} \\ \hline \qquad 21\frac{1}{2} \text{ pints} \end{array}$

30) $\begin{array}{l} 20\frac{1}{2} - 7\frac{1}{4} : 20\frac{2}{4} \\ \qquad - 7\frac{1}{4} \\ \hline \qquad 13\frac{1}{4} \text{ pounds} \end{array}$

Review Set 3 from pages 19–20

1) $\frac{1}{40}$ **2)** $\frac{36}{125}$ **3)** $\frac{35}{48}$ **4)** $\frac{3}{100}$ **5)** 3 **6)** $1\frac{2}{3}$ **7)** $\frac{4}{5}$ **8)** $6\frac{8}{15}$ **9)** $\frac{1}{2}$ **10)** $23\frac{19}{36}$ **11)** $\frac{3}{32}$ **12)** $254\frac{1}{6}$ **13)** 3 **14)** $1\frac{34}{39}$ **15)** $\frac{3}{14}$ **16)** $\frac{1}{11}$ **17)** $\frac{1}{2}$ **18)** $\frac{1}{30}$ **19)** $3\frac{1}{3}$ **20)** $\frac{3}{20}$ **21)** $\frac{1}{3}$ **22)** $\frac{7}{12}$ **23)** $1\frac{1}{9}$ **24)** 60 calories **25)** 560 seconds **26)** 40 doses **27)** $31\frac{1}{2}$ tablets **28)** 1,275 milliliters **29)** $52\frac{1}{2}$ ounces **30)** 6 full days

Solutions—Review Set 3

3) $\frac{5}{8} \times 1\frac{1}{6} = \frac{5}{8} \times \frac{7}{6} = \frac{35}{48}$

5) $\frac{\frac{1}{6}}{\frac{1}{4}} \times \frac{\frac{3}{1}}{\frac{2}{3}} = \left(\frac{1}{6} \times \frac{4}{1}\right) \times \left(\frac{3}{1} \times \frac{3}{2}\right) = \frac{\overset{2}{\cancel{4}}}{\underset{3}{\cancel{6}}} \times \frac{9}{2} = \frac{\overset{3}{\cancel{18}}}{\underset{1}{\cancel{6}}} = 3$

16) $\frac{1}{33} \div \frac{1}{3} = \frac{1}{33} \times \frac{3}{1} = \frac{\overset{1}{\cancel{3}}}{\underset{11}{\cancel{33}}} = \frac{1}{11}$

19) $2\frac{1}{2} \div \frac{3}{4} = \frac{5}{2} \div \frac{3}{4} = \frac{5}{2} \times \frac{\overset{2}{\cancel{4}}}{\underset{1}{3}} = \frac{10}{3} = 3\frac{1}{3}$

27) $3 \times 7 = 21$ doses

$21 \times 1\frac{1}{2} = 21 \times \frac{3}{2} = \frac{63}{2} = 31\frac{1}{2}$ tablets

28) $850 \div \frac{2}{3} = \frac{\overset{425}{\cancel{850}}}{1} \times \frac{3}{\underset{1}{\cancel{2}}} = 1,275$ milliliters

30)

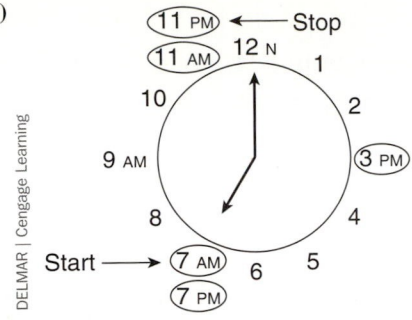

Start → 7 AM, 7 PM
Stop ← 11 PM, 11 AM

DELMAR | Cengage Learning

Daily doses would be taken at: 7 AM, 11 AM, 3 PM, 7 PM, and 11 PM for 5 doses/day.

5 doses/day $\times \frac{1}{2}$ fluid ounce/dose $= \frac{5}{2} =$

$2\frac{1}{2}$ fluid ounces/day

16 fluid ounces $\div 2\frac{1}{2}$ fluid ounces/day $= \frac{16}{1} \div \frac{5}{2} =$

$\frac{16}{1} \times \frac{2}{5} = \frac{32}{5} = 6\frac{2}{5}$ days or 6 full days

Review Set 4 from pages 26–27

1) 0.2, two tenths **2)** $\frac{17}{20}$, 0.85 **3)** $1\frac{1}{20}$, one and five hundredths **4)** $\frac{3}{500}$, six thousandths **5)** 10.015, ten and fifteen thousandths **6)** $1\frac{9}{10}$, one and nine tenths **7)** $5\frac{1}{10}$, 5.1 **8)** 0.8, eight tenths **9)** $250\frac{1}{2}$, two hundred fifty and five tenths **10)** 33.03, thirty-three and three hundredths **11)** $\frac{19}{20}$, ninety-five hundredths **12)** 2.75, two and seventy-five hundredths **13)** $7\frac{1}{200}$, 7.005 **14)** 0.084, eighty-four thousandths **15)** $12\frac{1}{8}$, twelve and one hundred twenty-five thousandths **16)** $20\frac{9}{100}$, twenty and nine hundredths **17)** $22\frac{11}{500}$, 22.022 **18)** $\frac{3}{20}$, fifteen hundredths **19)** 1,000.005, one thousand and five thousandths **20)** $4,085\frac{3}{40}$, 4,085.075 **21)** 0.0170 **22)** 0.25 **23)** 0.75 **24)** $\frac{9}{200}$ **25)** 0.12 **26)** 0.063 **27)** False **28)** False **29)** True **30)** 0.8 gram and 1.25 grams

Solutions—Review Set 4

4) $0.006 = \frac{6}{1,000} = \frac{3}{500}$

8) $\frac{4}{5} = 5\overline{)4.0}$ quotient 0.8

14) $\frac{21}{250} = 250\overline{)21.000}$
$\quad\quad\quad\quad\quad 0.084$
$\quad\quad\quad\quad 20\ 00$
$\quad\quad\quad\quad\quad 1\ 000$
$\quad\quad\quad\quad\quad 1\ 000$

15) $12.125 = 12\frac{125}{1,000} = 12\frac{1}{8}$

18) $0.15 = \frac{15}{100} = \frac{3}{20}$

30)   0.5 gram is less than or equal to safe dose is less than or equal to 2 grams

Safe doses: 0.8 gram and 1.25 grams

Review Set 5 from pages 28–29

1) 22.585 **2)** 44.177 **3)** 12.309 **4)** 11.3 **5)** 175.199 **6)** 25.007 **7)** 0.518 **8)** $9.48 **9)** $18.91 **10)** $22.71 **11)** 6.403 **12)** 0.27 **13)** 4.15 **14)** 1.51 **15)** 10.25 **16)** 2.517 **17)** 374.35 **18)** 604.42 **19)** 27.449 **20)** 23.619 **21)** 0.697 gram **22)** 188.25 milliliters **23)** $2,058.06 **24)** 10.3 grams **25)** 8.1 hours

Solutions—Review Set 5

2)
$\quad$ 7.517
$\quad$ 3.200
$\quad$ 0.160
$\quad$ 33.300
$\quad$ ——
$\quad$ 44.177

9)
$\quad$ 8 9 10
$\quad$ $19.00
$\quad$ − 0.09
$\quad$ ——
$\quad$ $18.91

25)
$\quad$ 3 h 20 min
$\quad\quad\quad$ 40 min
$\quad$ 3 h 30 min
$\quad\quad\quad$ 24 min
$\quad$ + $\quad$ 12 min
$\quad$ ——
$\quad$ 6 h 126 min = 8 h 6 min (60 minutes/hour)
$\quad\quad\quad\quad = 8\frac{6}{60} = 8\frac{1}{10} = 8.1$ hours

Review Set 6 from page 34

1) 5.83 **2)** 2.2 **3)** 42.75 **4)** 0.15 **5)** 403.14 **6)** 75,100.75 **7)** 32.86 **8)** 2.78 **9)** 348.58 **10)** 0.02 **11)** 400 **12)** 3.74 **13)** 5 **14)** 2.98 **15)** 4,120 **16)** 5.45 **17)** 272.67 **18)** 1.5 **19)** 50,020 **20)** 300 **21)** 562.50. = 56,250 **22)** 16.0. = 160 **23)** .025. = 0.025 **24)** .032.005 = 0.032005 **25)** .00.125 = 0.00125 **26)** 23.2.5 = 232.5 **27)** 71.7.717 = 71.7717 **28)** 83.1.6 = 831.6 **29)** 0.33. = 33 **30)** 14.106. = 14,106

Solutions—Review Set 6

2) $0.314 \times 7 = 2.198 = 2.20 = 2.2$ **10)** $1.14 \times 0.014 = 0.01596 = 0.02$ **14)** $45.5 \div 15.25 = 2.983 = 2.98$

Practice Problems—Chapter 1 from pages 34–36

1) $\frac{7}{20}$ **2)** 0.375 **3)** LCD = 21 **4)** LCD = 55 **5)** LCD = 18 **6)** LCD = 15 **7)** $3\frac{7}{15}$ **8)** $7\frac{29}{60}$ **9)** $\frac{1}{2}$ **10)** $2\frac{7}{24}$ **11)** $\frac{7}{27}$ **12)** $10\frac{1}{8}$ **13)** $4\frac{4}{17}$ **14)** $\frac{39}{80}$ **15)** $5\frac{1}{55}$ **16)** $5\frac{5}{18}$ **17)** $2\frac{86}{87}$ **18)** $\frac{3}{20}$ **19)** $\frac{1}{3,125}$ **20)** $\frac{1}{4}$ **21)** $1\frac{5}{7}$ **22)** $16\frac{1}{32}$ **23)** 60.27 **24)** 66.74 **25)** 42.98 **26)** 4,833.92 **27)** 190.8 **28)** 19.17 **29)** 9.48 **30)** 7.7 **31)** 42.75 **32)** 300 **33)** 12,930.43 **34)** 3,200.63 **35)** 2 **36)** 150.96 **37)** 9.716. = 9,716 **38)** .50.25 = 0.5025 **39)** 0.25. = 25 **40)** 5.750. = 5,750 **41)** .0.25 = 0.025 **42)** 11.5.25 = 115.25 **43)** 147 fluid ounces **44)** 138 nurses; 46 maintenance/cleaners; 92 technicians; 92 others **45)** False **46)** $1,082.79 **47)** $1.46 **48)** 0.31 gram **49)** 800 milliliters **50)** 2.95 kilograms

Solutions—Practice Problems—Chapter 1

43) $3\frac{1}{2}$ fluid ounces/feeding $\times$ 6 feedings/day =
21 fluid ounces/day, and 21 fluid ounces/day $\times$
7 days/week = 147 fluid ounces in one week

44) $\frac{3}{8} \times 368 = 138$ nurses
$\frac{1}{8} \times 368 = 46$ maintenance/cleaners
$\frac{1}{4} \times 368 = 92$ technicians and 92 others

45) $1\frac{2}{32} = 1.0625$; False, it's greater than normal.

46)   40 hours $\times$ $20.43/hour = $817.20
6.5 hours overtime $\times$ $40.86 =   + 265.59
(Overtime rate = $20.43 $\times$ 2 = 40.86) $1,082.79

47)   A case of 12 boxes with 12 catheters/box =
144 catheters
By case: $975 \div 144 = $6.77/catheter
By box: $98.76 \div 12 = $8.23/catheter
$8.23
$\underline{- 6.77}$
$1.46 savings/catheter

48)   0.065 gram/ounce $\times$ 4.75 ounces = 0.31 gram

49) $1{,}200 \text{ milliliters} \times \frac{2}{3} = \frac{\overset{400}{\cancel{1{,}200}}}{1} \times \frac{2}{\underset{1}{\cancel{3}}} = 800$ milliliters

50)   6.65 kilograms
$\underline{- 3.70 \text{ kilograms}}$
2.95 kilograms gained

Review Set 7 from pages 41–42

1) $\frac{1}{50}$ **2)** $\frac{3}{5}$ **3)** $\frac{1}{3}$ **4)** $\frac{4}{7}$ **5)** $\frac{3}{4}$ **6)** 0.5 **7)** 0.15 **8)** 0.14 **9)** 0.07 **10)** 0.24 **11)** 25% **12)** 40% **13)** 12.5% **14)** 70% **15)** 50% **16)** $\frac{9}{20}$ **17)** $\frac{3}{5}$ **18)** $\frac{1}{200}$ **19)** $\frac{1}{100}$ **20)** $\frac{2}{3}$ **21)** 0.03 **22)** 0.05 **23)** 0.06 **24)** 0.33 **25)** 0.01 **26)** 4:25 **27)** 1:4 **28)** 1:2 **29)** 9:20 **30)** 3:50 **31)** 0.9 **32)** $\frac{1}{5}$ **33)** 0.25% **34)** 0.5 **35)** $\frac{1}{100}$

Solutions—Review Set 7

1) $\dfrac{3}{150} = \dfrac{\overset{1}{\cancel{\frac{3}{2}}}}{\underset{50}{\cancel{150}}} = \dfrac{1}{50}$

3) $\dfrac{\overset{1}{\cancel{0.05}}}{\underset{3}{\cancel{0.15}}} = \dfrac{1}{3}$

7) $\dfrac{\frac{1}{1,000}}{\frac{1}{150}} = \dfrac{1}{\cancel{1,000}} \times \dfrac{\overset{15}{\cancel{150}}}{1} = \dfrac{15}{100} = 0.15. = 0.15$

12) $2:5 = \dfrac{2}{5} = 0.4;\ 0.4 = \dfrac{4}{10} = \dfrac{40}{100} = 40\%$

13) $0.08 : 0.64 = \dfrac{0.08}{0.64} = \dfrac{1}{8} = 0.125;$

$0.125 = \dfrac{125}{1,000} = \dfrac{12.5}{100} = 12.5\%$

17) $60\% = \dfrac{60}{100} = \dfrac{3}{5}$

18) $0.5\% = \dfrac{0.5}{100} = 0.5 \div 100 = 0.00.5 = 0.005 = \dfrac{5}{1,000} = \dfrac{1}{200}$

21) $2.94\% = \dfrac{2.94}{100} = 2.94 \div 100 = 0.02.94 = 0.0294 = 0.03$

30) $6\% = \dfrac{6}{100} = \dfrac{3}{50} = 3:50$

31) Convert to decimals and compare:

$0.9\% = 0.009$

$0.9 = 0.900$ (largest)

$1:9 = 0.111$

$1:90 = 0.011$

Review Set 8 from pages 45–46

1) 3 **2)** 3.3 **3)** 1.25 **4)** 5.33 **5)** 0.56 **6)** 1.8 **7)** 0.64 **8)** 12.6 **9)** 40 **10)** 0.48 **11)** 1 **12)** 0.96 **13)** 4.5 **14)** 0.94 **15)** 10 **16)** 0.4 **17)** 1.5 **18)** 10 **19)** 20 **20)** 1.8

Solutions—Review Set 8

2) $\dfrac{\frac{3}{4}}{\frac{1}{2}} \times 2.2 = X$

$\dfrac{3}{4} \div \dfrac{1}{2} \times \dfrac{2.2}{1} = X$

$\dfrac{3}{\underset{2}{\cancel{4}}} \times \dfrac{\overset{1}{\cancel{2}}}{1} \times \dfrac{2.2}{1} = X$

$\dfrac{6.6}{2} = X$

$X = 3.3$

4) $\dfrac{40\%}{60\%} \times 8 = X$

$\dfrac{\overset{2}{\cancel{0.4}}}{\underset{3}{\cancel{0.6}}} \times 8 = X$

$\dfrac{2}{3} \times \dfrac{8}{1} = X$

$\dfrac{16}{3} = X$

$X = 5.33\overline{3}$

$X = 5.33$

6) $\dfrac{0.15}{0.1} \times 1.2 = X$

$\dfrac{\overset{3}{\cancel{0.15}}}{\underset{2}{\cancel{0.10}}} \times \dfrac{1.2}{1} = X$

$\dfrac{3}{2} \times \dfrac{1.2}{1} = X$

$\dfrac{3.6}{2} = X$

$X = 1.8$

8) $\dfrac{\overset{3}{\cancel{1,200,000}}}{\underset{1}{\cancel{400,000}}} \times 4.2 = X$

$\dfrac{3}{1} \times \dfrac{4.2}{1} = X$

$\dfrac{12.6}{1} = X$

$X = 12.6$

10) $\dfrac{\overset{3}{\cancel{30}}}{\underset{5}{\cancel{50}}} \times 0.8 = X$

$\dfrac{3}{5} \times \dfrac{0.8}{1} = X$

$\dfrac{2.4}{5} = X$

$X = 0.48$

14) $\dfrac{\overset{1}{\cancel{250,000}}}{\underset{8}{\cancel{2,000,000}}} \times 7.5 = X$

$\dfrac{1}{8} \times \dfrac{7.5}{1} = X$

$\dfrac{7.5}{8} = X$

$X = 0.937$

$X = 0.94$

20) $\dfrac{\frac{1}{100}}{\frac{1}{150}} \times 1.2 = X$

$\dfrac{1}{100} \div \dfrac{1}{150} \times \dfrac{1.2}{1} = X$

$\dfrac{1}{\underset{2}{\cancel{100}}} \times \dfrac{\overset{3}{\cancel{150}}}{1} \times \dfrac{1.2}{1} = X$

$\dfrac{1}{2} \times \dfrac{3}{1} \times \dfrac{1.2}{1} = X$

$\dfrac{3.6}{2} = X$

$X = 1.8$

Review Set 9 from pages 49–50

1) 0.25 **2)** 1 **3)** 0.56 **4)** 1,000 **5)** 0.7 **6)** 8 **7)** 21.43 **8)** 500 **9)** 200 **10)** 10.5 **11)** 3 **12)** 0.63 **13)** 10 **14)** 0.67 **15)** 1.25
16) 31.25 **17)** 16.67 **18)** 240 **19)** 0.75 **20)** 2.27 **21)** 1 **22)** 6 **23)** 108 nurses **24)** 72 calories **25)** 81.82 milligrams/hour

Solutions—Review Set 9

4)
$$\frac{0.5}{2} \times \frac{250}{X}$$
$$0.5X = 500$$
$$\frac{0.5X}{0.5} = \frac{500}{0.5}$$
$$X = 1,000$$

6)
$$\frac{40}{X} \times 12 = 60$$
$$\frac{40}{X} \times \frac{12}{1} = 60$$
$$\frac{480}{X} \times \frac{60}{1}$$
$$60X = 480$$
$$\frac{60X}{60} = \frac{480}{60}$$
$$X = 8$$

9)
$$\frac{15}{500} \times X = 6$$
$$\frac{15X}{500} \times \frac{6}{1}$$
$$15X = 3,000$$
$$\frac{15X}{15} = \frac{3,000}{15}$$
$$X = 200$$

10)
$$\frac{5}{X} \times \frac{10}{21}$$
$$10X = 105$$
$$\frac{10X}{10} = \frac{105}{10}$$
$$X = 10.5$$

11)
$$\frac{250}{1} \times \frac{750}{X}$$
$$250X = 750$$
$$\frac{250X}{250} = \frac{750}{250}$$
$$X = 3$$

14)
$$\frac{\frac{1}{100}}{1} \times \frac{\frac{1}{150}}{X}$$
$$\frac{1}{100}X = \frac{1}{150}$$
$$\frac{\frac{1}{100}X}{\frac{1}{100}} = \frac{\frac{1}{150}}{\frac{1}{100}}$$
$$X = \frac{1}{150} \div \frac{1}{100}$$
$$X = \frac{1}{\underset{3}{\cancel{150}}} \times \frac{\overset{2}{\cancel{100}}}{1}$$
$$X = \frac{2}{3} = 0.666 = 0.67$$

22)
$$\frac{25\%}{30\%} = \frac{5}{X}$$
$$\frac{0.25}{0.3} \times \frac{5}{X}$$
$$0.25X = 1.5$$
$$\frac{0.25X}{0.25} = \frac{1.5}{0.25}$$
$$X = 6$$

23)
$$\frac{45}{100} \times \frac{X}{240}$$
$$100X = 10,800$$
$$\frac{100X}{100} = \frac{10,800}{100}$$
$$X = 108$$

Review Set 10 from page 51

1) 1.3 **2)** 4.75 **3)** 56 **4)** 0.43 **5)** 26.67 **6)** 15 **7)** 0.8 **8)** 2.38 **9)** 37.5 **10)** 112.5 **11)** 8 pills **12)** 720 milliliters
13) $3,530.21 **14)** 7.2 ounces **15)** 700 calories

Solutions—Review Set 10

1) $0.0025 \times 520 = 1.3$

8) $0.07 \times 34 = 2.38$

11) 0.4×20 pills $= 8$ pills

13) 80% of $17,651.07 $= 0.8 \times \$17,651.07 = \$14,120.86$

    $17,651.07 total bill
    − 14,120.86 paid by insurance co.
    $3,530.21 paid by patient

14) 0.4×18 ounces $= 7.2$ ounces

15) $0.2 \times 3,500$ calories $= 700$ calories

Practice Problems—Chapter 2 from pages 52–53

1) 0.4, 40%, 2:5 **2)** $\frac{1}{20}$, 5%, 1:20 **3)** 0.17, $\frac{17}{100}$, 17:100 **4)** 0.25, $\frac{1}{4}$, 25% **5)** 0.06, $\frac{3}{50}$, 3:50 **6)** 0.17, 17%, 1:6 **7)** 0.5, $\frac{1}{2}$, 1:2
8) 0.01, $\frac{1}{100}$, 1% **9)** $\frac{9}{100}$, 9%, 9:100 **10)** 0.38, 38%, 3:8 **11)** 0.67, $\frac{2}{3}$, 67% **12)** 0.33, 33%, 1:3 **13)** $\frac{13}{25}$, 52%, 13:25

14) 0.45, $\frac{9}{20}$, 45% **15)** 0.86, 86%, 6:7 **16)** 0.3, $\frac{3}{10}$, 30% **17)** 0.02, 2%, 1:50 **18)** $\frac{3}{5}$, 60%, 3:5 **19)** $\frac{1}{25}$, 4%, 1:25

20) 0.1, $\frac{1}{10}$, 1:10 **21)** 0.04 **22)** 1:40 **23)** 7.5% **24)** $\frac{1}{2}$ **25)** 3:4 **26)** 262.5 **27)** 3.64 **28)** 1.97 **29)** 1:4 **30)** 1:10 **31)** 84

32) 90,000 **33)** 1 **34)** 1.1 **35)** 100 **36)** 39 **37)** 0.75 **38)** 21 **39)** 120 **40)** 90 **41)** 25 grams protein; 6.25 grams fat

42) 231 points **43)** 60 minutes **44)** 50 milliliters **45)** 27 milligrams **46)** 5.4 grams **47)** 283.5 milligrams **48)** 6.5 pounds

49) \$10.42 **50)** 6 total doses

Solutions—Practice Problems—Chapter 2

36)

$$\frac{3}{9} \underset{\diagdown}{\overset{\diagup}{\times}} \frac{X}{117}$$

$$9X = 351$$

$$\frac{9X}{9} = \frac{351}{9}$$

$$X = 39$$

41)

$$125 \times 0.2 = 25 \text{ grams protein}$$

$$125 \times 0.05 = 6.25 \text{ grams fat}$$

$$\begin{array}{r} 125 \\ \times\ 0.2 \\ \hline 25.0 = 25 \end{array}$$

$$\begin{array}{r} 125 \\ \times\ 0.05 \\ \hline 6.25 \end{array}$$

43)

$$\frac{90}{27} \underset{\diagdown}{\overset{\diagup}{\times}} \frac{200}{X}$$

$$90X = 5,400$$

$$\frac{90X}{90} = \frac{5,400}{90}$$

$$X = 60$$

45)

$$60 \times 0.45 = 27 \text{ milligrams}$$

$$\begin{array}{r} 60 \\ \times\ 0.45 \\ \hline 300 \\ 240 \\ \hline 27.00 = 27 \end{array}$$

46)

$$\frac{3}{4} = 0.75$$

$$1\frac{1}{2} = 1.5$$

$$\frac{2.7}{0.75} \underset{\diagdown}{\overset{\diagup}{\times}} \frac{X}{1.5}$$

$$0.75X = 4.05$$

$$\frac{0.75X}{0.75} = \frac{4.05}{0.75}$$

$$X = 5.4$$

47)

$$\frac{6.75}{1} \underset{\diagdown}{\overset{\diagup}{\times}} \frac{X}{42}$$

$$X = 283.5$$

48)

$$130 \times 0.05 = 6.5 \text{ pounds}$$

$$\begin{array}{r} 130 \\ \times\ 0.05 \\ \hline 6.50 = 6.5 \end{array}$$

49)

$$0.17 \times \$12.56 = \$2.14$$

$$\begin{array}{r} \$12.56 \\ -\ 2.14 \\ \hline \$10.42 \end{array}$$

50)

$$10\% \text{ of } 150 = 0.10 \times 150 = 15$$

$$\begin{array}{ll} 150 \text{ mg} & \text{first dose} \\ -\ \ 15 \\ \hline 135 \text{ mg} & \text{second dose} \\ -\ \ 15 \\ \hline 120 \text{ mg} & \text{third dose} \\ -\ \ 15 \\ \hline 105 \text{ mg} & \text{fourth dose} \\ -\ \ 15 \\ \hline 90 \text{ mg} & \text{fifth dose} \\ -\ \ 15 \\ \hline 75 \text{ mg} & \text{sixth dose} \end{array}$$

6 total doses

Section 1—Self-Evaluation from pages 54–55

1) 3.05 **2)** 4,002.5 **3)** 0.63 **4)** 723.27 **5)** LCD = 12 **6)** LCD = 110 **7)** $\frac{11}{12}$ **8)** $\frac{47}{63}$ **9)** 1 **10)** $\frac{1}{2}$ **11)** 45.78 **12)** 0.02

13) 59.24 **14)** 0.09 **15)** 12 **16)** $\frac{2}{3}$ **17)** $\frac{1}{2}$ **18)** 0.64 **19)** $\frac{1}{10}, \frac{1}{6}, \frac{1}{5}, \frac{1}{3}, \frac{1}{2}$ **20)** $\frac{2}{3}, \frac{3}{4}, \frac{5}{6}, \frac{7}{8}, \frac{9}{10}$ **21)** 0.009, 0.125, 0.1909, 0.25, 0.3

22) $\frac{1}{2}$%, 0.9%, 50%, 100%, 500% **23)** 1:3 **24)** 1:600 **25)** 0.01 **26)** 0.04 **27)** 0.9% **28)** $\frac{1}{3}$ **29)** 5:9 **30)** $\frac{1}{20}$ **31)** 1:200 **32)** $\frac{2}{3}$

33) 75% **34)** 40% **35)** 0.17 **36)** 1.21 **37)** 1.3 **38)** 2.5 **39)** 0.67 **40)** 100 **41)** 4 **42)** 20,000 **43)** 3.3 **44)** 300 **45)** 8.33

46) 24 participants **47)** 2 holidays **48)** \$2.42 **49)** 12 cans of water **50)** 8 centimeters

Solutions—Section 1—Self-Evaluation

16) $\frac{1}{150} \div \frac{1}{100} = \frac{1}{150} \times \frac{100}{1} = \frac{\overset{2}{\cancel{100}}}{\underset{3}{\cancel{150}}} = \frac{2}{3}$

18) $\frac{16\%}{\frac{1}{4}} = 16\% \times \frac{4}{1} = 0.16 \times 4 = 0.64$

33) $3:4 = \frac{3}{4} = 4\overline{)3.0}^{\,0.75} = 75\%$

37) $\frac{0.3}{2.6} \diagdown \frac{0.15}{X}$

$0.3X = 2.6 \times 0.15$

$0.3X = 0.39$

$\frac{0.3X}{0.3} = \frac{0.39}{0.3}$

$X = 1.3$

42) $\frac{10\%}{\frac{1}{2}\%} \times 1,000 = X$

$\frac{0.1}{0.005} \times \frac{1,000}{1} = X$

$\frac{100}{0.005} = X$

$X = 20,000$

46) $600 \times 0.04 = 24$ participants

$$\begin{array}{r} 600 \\ \times\ 0.04 \\ \hline 24.00 \end{array} = 24$$

Review Set 11 from pages 62–63

1) metric **2)** volume **3)** weight **4)** length **5)** $\frac{1}{1,000}$ or 0.001 **6)** 1,000 **7)** microgram **8)** kilogram **9)** milligram **10)** 1,000 **11)** 1 **12)** 1,000 **13)** 10 **14)** 0.3 g **15)** 1.33 mL **16)** 5 kg **17)** 1.5 mm **18)** 10 mg **19)** microgram **20)** milliliter **21)** milligram **22)** gram **23)** millimeter **24)** kilogram **25)** centimeter

Review Set 12 from page 68

1) 20 drops **2)** 10 pounds **3)** 10 milliequivalents **4)** 4 grains **5)** 10 tablespoons **6)** 4 gtt **7)** 30 mEq **8)** 5 T **9)** $1\frac{1}{2}$ t **10)** gr x **11)** False **12)** False **13)** False **14)** units **15)** 3 **16)** 2 **17)** 1 **18)** 1 **19)** 1 **20)** milliequivalent, mEq

Practice Problems—Chapter 3 from pages 70–72

1) milli **2)** micro **3)** centi **4)** kilo **5)** 1 milligram **6)** 1 kilogram **7)** 1 microgram **8)** 1 centimeter **9)** meter **10)** gram **11)** liter **12)** drop **13)** fluid ounce **14)** ounce **15)** grain **16)** milligram **17)** microgram **18)** pound **19)** milliequivalent **20)** teaspoon **21)** quart **22)** milliliter **23)** pint **24)** tablespoon **25)** millimeter **26)** gram **27)** centimeter **28)** liter **29)** meter **30)** kilogram **31)** 3 **32)** 325 mcg **33)** gr $\frac{1}{2}$ **34)** 2 t **35)** $\frac{1}{3}$ fl oz **36)** 5,000,000 units **37)** 0.5 L **38)** gr $\frac{1}{4}$ **39)** gr $\frac{1}{200}$ **40)** 0.05 mg **41)** eight and one-quarter ounces **42)** three hundred seventy-five grams **43)** one quarter of a grain **44)** two and six tenths milliliters **45)** twenty milliequivalents **46)** four tenths of a liter **47)** one four hundredth of a grain **48)** seventeen hundredths of a milligram

49) **Prevention:** This type of error can be prevented by avoiding the use of a decimal point or trailing zero when not necessary. In this instance the decimal point and zero serve no purpose and can easily be misinterpreted, especially if the decimal point is difficult to see. Question any order that is unclear or unreasonable.

50) **Prevention:** This is both an error in notation and transcription. One grain should have been written *gr i*. Health care facilities would be wise to require the use of metric notation, especially for narcotics. With knowledge of correct notation, as well as common dosages for pain medication, the nurse should have noticed a problem. Question any order that is unclear or unreasonable.

Review Set 13 from page 82

1) 0.5 **2)** 15 **3)** 0.008 **4)** 0.01 **5)** 0.06 **6)** 0.3 **7)** 200 **8)** 1,200 **9)** 2.5 **10)** 65 **11)** 5 **12)** 1,500 **13)** 0.1 **14)** 0.25 **15)** 2,000

16) 750 **17)** 5 **18)** 1,000 **19)** 1,000 **20)** 3 **21)** 0.023 **22)** 0.00105 **23)** 0.018 **24)** 400 **25)** 2.625 **26)** 0.5 **27)** 10,000

28) 0.45 **29)** 0.005 **30)** 30,000

Solutions—Review Set 13

2) $\dfrac{1\text{ g}}{1{,}000\text{ mg}} \times \dfrac{0.015\text{ g}}{X\text{ mg}}$

$$X = 1{,}000 \times 0.015$$
$$X = 15\text{ mg}$$

3) $\dfrac{1\text{ g}}{1{,}000\text{ mg}} \times \dfrac{X\text{ g}}{8\text{ mg}}$

$$1{,}000X = 8$$
$$\dfrac{1{,}000X}{1{,}000} = \dfrac{8}{1{,}000}$$
$$X = 0.008\text{ g}$$

9) $\dfrac{1\text{ kg}}{1{,}000\text{ g}} \times \dfrac{0.0025\text{ kg}}{X\text{ g}}$

$$X = 1{,}000 \times 0.0025$$
$$X = 2.5\text{ g}$$

16) $\dfrac{1\text{ L}}{1{,}000\text{ mL}} \times \dfrac{0.75\text{ L}}{X\text{ mL}}$

$$X = 0.75 \times 1{,}000$$
$$X = 750\text{ mL}$$

20) $\dfrac{1\text{ L}}{1{,}000\text{ mL}} \times \dfrac{X\text{ L}}{3{,}000}$

$$1{,}000X = 3{,}000$$
$$\dfrac{1{,}000X}{1{,}000} = \dfrac{3{,}000}{1{,}000}$$
$$X = 3\text{ L}$$

23) $\dfrac{1\text{ mg}}{1{,}000\text{ mcg}} \times \dfrac{X\text{ mg}}{18\text{ mcg}}$

$$1{,}000X = 18$$
$$\dfrac{1{,}000X}{1{,}000} = \dfrac{18}{1{,}000}$$
$$X = 0.018\text{ mg}$$

Review Set 14 from pages 86–87

1) 30, gr i = 60 mg **2)** 45, gr i = 60 mg **3)** 0.003, 1 kg = 1,000 g **4)** 0.4, gr i = 60 mg **5)** 600, gr i = 60 mg **6)** $\frac{1}{4}$, gr i = 60 mg **7)** 65, 1 t = 5 mL **8)** $\frac{1}{2}$, 1 fl oz = 30 mL **9)** 75, 1 fl oz = 30 mL **10)** $1\frac{1}{2}$, 1 pt = 500 mL **11)** 4, 1 t = 5 mL **12)** 60, 1 T = 15 mL **13)** 19.8, 1 kg = 2.2 lb **14)** 113.6, 1 kg = 2.2 lb **15)** 96, 1 L = 32 fl oz **16)** 121, 1 kg = 2.2 lb **17)** 30, 1 in = 2.5 cm **18)** 2, 1 qt = 1 L **19)** 15, 1 t = 5 mL **20)** 45, 1 kg = 2.2 lb **21)** 300, gr i = 60 mg; or 325, gr i = 65 mg (in select cases) **22)** $\frac{1}{2}$, gr i = 60 mg **23)** 500, 1 pt = 500 mL **24)** 600, gr i = 60 mg; or 650, gr i = 65 mg (in select cases) **25)** v, gr i = 60 mg **26)** 12, 1 in = 2.5 cm **27)** i $\frac{1}{2}$, gr i = 60 mg **28)** 2, 1 fl oz = 30 mL **29)** 10, gr i = 60 mg **30)** i, gr i = 65 mg (only in select cases) **31)** 80, 1 in = 2.5 cm **32)** 14, 1 in = 2.5 cm, 1 cm = 10 mm **33)** 3, 1 in = 2.5 cm **34)** 50, 1 in = 2.5 cm, 1 cm = 10 mm **35)** 88, 1 kg = 2.2 lb **36)** 7,160, 1 kg = 1,000 g **37)** 50, 1 kg = 2.2 lb **38)** 7.7, 1 kg = 2.2 lb **39)** 28.64, 1 kg = 2.2 lb **40)** 53.75 **41)** 4, $\frac{1}{2}$ **42)** yes **43)** 2,430 **44)** 1.25 **45)** 10 **46)** Dissolve 2 teaspoons of Betadine concentrate in 1 pint or 2 cups of warm water. **47)** 2 **48)** 3 **49)** 16 **50)** 93.64

Solutions—Review Set 14

2) $\dfrac{\text{gr }1}{60\text{ mg}} \times \dfrac{\text{gr }\frac{3}{4}}{X\text{ mg}}$

$$X = 60 \times \frac{3}{4}$$
$$X = 45\text{ mg}$$

4) $\dfrac{\text{gr }1}{60\text{ mg}} \times \dfrac{\text{gr }\frac{1}{150}}{X\text{ mg}}$

$$X = 60 \times \frac{1}{150}$$
$$X = 0.4\text{ mg}$$

5) $\dfrac{\text{gr }1}{60\text{ mg}} \times \dfrac{\text{gr }10}{X\text{ mg}}$

$$X = 60 \times 10$$
$$X = 600\text{ mg}$$

6) $\dfrac{\text{gr }1}{60\text{ mg}} \times \dfrac{\text{gr }X}{15\text{ mg}}$

$$60X = 15$$
$$\dfrac{60X}{60} = \dfrac{15}{60}$$
$$X = \text{gr }\frac{1}{4}$$

9)
$$\frac{1 \text{ fl oz}}{30 \text{ mL}} \times \frac{2\frac{1}{2}\text{fl oz}}{X \text{ mL}}$$

$$X = 30 \times 2.5$$

$$X = 75 \text{ mL}$$

11)
$$\frac{1 \text{ t}}{5 \text{ mL}} \times \frac{X \text{ t}}{20 \text{ mL}}$$

$$5X = 20$$

$$\frac{5X}{5} = \frac{20}{5}$$

$$X = 4 \text{ t}$$

16)
$$\frac{1 \text{ kg}}{2.2 \text{ lb}} \times \frac{55 \text{ kg}}{X \text{ lb}}$$

$$X = 2.2 \times 55$$

$$X = 121 \text{ lb}$$

20)
$$\frac{1 \text{ kg}}{2.2 \text{ lb}} \times \frac{X \text{ kg}}{99 \text{ lb}}$$

$$2.2X = 99$$

$$\frac{2.2X}{2.2} = \frac{99}{2.2}$$

$$X = 45 \text{ kg}$$

24)
$$\frac{\text{gr } 1}{60 \text{ mg}} \times \frac{\text{gr } 10}{X \text{ mg}}$$

$$X = 600 \text{ mg}$$

28)
$$\frac{1 \text{ fl oz}}{30 \text{ mL}} \times \frac{X \text{ fl oz}}{60 \text{ mL}}$$

$$30X = 60$$

$$\frac{30X}{30} = \frac{60}{30}$$

$$X = 2 \text{ fl oz}$$

34)
$$\frac{1 \text{ in}}{2.5 \text{ cm}} \times \frac{2 \text{ in}}{X \text{ cm}}$$

$$X = 2.5 \times 2$$

$$X = 5 \text{ cm}$$

$$\frac{1 \text{ cm}}{10 \text{ mm}} \times \frac{5 \text{ cm}}{X \text{ mm}}$$

$$X = 50 \text{ mm}$$

41)
$$\frac{1 \text{ fl oz}}{30 \text{ mL}} \times \frac{X \text{ fl oz}}{120 \text{ mL}}$$

$$30X = 120$$

$$\frac{30X}{30} = \frac{120}{30}$$

$$X = 4 \text{ fl oz}$$

$$\frac{1 \text{ cup}}{8 \text{ fl oz}} \times \frac{X \text{ cups}}{4 \text{ fl oz}}$$

$$8X = 4$$

$$\frac{8X}{8} = \frac{4}{8}$$

$$X = \frac{1}{2} \text{ cup}$$

42)
$$\frac{1 \text{ kg}}{2.2 \text{ lb}} \times \frac{108 \text{ kg}}{X \text{ lb}}$$

$$X = 108 \times 2.2$$

$$X = 237.6 \text{ lb}$$

$$250 \text{ lb} - 237.6 \text{ lb} = 12.4 \text{ lb}$$

Yes. He has met weight loss goal of 10 lb.

43)   Add up the fluid ounces: 81 fluid ounces

$$\frac{1 \text{ fl oz}}{30 \text{ ml}} \times \frac{81 \text{ fl oz}}{X \text{ ml}}$$

$$X = 2,430 \text{ mL}$$

44)
$$\frac{1 \text{ kg}}{2.2 \text{ lb}} \times \frac{X \text{ kg}}{55 \text{ lb}}$$

$$2.2X = 55$$

$$\frac{2.2X}{2.2} = \frac{55}{2.2}$$

$$X = 25 \text{ kg}$$

$$\frac{1 \text{ kg}}{0.05 \text{ mg}} \times \frac{25 \text{ kg}}{X \text{ mg}}$$

$$X = 0.05 \times 25$$

$$X = 1.25 \text{ mg}$$

45)   Find the total number of mL per day and the total number of mL per bottle.

mL per day for 4 doses:

$$\frac{12 \text{ mL}}{1 \text{ dose}} \times \frac{X \text{ mL}}{4 \text{ doses}}$$

$$X = 48 \text{ mL}$$

mL per bottle:

$$\frac{1 \text{ fl oz}}{30 \text{ mL}} \times \frac{16 \text{ fl oz}}{X \text{ mL}}$$

$$X = 480 \text{ mL (per bottle)}$$

How many days will 480 mL (or 16 ounces) last?

$$\frac{1 \text{ day}}{48 \text{ mL}} \times \frac{X \text{ days}}{480 \text{ mL}}$$

$$48X = 480$$

$$\frac{48X}{48} = \frac{480}{48}$$

$$X = 10 \text{ days}$$

46)
$$\frac{1 \text{ t}}{5 \text{ mL}} \times \frac{X \text{ t}}{10 \text{ mL}}$$

$$5X = 10$$

$$\frac{5X}{5} = \frac{10}{5}$$

$$X = 2 \text{ t}$$

500 mL = 1 pt or 2 cups water

Use 2 t Betadine concentrate in 1 pint or 2 cups of water

48) 1 qt = 32 fl oz (per container)

At 1 feeding every 3 hours, how many feedings does the infant require during 24 hours or per day?

$$\frac{1 \text{ feeding}}{3 \text{ hours}} \times \frac{X \text{ feedings}}{24 \text{ hours}}$$

$$3X = 24$$

$$\frac{3X}{3} = \frac{24}{3}$$

$$X = 8 \text{ feedings}$$

How many ounces will the infant consume for 8 feedings or per day?

$$\frac{1 \text{ feeding}}{4 \text{ fl oz}} \times \frac{8 \text{ feedings}}{X \text{ fl oz}}$$

$$X = 32 \text{ fl oz (per day)}$$

Each container holds 1 quart or 32 fluid ounces (equivalent: 1 qt = 32 fl oz), so you know she needs 3 containers of formula for 3 days.

Practice Problems—Chapter 4 from pages 88–90

1) 500 **2)** 10 **3)** 0.0075 **4)** 3 **5)** 4,000 **6)** 0.5 **7)** $\frac{1}{2}$ **8)** 0.3 **9)** 70 **10)** 149.6 **11)** 180 **12)** 105 **13)** 0.3 **14)** 15 **15)** 6 **16)** 90 **17)** 32.05 **18)** 7.99 **19)** 0.008 **20)** 0.45 **21)** 95 **22)** 500 **23)** 600 **24)** 0.67 **25)** 68.18 **26)** i **27)** 10 **28)** 500 **29)** 2 **30)** 3 **31)** 0.375 **32)** 30 **33)** 1 **34)** 1 **35)** 1 **36)** 1,500 **37)** 45 **38)** $1\frac{1}{2}$ **39)** $\frac{1}{6}$ **40)** 0.025 **41)** 4,300 **42)** 0.06 **43)** 15 **44)** 3 **45)** 250 **46)** 9 **47)** 8 **48)** 840 **49)** 100%; all of it

50) **Prevention:** The nurse didn't use the conversion rules correctly. The nurse divided instead of multiplied. This type of medication error is avoided by double-checking your dosage calculations and asking yourself, "Is this dosage reasonable?" Certainly you know if there are 1,000 mg in 1 g, and you want to give 2 g, then you need *more* than 1,000 milligrams, not less. The correct calculations are:

Convert:

$$\frac{1 \text{ g}}{1,000 \text{ mg}} = \frac{2 \text{ g}}{X \text{ mg}}$$

$$X = 2 \times 1,000$$

$$X = 2,000 \text{ mg}$$

Calculate:

$$\frac{1,000 \text{ mg}}{10 \text{ mL}} = \frac{2,000 \text{ mg}}{X \text{ mL}}$$

$$1,000X = 20,000$$

$$\frac{1,000X}{1,000} = \frac{20,000}{1,000}$$

$$X = 20 \text{ mL}$$

To give 2,000 mg you would need twice the amount of the available strength. Therefore, you would need 20 mL of the 1,000 mg per 10 mL strength.

Solutions—Practice Problems—Chapter 4

46) Per bottle:

$$\frac{1 \text{ fl oz}}{30 \text{ mL}} \times \frac{4 \text{ fl oz}}{X \text{ mL}}$$

$$X = 120 \text{ mL}$$

Each dose:

$$\frac{1 \text{ t}}{5 \text{ mL}} \times \frac{2\frac{1}{2} \text{ t}}{X \text{ mL}}$$

$$X = 12.5 \text{ mL}$$

Bottle holds 120 mL; each dose is 12.5 mL

$$\frac{1 \text{ dose}}{12.5 \text{ mL}} \times \frac{X \text{ doses}}{120 \text{ mL}}$$

$$12.5X = 120$$

$$\frac{12.5X}{12.5} = \frac{120}{12.5}$$

$$X = 9.6 \text{ doses or 9 full doses}$$

47) $$\frac{1 \text{ dose}}{15 \text{ mL}} \times \frac{X \text{ doses}}{120 \text{ mL}}$$

$$15X = 120$$

$$\frac{15X}{15} = \frac{120}{15}$$

$$X = 8 \text{ doses}$$

48) 4 + 8 + 6 + 10 = 28 fluid ounces

$$\frac{1 \text{ fl oz}}{30 \text{ mL}} \times \frac{28 \text{ fl oz}}{X \text{ mL}}$$

$$X = 840 \text{ mL}$$

49) $$\frac{\text{gr } 1}{60 \text{ mg}} \times \frac{\text{gr } \frac{1}{6}}{X \text{ mg}}$$

$$X = 60 \times \frac{1}{6}$$

$$X = 10 \text{ mg}$$

The ampule contains 10 mg, and the doctor orders gr $\frac{1}{6}$ or 10 mg; therefore, the patient should receive all of the solution in the ampule.

Review Set 15 from page 94

1) 12:32 AM 2) 7:30 AM 3) 4:40 PM 4) 9:21 PM 5) 11:59 PM 6) 12:15 PM 7) 2:20 AM 8) 10:10 AM 9) 1:15 PM
10) 6:25 PM 11) 1330 12) 0004 13) 2145 14) 1200 15) 2315 16) 0345 17) 2400 18) 1530 19) 0620 20) 1745
21) *zero six twenty-three* 22) *zero-zero forty-one* 23) *nineteen zero three* 24) *twenty-three eleven* 25) *zero three hundred*

Review Set 16 from page 96–97

1) 38 2) 101.1 3) 97.2 4) 89.6 5) 37 6) 37.2 7) 39.8 8) 104 9) 102 10) 97.5 11) 37.8 12) 102.2 13) 99.3 14) 34.6
15) 39.3 16) 35.3 17) 44.6 18) 31.1 19) 98.6 20) 39.7

Solutions—Review Set 16

1)
$$°C = \frac{°F - 32}{1.8}$$
$$°C = \frac{100.4 - 32}{1.8}$$
$$°C = \frac{68.4}{1.8}$$
$$°C = 38°$$

2)
$$°F = 1.8°C + 32$$
$$°F = (1.8 \times 38.4) + 32$$
$$°F = 69.12 + 32$$
$$°F = 101.12 \cong 101.1°$$

Practice Problems—Chapter 5 from pages 98–99

1) 2:57 AM 2) 0310 3) 1622 4) 8:01 PM 5) 11:02 AM 6) 0033 7) 0216 8) 4:42 PM 9) 11:56 PM 10) 0420 11) 1931
12) 2400 or 0000 13) 0645 14) 9:15 AM 15) 9:07 PM 16) 6:23 PM 17) 5:40 AM 18) 1155 19) 2212 20) 2106 21) 4 h
22) 7 h 23) 8 h 30 min 24) 12 h 15 min 25) 14 h 50 min 26) 4 h 12 min 27) 4 h 48 min 28) 3 h 41 min 29) 6 h 30 min
30) 16 h 38 min 31) False 32) a. AM; b. PM; c. AM; d. PM 33) 37.6 34) 97.7 35) 102.6 36) 37.9 37) 36.7 38) 99.3
39) 100.8 40) 40 41) 36.6 42) 95.7 43) 39.7 44) 102.2 45) 98.4 46) 38.6 47) 36.2 48) 37.2, 99 (98.96° rounds to 99.0°F)
49) True

50) **Prevention:** Such situations can be easily prevented by accurately applying the complete formula for temperature conversion. Guessing is not acceptable in medical and health care calculations. Temperature conversion charts are readily available in most health care settings, but, when they are not, the conversion formulas should be used. It may be wise to try to memorize the common fever temperature conversions between 98.6°F (37°C) and 104°F (40°C).

Solutions—Practice Problems—Chapter 5

24)
$$\begin{array}{r} 2150 \\ -\ 0935 \\ \hline 1215 \end{array} = 12\ h\ 15\ min$$

26) 2316 = 11:16 PM, 0328 = 3:28 AM
11:16 PM → 3:16 AM = 4 h
3:16 AM → 3:28 AM = 12 min
4 h 12 min

28) 4:35 PM → 7:35 PM = 3 h
7:35 PM → 8:16 PM = 41 min
3 h 41 min

48) $\dfrac{37.6 + 35.5 + 38.1 + 37.6}{4} = \dfrac{148.8}{4} = 37.2°C$ (average)
$°F = 1.8(37.2) + 32 = 99°$

Review Set 17 from pages 110–112

1) 1 mL (tuberculin) 2) Round 1.25 to 1.3 and measure on the mL scale as 1.3 mL. 3) No 4) 0.5 mL 5) a. False;
b. The size of the drop varies according to the diameter of the tip of the dropper. 6) No 7) Measure the oral liquid in a
3 mL syringe, which is not intended for injections. 8) 5 9) Discard the excess prior to injecting the patient. In some cases,
such as for controlled substances, the nurse may need a witness to observe discarding the excess. 10) To prevent needlestick injury.

11)

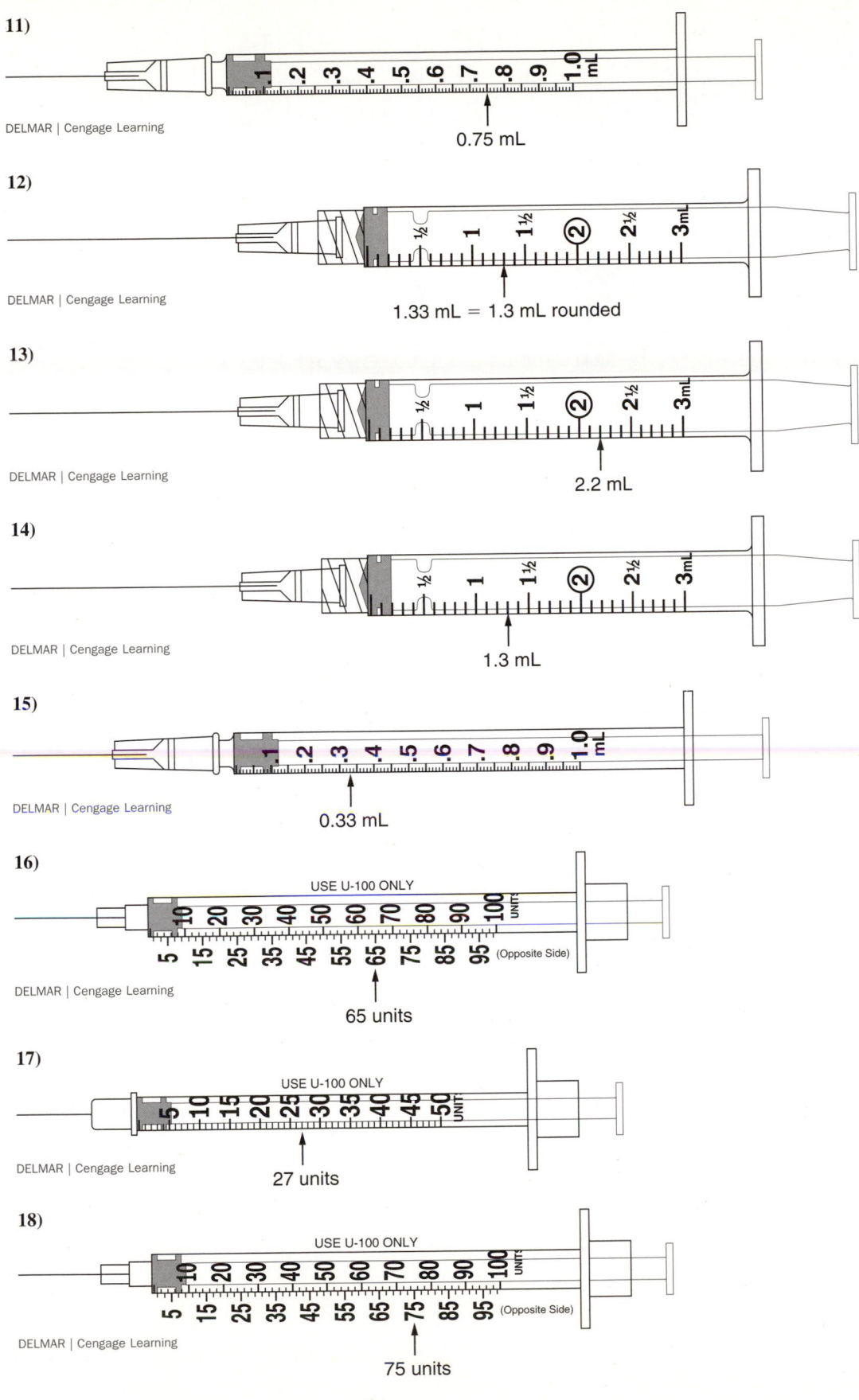

DELMAR | Cengage Learning

0.75 mL

12)

DELMAR | Cengage Learning

1.33 mL = 1.3 mL rounded

13)

DELMAR | Cengage Learning

2.2 mL

14)

DELMAR | Cengage Learning

1.3 mL

15)

DELMAR | Cengage Learning

0.33 mL

16)

USE U-100 ONLY

(Opposite Side)

DELMAR | Cengage Learning

65 units

17)

USE U-100 ONLY

DELMAR | Cengage Learning

27 units

18)

USE U-100 ONLY

(Opposite Side)

DELMAR | Cengage Learning

75 units

19)

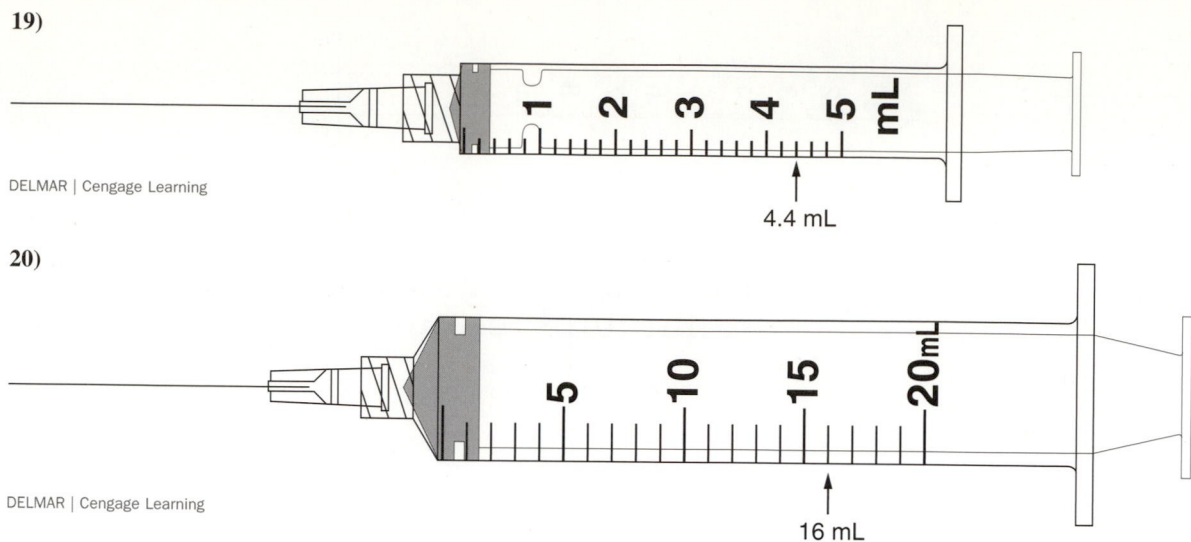

DELMAR | Cengage Learning

4.4 mL

20)

DELMAR | Cengage Learning

16 mL

21) 0.2 mL   **22)** 1 mL   **23)** 0.2 mL

Practice Problems—Chapter 6 from pages 113–116

1) 1   **2)** hundredths or 0.01   **3)** No. The tuberculin syringe has a maximum capacity of 1 mL.   **4)** Round to 1.3 mL and measure at 1.3 mL.   **5)** 30; 1   **6)** 1 mL   **7)** 0.75   **8)** False   **9)** False   **10)** True   **11)** To prevent accidental needle sticks during intravenous administration   **12)** top ring   **13)** 10   **14)** False   **15)** 3 mL, 1 mL, and insulin

16)

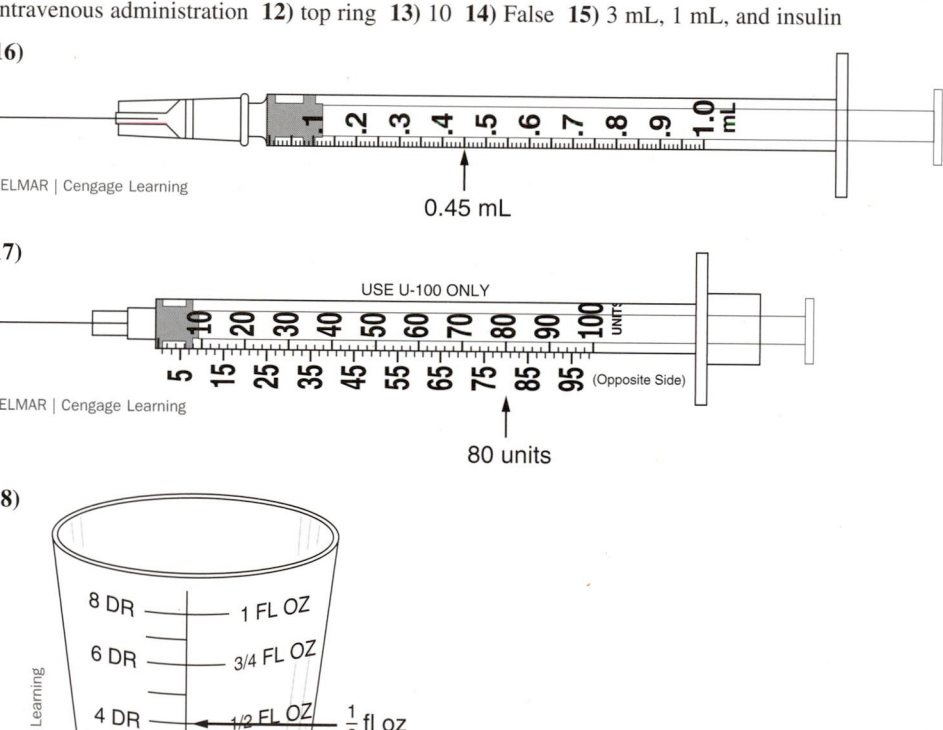

DELMAR | Cengage Learning

0.45 mL

17)

USE U-100 ONLY

(Opposite Side)

DELMAR | Cengage Learning

80 units

18)

8 DR ——— 1 FL OZ
6 DR ——— 3/4 FL OZ
4 DR ——— 1/2 FL OZ   ← $\frac{1}{2}$ fl oz
2 DR ——— 1/4 FL OZ
1 DR ——— 1/8 FL OZ

DELMAR | Cengage Learning

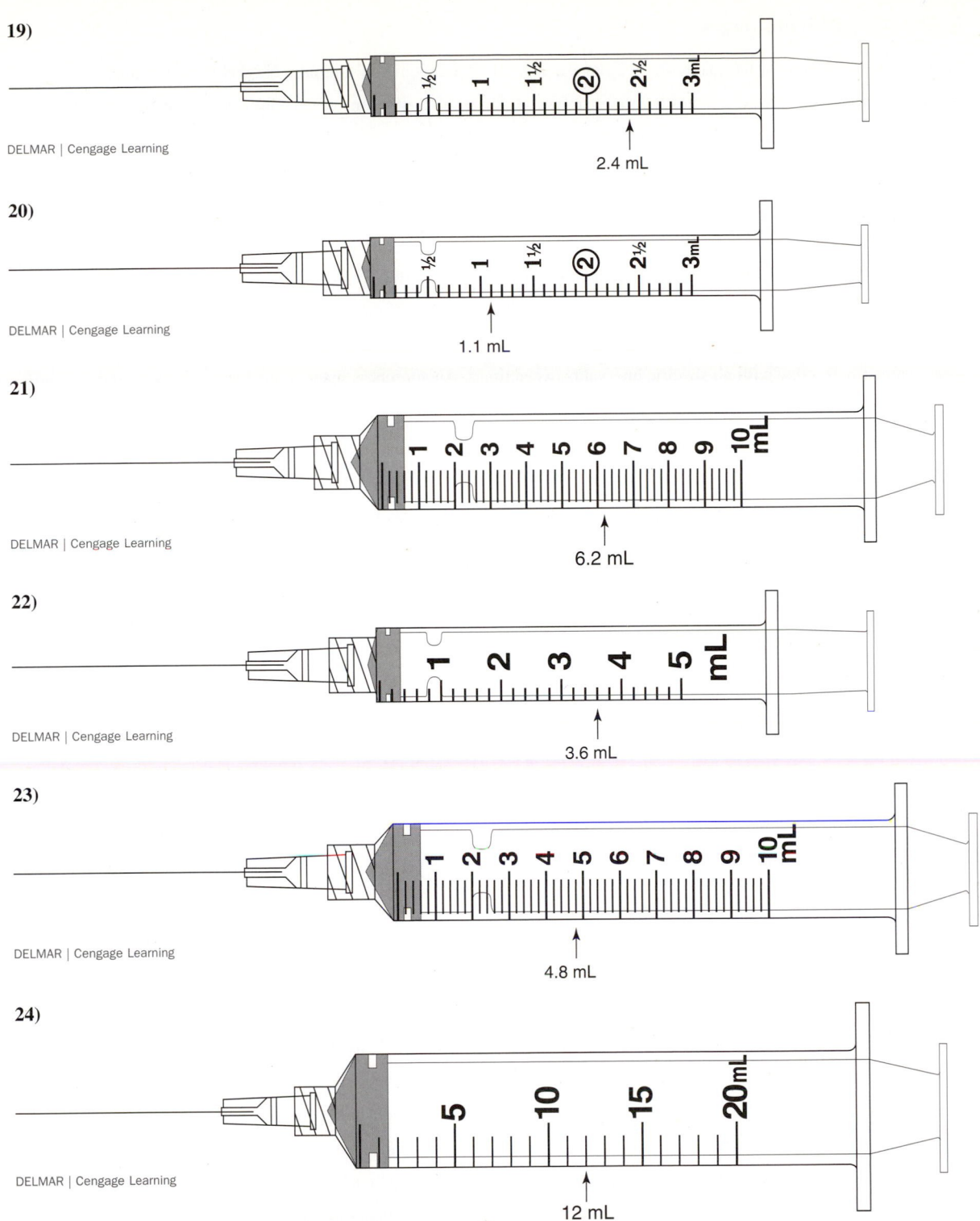

19)

DELMAR | Cengage Learning

2.4 mL

20)

DELMAR | Cengage Learning

1.1 mL

21)

DELMAR | Cengage Learning

6.2 mL

22)

DELMAR | Cengage Learning

3.6 mL

23)

DELMAR | Cengage Learning

4.8 mL

24)

DELMAR | Cengage Learning

12 mL

25) Prevention: This error could have been avoided by following a simple principle: Don't put oral drugs in syringes intended for injection. Instead, place the medication in an oral syringe to which a needle cannot be attached. In addition, the medication should have been labeled for oral use only. The medication was ordered orally, not by injection. An alert nurse would have noticed the discrepancy. Finally, but just as important, a medication should be administered only by the nurse who prepared it. **26) Prevention:** The nurse should ask for assistance to learn how to use unfamiliar equipment. Do not put the patient at risk. The nurse must remove the cap on the oral syringe prior to administering the medication, so that the child cannot choke on the cap.

Review Set 18 from pages 120–121

1) Give 250 milligrams of naproxen orally 2 times a day. 2) Give 30 units of Humulin N NPH U-100 insulin subcutaneously every day 30 minutes before breakfast. 3) Give 500 milligrams of cefaclor orally immediately, and then give 250 milligrams every 8 hours. 4) Give 25 micrograms of Synthroid orally once a day. 5) Give 10 milligrams of Ativan intramuscularly every 4 hours as necessary for agitation. 6) Give 20 milligrams of furosemide intravenously (slowly) immediately. 7) Give 10 milliliters of Mylanta orally after meals and at bedtime. 8) Instill 2 drops of 1% atropine sulfate ophthalmic in the right eye every 15 minutes for 4 applications. 9) Give $\frac{1}{4}$ grain of morphine sulfate intramuscularly every 3 hours as needed for pain. 10) Give 0.25 milligram of digoxin orally once a day. 11) Give 250 milligrams of tetracycline orally 4 times a day. 12) Give $\frac{1}{400}$ grain of nitroglycerin sublingually immediately. 13) Instill 2 drops of Cortisporin otic suspension in both ears 3 times a day and at bedtime. 14) The abbreviation t.i.d. means three times a day with no specific interval between times. An attempt is made to give the 3 doses during waking hours. The abbreviation q.8h means every 8 hours. These doses would be given around the clock at 8-hour intervals. For example, administration times for t.i.d. might be 0800, 1200, 1700; administration times for q.8h could be 0600, 1400, 2200. 15) Contact the physician for clarification. 16) No, q.i.d. orders are given 4 times in 24 hours with no specific interval between times indicated in order, typically during waking hours; whereas q.4h orders are given 6 times in 24 hours at 4-hour intervals. 17) They are determined by hospital or institutional policy. 18) Patient, drug, dosage, route, frequency, date and time written, signature of physician/prescriber. 19) Parts 1–5: patient's name, drug, dosage, route, frequency 20) The right patient must receive the right drug in the right amount by the right route at the right time, followed by the right documentation.

Review Set 19 from pages 126–127

1) 9 AM, 9 PM 2) 9 AM 3) 7:30 AM, 11:30 AM, 4:30 PM, 9 PM 4) 9 AM, 9 PM 5) every 6 hours, as needed for severe pain 6) 9/7/xx at 0900 or 9 AM 7) sublingual, under the tongue 8) once a day 9) 125 mcg 10) nitroglycerin, Darvocet-N 100, ketoralac 11) subcutaneous injection 12) once 13) Cephalexin 14) before breakfast (at 7:30 AM) 15) milliequivalent 16) Cephalexin and K-Dur 17) Tylenol 18) twice 19) 0900 and 2100 20) 2400, 0600, 1200, and 1800 21) In the "One-Time Medication Dosage" section, lower left corner.

Practice Problems—Chapter 7 from pages 128–132

1) twice a day 2) per rectum 3) before meals 4) after 5) 3 times a day 6) every 4 hours 7) when necessary 8) by mouth, orally 9) intravenous 10) four times a day 11) immediately 12) freely, as desired 13) after meals 14) intramuscular 15) without 16) noct 17) gtt 18) mL 19) gr 20) g 21) q.i.d. 22) $\bar{c}$ 23) subcut 24) t 25) b.i.d. 26) q.3h 27) p.c. 28) $\bar{a}$ 29) kg 30) Give 60 milligrams of Toradol intravenously immediately and every 6 hours when necessary for pain. 31) Give 300,000 units of procaine penicillin G intravenously 4 times a day. 32) Give 5 milliliters of Mylanta orally 1 hour before and 1 hour after meals, at bedtime, and every 2 hours as needed at night for gastric upset. 33) Give 25 milligrams of Librium orally every 6 hours when necessary for agitation. 34) Give 5,000 units of heparin subcutaneously immediately. 35) Give 5 milligrams of morphine sulfate intravenously every 4 hours when necessary for moderate to severe pain. 36) Give 0.25 milligram of digoxin orally every day. 37) Instill 2 drops of 10% Neo-Synephrine ophthalmic to the left eye every 30 minutes for 2 applications. 38) Give 40 milligrams of Lasix intramuscularly immediately. 39) Give 4 milligrams of Decadron intravenously twice a day. 40) 12:00 midnight, 8:00 AM, 4:00 PM 41) 20 units 42) subcut: subcutaneous 43) Give 500 milligrams of Cipro orally every 12 hours. 44) 8:00 AM, 12:00 noon, 6:00 PM 45) digoxin (Lanoxin) 0.125 mg p.o. daily 46) with, $\bar{c}$ 47) Give 150 milligrams of ranitidine tablets orally twice daily with breakfast and supper. 48) Vancomycin 49) 12 hours 50) **Prevention:** This error could have been avoided by paying careful attention to the ordered frequency and by writing the frequency on the MAR.

Review Set 20 from pages 142–144

1) B **2)** D **3)** C **4)** A **5)** E **6)** F **7)** G **8)** 5 mL **9)** oral **10)** A, B, C, D, E, F, G **11)** Filmtab means *film sealed tablet.*
12) 1 mg/mL **13)** 2 tablets **14)** D **15)** It is a Schedule IV drug. It has limited potential for abuse and is clinically useful.
16) penicillin G potassium **17)** Pfizerpen **18)** 5,000,000 units per vial; reconstituted to 250,000 units/mL, 500,000 units/mL,
or 1,000,000 units/mL **19)** IM or IV **20)** 0049-0520-83 **21)** Pfizer-Roerig **22)** 1 **23)** 0.01 g per 1 mL **24)** 10

Practice Problems—Chapter 8 from pages 145–148

1) 50 mEq per 50 mL (or 1 mEq/mL) **2)** 0517-1550-25 **3)** 4,200 per 50 mL (or 84 mg/mL) **4)** cefpodoxime proxetil
5) "Shake bottle to loosen granules. Add approximately $\frac{1}{2}$ the total amount of distilled water required for constitution
(total water = 29 mL). Shake vigorously to wet the granules. Add remaining water and shake vigorously." **6)** Pharmacia
and Upjohn **7)** 10 mL **8)** 250 mg per 10 mL (25 mg/mL) **9)** 1 mL **10)** Depo-Provera **11)** medroxyprogesterone acetate
12) 0009-0626-01 **13)** injection solution **14)** 10 mL **15)** intramuscular **16)** Akrimax Pharmaceuticals LLC **17)** capsule
18) 20° to 25°C (68°–77°F) **19)** 1 mg per 4 mL (or 0.25 mg/mL) **20)** 1 mg (per 4 mL vial) **21)** I **22)** H **23)** H **24)** oral
25) 401803C **26)** III **27)** 2% **28)** 2/100; 20 **29) Prevention:** This error could have been prevented by carefully
comparing the drug label and dosage to the MAR drug and dosage three times while preparing the medication. In this
instance both the incorrect drug and the incorrect dosage strength sent by the pharmacy should have been noted by the
nurse. Further, the nurse should have asked for clarification of the order. **30a) Prevention:** The nurse should have recognized
that the patient was still complaining of signs and symptoms that the medication was ordered to treat. **30b)** If the order was
difficult to read, the physician should have been called to clarify the order. Was the dosage of 100 mg a usual dosage for
Celexa? The nurse should have consulted a drug guide to ensure that the dosage was appropriate. Also, if the patient wasn't
complaining of or diagnosed with depression, the nurse should have questioned why Celexa was ordered.

Review Set 21 from page 160–161

1) Right patient, right drug, right amount (dosage or dose), right route, right time, right documentation **2)** *NPH insulin
20 units subcut daily* **3)** After preparing the drug, just prior to administration **4)** To ensure patient safety and to prevent
medication errors, patient injury, patient death, increased health care costs, unnecessary liability, stress, and costs to
health care practitioners **5)** True **6)** Verify the drug order by consulting a reputable drug reference resource; e.g.,
the *Hospital Formulary.* **7)** Insulins **8)** To ensure dispensing and administration of the correct medication to the right
patient **9)** $93 billion ($93,000,000,000) **10)** Write the order down on the patient's chart or enter it into the computer
record, then read the order back, and finally get confirmation from the prescriber that it is correct. Before administering
the medication, verify the safety of the order by consulting a reputable drug reference, if you are unfamiliar with
the order.

Practice Problems—Chapter 9 from pages 162–163

1) 44,000–98,000 **2)** False **3)** True **4)** True **5)** True **6)** Patient, drug (or medication), amount (or dosage or dose), route,
time, documentation **7)** Prescription, transcription, administration **8)** Upon first contact with the drug, while measuring
the dosage, and just prior to administration **9)** 0.75 mg **10)** Write out the order, read it back, and get confirmation from
the prescriber. **11)** Any four of these: patient injury; loss of life; increased health care costs; additional technology
expenses to prevent error; liability defense; increased length of stay; harm to the nurse involved in regard to his or her
personal and professional status, confidence, and practice **12) Prevention:** The health care professional originating the
order should not have used q.d. to indicate the frequency of administration. The employee transcribing the order and the
nurse signing off the order should have been alert to the risk of errors associated with the use of this notation and should
have been especially cautious in transcribing the order correctly.

Section 2—Self-Evaluation from pages 165–168

1) gr $\frac{2}{3}$ **2)** 4 t **3)** gr $\frac{1}{300}$ **4)** 0.5 mL **5)** $\frac{1}{2}$ fl oz **6)** four drops **7)** four hundred fifty milligrams **8)** one one hundredth of a grain **9)** seven and one-half grains **10)** twenty-five hundredths of a liter **11)** 7,130 **12)** 0.925 **13)** 0.125 **14)** 165 **15)** 10; 0.01 **16)** 0.02; $\frac{1}{3}$ **17)** 12; 60 **18)** 150; 0.15 **19)** 37.5; 375 **20)** 5.62; 2.25 or $2\frac{1}{4}$ **21)** 90; 90,000 **22)** 11,590; 25.5 or $25\frac{1}{2}$ **23)** iii **24)** 360 **25)** 0.2 **26)** 6 **27)** 480 **28)** 2335 **29)** 6:44 PM **30)** 0417 **31)** 8:03 AM **32)** 100.4 **33)** 38.6 **34)** 99

35)

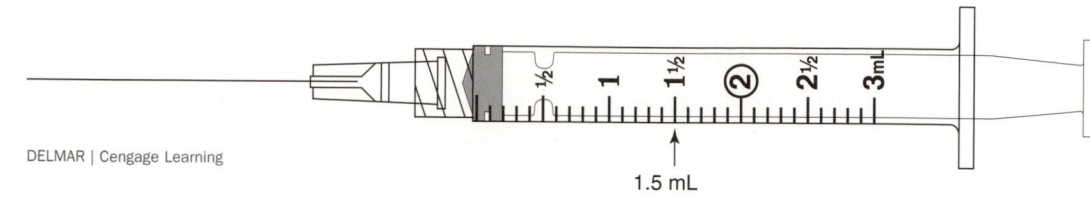

1.5 mL

36)

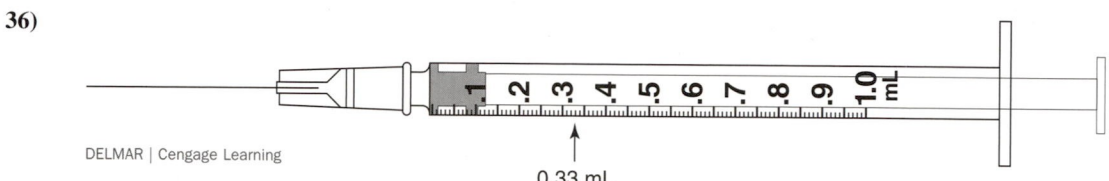

0.33 mL

37)

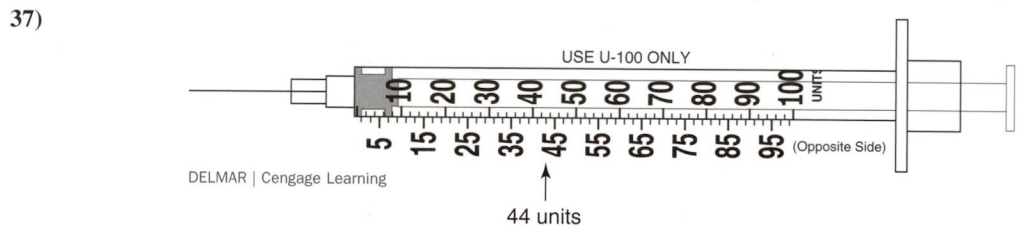

44 units

38)

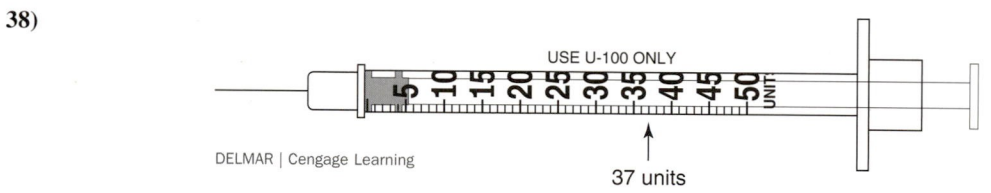

37 units

39)

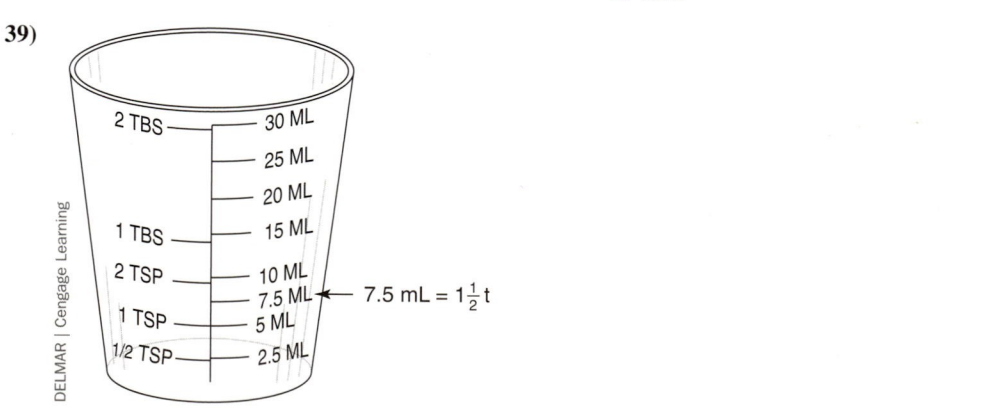

7.5 mL = $1\frac{1}{2}$ t

40) nitroglycerin **41)** under the tongue **42)** 100 tablets **43)** Give 400 micrograms of nitroglycerin by the sublingual route immediately. **44)** 5,000 units per mL **45)** 63323-047-10 **46)** Give 3,750 units of heparin subcutaneously every 8 hours. **47)** neomycin sulfate **48)** 125 mg per 5 mL **49)** *heparin 5,000 units subcut daily* **50)** The right patient must receive the right drug, in the right amount, by the right route, at the right time, with the right documentation.

Solutions—Section 2—Self-Evaluation

15)
$$\frac{\text{gr } 1}{60 \text{ mg}} \diagdown \frac{\text{gr } \frac{1}{6}}{\text{X mg}}$$

$$X = 60 \times \frac{1}{6}$$

$$X = 10 \text{ mg}$$

$$\frac{1 \text{ g}}{1{,}000 \text{ mg}} \diagdown \frac{\text{X g}}{10 \text{ mg}}$$

$$1{,}000X = 10$$

$$\frac{1{,}000X}{1{,}000} = \frac{10}{1{,}000}$$

$$X = 0.01 \text{ g}$$

21)
$$\frac{1 \text{ kg}}{2.2 \text{ lb}} \diagdown \frac{\text{X kg}}{198 \text{ lb}}$$

$$2.2X = 198$$

$$\frac{2.2X}{2.2} = \frac{198}{2.2}$$

$$X = 90 \text{ kg}$$

$$\frac{1 \text{ kg}}{1{,}000 \text{ g}} \diagdown \frac{90 \text{ kg}}{\text{X g}}$$

$$X = 90{,}000 \text{ g}$$

24)
$$\frac{\text{gr } 1}{60 \text{ mg}} \diagdown \frac{\text{gr } \frac{3}{4}}{\text{X mg}}$$

$$X = 60 \times \frac{3}{4}$$

$$X = 45 \text{ mg}$$

q.3h = 8 doses per 24 hours

$$\frac{1 \text{ dose}}{45 \text{ mg}} \diagdown \frac{8 \text{ doses}}{\text{X mg}}$$

$$X = 360 \text{ mg}$$

27)
$$\frac{1 \text{ fl oz}}{30 \text{ mL}} \diagdown \frac{16 \text{ fl oz}}{\text{X mL}}$$

$$X = 480 \text{ mL}$$

Review Set 22 from pages 182-185

1) 1 **2)** 1 **3)** $1\frac{1}{2}$ **4)** $\frac{1}{2}$ **5)** $\frac{1}{2}$ **6)** 3 **7)** 2 **8)** 2 **9)** 2 **10)** 2 **11)** 1 **12)** $\frac{1}{2}$ **13)** 2 **14)** 2 **15)** 2 **16)** $1\frac{1}{2}$ **17)** 2.5, 2

18) 10 and 5, 1 of each, 4 **19)** 15, 1 **20)** 60, 1 **21)** B, 1 caplet **22)** I, 2 tablets **23)** F, 1 tablet **24)** H, 2 tablets

25) G, $1\frac{1}{2}$ tablets **26)** E, 2 tablets **27)** D, 2 tablets **28)** G, 2 tablets **29)** A, 1 capsule **30)** C, 1 tablet

Solutions—Review Set 22

1) Order: 0.1 g

Convert:

$$\frac{1 \text{ g}}{1{,}000 \text{ mg}} \diagdown \frac{0.1 \text{ g}}{\text{X mg}}$$

$$X = 1{,}000 \times 0.1$$

$$X = 100 \text{ mg}$$

Supply: 100 mg/tab

Think: Now it is obvious that you want to give 1 tablet.

Calculate:

$$\frac{100 \text{ mg}}{1 \text{ tab}} \diagdown \frac{100 \text{ mg}}{\text{X tab}}$$

$$X = 1 \text{ tab}$$

5) Order: 0.125 mg

Supply 0.25 mg/tab

$$\frac{0.25 \text{ mg}}{1 \text{ tab}} \diagdown \frac{0.125 \text{ mg}}{\text{X tab}}$$

$$0.25X = 0.125$$

$$\frac{0.25X}{0.25} = \frac{0.125}{0.25}$$

$$X = \frac{1}{2} \text{ tab}$$

10) Order: 5 mg

Supply: 2.5 mg/tab

$$\frac{2.5 \text{ mg}}{1 \text{ tab}} \diagdown \frac{5 \text{ mg}}{\text{X tab}}$$

$$2.5X = 5$$

$$\frac{2.5X}{2.5} = \frac{5}{2.5}$$

$$X = 2 \text{ tab}$$

14) Order: 0.1 mg

$$\frac{1 \text{ mg}}{1{,}000 \text{ mcg}} \diagdown \frac{0.1 \text{ mg}}{\text{X mcg}}$$

$$X = 1{,}000 \times 0.1$$

$$X = 100 \text{ mcg}$$

Supply: 50 mcg/tab

$$\frac{50 \text{ mcg}}{1 \text{ tab}} \diagdown \frac{100 \text{ mcg}}{\text{X tab}}$$

$$50X = 100$$

$$\frac{50X}{50} = \frac{100}{50}$$

$$X = 2 \text{ tab}$$

19)   Order gr $\frac{1}{4}$

Convert:

$$\frac{gr\ 1}{60\ mg} \times \frac{gr\ \frac{1}{4}}{X\ mg}$$

$$X = 60 \times \frac{1}{4}$$

$$X = 15\ mg$$

Supply: 15 mg, 30 mg, and 60 mg/tab

Think: It is obvious that you should select the 15 mg tablet and give one.

$$\frac{15\ mg}{1\ tablet} \times \frac{15\ mg}{X\ tablets}$$

$$15X = 15$$

$$\frac{15X}{15} = \frac{15}{15}$$

$$X = 1\ tab$$

Select 15 mg tablet and give 1 tablet.

28)   Order: 0.5 mg

$$\frac{1\ mg}{1,000\ mcg} \times \frac{0.5\ mg}{X\ mcg}$$

$$X = 500\ mcg$$

Supply: 250 mcg/tab

$$\frac{250\ mcg}{1\ tab} \times \frac{500\ mcg}{X\ tab}$$

$$250X = 500$$

$$\frac{250X}{250} = \frac{500}{250}$$

$$X = 2\ tab$$

Review Set 23 from pages 189–192

1) 7.5 **2)** 5 **3)** 20 **4)** 2.5 **5)** 1 **6)** 20 **7)** 2 **8)** 7.5 **9)** 3 **10)** 10 **11)** 45 **12)** 7.5 **13)** 2 **14)** 2.5 **15)** 5 **16)** 1 **17)** $1\frac{1}{2}$ **18)** 1 **19)** 10 **20)** 1 **21)** 2 **22)** B; 10 mL **23)** C; 10 mL **24)** A; 2 mL **25)** 5 **26)** 0.75 **27)** 10; 48 **28)** 3 **29)** 4 **30)** 0900, 1300, 1900

Solutions—Review Set 23

2)   Order: gr $\frac{1}{6}$

$$\frac{gr\ 1}{60\ mg} \times \frac{gr\ \frac{1}{6}}{X\ mg}$$

$$X = 60 \times \frac{1}{6}$$

$$X = 10\ mg$$

Supply: 10 mg per 5 mL

Think: It is obvious you want to give 5 mL.

$$\frac{10\ mg}{5\ mL} \times \frac{10\ mg}{X\ mL}$$

$$10X = 50$$

$$\frac{10X}{10} = \frac{50}{10}$$

$$X = 5\ mL$$

4)   Order: 100 mg

Supply: 200 mg per 5 mL

$$\frac{200\ mg}{5\ mL} \times \frac{100\ mg}{X\ mL}$$

$$200X = 500$$

$$\frac{200X}{200} = \frac{500}{200}$$

$$X = 2.5\ mL$$

6)   Order: 25 mg

Supply: 6.25 mg/t or 6.25 mg per 5 mL (1 t = 5 mL)

$$\frac{6.25\ mg}{5\ mL} \times \frac{25\ mg}{X\ mL}$$

$$6.25X = 125$$

$$\frac{6.25X}{6.25} = \frac{125}{6.25}$$

$$X = 20\ mL$$

7)   Order: 125 mg

Supply: 62.5 mg per 5 mL or 62.5 mg/1 t (1 t = 5 mL)

$$\frac{62.5\ mg}{1\ t} \times \frac{125\ mg}{X\ t}$$

$$62.5\ X = 125$$

$$\frac{62.5X}{62.5} = \frac{125}{62.5}$$

$$X = 2\ t$$

11)   Order: 0.24 g

$$\frac{1\ g}{1,000\ mg} \times \frac{0.24\ g}{X\ mg}$$

$$X = 1,000 \times 0.24$$

$$X = 240\ mg$$

Supply: 80 mg per 15 mL

$$\frac{80 \text{ mg}}{15 \text{ mL}} \times \frac{240 \text{ mg}}{X \text{ mL}}$$

$$80X = 3,600$$

$$\frac{80X}{80} = \frac{3,600}{80}$$

$$X = 45 \text{ mL}$$

15)   Order: 0.25 mg

$$\frac{1 \text{ mg}}{1,000 \text{ mcg}} \times \frac{0.25 \text{ mg}}{X \text{ mcg}}$$

$$X = 1,000 \times 0.25$$

$$X = 250 \text{ mcg}$$

Supply: 50 mcg/mL

$$\frac{50 \text{ mcg}}{1 \text{ mL}} \times \frac{250 \text{ mcg}}{X \text{ mL}}$$

$$50X = 250$$

$$\frac{50X}{50} = \frac{250}{50}$$

$$X = 5 \text{ mL}$$

17)   Order: 375 mg

Supply: 250 mg per 5 mL

$$\frac{250 \text{ mg}}{5 \text{ mL}} \times \frac{375 \text{ mg}}{X \text{ mL}}$$

$$250X = 1,875$$

$$\frac{250X}{250} = \frac{1,875}{250}$$

$$X = 7.5 \text{ mL}$$

$$5 \text{ mL} = 1 \text{ t}$$

$$\frac{1 \text{ t}}{5 \text{ mL}} \times \frac{X \text{ t}}{7.5 \text{ mL}}$$

$$5X = 7.5$$

$$\frac{5X}{5} = \frac{7.5}{5}$$

$$X = 1\frac{1}{2} \text{ t}$$

19)   Order: 1.2 g

$$\frac{1 \text{ g}}{1,000 \text{ mg}} \times \frac{1.2 \text{ g}}{X \text{ mg}}$$

$$X = 1,000 \times 1.2$$

$$X = 1,200 \text{ mg}$$

Supply: 600 mg per 5 mL

$$\frac{600 \text{ mg}}{5 \text{ mL}} \times \frac{1,200 \text{ mg}}{X \text{ mL}}$$

$$600X = 6,000$$

$$\frac{600X}{600} = \frac{6,000}{600}$$

$$X = 10 \text{ mL}$$

20)   Order: 0.25 g

$$\frac{1 \text{ g}}{1,000 \text{ mg}} \times \frac{0.25 \text{ g}}{X \text{ mg}}$$

$$X = 1,000 \times 0.25$$

$$X = 250 \text{ mg}$$

Supply: 125 mg per 2.5 mL

$$\frac{125 \text{ mg}}{2.5 \text{ mL}} \times \frac{250 \text{ mg}}{X \text{ mL}}$$

$$125X = 625$$

$$\frac{125X}{125} = \frac{625}{125}$$

$$X = 5 \text{ mL} = 1 \text{ t (Equivalent: 1 t = 5 mL)}$$

21)   Order: 100 mg

Supply: 250 mg per 5 mL

$$\frac{250 \text{ mg}}{5 \text{ mL}} \times \frac{100 \text{ mg}}{X \text{ mL}}$$

$$250X = 500$$

$$\frac{250X}{250} = \frac{500}{250}$$

$$X = 2 \text{ mL}$$

Practice Problems—Chapter 10 from pages 196–204

1) $\frac{1}{2}$ 2) 2 3) $\frac{1}{2}$ 4) 2.5 5) 10 6) 2 7) 8 8) $1\frac{1}{2}$ 9) 1 10) $\frac{1}{2}$ 11) $1\frac{1}{2}$ 12) 1 13) $1\frac{1}{2}$ 14) 1 15) 2 16) 5; $1\frac{1}{2}$ 17) 7.5

18) 2 19) 2 20) 1.5 21) 0.75; 1 22) $\frac{1}{2}$ 23) 2 24) 2 25) 2 26) 2 27) 15 and 30; one of each 28) 2.4 29) 5 30) 3

31) D; 2 tablets 32) A; 1 capsule 33) C; 1 tablet 34) B; 1 capsule 35) I; 2 tablets 36) G; 2 tablets 37) F; 2 tablets

38) H; 1 tablet 39) M; 2 tablets 40) L; 2 tablets 41) E; 30 mL 42) K; 1 tablet 43) I; 2 tablets 44) N; 2 tablets

45) O; 1 tablet 46) Q; 2 tablets 47) P; 1 capsule 48) J; 1 tablet 49) R; 2 tablets

50)   **Prevention:** This medication error could have been prevented if the nurse had more carefully read the physician's order and the medication label. The doctor's order misled the nurse by noting the volume first and then the drug dosage. If confused by the order, the nurse should have clarified the intent with the physician. By focusing on the volume, the nurse failed to follow the steps in dosage calculation. Had the nurse noted 250 mg as the desired dosage and the supply (or on-hand) dosage as 125 mg per 5 mL, the correct amount to be administered would have been clear. Slow down and take time to compare the order with the labels. Calculate each dose carefully before preparing and administering both solid- and liquid-form medications.

Solutions—Practice Problems—Chapter 10

2) Order: gr $\frac{1}{2}$

$$\frac{gr\ 1}{60\ mg} \diagdown \frac{gr\ \frac{1}{2}}{X\ mg}$$

$$X = 60 \times \frac{1}{2}$$

$$X = 30\ mg$$

Supply: 15 mg/tab

$$\frac{15\ mg}{1\ tab} \diagdown \frac{30\ mg}{X\ tab}$$

$$15X = 30$$

$$\frac{15X}{15} = \frac{30}{15}$$

$$X = 2\ tab$$

3) Order: 0.075 mg

$$\frac{1\ mg}{1,000\ mcg} \diagdown \frac{0.075\ mg}{X\ mcg}$$

$$X = 75\ mcg$$

Supply: 150 mcg/tab

$$\frac{150\ mcg}{1\ tab} \diagdown \frac{75\ mcg}{X\ tab}$$

$$150X = 75$$

$$\frac{150X}{150} = \frac{75}{150}$$

$$X = \frac{1}{2}\ tab$$

8) Order: 150 mg

Supply: 100 mg/tab

$$\frac{1\ g}{1,000\ mg} \diagdown \frac{0.1\ g}{X\ mg}$$

$$X = 1,000 \times 0.1$$

$$X = 100\ mg$$

$$\frac{100\ mg}{1\ tab} \diagdown \frac{150\ mg}{X\ tab}$$

$$100X = 150$$

$$\frac{100X}{100} = \frac{150}{100}$$

$$X = 1\frac{1}{2}\ tab$$

9) Order: gr v = gr 5

$$\frac{gr\ 1}{60\ mg} \diagdown \frac{gr\ 5}{X\ mg}$$

$$X = 300\ mg$$

Supply: 325 mg/tab

$$\frac{325\ mg}{1\ tab} \diagdown \frac{300\ mg}{X\ tab}$$

$$325X = 300$$

$$\frac{325X}{325} = \frac{300}{325}$$

$$X = 0.92\ tab$$

0.92 tablets is not a reasonable dosage. Remember, in some instances gr i = 65 mg is more appropriate for conversion from grains to milligrams.

$$\frac{gr\ 1}{65\ mg} \diagdown \frac{gr\ 5}{X\ mg}$$

$$X = 325\ mg$$

Supply: 325 mg/tab

$$\frac{325\ mg}{1\ tab} \diagdown \frac{325\ mg}{X\ tab}$$

$$325X = 325$$

$$\frac{325X}{325} = \frac{325}{325}$$

$$X = 1\ tab$$

14) Order: gr $\frac{1}{8}$

$$\frac{gr\ 1}{60\ mg} \diagdown \frac{gr\ \frac{1}{8}}{X\ mg}$$

$$X = 60 \times \frac{1}{8}$$

$$X = 7.5\ mg$$

Supply: 7.5 mg/tab

Think: It is obvious that you want to give 1 tablet.

$$\frac{7.5\ mg}{1\ tab} \diagdown \frac{7.5\ mg}{X\ tab}$$

$$7.5X = 7.5$$

$$\frac{7.5X}{7.5} = \frac{7.5}{7.5}$$

$$X = 1\ tab$$

19) Order: 0.25 mg

Supply: 0.125 mg/tab

$$\frac{0.125\ mg}{1\ tab} \diagdown \frac{0.25\ mg}{X\ tab}$$

$$0.125X = 0.25$$

$$\frac{0.125X}{0.125} = \frac{0.25\ mg}{0.125}$$

$$X = 2\ tab$$

27) Order: gr $\frac{3}{4}$

$$\frac{gr\ 1}{60\ mg} \diagdown \frac{gr\ \frac{3}{4}}{X\ mg}$$

$$X = 60 \times \frac{3}{4}$$

$$X = 45\ mg$$

Supply: 15 mg, 30 mg, and 60 mg tablets

Select: One 15 mg tablet and one 30 mg tablet for 45 mg total dosage

Remember: If you have a choice, give whole tablets and as few as possible

Review Set 24 from pages 212–218

1) 2.5

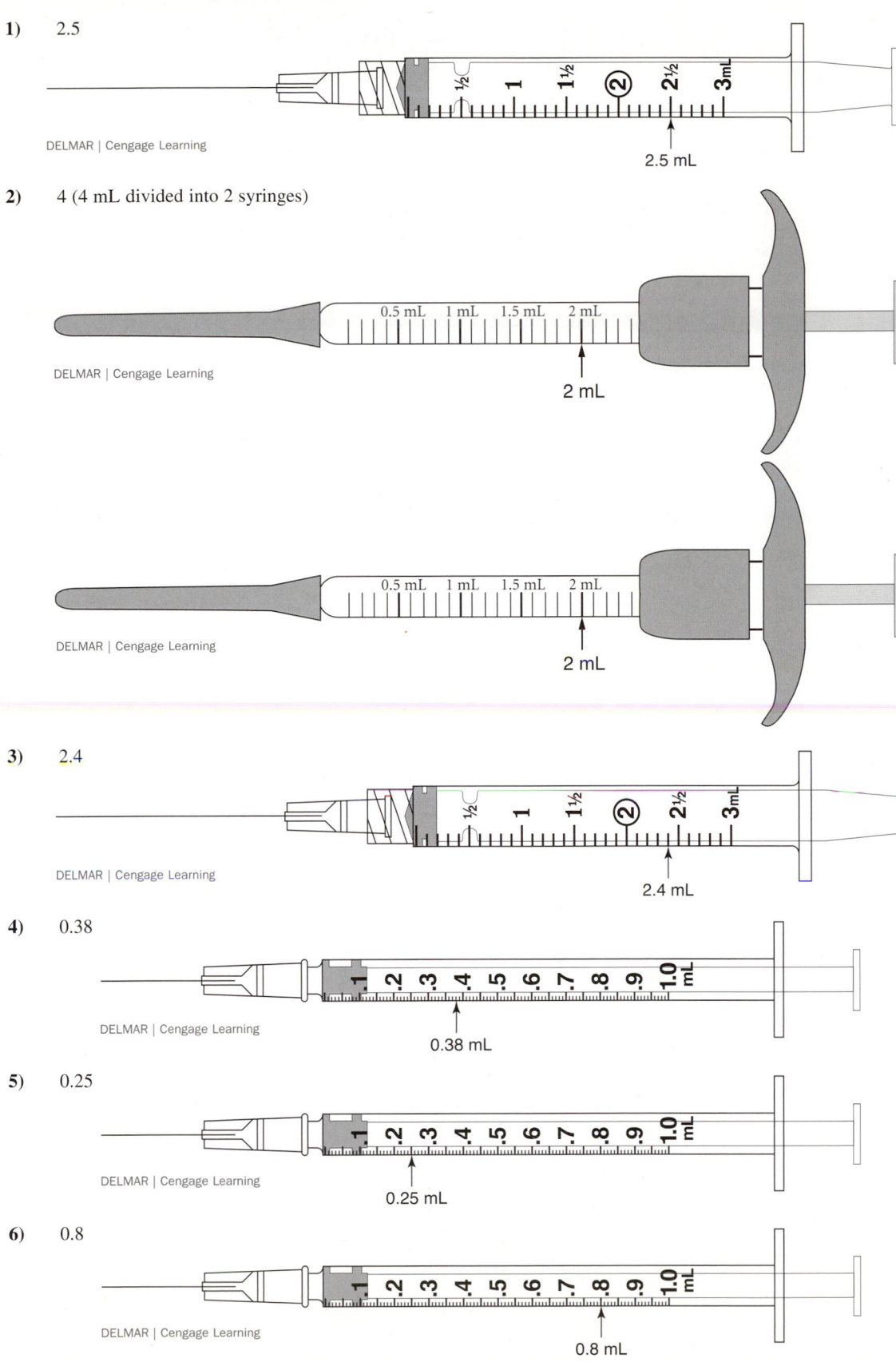

2.5 mL

2) 4 (4 mL divided into 2 syringes)

2 mL

2 mL

3) 2.4

2.4 mL

4) 0.38

0.38 mL

5) 0.25

0.25 mL

6) 0.8

0.8 mL

7) 1.5

8) 0.6

9) 2

10) 1

11) 1.2

12) 0.9

13) 0.5

14) 0.4

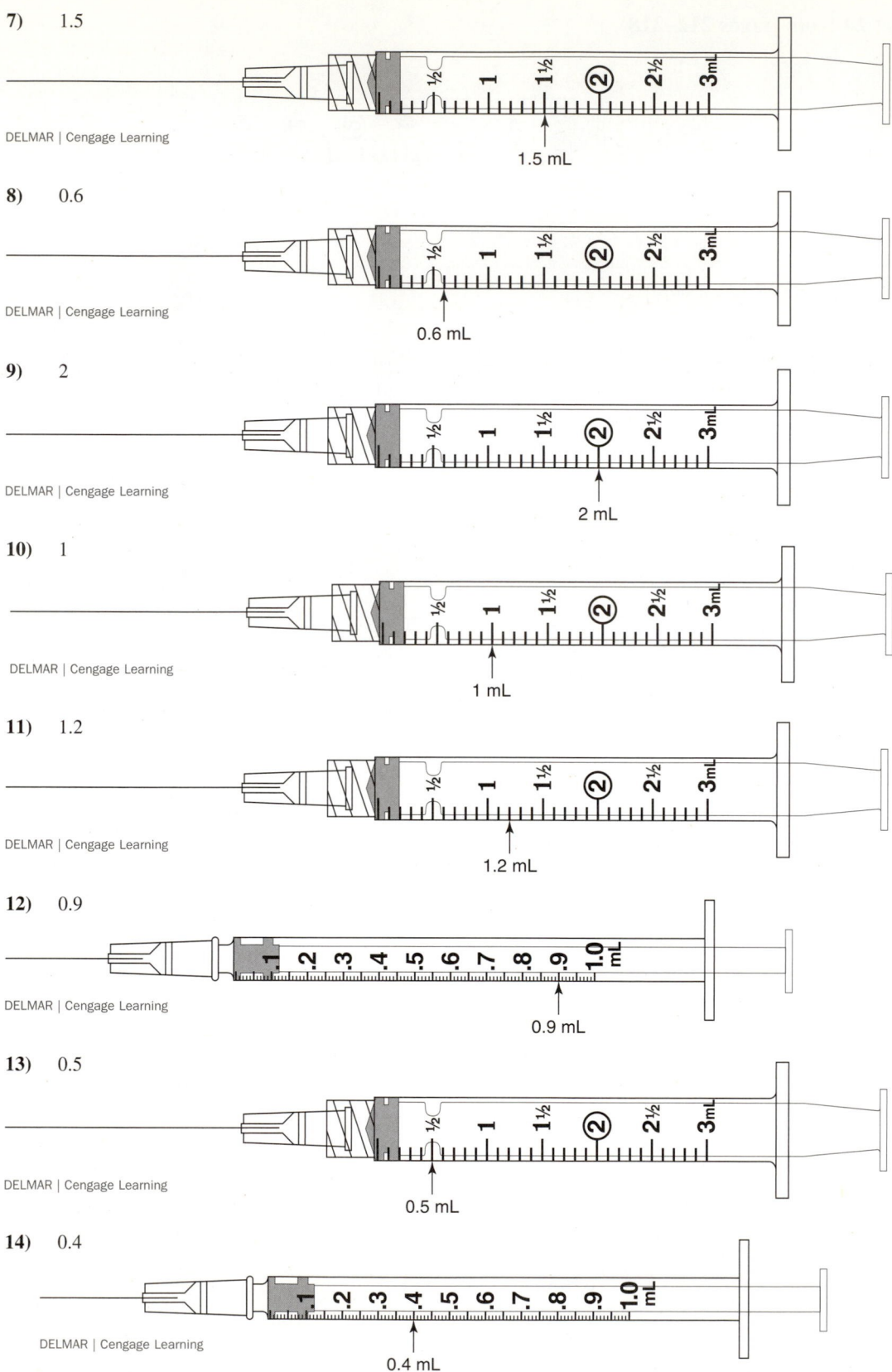

The route is IM; the needle may need to be changed to an appropriate gauge and length.

15)   3

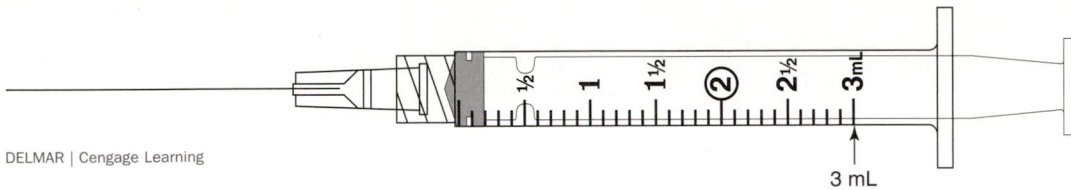

3 mL

16)   0.1

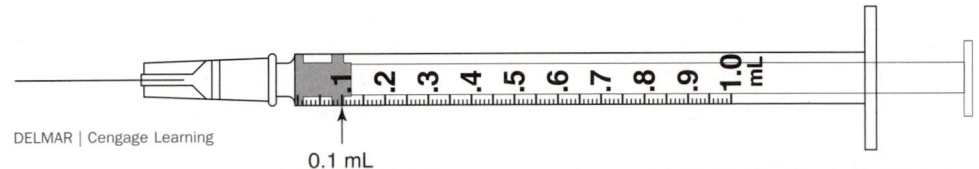

0.1 mL

The route is IM. Because this is such a small dose (0.1 mL), change the needle to IM gauge and length before drawing up the medication. Otherwise some of the medication will be trapped in the needle, and the patient may not receive the full intended dose.

17)   4

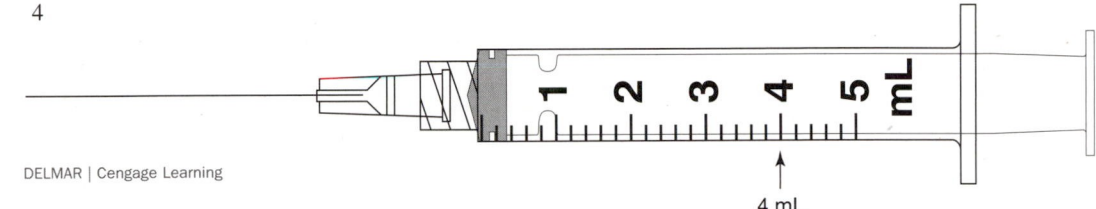

4 mL

18)   0.8

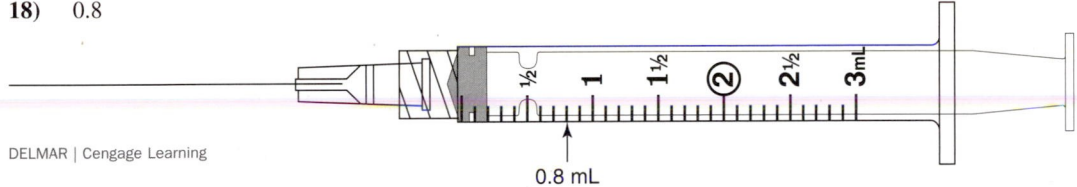

0.8 mL

19)   0.25

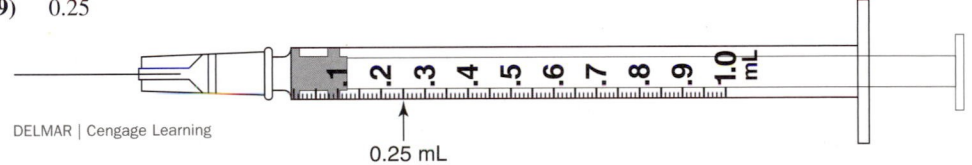

0.25 mL

The route is IM; the needle may need to be changed to an appropriate gauge and length.

20)   1.5

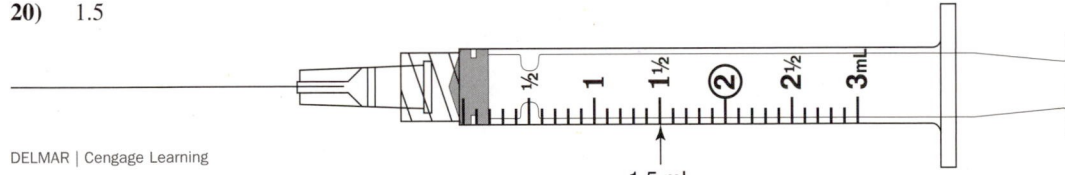

1.5 mL

Solutions—Review Set 24

1)   Order: 1 g = 1,000 mg

Supply: 400 mg/mL

$$\frac{400 \text{ mg}}{1 \text{ mL}} \diagtimes \frac{1,000 \text{ mg}}{X \text{ mL}}$$

$$400X = 1,000$$

$$\frac{400X}{400} = \frac{1,000}{400}$$

$$X = 2.5 \text{ mL}$$

2)   Order: 2,400,000 units

Supply: 1,200,000 units per 2 mL

$$\frac{1,200,000 \text{ units}}{2 \text{ mL}} \diagtimes \frac{2,400,000 \text{ units}}{X \text{ mL}}$$

$$1,200,000X = 4,800,000$$

$$\frac{1,200,000X}{1,200,000} \diagtimes \frac{4,800,000}{1,200,000}$$

$$X = 4 \text{ mL divided into 2 doses}$$

of 2 mL each

3) Order: 600 mcg

Supply: 250 mcg/mL

$$\frac{250 \text{ mcg}}{1 \text{ mL}} \diagdown \frac{600 \text{ mcg}}{X \text{ mL}}$$

$$250X = 600$$

$$\frac{250X}{250} \diagdown \frac{600}{250}$$

$$X = 2.4 \text{ mL}$$

5) Order: 250 mcg

Supply: 1 mg/mL

1 mg = 1,000 mcg

$$\frac{1,000 \text{ mcg}}{1 \text{ mL}} \diagdown \frac{250 \text{ mcg}}{X \text{ mL}}$$

$$1,000X = 250$$

$$\frac{1,000X}{1,000} = \frac{250}{1,000}$$

$$X = 0.25 \text{ mL}$$

6) Order: 4,000 units

Supply: 5,000 units/mL

$$\frac{5,000 \text{ units}}{1 \text{ mL}} \diagdown \frac{4,000 \text{ units}}{X \text{ mL}}$$

$$5,000X = 4,000$$

$$\frac{5,000X}{5,000} \diagdown \frac{4,000}{5,000}$$

$$X = 0.8 \text{ mL}$$

10) Order: gr $\frac{1}{4}$

$$\frac{\text{gr } 1}{60 \text{ mg}} \diagdown \frac{\text{gr } \frac{1}{4}}{X \text{ mg}}$$

$$X = 60 \times \frac{1}{4}$$

$$X = 15 \text{ mg}$$

Supply: 15 mg/mL

Think: It is obvious that you want to give 1 mL.

$$\frac{15 \text{ mg}}{1 \text{ mL}} \diagdown \frac{15 \text{ mg}}{X \text{ mL}}$$

$$15X = 15$$

$$\frac{15X}{15} = \frac{15}{15}$$

$$X = 1 \text{ mL}$$

11) Order: 30 mg

Supply: 25 mg/mL

$$\frac{25 \text{ mg}}{1 \text{ mL}} \diagdown \frac{30 \text{ mg}}{X \text{ mL}}$$

$$25X = 30$$

$$\frac{25X}{25} = \frac{30}{25}$$

$$X = 1.2 \text{ mL}$$

19) Order: 12.5 mg

Supply: 50 mg/mL

$$\frac{50 \text{ mg}}{1 \text{ mL}} \diagdown \frac{12.5 \text{ mg}}{X \text{ mL}}$$

$$50X = 12.5$$

$$\frac{50X}{50} = \frac{12.5}{50}$$

$$X = 0.25 \text{ mL}$$

Review Set 25 from pages 229–233

1) Humulin R, regular, short-acting, 100 units/mL, U-100 insulin syringe **2)** Novolin N, NPH, intermediate-acting, 100 units/mL, U-100 insulin syringe **3)** NovoLog, aspart, rapid-acting, 100 units/mL, U-100 insulin syringe

4) Humalog, lispro, rapid-acting, 100 units/mL, U-100 insulin syringe **5)** Humulin R, regular, short-acting, 500 units/mL, 1 mL syringe **6)** Lantus, glargine, long-acting, 100 units/mL, U-100 insulin syringe **7)** Standard, dual-scale 100 unit/mL U-100 syringe; Lo-dose, 50 unit/0.5 mL U-100 syringe; Lo-dose, 30 unit/0.3 mL U-100 syringe **8)** Lo-dose, 50 unit U-100 syringe **9)** 0.6 **10)** 0.25 **11)** Standard, dual-scale 100 unit U-100 syringe **12)** False **13)** 68 **14)** 15 **15)** 23 **16)** 57

17)

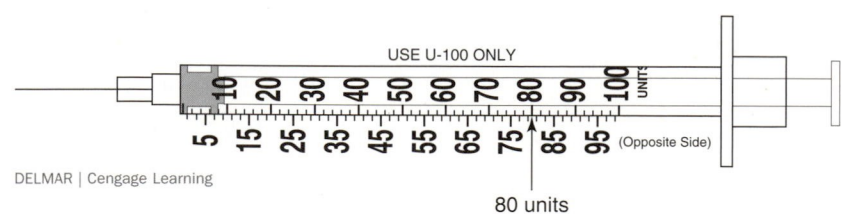

80 units

18)

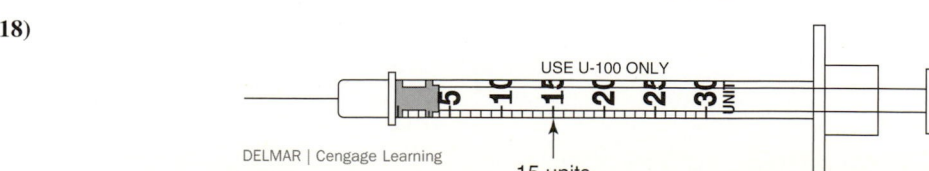

15 units

19)

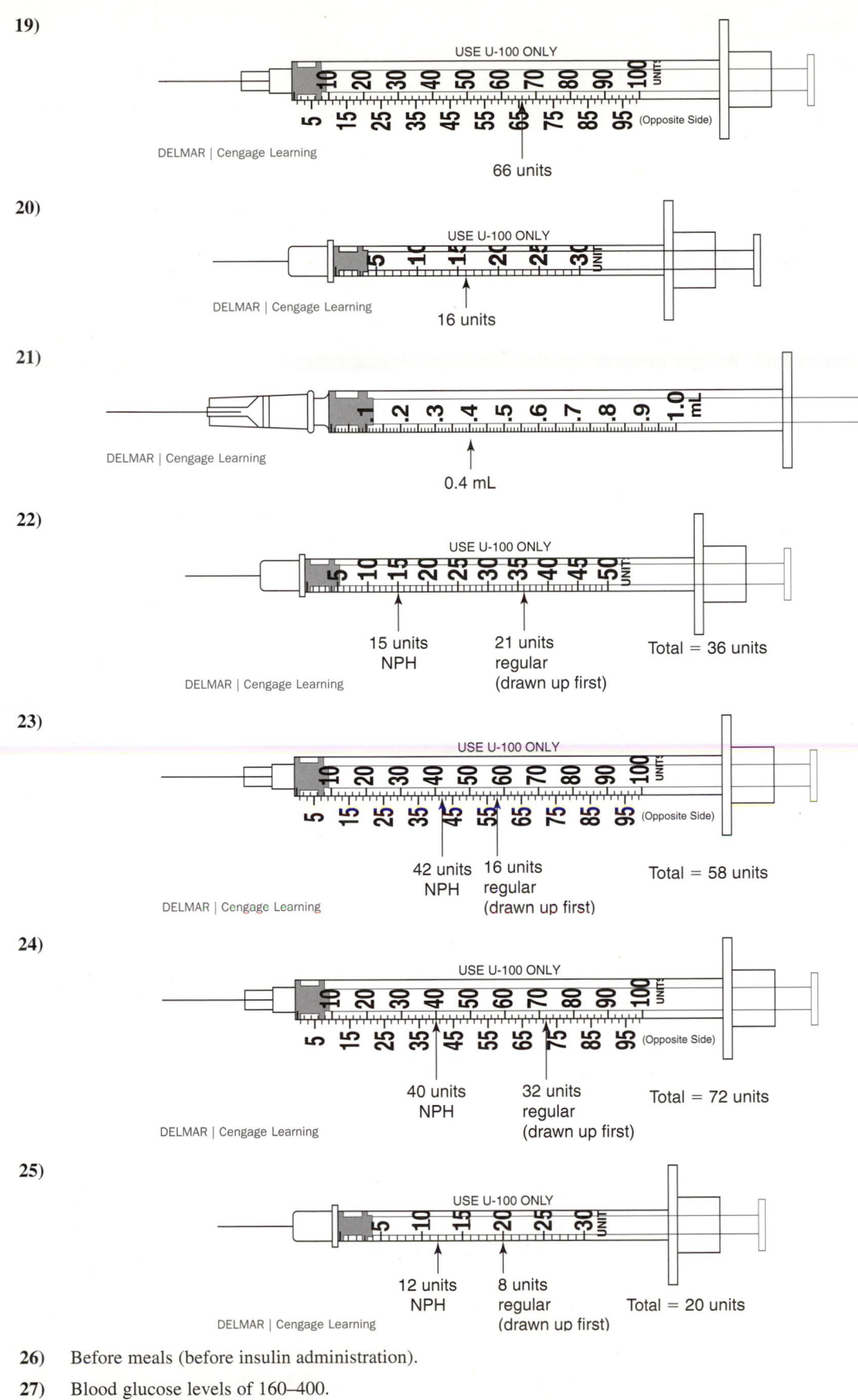

20)

16 units

21)

0.4 mL

22)

| 15 units NPH | 21 units regular (drawn up first) | Total = 36 units |

23)

| 42 units NPH | 16 units regular (drawn up first) | Total = 58 units |

24)

| 40 units NPH | 32 units regular (drawn up first) | Total = 72 units |

25)

| 12 units NPH | 8 units regular (drawn up first) | Total = 20 units |

26) Before meals (before insulin administration).

27) Blood glucose levels of 160–400.

28) Administer 4 units of Humulin R regular U-100 insulin.

29) None, do not administer insulin.

30) Contact the physician immediately for further instructions.

Solutions—Review Set 25

9)   Recall that U-100 = 100 units/mL

$$\frac{\text{Dosage on hand}}{\text{Amount on hand}} = \frac{\text{Dosage desired}}{\text{X Amount desired}}$$

$$\frac{100 \text{ units}}{1 \text{ mL}} \diagdown \frac{60 \text{ units}}{\text{X mL}}$$

$$100X = 60$$

$$\frac{100X}{100} = \frac{60}{100}$$

$$X = 0.6 \text{ mL}$$

This problem demonstrates that 60 units of U-100 insulin equal 0.6 mL. But, you would measure this dose as *60 units in a U-100 insulin syringe.*

10)   Recall that U-500 = 500 units/mL

$$\frac{\text{Dosage on hand}}{\text{Amount on hand}} = \frac{\text{Dosage desired}}{\text{X Amount desired}}$$

$$\frac{500 \text{ units}}{1 \text{ mL}} \diagdown \frac{125 \text{ units}}{\text{X mL}}$$

$$500X = 125$$

$$\frac{500X}{500} = \frac{125}{500}$$

$$X = 0.25 \text{ mL}$$

Measure 0.25 mL of U-500 insulin in a 1 mL syringe to administer 125 units.

21)   Recall that U-500 = 500 units/mL

$$\frac{\text{Dosage on hand}}{\text{Amount on hand}} = \frac{\text{Dosage desired}}{\text{X Amount desired}}$$

$$\frac{500 \text{ units}}{1 \text{ mL}} \diagdown \frac{200 \text{ units}}{\text{X mL}}$$

$$500X = 200$$

$$\frac{500X}{500} = \frac{200}{500}$$

$$X = 0.4 \text{ mL}$$

Measure 0.4 mL of U-500 insulin in a 1 mL syringe to administer 200 units.

Practice Problems—Chapter 11 from pages 235–243

1)   0.4; 1 mL

2)   1.5; 3 mL

3)   2.4; 3 mL

4)   0.6; 1 mL or 3 mL

5)   2; 3 mL

6)   10; 10 mL

7)   0.8; 1 mL or 3 mL

8)   1; 3 mL

9)   1; 3 mL

10)   2; 3 mL

11)   1.5; 3 mL

12)   0.6; 1 mL or 3 mL

13)   0.6; 1 mL or 3 mL

14)   1.9; 3 mL

15)   0.6; 1 mL or 3 mL

16)   1; 3 mL

17)   0.67; 1 mL

18)   1; 3 mL

19)   0.3; 1 mL

20)   1.6; 3 mL

21)   0.75; 1 mL

The route is IM; the needle may need to be changed to an appropriate gauge and length.

22)   1.5; 3 mL

23)   0.7; 1 mL or 3 mL

24)   0.8; 1 mL or 3 mL

25)   1.3; 3 mL

26)   1.6; 3 mL

27)   6; 10 mL

28)   0.8; 1 mL or 3 mL

29)   1.5; 3 mL

30)   2.5; 3 mL

31)   1.6; 3 mL

32)   0.7; 1 mL or 3 mL

33)   1; 3 mL

34)   10; 10 mL

35)   16; Lo-Dose 30 units U-100 insulin

36)   25; Lo-Dose 50 units U-100 insulin

37)   1.5

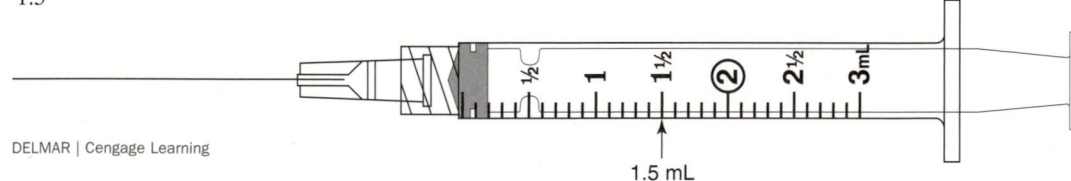

1.5 mL

38)   1.3

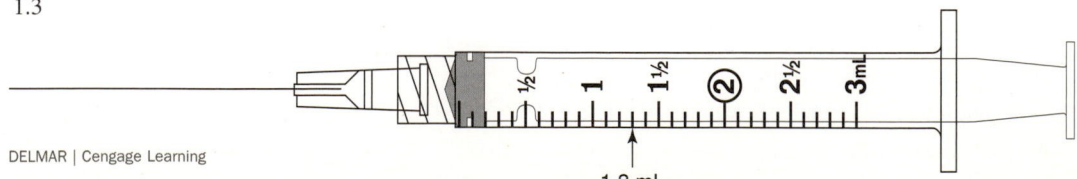

1.3 mL

39) 0.4

40) 1.5

41) 0.5

42) 22

43) 0.8

44) 0.6

45) 5

46) 0.25

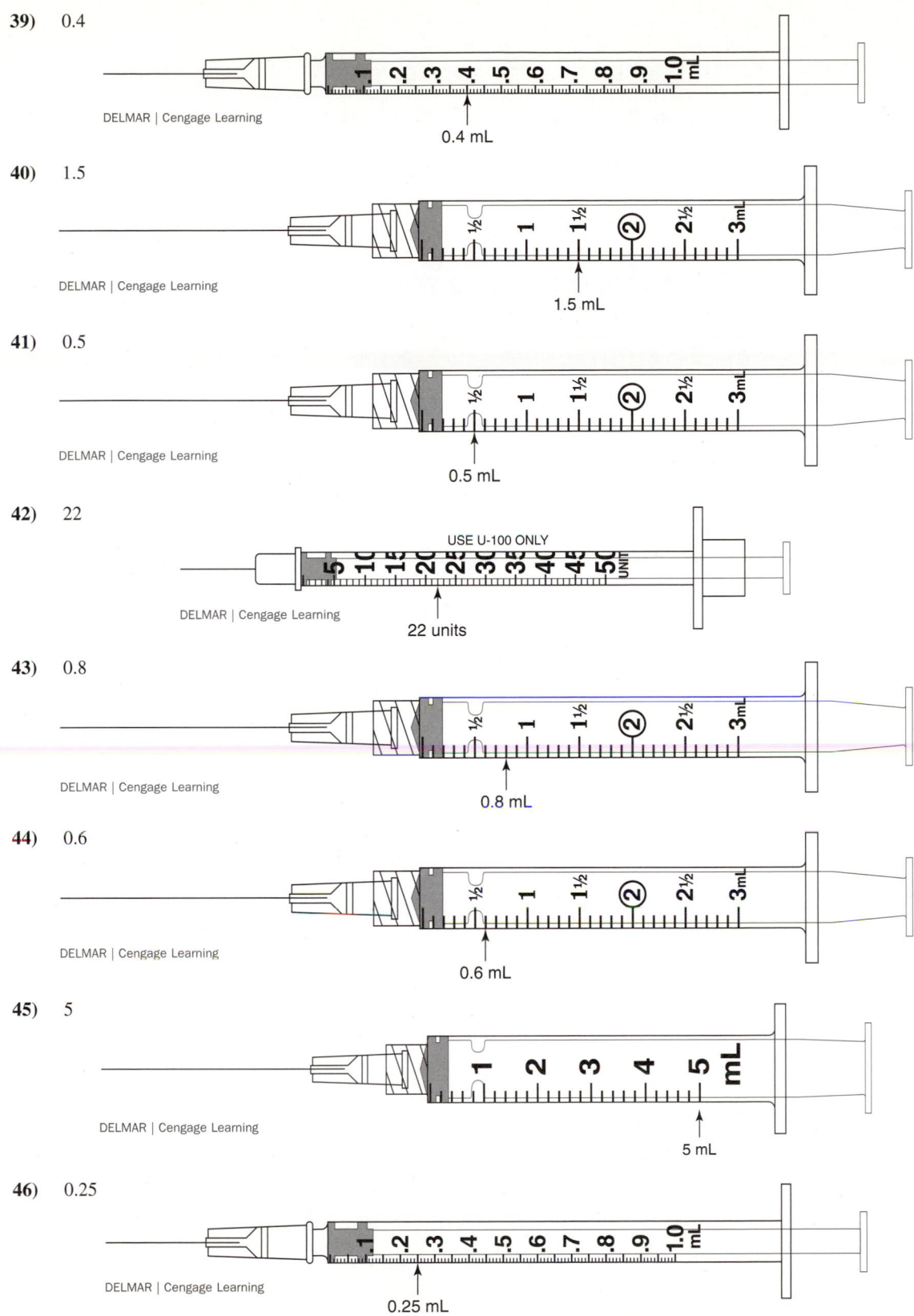

The route is IM. Because this is such a small dose (0.25 mL), change the needle to IM gauge and length before drawing up the medication. Otherwise some of the medication will be trapped in the needle, and the patient may not receive the full intended dose.

47) 86

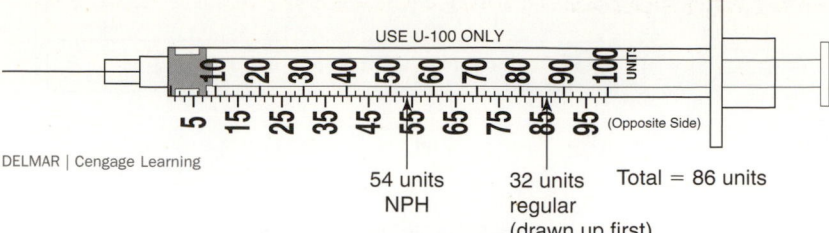

54 units   32 units   Total = 86 units
NPH   regular
(drawn up first)

48) 46

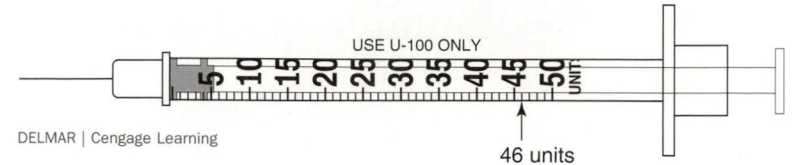

46 units

49) **Prevention:** This error could have been avoided had the nurse been more careful checking the label of the insulin vial and comparing the label to the order. The nurse should have checked the label three times. In addition, the nurse should have asked another nurse to double-check her as she was drawing up the insulin, as required. Such hospital policies and procedures are written to protect the patient and the nurse.

50) **Prevention:** This insulin error should never occur. It is obvious that the nurse did not use Step 2 of the three-step method. The nurse did not stop to think of the reasonable dosage. If so, the nurse would have realized that the supply dosage of U-100 insulin is 100 units/mL, not 10 units/mL.

    If you are unsure of what you are doing, you need to ask before you act. Insulin should only be given in an insulin syringe. The likelihood of the nurse needing to give insulin in a tuberculin syringe because an insulin syringe was unavailable is almost nonexistent today. The nurse chose the incorrect syringe. Whenever you are in doubt, you should ask for help. Further, if the nurse had asked another nurse to double-check the dosage, as required, the error could have been found before the patient received the wrong dosage of insulin. After giving the insulin, it is too late to rectify the error.

Solutions—Practice Problems—Chapter 11

3) Order: 0.6 mg

$$\frac{1 \text{ mg}}{1,000 \text{ mcg}} \times \frac{0.6 \text{ mg}}{X \text{ mcg}}$$

$$X = 1,000 \times 0.6$$

$$X = 600 \text{ mcg}$$

Supply: 500 mcg per 2 mL

$$\frac{500 \text{ mcg}}{2 \text{ mL}} \times \frac{600 \text{ mcg}}{X \text{ mL}}$$

$$500X = 1,200$$

$$\frac{500X}{500} = \frac{1,200}{500}$$

$$X = 2.4 \text{ mL}$$

6) Order: 50 mg

Supply: 5 mg/mL

$$\frac{5 \text{ mg}}{1 \text{ mL}} \times \frac{50 \text{ mg}}{X \text{ mL}}$$

$$5X = 50$$

$$\frac{5X}{5} = \frac{50}{5}$$

$$X = 10 \text{ mL}$$

Note: route is IV so this large dose is acceptable

11) Order: gr $\frac{1}{100}$

$$\frac{\text{gr } 1}{60 \text{ mg}} \times \frac{\text{gr } \frac{1}{100}}{X \text{ mg}}$$

$$X = 60 \times \frac{1}{100}$$

$$X = 0.6 \text{ mg}$$

Supply: 0.4 mg/mL

$$\frac{0.4 \text{ mg}}{1 \text{ mL}} \times \frac{0.6 \text{ mg}}{X \text{ mL}}$$

$$0.4X = 0.6$$

$$\frac{0.4X}{0.4} = \frac{0.6}{0.4}$$

$$X = 1.5 \text{ mL}$$

14) Order: 75 mg

Supply: 40 mg/mL

$$\frac{40 \text{ mg}}{1 \text{ mL}} \times \frac{75 \text{ mg}}{X \text{ mL}}$$

$$40X = 75$$

$$\frac{40X}{40} = \frac{150}{40}$$

$$X = 1.9 \text{ mL}$$

15) Order: gr $\frac{1}{10}$

$$\frac{\text{gr }1}{60\text{ mg}} \diagdown \frac{\text{gr }\frac{1}{10}}{\text{X mg}}$$

$$X = 60 \times \frac{1}{10}$$

$$X = 6\text{ mg}$$

Supply: 10 mg/mL

$$\frac{10\text{ mg}}{1\text{ mL}} \diagdown \frac{6\text{ mg}}{\text{X mL}}$$

$$10X = 6$$

$$\frac{10X}{10} = \frac{6}{10}$$

$$X = 0.6\text{ mL}$$

19) Order: 3 mg

Supply: 10 mg/mL

$$\frac{10\text{ mg}}{1\text{ mL}} \diagdown \frac{3\text{ mg}}{\text{X mL}}$$

$$10X = 3$$

$$\frac{10X}{10} = \frac{3}{10}$$

$$X = 0.3\text{ mL}$$

26) Order: 0.4 mg

Supply: 500 mcg per 2 mL

$$\frac{1\text{ mg}}{1,000\text{ mcg}} \diagdown \frac{0.4\text{ mg}}{\text{X mcg}}$$

$$X = 400\text{ mcg}$$

$$\text{Order} = 400\text{ mcg}$$

$$\frac{500\text{ mcg}}{2\text{ mL}} \diagdown \frac{400\text{ mcg}}{\text{X mL}}$$

$$500X = 800$$

$$\frac{500X}{500} = \frac{800}{500}$$

$$X = 1.6\text{ mL}$$

30) Order: 50 mg

Supply: 2% = 2 g per 100 mL

$$\frac{1\text{ g}}{1,000\text{ mg}} \diagdown \frac{2\text{ g}}{\text{X mg}}$$

$$X = 2,000\text{ mg}$$

$$\frac{2,000\text{ mg}}{100\text{ mL}} \diagdown \frac{50\text{ mg}}{\text{X mL}}$$

$$2,000X = 5,000$$

$$\frac{2,000X}{2,000} = \frac{5,000}{2,000}$$

$$X = 2.5\text{ mL}$$

33) Order: 0.5 mg

Supply: 1:2,000 = 1 g per 2,000 mL =
1,000 mg per 2,000 mL

$$\frac{1,000\text{ mg}}{2,000\text{ mL}} \diagdown \frac{0.5\text{ mg}}{\text{X mL}}$$

$$1,000X = 1,000$$

$$\frac{1,000X}{1,000} = \frac{1,000}{1,000}$$

$$X = 1\text{ mL}$$

41) Order: 0.2 mg

Supply: 0.4 mg/mL

$$\frac{0.4\text{ mg}}{1\text{ mL}} \diagdown \frac{0.2\text{ mg}}{\text{X mL}}$$

$$0.4X = 0.2$$

$$\frac{0.4X}{0.4} = \frac{0.2}{0.4}$$

$$X = 0.5\text{ mL}$$

Review Set 26 from pages 264–275

1) 4.8; 100; 4; 1

Reconstitution label

2/6/xx, 0800, reconstituted as IV solution
100 mg/mL. Expires 2/9/xx, 0800.
Keep refrigerated. G.D.P.

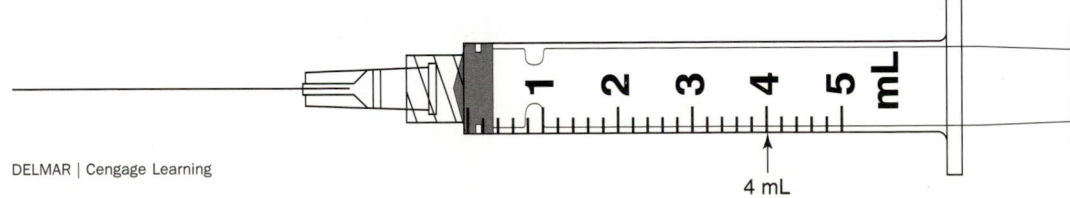

DELMAR | Cengage Learning

4 mL

2) 23; 200,000; 0.75

18; 250,000; 0.6

8; 500,000; 0.3

3; 1,000,000; 0.15

250,000; 0.6

The 250,000 units/mL concentration can be measured at 0.6 mL exactly in a 3 mL syringe, and 0.6 mL is a reasonable dose amount to measure in a 3 mL syringe. The 0.75 mL dose would require rounding to measure in a 3 mL syringe. The 0.75, 0.3, and 0.15 mL doses are more risky to measure in a 3 mL syringe. The nurse could measure them in a 1 mL syringe, but this would not be necessary with the solution strength choices available. 33 full doses are available. At 2 doses per day, 14 doses will be used before expiration.

Reconstitution label

2/6/XX, 0800, reconstituted as 250,000 units/mL. Expires 2/13/XX, 0800. Keep refrigerated. G.D.P.

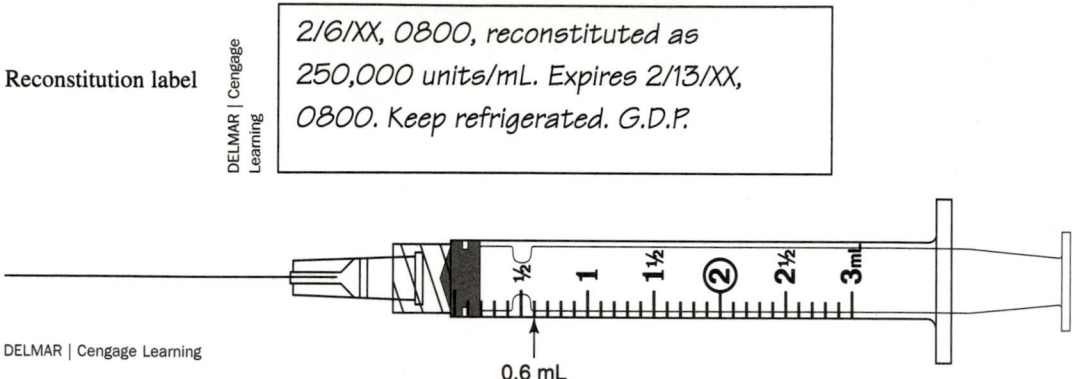

0.6 mL

DELMAR | Cengage Learning

3) 1.7; 250; 1.5

One full dose is available. No reconstitution label would be needed because there is only 1 full dose available and the alert says to use solution within 1 hour; the next dose is not due for 6 more hours.

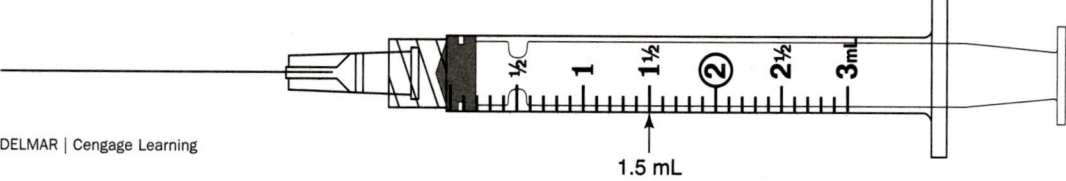

1.5 mL

DELMAR | Cengage Learning

4) 4.8; 100; 5; 1

No reconstitution label is required; all of the medication will be used for 1 dose.

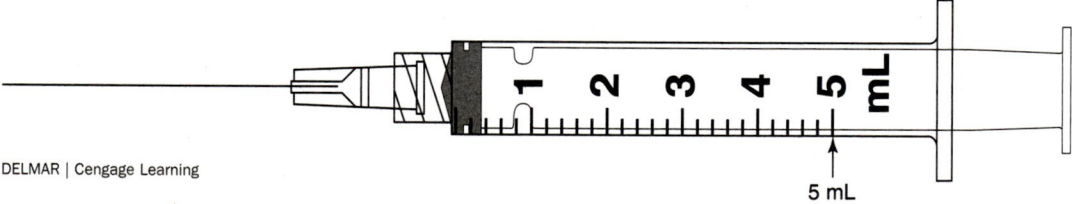

5 mL

DELMAR | Cengage Learning

5) 2.1; 350; 2.1; 1

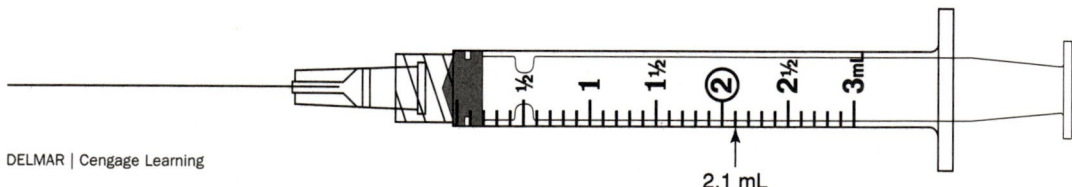

2.1 mL

DELMAR | Cengage Learning

6) 18.2; 250,000; 4

8.2; 500,000; 2

3.2; 1,000,000; 1

Select 1,000,000 units per mL and give 1 mL. Select this reconstitution concentration because the amount to give is then obvious. No calculation is necessary.

Five full doses are available in vial.

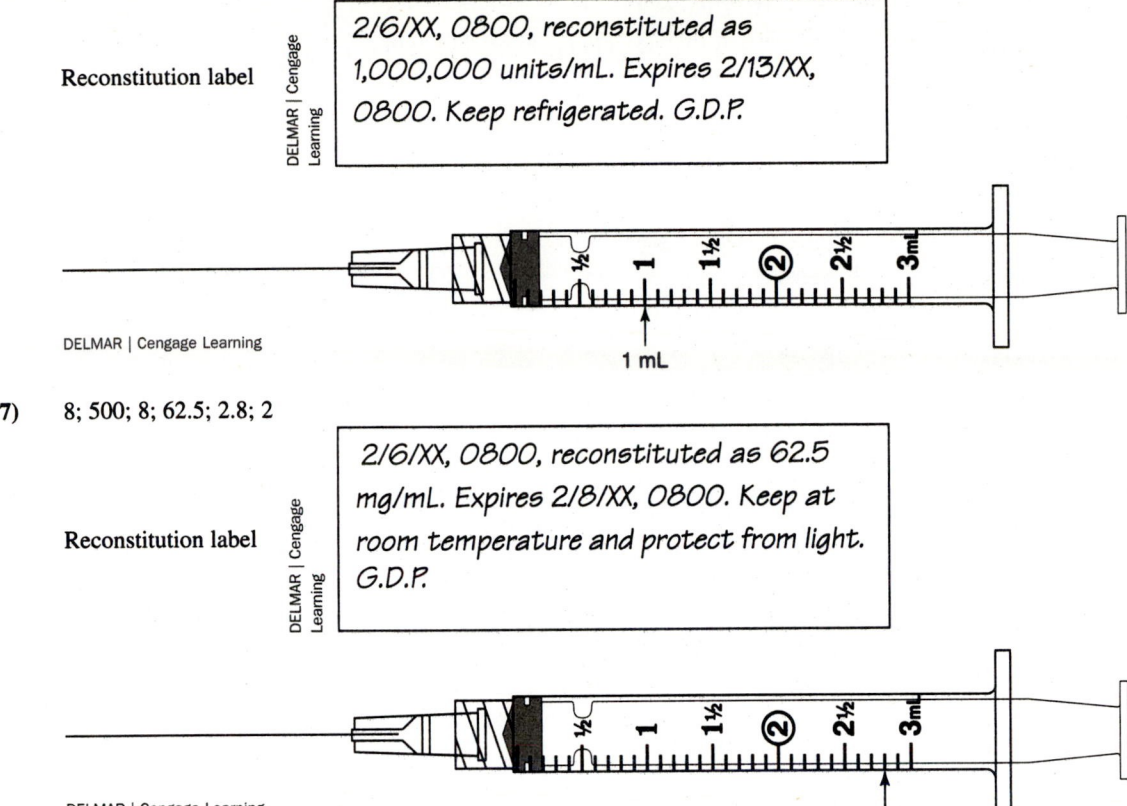

7)   8; 500; 8; 62.5; 2.8; 2

8)   10; 50; 4; 2

9)   20; 50,000; 10

10; 100,000; 5

4; 250,000; 2

1.8; 500,000; 1

Select 500,000 units/mL and give 1 mL. As this is an IV route, the dose would require further dilution before IV administration.

2 doses available

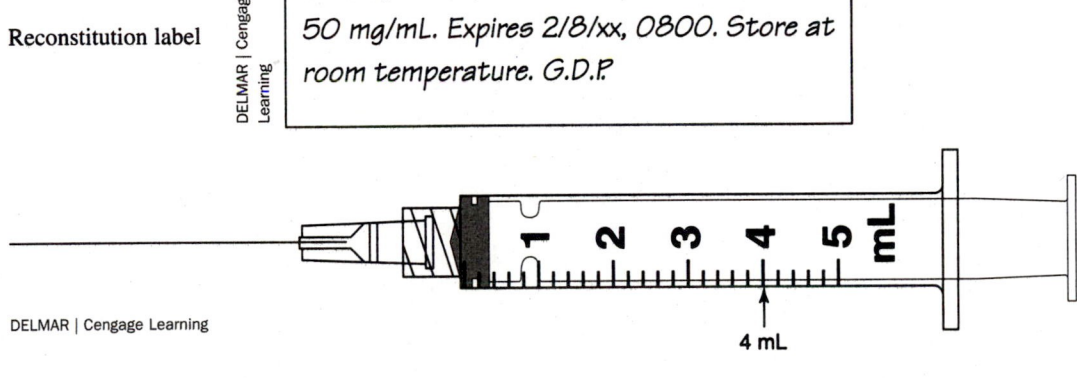

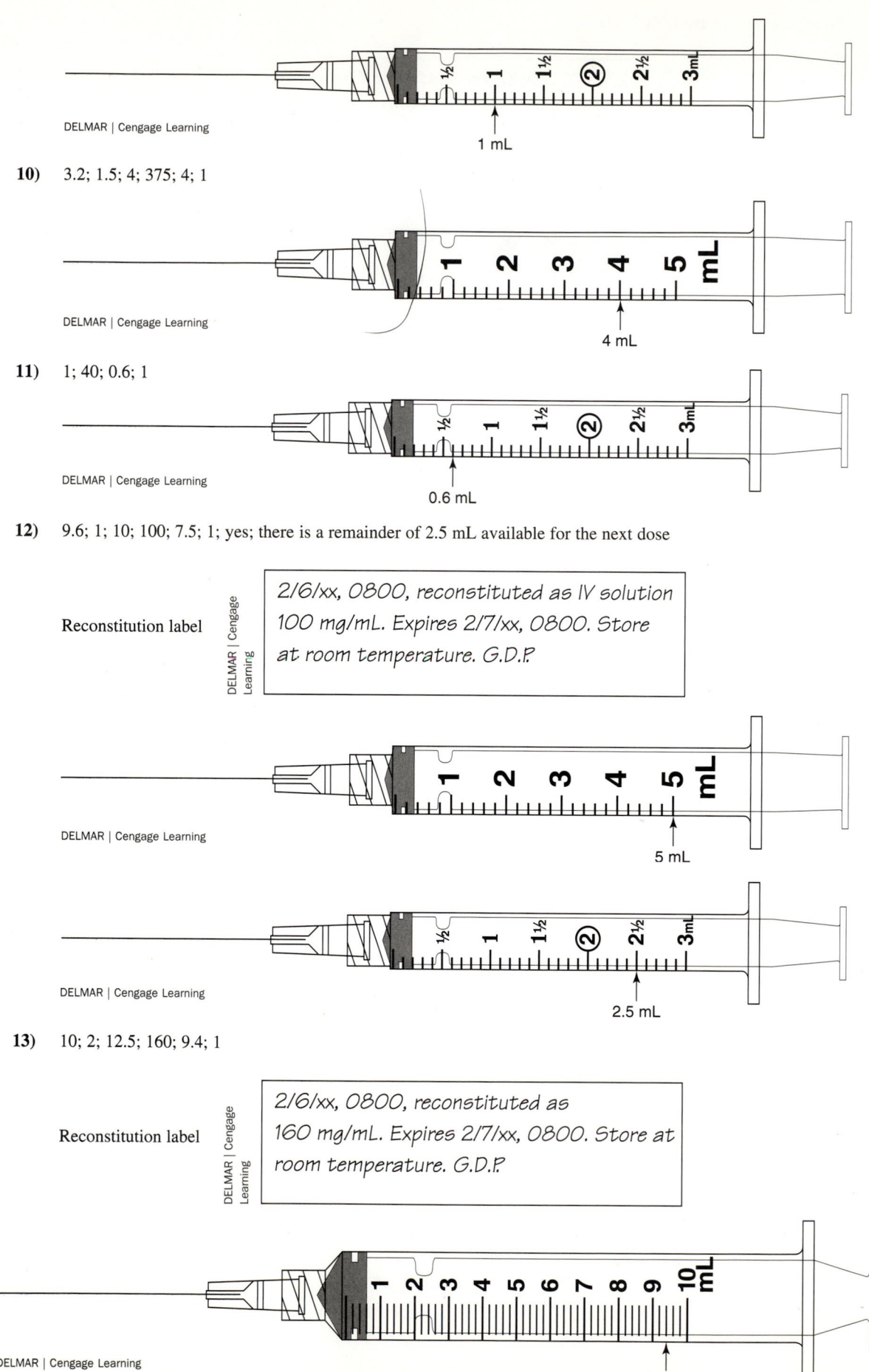

10) 3.2; 1.5; 4; 375; 4; 1

11) 1; 40; 0.6; 1

12) 9.6; 1; 10; 100; 7.5; 1; yes; there is a remainder of 2.5 mL available for the next dose

Reconstitution label

2/6/xx, 0800, reconstituted as IV solution 100 mg/mL. Expires 2/7/xx, 0800. Store at room temperature. G.D.P.

13) 10; 2; 12.5; 160; 9.4; 1

Reconstitution label

2/6/xx, 0800, reconstituted as 160 mg/mL. Expires 2/7/xx, 0800. Store at room temperature. G.D.P.

14) 5; 50; 5; 1

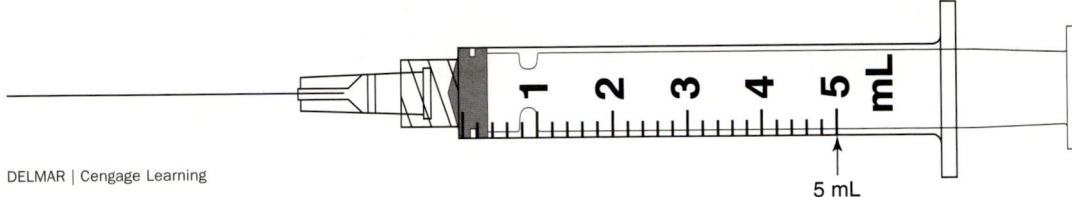

DELMAR | Cengage Learning

5 mL

15) 2; 225; 1.1; 2

Reconstitution label

DELMAR | Cengage Learning

2/6/XX, 0800, reconstituted as 225 mg/mL. Expires 2/7/XX, 0800 when kept at room temperature. G.D.P.

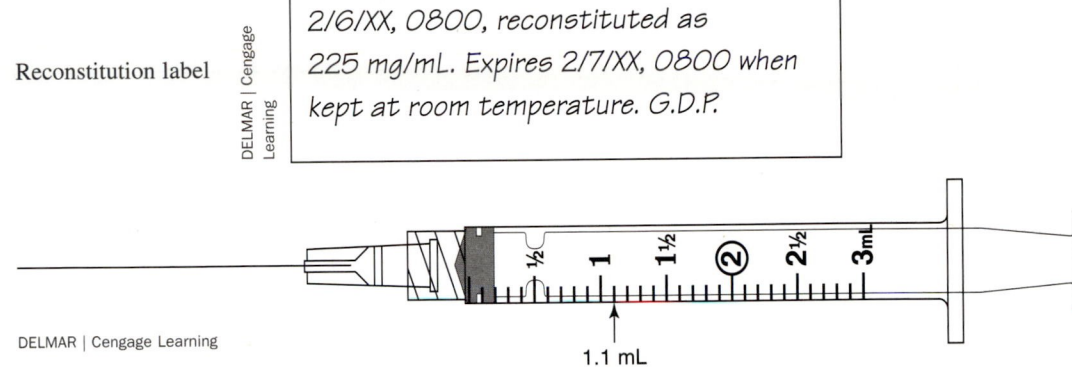

DELMAR | Cengage Learning

1.1 mL

Solutions—Review Set 26

1) Order: 400 mg

Supply: 100 mg/mL

$$\frac{\text{Dosage on hand}}{\text{Amount on hand}} = \frac{\text{Dosage desired}}{\text{X Amount desired}}$$

$$\frac{100 \text{ mg}}{1 \text{ mL}} \times \frac{400 \text{ mg}}{\text{X mL}}$$

$$100X = 400$$

$$\frac{100X}{100} = \frac{400}{100}$$

$$X = 4 \text{ mL}$$

$$\frac{400 \text{ mg}}{1 \text{ dose}} \times \frac{500 \text{ mg}}{\text{X doses}}$$

$$400X = 500$$

$$\frac{400X}{400} = \frac{500}{400}$$

$$X = 1.25 \text{ doses (per vial or 1 full dose)}$$

2) Order: 150,000 units

Supply: 250,000 units/mL

$$\frac{\text{Dosage on hand}}{\text{Amount on hand}} = \frac{\text{Dosage desired}}{\text{X Amount desired}}$$

$$\frac{250,000 \text{ units}}{1 \text{ mL}} \times \frac{150,000 \text{ units}}{\text{X mL}}$$

$$250,000X = 150,000$$

$$\frac{250,000X}{250,000} = \frac{150,000}{250,000}$$

$$X = 0.6 \text{ mL}$$

$$\frac{150,000 \text{ units}}{1 \text{ dose}} \times \frac{5,000,000 \text{ units}}{\text{X doses}}$$

$$150,000X = 5,000,000$$

$$\frac{150,000X}{150,000} = \frac{5,000,000}{150,000}$$

$$X = 33.33 \text{ doses (per vial or 33 full doses)}$$

$$\frac{2 \text{ doses}}{1 \text{ day}} = \frac{\text{X doses}}{7 \text{ days}}$$

$$X = 14 \text{ doses (will be used before expiration)}$$

3) Order: 375 mg

Supply: 250 mg/mL

$$\frac{\text{Dosage on hand}}{\text{Amount on hand}} = \frac{\text{Dosage desired}}{\text{X Amount desired}}$$

$$\frac{250 \text{ mg}}{1 \text{ mL}} \times \frac{375 \text{ mg}}{\text{X mL}}$$

$$250X = 375$$

$$\frac{250X}{250} = \frac{375}{250}$$

$$X = 1.5 \text{ mL}$$

$$\frac{375 \text{ mg}}{1 \text{ dose}} \times \frac{500 \text{ mg}}{\text{X doses}}$$

$$375X = 500$$

$$\frac{375X}{375} = \frac{500}{375}$$

$$X = 1.33 \text{ doses (per vial or 1 full dose)}$$

5) Order: 750 mg

Supply: 350 mg/mL

$$\frac{\text{Dosage on hand}}{\text{Amount on hand}} = \frac{\text{Dosage desired}}{\text{X Amount desired}}$$

$$\frac{350 \text{ mg}}{1 \text{ mL}} \diagdown \frac{750 \text{ mg}}{\text{X mL}}$$

$$350\text{X} = 750$$

$$\frac{350\text{X}}{350} = \frac{750}{350}$$

$$\text{X} = 2.1 \text{ mL}$$

$$\frac{750 \text{ mg}}{1 \text{ dose}} \diagdown \frac{1,000 \text{ mg}}{\text{X doses}}$$

$$750\text{X} = 1,000$$

$$\frac{750\text{X}}{750} = \frac{1,000}{750}$$

$$\text{X} = 1.33 \text{ doses (per vial or 1 full dose)}$$

6) Order: 1,000,000 units

Supply: 250,000 units/mL

$$\frac{250,000 \text{ units}}{1 \text{ mL}} \diagdown \frac{1,000,000 \text{ units}}{\text{X mL}}$$

$$250,000\text{X} = 1,000,000$$

$$\frac{250,000\text{X}}{250,000} \diagdown \frac{1,000,000}{250,000}$$

$$\text{X} = 4 \text{ mL}$$

Order: 1,000,000 units

Supply: 500,000 units/mL

$$\frac{500,000 \text{ units}}{1 \text{ mL}} \diagdown \frac{1,000,000 \text{ units}}{\text{X mL}}$$

$$500,000\text{X} = 1,000,000$$

$$\frac{500,000\text{X}}{500,000} = \frac{1,000,000}{500,000}$$

$$\text{X} = 2 \text{ mL}$$

Order: 1,000,000 units

Supply: 1,000,000 units/mL

It is obvious that dose is 1 mL.

$$\frac{1,000,000 \text{ units}}{1 \text{ dose}} \diagdown \frac{5,000,000 \text{ units}}{\text{X doses}}$$

$$1,000,000\text{X} = 5,000,000$$

$$\frac{1,000,000\text{X}}{1,000,000} \diagdown \frac{5,000,000}{1,000,000}$$

$$\text{X} = 5 \text{ doses (available per vial)}$$

7) Order: 175 mg

Supply: 500 mg per 8 mL

$$\frac{500 \text{ mg}}{8 \text{ mL}} \diagdown \frac{\text{X mg}}{1 \text{ mL}}$$

$$8\text{X} = 500$$

$$\frac{8\text{X}}{8} = \frac{500}{8}$$

$$\text{X} = 62.5 \text{ mg}$$

$$\frac{62.5 \text{ mg}}{1 \text{ mL}} \diagdown \frac{175 \text{ mg}}{\text{X mL}}$$

$$62.5\text{X} = 175$$

$$\frac{62.5\text{X}}{62.5} = \frac{175}{62.5}$$

$$\text{X} = 2.8 \text{ mL}$$

$$\frac{175 \text{ mg}}{1 \text{ dose}} = \frac{500 \text{ mg}}{\text{X doses}}$$

$$175\text{X} = 500$$

$$\frac{175\text{X}}{175} = \frac{500}{175}$$

$$\text{X} = 2.85 \text{ or 2 full doses}$$

8) Order: 200 mg

Supply: 50 mg/mL

$$\frac{50 \text{ mg}}{1 \text{ mL}} \diagdown \frac{200 \text{ mg}}{\text{X mL}}$$

$$50\text{X} = 200$$

$$\frac{50\text{X}}{50} = \frac{200}{50}$$

$$\text{X} = 4 \text{ mL}$$

$$\frac{200 \text{ mg}}{1 \text{ dose}} \diagdown \frac{500 \text{ mg}}{\text{X doses}}$$

$$200\text{X} = 500$$

$$\frac{200\text{X}}{200} = \frac{500}{200}$$

$$\text{X} = 2.5 \text{ doses (per vial or 2 full doses)}$$

12) Order: 750 mg

Supply: 100 mg/mL

$$\frac{100 \text{ mg}}{1 \text{ mL}} \diagdown \frac{750 \text{ mg}}{\text{X mL}}$$

$$100\text{X} = 750$$

$$\frac{100\text{X}}{100} = \frac{750}{100}$$

$$\text{X} = 7.5 \text{ mL}$$

$$\frac{750 \text{ mg}}{1 \text{ dose}} \diagdown \frac{1,000 \text{ mg}}{\text{X doses}}$$

$$750\text{X} = 1,000$$

$$\frac{750\text{X}}{750} = \frac{1,000}{750}$$

$$\text{X} = 1.33 \text{ doses (per vial or 1 full dose)}$$

13) Order: 1,500 mg

Supply: 160 mg/mL

$$\frac{160 \text{ mg}}{1 \text{ mL}} \diagdown \frac{1,500 \text{ mg}}{\text{X mL}}$$

$$160\text{X} = 1,500$$

$$\frac{160\text{X}}{160} = \frac{1,500}{160}$$

$$\text{X} = 9.375 \text{ mL} = 9.4 \text{ mL}$$

$$\frac{1,500 \text{ mg}}{1 \text{ dose}} \times \frac{2,000 \text{ mg}}{X \text{ doses}}$$

$$1,500X = 2,000$$

$$\frac{1,500X}{1,500} = \frac{2,000}{1,500}$$

$$X = 1.33 \text{ doses (per vial or 1 full dose)}$$

14)   Order: 250 mg

Supply: 250 mg per 5 mL

$$\frac{250 \text{ mg}}{5 \text{ mL}} \times \frac{X \text{ mg}}{1 \text{ mL}}$$

$$5X = 250$$

$$\frac{5X}{5} = \frac{250}{5}$$

$$X = 50 \text{ mg (50 mg/mL)}$$

You will give all of the 250 mg reconstituted with

5 mL diluent; give 5 mL. One full dose is available.

Review Set 27 from page 280–281

1)   160 mL hydrogen peroxide (solute) + 320 mL saline (solvent) = 480 mL $\frac{1}{3}$ strength solution.

2)   1 fl oz hydrogen peroxide + 3 fl oz saline = 4 fl oz $\frac{1}{4}$ strength solution.

3)   180 mL hydrogen peroxide + 60 mL saline = 240 mL $\frac{3}{4}$ strength solution.

4)   8 fl oz hydrogen peroxide + 8 fl oz saline = 16 fl oz $\frac{1}{2}$ strength solution.

5)   300 mL Ensure + 600 mL water = 900 mL $\frac{1}{3}$ strength Ensure; one 12 fl oz can. Discard 2 fl oz (60 mL).

6)   6 fl oz (180 mL) Isomil + 18 fl oz (540 mL) water = 24 fl oz (720 mL) $\frac{1}{4}$ strength Isomil; one 6 fl oz can.

   None discarded.

7)   1,200 mL needed for daily supply. 800 mL Sustacal + 400 mL water = 1,200 mL $\frac{2}{3}$ strength Sustacal; three

   10 fl oz cans. Discard 100 mL.

8)   13 fl oz Ensure + 13 fl oz water = 26 fl oz $\frac{1}{2}$ strength Ensure; one 12 fl oz can + one 4 fl oz can. Discard 3 fl oz (90 mL).

9)   1,000 mL needed for daily supply. 500 mL Sustacal + 500 mL water = 1,000 mL $\frac{1}{2}$ strength Sustacal;

   two 10 fl oz cans. Discard 100 mL.

10)   36 fl oz Isomil + 12 fl oz water = 48 fl oz $\frac{3}{4}$ strength Isomil; use three 12 fl oz cans. None discarded.

11)   4 fl oz Ensure + 2 fl oz water = 6 fl oz $\frac{2}{3}$ strength Ensure; use one 4 fl oz can. None discarded.

12)   4 fl oz Ensure + 12 fl oz water = 16 fl oz (1 pt) $\frac{1}{4}$ strength Ensure; use one 4 fl oz can. None discarded.

Solutions—Review Set 27

1) $\frac{1}{3} \times \frac{X \text{ mL}}{480 \text{ mL}}$

$$3X = 480$$

$$\frac{3X}{3} = \frac{480}{3}$$

$$X = 160 \text{ mL (solute)}$$

480 mL (quantity of solution desired) − 160 mL

(solute) = 320 mL (solvent)

5) $\frac{1}{3} \times \frac{X \text{ mL}}{900 \text{ mL}}$

$$3X = 900$$

$$\frac{3X}{3} = \frac{900}{3}$$

$$X = 300 \text{ mL (Ensure)}$$

900 mL (total solution) − 300 mL (Ensure) =

600 mL (water)

$$\frac{1 \text{ fl oz}}{30 \text{ mL}} \times \frac{12 \text{ fl oz}}{X \text{ mL}}$$

$$X = 360 \text{ mL (per can)}$$

360 mL (full can) − 300 mL (Ensure needed) =

60 mL (discarded)

6) $\frac{1}{4} \times \frac{X \text{ fl oz}}{24 \text{ fl oz}}$

$$4X = 24$$

$$\frac{4X}{4} = \frac{24}{4}$$

$$X = 6 \text{ fl oz (Isomil)}$$

24 fl oz (solution) − 6 fl oz (Isomil) = 18 fl oz

(water); use one 6-fl oz can

12) $\frac{1}{4} \times \frac{X \text{ fl oz}}{16 \text{ fl oz}}$

$$4X = 16$$

$$\frac{4X}{4} = \frac{16}{4}$$

$$X = 4 \text{ fl oz (Ensure)}$$

16 fl oz (solution) − 4 fl oz (Ensure) = 12 fl oz (water);

use one 4-fl oz can of Ensure; none discarded

Practice Problems—Chapter 12 from pages 283–290

1) 3.375; 5; 3.7; 5 mL **2)** 2; 3 mL **3)** 1.5; 3 mL **4)** 9.6; 100; 9; 1; 10 mL

5) 1.8; 3 mL; 2 (Dilute further for IV administration)

> *2/6/XX, 0800, reconstituted as 280 mg/mL.*
> *Expires 2/13/XX, 0800. Keep refrigerated. G.D.P.*

6) 3.8; 5 mL; 1 **7)** 2; 225; 1.3; 3 mL; 1; Yes **8)** 8; 500; 8; 62.5; 3.2; 5; 2; Yes **9)** 19.2; 100; 12.5; 20 mL; 1; Yes **10)** 3; 1,000,000; 0.5; 3 mL; 10; Yes **11)** 0.9; 250; 0.8; 3; 1; No it would be too difficult to withdraw the small remainder for the next dose. **12)** 29; 20; 10; 5; Yes **13)** 2; 225; 1.8; 3 mL; 1; Yes **14)** 3.2; 1,000,000; 2; 3 mL; 2; Yes **15)** 1.8; 500,000; 2; 3 mL; 1; No

16)   2 fl oz hydrogen peroxide + 14 fl oz normal saline = 16 fl oz of the $\frac{1}{8}$ strength solution

17)   120 mL hydrogen peroxide + 200 mL normal saline = 320 mL of the $\frac{3}{8}$ strength solution

18)   50 mL hydrogen peroxide + 30 mL normal saline = 80 mL of the $\frac{5}{8}$ strength solution

19)   12 fl oz hydrogen peroxide + 6 fl oz normal saline = 18 fl oz of the $\frac{2}{3}$ strength solution

20)   14 fl oz hydrogen peroxide + 2 fl oz normal saline = 16 fl oz (1 pt) of the $\frac{7}{8}$ strength solution

21)   250 mL hydrogen peroxide + 750 mL normal saline = 1,000 mL (1 L) of the $\frac{1}{4}$ strength solution

22)   30 mL Enfamil + 90 mL water = 120 mL of the $\frac{1}{4}$ strength Enfamil; one *3 fl oz* bottle. Discard 2 fl oz (60 mL).

23)   270 mL Sustacal + 90 mL water = 360 mL of the $\frac{3}{4}$ strength Sustacal; one *10 fl oz* can. Discard 1 fl oz (30 mL).

24)   300 mL Ensure + 150 mL water = 450 mL of the $\frac{2}{3}$ strength Ensure; two *8 fl oz* cans. Discard 6 fl oz (180 mL).

25)   36 fl oz Enfamil + 60 fl oz water = 96 fl oz of the $\frac{3}{8}$ strength Enfamil; six *6 fl oz* bottles. None discarded.

26)   20 mL Ensure + 140 mL water = 160 mL of the $\frac{1}{8}$ strength Ensure; one *4 fl oz* can. Discard 100 mL.

27)   275 mL Ensure + 275 mL water = 550 mL of the $\frac{1}{2}$ strength Ensure; one *12 fl oz* can. Discard 85 mL.

28)   2 cans are needed; $1\frac{1}{2}$ cans are used (*12 fl oz* Enfamil)

29)   36

30)   **Prevention:** This type of error could have been prevented had the nurse read the label carefully for the correct amount of diluent for the dosage of medication to be prepared. Had the nurse read the label carefully before the medication was prepared, medication, valuable time, health care resources, and patient expense charges would have been saved. Additionally, if the nurse had used Step 2 (Think) of the three-step method, the nurse would have realized earlier (before preparing it) that 4 mL would be an unreasonable volume for an IM injection.

Solutions—Practice Problems—Chapter 12

1)   Concentration is 3.375 g per 5 mL

Order: 2.5 g

Supply: 3.375 g per 5 mL

$$\frac{3.375\text{ g}}{5\text{ mL}} \times\!\!\!\!\diagup \frac{2.5\text{ g}}{\text{X mL}}$$

$$3.375\text{X} = 12.5$$

$$\frac{3.375\text{X}}{3.375} = \frac{12.5}{3.375}$$

$$\text{X} = 3.7\text{ mL}$$

4)   Order: 900 mg

Supply: 100 mg/mL

$$\frac{100\text{ mg}}{1\text{ mL}} \times\!\!\!\!\diagup \frac{900\text{ mg}}{\text{X mL}}$$

$$100\text{X} = 900$$

$$\frac{100\text{X}}{100} = \frac{900}{100}$$

$$\text{X} = 9\text{ mL}$$

Vial has 1 g Rocephin. Order is for 900 mg/dose.

$$\frac{900\text{ mg}}{1\text{ dose}} \times\!\!\!\!\diagup \frac{1,000\text{ mg}}{\text{X doses}}$$

$$900\text{X} = 1,000$$

$$\frac{900\text{X}}{900} = \frac{1,000}{900}$$

$$\text{X} = 1.1\text{ doses (per vial or 1 full dose per vial)}$$

6) Order: 375 mg

Supply: 100 mg/mL

$$\frac{100 \text{ mg}}{1 \text{ mL}} \diagdown \frac{375 \text{ mg}}{X \text{ mL}}$$

$$100X = 375$$

$$\frac{100X}{100} = \frac{375}{100}$$

$$X = 3.75 \text{ mL} = 3.8 \text{ mL}$$

$$\frac{375 \text{ mg}}{1 \text{ dose}} \diagdown \frac{500 \text{ mg}}{X \text{ dose}}$$

$$375X = 500$$

$$\frac{375X}{375} = \frac{500}{375}$$

$$X = 1.3 \text{ doses (per vial or 1 full dose per vial)}$$

8) Order: 200 mg

Supply: 62.5 mg/mL

$$\frac{62.5 \text{ mg}}{1 \text{ mL}} \diagdown \frac{200 \text{ mg}}{X \text{ mL}}$$

$$62.5X = 200$$

$$\frac{62.5X}{62.5} = \frac{200}{62.5}$$

$$X = 3.2 \text{ mL}$$

$$\frac{200 \text{ mg}}{1 \text{ dose}} \diagdown \frac{500 \text{ mg}}{X \text{ doses}}$$

$$200X = 500$$

$$\frac{200X}{200} = \frac{500}{200}$$

$$X = 2.5 \text{ doses (per vial or 2 full doses per vial)}$$

9) Order: 1.25 g

Supply: 100 mg/mL

$$\frac{1,000 \text{ mg}}{1 \text{ g}} \diagdown \frac{X \text{ mg}}{1.25 \text{ g}}$$

$$1X = 1,250$$

$$X = 1,250 \text{ mg}$$

$$\frac{100 \text{ mg}}{1 \text{ mL}} \diagdown \frac{1,250 \text{ mg}}{X \text{ mL}}$$

$$100X = 1,250$$

$$\frac{100X}{100} = \frac{1,250}{100}$$

$$X = 12.5 \text{ mL}$$

$$\frac{1,250 \text{ mg}}{1 \text{ dose}} \diagdown \frac{2,000 \text{ mg}}{X \text{ doses}}$$

$$1,250X = 2,000$$

$$\frac{1,250X}{1,250} = \frac{2,000}{1,250}$$

$$X = 1.6 \text{ doses (per vial or 1 full dose per vial)}$$

11) Order: 200 mg

Supply: 250 mg/mL

$$\frac{250 \text{ mg}}{1 \text{ mL}} \diagdown \frac{200 \text{ mg}}{X \text{ mL}}$$

$$250X = 200$$

$$\frac{250X}{250} = \frac{200}{250}$$

$$X = 0.8 \text{ mL}$$

$$\frac{200 \text{ mg}}{1 \text{ dose}} \diagdown \frac{250 \text{ mg}}{X \text{ doses}}$$

$$200X = 250$$

$$\frac{200X}{200} = \frac{250}{200}$$

$$X = 1.25 \text{ doses (per vial or 1 full dose per vial)}$$

15) Order: 1,000,000 units

Supply: 50,000 units/mL

$$\frac{50,000 \text{ units}}{1 \text{ mL}} \diagdown \frac{1,000,000 \text{ units}}{X \text{ mL}}$$

$$50,000X = 1,000,000$$

$$\frac{50,000X}{50,000} = \frac{1,000,000}{50,000}$$

$$X = 20 \text{ mL (too much for an IM dose)}$$

Order: 1,000,000 units

Supply: 100,000 units/mL

$$\frac{100,000 \text{ units}}{1 \text{ mL}} \diagdown \frac{1,000,000 \text{ units}}{X \text{ mL}}$$

$$100,000X = 1,000,000$$

$$\frac{100,000X}{100,000} = \frac{1,000,000}{100,000}$$

$$X = 10 \text{ mL (too much for an IM dose)}$$

Order: 1,000,000 units

Supply: 250,000 units/mL

$$\frac{250,000 \text{ units}}{1 \text{ mL}} \diagdown \frac{1,000,000 \text{ units}}{X \text{ mL}}$$

$$250,000X = 1,000,000$$

$$\frac{250,000X}{250,000} = \frac{1,000,000}{250,000}$$

X = 4 mL (too much for an IM dose − 3 mL or less

is preferred)

Order: 1,000,000 units

Supply: 500,000 units/mL

$$\frac{500,000 \text{ units}}{1 \text{ mL}} \diagdown \frac{1,000,000 \text{ units}}{X \text{ mL}}$$

$$500,000X = 1,000,000$$

$$\frac{500,000X}{500,000} = \frac{1,000,000}{500,000}$$

$$X = 2 \text{ mL (acceptable IM dose)}$$

22) 12 mL every hour for 10 hours = $12 \times 10 =$

120 mL total:

$$\frac{1}{4} \diagdown \frac{X \text{ mL}}{120 \text{ mL}}$$

$4X = 120$

$$\frac{4X}{4} = \frac{120}{4}$$

X = 30 mL (Enfamil)

120 mL (solution) − 30 mL (Enfamil) = 90 mL

(water); one 3 fl oz bottle = 90 mL

90 mL (full bottle) − 30 mL (Enfamil needed) =

60 mL (1 fl oz = 30 mL; 2 fl oz = 60 mL; therefore,

2 fl oz discarded)

28)

$$\frac{1}{4} \diagdown \frac{X \text{ fl oz}}{48 \text{ fl oz}}$$

$4X = 48$

$$\frac{4X}{4} = \frac{48}{4}$$

X = 12 fl oz (Enfamil)

$$\frac{1 \text{ can}}{8 \text{ fl oz}} \diagdown \frac{X \text{ cans}}{12 \text{ fl oz}}$$

$8X = 12$

$$\frac{8X}{8} = \frac{12}{8}$$

$X = 1\frac{1}{2}$ cans

Need $1\frac{1}{2}$ cans (8 fl oz/can) of Enfamil for each infant.

29) 48 fl oz solution − 12 fl oz (Enfamil) = 36 fl oz

(water)

Review Set 28 from page 293–294

1) 0.05, 1 L = 1,000 mL **2)** 5, gr i = 60 mg **3)** 38.18, 1 kg = 2.2 lb **4)** 600, gr i = 60 mg **5)** 7.5, gr i = 60 mg **6)** $2\frac{1}{2}$, 1 fl oz = 30 mL **7)** 0.75, 1 L = 1,000 mL **8)** 45, 1 fl oz = 30 mL **9)** $\frac{1}{4}$, gr i = 60 mg **10)** 0.625, 1 mg = 1,000 mcg **11)** $\frac{1}{2}$, 1 t = 5 mL **12)** 30, gr i = 60 mg **13)** $\frac{1}{6}$, gr i = 60 mg **14)** $\frac{1}{100}$, gr i = 60 mg **15)** 3, 1 in = 2.5 cm **16)** 16,000, 1 g = 1,000 mg **17)** $\frac{1}{2}$, 1 fl oz = 30 mL **18)** 0.2, 1 lb = 16 oz **19)** 2, 1 qt = 1 L **20)** 33, 1 kg = 2.2 lb **21)** 5, 1 fl oz = 30 mL **22)** 1, 1 t = 5 mL **23)** 8, 1 L = 1,000 mL, 1 qt = 1 L, 1 qt = 32 fl oz **24)** 3; 1 t = 5 mL **25)** 15, gr i = 60 mg

Solutions—Review Set 28

1) mL → L; Smaller ↑ Larger → (÷)

.050.mL = 0.050 = 0.05 L

3) lb → kg; Smaller ↑ Larger → (÷)

84 lb ÷ 2.2 lb/kg = 38.18 kg

5) gr → mg; Larger ↓ Smaller → (×)

gr $\frac{1}{8}$ × 60 mg/gr = 7.5 mg

7) mL → L; Smaller ↑ Larger → (÷)

.750.mL = 0.750 = 0.75 L

14) mL → L; Smaller ↑ Larger → (÷)

0.6 mg ÷ 60 mg/gr = 0.01 = gr $\frac{1}{100}$

23) fl oz → mL; Larger ↓ Smaller → (×)

8 fl oz × 30 mL/fl oz = 240 mL

2000 mL ÷ 240 mL/glass = 8.3 or 8 full glasses per day

Review Set 29 from page 297–298

1) 2 **2)** 2.5 **3)** 0.8 **4)** 1.3 **5)** 7.5 **6)** 0.6 **7)** $1\frac{1}{2}$ **8)** 3 **9)** 30 **10)** 1.6 **11)** 3 **12)** 0.5 **13)** 2 **14)** 250 mg; $\frac{1}{2}$ of 250 mg tab **15)** 2.4 **16)** 2 **17)** 18 **18)** 1.3 **19)** 16 **20)** 7

Solutions—Review Set 29

2) Order: 150 mg

Supply: 300 mg per 5 mL

$$\frac{D}{H} \times Q = \frac{\overset{1}{\cancel{150}} \text{ mg}}{\underset{2}{\cancel{300}} \text{ mg}} \times 5 \text{ mL} = \frac{5}{2} \text{ mL} = 2.5 \text{ mL}$$

5) Order: 450 mg

Supply: 300 mg per 5 mL

$$\frac{D}{H} \times Q = \frac{\overset{3}{\cancel{450}} \text{ mg}}{\underset{2}{\cancel{300}} \text{ mg}} \times 5 \text{ mL} = \frac{15}{2} \text{ mL} = 7.5 \text{ mL}$$

6) Order: 2.4 mg

Supply: 4 mg per 1 mL = 4.0 mg per 1 mL

$$\frac{D}{H} \times Q = \frac{2.4 \text{ mg}}{4.0 \text{ mg}} \times 1 \text{ mL} = 0.6 \text{ mL}$$

9) Order: 160 mg

Supply: 80 mg per 15 mL

$$\frac{D}{H} \times Q = \frac{\overset{2}{\cancel{160}} \text{ mg}}{\underset{1}{\cancel{80}} \text{ mg}} \times 15 \text{ mL} = \frac{30}{1} \text{ mL} = 30 \text{ mL}$$

13) Order: gr ½

Supply: 15 mg/tab

gr → mg; Larger ↓ Smaller → (×)

$g\cancel{r} \dfrac{1}{2} \times 60 \text{ mg/}g\cancel{r} = 30 \text{ mg}$

$\dfrac{D}{H} \times Q = \dfrac{\overset{2}{\cancel{30 \text{ mg}}}}{\underset{1}{\cancel{15 \text{ mg}}}} \times 1 \text{ tab} = 2 \text{ tab}$

16) Order: 0.15 mg

Supply: 75 mcg/tab

mg → mcg; Larger ↓ Smaller → (×)

0.150. mg = 150 mcg

$\dfrac{D}{H} \times Q = \dfrac{\overset{2}{\cancel{150 \text{ mcg}}}}{\underset{1}{\cancel{75 \text{ mcg}}}} \times 1 \text{ tab} = 2 \text{ tab}$

18) Order: 100 mg

Supply: 80 mg per 1 mL

$\dfrac{D}{H} \times Q = \dfrac{100 \text{ mg}}{80 \text{ mg}} \times 1 \text{ mL} = 1.25 \text{ mL} = 1.3 \text{ mL}$

19) Order: 8 mg

Supply: 2.5 mg per 5 mL

$\dfrac{D}{H} \times Q = \dfrac{8 \text{ mg}}{2.5 \text{ mg}} \times 5 \text{ mL} = \dfrac{40}{2.5} \text{ mL} = 16 \text{ mL}$

Review Set 30 from pages 308–309

1) 0.5 **2)** 3 **3)** 34 **4)** 12 **5)** 10 **6)** 13 **7)** $1\dfrac{1}{2}$ **8)** 2 **9)** 2 **10)** 3 **11)** 1.7 **12)** 0.91 **13)** 0.3 **14)** 7.5 **15)** 0.75 **16)** 6 **17)** 3.2

18) 1.2 **19)** 4.4 **20)** 6.2

Solutions—Review Set 30

1) $\text{X mL} = \dfrac{1 \text{ mL}}{10{,}000 \text{ units}} \times 5{,}000 \text{ units} = 0.5 \text{ mL}$

3) $\text{X mL} = \dfrac{5 \text{ mL}}{250 \text{ mg}} \times \dfrac{15 \text{ mg}}{1 \text{ kg}} \times \dfrac{1 \text{ kg}}{2.2 \text{ lb}} \times 250 \text{ lb} = 34 \text{ mL}$

6) $\text{X mL} = \dfrac{5 \text{ mL}}{250 \text{ mg}} \times \dfrac{1{,}000 \text{ mg}}{1 \text{ g}} \times \dfrac{0.01 \text{ g}}{1 \text{ kg}} \times \dfrac{1 \text{ kg}}{2.2 \text{ lb}} \times 143 \text{ lb} = 13 \text{ mL}$

11) $\text{X mL} = \dfrac{1 \text{ mL}}{0.2 \text{ mg}} \times \dfrac{1 \text{ mg}}{1{,}000 \text{ mcg}} \times \dfrac{4 \text{ mcg}}{1 \text{ kg}} \times \dfrac{1 \text{ kg}}{2.2 \text{ lb}} \times 185 \text{ lb} = 1.68 \text{ mL} = 1.7 \text{ mL}$

12) $\text{X mL} = \dfrac{1 \text{ mL}}{10{,}000 \text{ units}} \times \dfrac{150 \text{ units}}{1 \text{ kg}} \times \dfrac{1 \text{ kg}}{2.2 \text{ lb}} \times 133 \text{ lb} = 0.906 \text{ mL} = 0.91 \text{ mL}$

13) $\text{X mL} = \dfrac{1 \text{ mL}}{2 \text{ mg}} \times \dfrac{1 \text{ mg}}{1{,}000 \text{ mcg}} \times \dfrac{50 \text{ mcg}}{1 \text{ kg}} \times \dfrac{1 \text{ kg}}{2.2 \text{ lb}} \times 27 \text{ lb} = 0.3 \text{ mL}$

15) $\text{X mL} = \dfrac{1 \text{ mL}}{0.2 \text{ mg}} \times \dfrac{1 \text{ mg}}{1{,}000 \text{ mcg}} \times 150 \text{ mcg} = 0.75 \text{ mL}$

17) $\text{X mL} = \dfrac{1 \text{ mL}}{2 \text{ mg}} \times \dfrac{1 \text{ mg}}{1{,}000 \text{ mcg}} \times \dfrac{80 \text{ mcg}}{1 \text{ kg}} \times 80 \text{ kg} = 3.2 \text{ mL}$

19) $\text{X mL} = \dfrac{5 \text{ mL}}{375 \text{ mg}} \times \dfrac{990 \text{ mg}}{1 \text{ day}} \times \dfrac{1 \text{ day}}{24 \text{ h}} \times 8 \text{ h} = 4.4 \text{ mL (per dose)}$

Practice Problems—Chapter 13 from pages 311–314

1) 45 **2)** 2 **3)** 2 **4)** $\dfrac{1}{2}$ **5)** 2.5 **6)** 16 **7)** 1.4 **8)** 0.7 **9)** 2.3 **10)** 0.13 (measured in a 1 mL syringe) **11)** 1.6 **12)** 1.5

13) 1.3 **14)** 2.5 **15)** 1.6 **16)** 7.5 **17)** 1.6 **18)** 2 **19)** 8 **20)** 4.5 **21)** 30 **22)** 1.4 **23)** 0.4 **24)** 20 **25)** 12

26) **Prevention:** This type of calculation error occurred because the nurse set up the formula incorrectly. In this

instance the nurse placed the *have-on-hand dosage* (H) in the numerator and the *desired dosage* (D) in the denominator.

The *desired dosage* should be in the numerator and the *dosage you have on hand* should be placed in the denominator.

$\dfrac{\text{D (desired)}}{\text{H (have)}} \times \text{Q (quantity)} = \times \text{(amount)}$

$\dfrac{D}{H} \times Q = \dfrac{50 \text{ mg}}{125 \text{ mg}} \times 5 \text{ mL} = \dfrac{\overset{2}{\cancel{250}}}{\underset{1}{\cancel{125}}} \text{ mL} = \dfrac{2}{1} \text{ mL} = 2 \text{ mL}$

In addition, **think first.** Then use the $\dfrac{D}{H} \times Q$ formula to calculate the dosage.

Solutions—Practice Problems—Chapter 13

1) Formula Method

Order: 30 g = 30.00 g

Supply: 3.33 g per 5 mL

$$\frac{D}{H} \times Q = \frac{30.00 \text{ g}}{3.33 \text{ g}} \times 5 \text{ mL} = 45 \text{ mL}$$

Dimensional Analysis

$$\text{X mL} = \frac{5 \text{ mL}}{3.33 \text{ g}} \times 30 \text{ g} = 45 \text{ mL}$$

2) Formula Method

Order: 500,000 units

Supply: 5,000,000 units per 20 mL

$$\frac{D}{H} \times Q = \frac{\overset{1}{500,000 \text{ units}}}{\underset{10}{5,000,000 \text{ units}}} \times 20 \text{ mL} = \frac{20}{10} \text{ mL} = 2 \text{ mL}$$

Dimensional Analysis

$$\text{X mL} = \frac{20 \text{ mL}}{5,000,000 \text{ units}} \times 500,000 \text{ units} = 2 \text{ mL}$$

6) Formula Method

Order: 40 mg

Supply: 12.5 mg per 5 mL

$$\frac{D}{H} \times Q = \frac{40 \text{ mg}}{12.5 \text{ mg}} \times 5 \text{ mL} = \frac{200}{12.5} \text{ mL} = 16 \text{ mL}$$

Dimensional Analysis

$$\text{X mL} = \frac{5 \text{ mL}}{12.5 \text{ mg}} \times 40 \text{ mg} = 16 \text{ mL}$$

7) Formula Method

Order: 350,000 units

Supply: 500,000 units per 2 mL

$$\frac{D}{H} \times Q = \frac{350,000 \text{ units}}{500,000 \text{ units}} \times 2 \text{ mL} = \frac{14}{10} \text{ mL} = 1.4 \text{ mL}$$

Dimensional Analysis

$$\text{X mL} = \frac{2 \text{ mL}}{500,000 \text{ units}} \times 350,000 \text{ units} = 1.4 \text{ mL}$$

8) Formula Method

Order: 3.5 mg

Supply: 10 mg per 2 mL

$$\frac{D}{H} \times Q = \frac{3.5 \text{ mg}}{10 \text{ mg}} \times 2 \text{ mL} = \frac{7}{10} \text{ mL} = 0.7 \text{ mL}$$

Dimensional Analysis

$$\text{X mL} = \frac{2 \text{ mL}}{10 \text{ mg}} \times 3.5 \text{ mg} = 0.7 \text{ mL}$$

9) Formula Method

Order: 90 mg

Supply: 80 mg per 2 mL

$$\frac{D}{H} \times Q = \frac{90 \text{ mg}}{80 \text{ mg}} \times 2 \text{ mL} = \frac{180}{80} \text{ mL} = 2.25 \text{ mL} = 2.3 \text{ mL}$$

Dimensional Analysis

$$\text{X mL} = \frac{2 \text{ mL}}{80 \text{ mg}} \times 90 \text{ mg} = 2.25 \text{ mL} = 2.3 \text{ mL}$$

13) Formula Method

Order: 500 mg

Supply: 1 g per 2.5 mL = 1,000 mg per 2.5 mL

$$\frac{D}{H} \times Q = \frac{\overset{1}{500 \text{ mg}}}{\underset{2}{1,000 \text{ mg}}} \times 2.5 \text{ mL} = \frac{2.5}{2} \text{ mL} = 1.25 \text{ mL} = 1.3 \text{ mL}$$

Dimensional Analysis

$$\text{X mL} = \frac{2.5 \text{ mL}}{1 \text{ g}} \times \frac{1 \text{ g}}{1,000 \text{ mg}} \times 500 \text{ mg} = 1.25 \text{ mL} = 1.3 \text{ mL}$$

16) Formula Method

Order: 10 mEq

Supply: 20 mEq per 15 mL

$$\frac{D}{H} \times Q = \frac{\overset{1}{10 \text{ mEq}}}{\underset{2}{20 \text{ mEq}}} \times 15 \text{ mL} = \frac{15}{2} \text{ mL} = 7.5 \text{ mL}$$

Dimensional Analysis

$$\text{X mL} = \frac{15 \text{ mL}}{20 \text{ mEq}} \times 10 \text{ mEq} = 7.5 \text{ mL}$$

18) Formula Method

Order: 150 mcg

Supply: 0.075 mg/tab

mg $\rightarrow$ mcg; Larger $\downarrow$ Smaller $\rightarrow$ $(\times)$

0.075. mg = 75 mcg

$$\frac{D}{H} \times Q = \frac{\overset{2}{150 \text{ mcg}}}{\underset{1}{75 \text{ mcg}}} \times 1 \text{ tab} = 2 \text{ tab}$$

Dimensional Analysis

$$\text{X tab} = \frac{1 \text{ tab}}{0.075 \text{ mg}} \times \frac{1 \text{ mg}}{1,000 \text{ mcg}} \times 150 \text{ mcg} = \frac{150}{75} = 2 \text{ tab}$$

Review Set 31 from pages 330–335

1) 25; 312.5; 78.1; 625; 156.3; Yes **2)** 10 **3)** 2.2; 110; 55; Yes **4)** 0.55 **5)** 15; 120; Yes **6)** 6; 8 **7)** 32; 320; 480; Yes

8) 15 **9)** 20; 500; 125; 1,000; 250; Yes **10)** 5 **11)** 5; 7.5; 9.5; Yes

12) 0.8

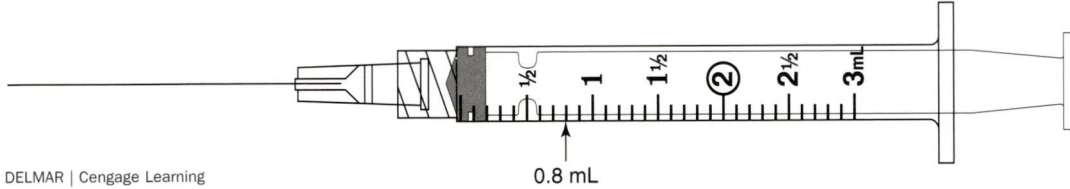

0.8 mL

DELMAR | Cengage Learning

13)   3.4; 51; 17; No

14)   The dosage of Kantrex 34 mg IV q.8h is higher than the recommended dosage. Therefore, the ordered dosage is not safe. The prescribing practitioner should be called and the order questioned.

15)   120; 60; 7.5; Yes

16)   7.5; $1\frac{1}{2}$

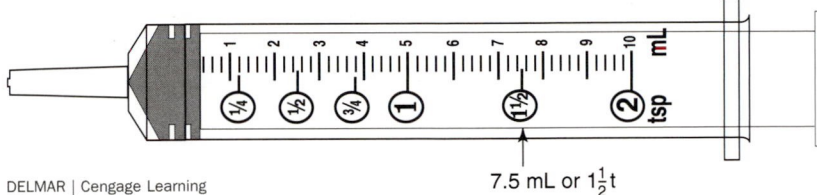

7.5 mL or $1\frac{1}{2}$t

DELMAR | Cengage Learning

17)   1.8; 4.5; No

18)   The ordered dosage is too high and ordered to be given too frequently. The recommended dosage is 4.5 mg q.12h. The ordered dosage is 40 mg q.8h. The prescribing practitioner should be notified and the order questioned.

19)   32.7; 818; 205; 1,635; 409; Yes

20)   1.6

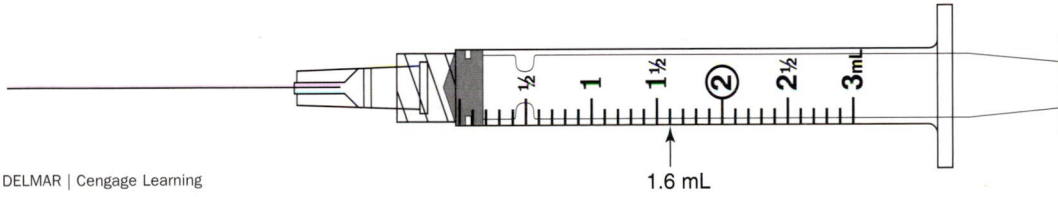

1.6 mL

DELMAR | Cengage Learning

21)   17.7; 354; 118; 708; 236; No

22)   The dosage ordered of 100 mg q.8h does not fall within the recommended dosage range of 118 to 236 mg/dose. It is an underdosage and would not produce a therapeutic effect. The physician should be called for clarification.

23)   25; 375; 125; 625; 208.3; No

24)   The ordered dosage of 100 mg q.8h does not fall within the recommended dosage range of 125 to 208.3 mg q.8h. It is an underdosage and the physician should be called for clarification.

25)   No, the ordered dosage is not safe. The label states a maximum of 250 mg per single daily injection for children older than 8 years of age. This child is only 7 and the order exceeds the maximum recommended dosage. The physician should be called to clarify the order.

26)   1 to 1.7 mg/kg IM/IV q.8h

27)   5 to 7 mg/kg IV q.24h

28)   59; 100

29)   296; 414

30)   Yes

Solutions—Review Set 31

1)

$$\frac{1 \text{ kg}}{2.2 \text{ lb}} \diagdown \frac{X \text{ kg}}{55 \text{ lb}}$$

$$2.2X = 55$$

$$\frac{2.2X}{2.2} = \frac{55}{2.2}$$

$$X = 25 \text{ kg}$$

Minimum daily dose: 12.5 mg/kg/day × 25 kg =

312.5 mg/day, or:

$$\frac{1 \text{ kg}}{12.5 \text{ mg}} \diagdown \frac{25 \text{ kg}}{X \text{ mg}}$$

$$X = 312.5 \text{ mg/day}$$

312.5 mg ÷ 4 doses = 78.12 mg/dose = 78.1 mg/dose

Maximum daily dose:

25 mg/kg/day × 25 kg = 625 mg/day or

$$\frac{1 \text{ kg}}{25 \text{ mg}} \diagdown \frac{25 \text{ kg}}{X \text{ mg}}$$

$$X = 625 \text{ mg/day}$$

625 mg ÷ 4 doses = 156.25 mg/dose = 156.3 mg/dose

Yes, dosage is safe.

2)

$$\frac{62.5 \text{ mg}}{5 \text{ mL}} \diagdown \frac{125 \text{ mg}}{X \text{ mL}}$$

$$62.5X = 625$$

$$\frac{62.5X}{62.5} = \frac{625}{62.5}$$

$$X = 10 \text{ mL}$$

3)

$$\frac{1 \text{ kg}}{1,000 \text{ g}} \diagdown \frac{X \text{ kg}}{2,200 \text{ g}}$$

$$1,000X = 2,200$$

$$\frac{1,000X}{1,000} = \frac{2,200}{1,000}$$

$$X = 2.2 \text{ kg}$$

Dose: 50 mg/kg/day × 2.2 kg = 110 mg/day, or:

$$\frac{1 \text{ kg}}{50 \text{ mg}} \diagdown \frac{2.2 \text{ kg}}{X \text{ mg}}$$

$$X = 110 \text{ mg (per day)}$$

110 mg ÷ 2 doses = 55 mg dose

Yes, dosage is safe.

4)

$$\frac{1,000 \text{ mg}}{10 \text{ mL}} \diagdown \frac{55 \text{ mg}}{X \text{ mL}}$$

$$1,000X = 550$$

$$\frac{1,000X}{1,000} = \frac{550}{1,000}$$

$$X = 0.55 \text{ mL}$$

6)

$$\frac{100 \text{ mg}}{5 \text{ mL}} \diagdown \frac{120 \text{ mg}}{X \text{ mL}}$$

$$100X = 600$$

$$\frac{100X}{100} = \frac{600}{100}$$

$$X = 6 \text{ mL}$$

50 mL ÷ 6 mL dose = 8.3 doses or 8 full doses

7) Minimum dose: 10 mg/kg/dose × 32 kg =

320 mg/dose, or:

$$\frac{1 \text{ kg}}{10 \text{ mg}} \diagdown \frac{32 \text{ kg}}{X \text{ mg}}$$

$$X = 320 \text{ mg (per dose)}$$

Maximum dose:

15 mg/kg/dose × 32 kg = 480 mg/dose, or:

$$\frac{1 \text{ kg}}{15 \text{ mg}} \diagdown \frac{32 \text{ kg}}{X \text{ mg}}$$

$$X = 480 \text{ mg (per dose)}$$

Dosage is the *maximum* dosage (480 mg) and is safe.

8)

$$\frac{160 \text{ mg}}{5 \text{ mL}} \diagdown \frac{480 \text{ mg}}{X \text{ mL}}$$

$$160X = 2,400$$

$$\frac{160X}{160} = \frac{2,400}{160}$$

$$X = 15 \text{ mL}$$

13)

$$\frac{1 \text{ lb}}{16 \text{ oz}} \diagdown \frac{X \text{ lb}}{8 \text{ oz}}$$

$$16X = 8$$

$$\frac{16X}{16} = \frac{8}{16}$$

$$X = \frac{1}{2} \text{ lb}$$

7 lb 8 oz = $7\frac{1}{2}$ lb

$$\frac{1 \text{ kg}}{2.2 \text{ lb}} \diagdown \frac{X \text{ kg}}{7.5 \text{ lb}}$$

$$2.2X = 7.5$$

$$\frac{2.2X}{2.2} = \frac{7.5}{2.2}$$

$$X = 3.40 \text{ kg} = 3.4 \text{ kg}$$

15 mg/kg/day × 3.4 kg = 51 mg/day, or:

$$\frac{1 \text{ kg}}{15 \text{ mg}} \diagdown \frac{3.4 \text{ kg}}{X \text{ mg}}$$

$$X = 51 \text{ mg (per day)}$$

51 mg ÷ 3 doses = 17 mg/dose, if administered q.8h

Ordered dosage of 34 mg q.8h exceeds

recommended dosage and is not safe.

19)

$$\frac{1 \text{ kg}}{2.2 \text{ lb}} \diagdown \frac{X \text{ kg}}{72 \text{ lb}}$$

$$2.2X = 72$$

$$\frac{2.2X}{2.2} = \frac{72}{2.2}$$

$$X = 32.72 \text{ kg} = 32.7 \text{ kg}$$

Minimum daily dosage:

25 mg/kg/day × 32.7 kg = 817.5 mg/day =

818 mg/day; or

$$\frac{25 \text{ mg/day}}{1 \text{ kg}} = \frac{X \text{ mg/day}}{32.7 \text{ kg}}$$

$$X = 817.5 \text{ mg/day} = 818 \text{ mg/day}$$

Minimum single dosage:

818 mg ÷ 4 doses = 204.5 mg/dose = 205 mg/dose

Maximum daily dosage:

50 mg/k̶g̶/day × 32.7 k̶g̶ = 1,635 mg/day; or

$$\frac{50 \text{ mg/day}}{1 \text{ kg}} = \frac{X \text{ mg/day}}{32.7 \text{ kg}}$$

$$X = 1,635 \text{ mg/day}$$

Maximum single dosage:

1,635 mg ÷ 4 doses = 408.7 mg/dose = 409 mg/dose

Yes, dosage is safe.

20) Order: 400 mg

Supply: 250 mg/mL

$$\frac{250 \text{ mg}}{1 \text{ mL}} \diagdown \frac{400 \text{ mg}}{X \text{ mL}}$$

$$250 \text{ X} = 400$$

$$\frac{250X}{250} = \frac{400}{250}$$

$$X = 1.6 \text{ mL}$$

21) $\frac{1 \text{ kg}}{2.2 \text{ lb}} \diagup\!\!\!\!\diagdown \frac{X \text{ kg}}{39 \text{ lb}}$

$$2.2X = 39$$

$$\frac{2.2X}{2.2} = \frac{39}{2.2}$$

$$X = 17.72 \text{ kg} = 17.7 \text{ kg}$$

Minimum daily dosage:

20 mg/k̶g̶/day × 17.7 k̶g̶ = 354 mg/day, or:

$$\frac{1 \text{ kg}}{20 \text{ mg}} \diagdown\!\!\!\diagup \frac{17.7 \text{ kg}}{X \text{ mg}}$$

$$X = 354 \text{ mg (per day)}$$

Minimum single dosage: 354 mg ÷ 3 doses = 118 mg/dose

Maximum daily dosage:

40 mg/k̶g̶/day × 17.7 k̶g̶ = 708 mg/day, or:

$$\frac{1 \text{ kg}}{40 \text{ mg}} \diagup\!\!\!\!\diagdown \frac{17.7 \text{ kg}}{X \text{ mg}}$$

$$X = 708 \text{ mg (per day)}$$

Maximum single dosage:

708 mg ÷ 3 doses = 236 mg/dose

The dosage of 100 mg q.8h is not safe. It is an underdosage, and would not produce a therapeutic effect, as the recommended dosage range is 118–236 mg/dose.

28) $\frac{1 \text{ kg}}{2.2 \text{ lb}} \diagup\!\!\!\!\diagdown \frac{X \text{ kg}}{130 \text{ lb}}$

$$2.2X = 130$$

$$\frac{2.2X}{2.2} = \frac{130}{2.2}$$

$$X = 59.1 \text{ kg}$$

$$\frac{1 \text{ mg/dose}}{1 \text{ kg}} = \frac{X \text{ mg/dose}}{59.1 \text{ kg}}$$

$$X = 59.1 \text{ mg/dose}$$

$$\frac{1.7 \text{ mg/dose}}{1 \text{ kg}} = \frac{X \text{ mg/dose}}{59.1 \text{ kg}}$$

$$X = 100 \text{ mg/dose}$$

29) $\frac{5 \text{ mg/dose}}{1 \text{ kg}} \diagup\!\!\!\!\diagdown \frac{X \text{ mg/dose}}{59.1 \text{ kg}}$

$$X = 296 \text{ mg/dose}$$

$$\frac{7 \text{ mg/dose}}{1 \text{ kg}} = \frac{X \text{ mg/dose}}{59.1 \text{ kg}}$$

$$X = 413.7 \text{ mg/dose} = 414 \text{ mg/dose}$$

Practice Problems—Chapter 14 from pages 337–348

1) 5.5 **2)** 3.8 **3)** 1.6 **4)** 2.3 **5)** 15.5 **6)** 3 **7)** 23.6 **8)** 0.9 **9)** 240 **10)** 80 **11)** 19.5; 39; 48.8; Yes

12) 1

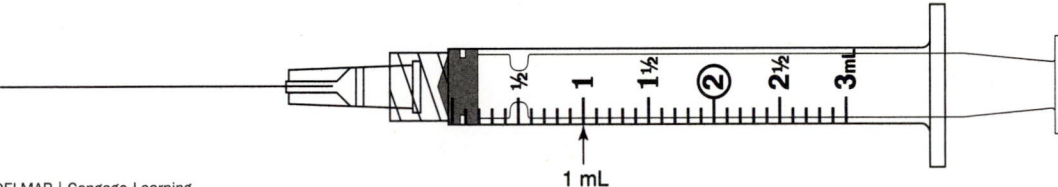

1 mL

13) 7.3; 3.7; 14.6; Yes

14) 1

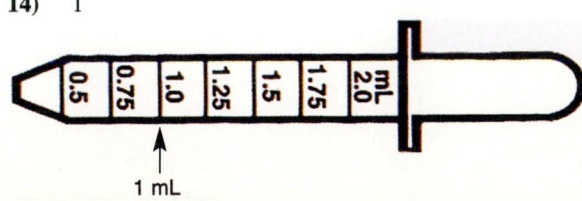

1 mL

15)   18.2; 182; 91; 364; 182; Yes

16)   7.5

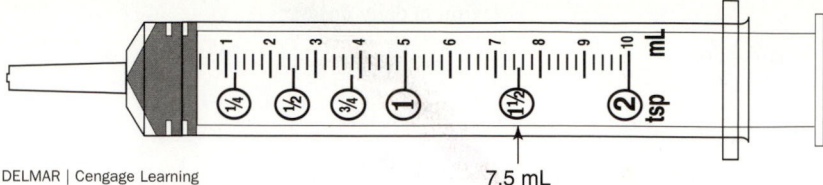

DELMAR | Cengage Learning   7.5 mL

17)   29.1; 291; 145.5; 436.5; 218.3; Yes

18)   3

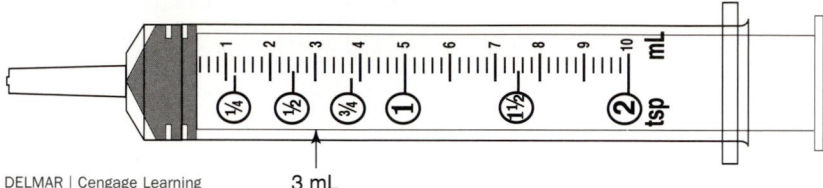

DELMAR | Cengage Learning   3 mL

19)   2.5; 125,000; 125,000; Yes

20)   18; 20; 250,000; 0.5

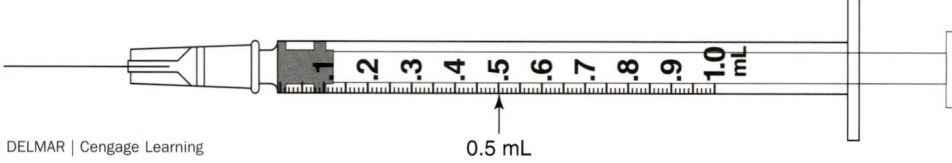

DELMAR | Cengage Learning   0.5 mL

21)   18.6; 372; 124; 744; 248; Yes

22)   6

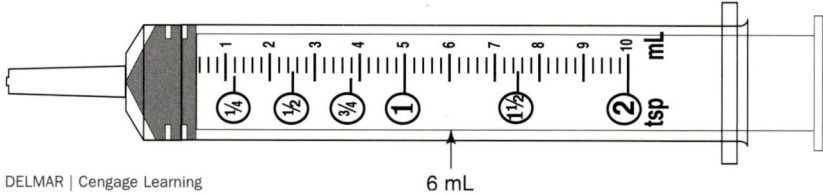

DELMAR | Cengage Learning   6 mL

23)   13.9; 556; 185.3; Yes, the ordered dosage is reasonably safe.

24)   5

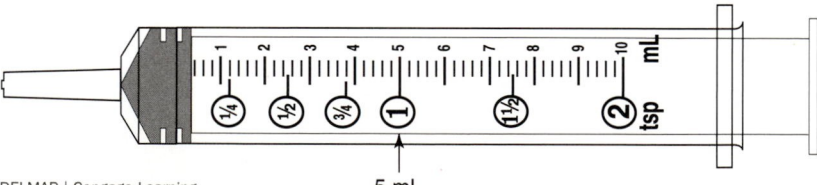

DELMAR | Cengage Learning   5 mL

25)   10; 0.1; Yes

26)   0.25

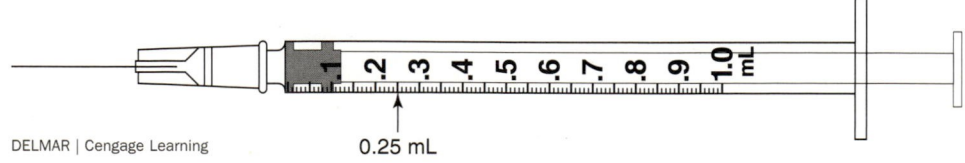

DELMAR | Cengage Learning   0.25 mL

27)   28; 35; Yes

28) 3.5

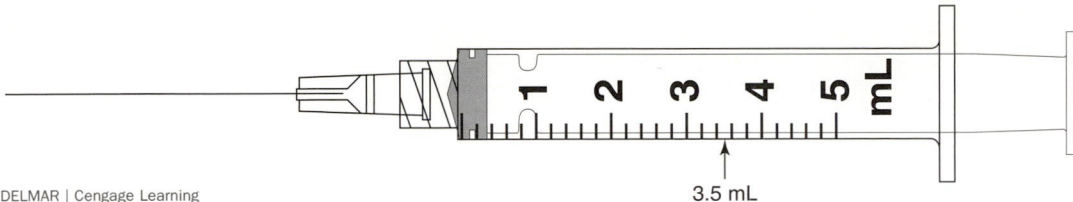

DELMAR | Cengage Learning

3.5 mL

29) 9.1; 455; 227.5; 682.5; 341.3; No

30) The ordered dosage of 1 g is not safe. The recommended dosage range for a child of this weight is 227.5 to 341.3 mg/dose. Physician should be called for clarification.

31) 25.1; 0.05; Yes

32) 0.25

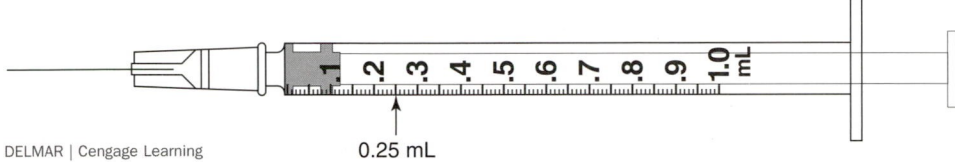

DELMAR | Cengage Learning

0.25 mL

Route is IM; may need to change needle to appropriate gauge and length.

33) 8.2; 1,200; 1.2; 410; 615; Yes

34) 9.6; 10; 100; 6

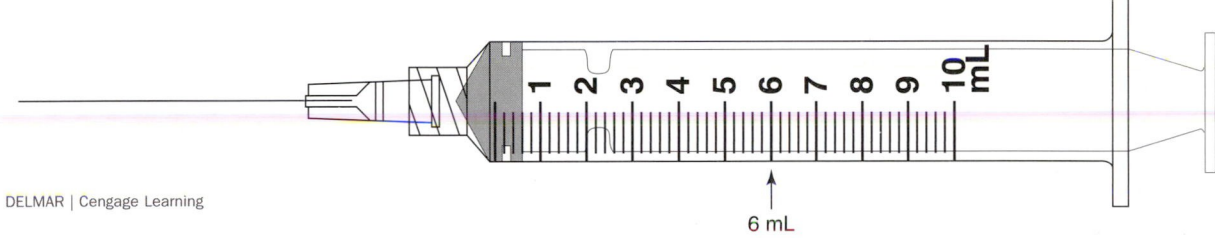

DELMAR | Cengage Learning

6 mL

35) 20.5; 512.5; 256.3; No

36) The dosage ordered is not safe. It is too low compared to the recommended dosage. Call the prescriber and clarify the order.

37) 8.2; 164; 54.7; No

38) Dosage ordered is not safe. Call prescriber for clarification because ordered dosage is higher than the recommended dosage.

39) 20.5; 200; 400; No

40) Dosage ordered is not safe based on recommended maximum daily dosage and on the frequency of the order. Call prescriber for clarification.

41) 23.2; 348; 174; Yes, dosage is reasonably safe.

42) 3.5

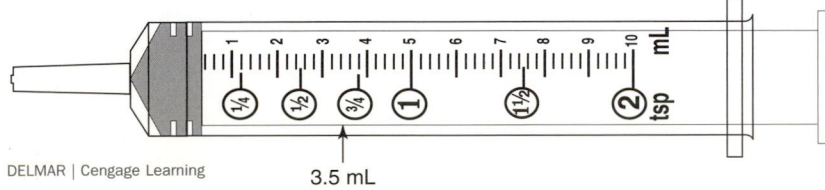

DELMAR | Cengage Learning

3.5 mL

43)   0.25

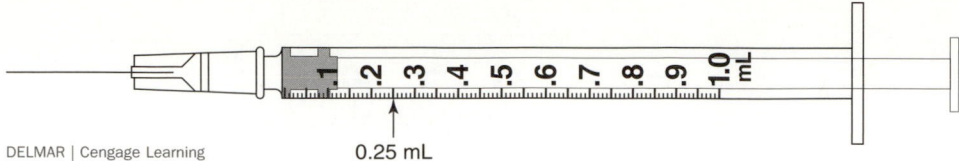

DELMAR | Cengage Learning   0.25 mL

44)   3.5

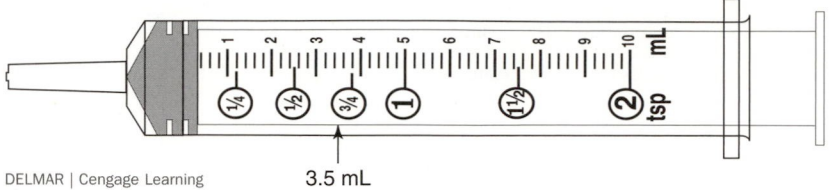

DELMAR | Cengage Learning   3.5 mL

45)   500,000; 0.9

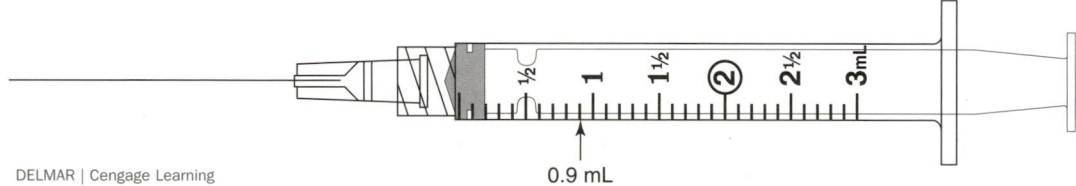

DELMAR | Cengage Learning   0.9 mL

46)   Dosage is not safe; this child is ordered a total of 2 mg/day, which is too high. Prescriber should be called to clarify.

47)   The ordered dosage of 1 mg IM stat is too high when compared to the recommended dosage range for a child of this weight. The order should be clarified with the prescriber.

48)   0.76; Route is IM; needle may need to be changed to appropriate gauge and length.

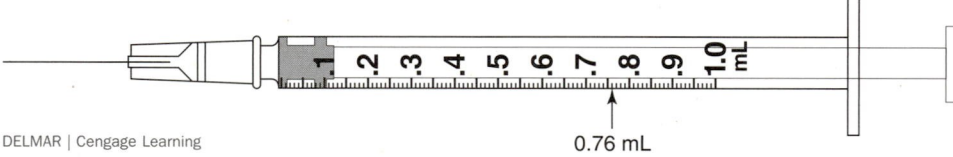

DELMAR | Cengage Learning   0.76 mL

49)   #45 (penicillin G potassium) and #48 (cefazolin). (Note: #43 methylprednisolone is a single-dose vial. Check package insert to determine if storage after mixing is safe.)

50)   **Prevention:** The child should have received 75 mg a day and no more than 25 mg per dose. The child received more than four times the safe dosage of tobramycin. Had the nurse calculated the safe dosage, the error would have been caught sooner, the resident would have been consulted, and the dosage could have been adjusted before the child ever received the first dose. The pharmacist also should have caught the error but did not. In this scenario the resident, pharmacist, and nurse all committed medication errors. If the resident had not noticed the error, one can only wonder how many doses the child would have received. The nurse is the last safety net for the child when it comes to a dosage error because the nurse administers the drug.

In addition, the nurse has to reconcile the fact that she actually gave the overdose. The nurse is responsible for whatever dosage is administered and must verify the safety of the order and the patient's Six Rights. We are all accountable for our actions. Taking shortcuts in administering medications to children can be disastrous. The time the nurse saved by not calculating the safe dosage was more than lost in the extra monitoring, not to mention the cost of follow-up to the medication error, and *most importantly*, the risk to the child.

Solutions—Practice Problems—Chapter 14

1) $\dfrac{1 \text{ kg}}{2.2 \text{ lb}} \diagdown \dfrac{X \text{ kg}}{12 \text{ lb}}$

$2.2X = 12$

$\dfrac{2.2X}{2.2} = \dfrac{12}{2.2}$

$X = 5.45 \text{ kg} = 5.5 \text{ kg}$

2) $8 \text{ lb } 4 \text{ oz} = 8\dfrac{4}{16} \text{ lb} = 8\dfrac{1}{4} \text{ lb} = 8.25 \text{ lb}$

$\dfrac{1 \text{ kg}}{2.2 \text{ lb}} \diagdown \dfrac{X \text{ kg}}{8.25 \text{ lb}}$

$2.2X = 8.25$

$\dfrac{2.2X}{2.2} = \dfrac{8.25}{2.2}$

$X = 3.75 \text{ kg} = 3.8 \text{ kg}$

3) $\dfrac{1 \text{ kg}}{1,000 \text{ g}} \diagdown \dfrac{X \text{ kg}}{1,570 \text{ g}}$

$1,000X = 1,570$

$\dfrac{1,000X}{1,000} = \dfrac{1,570}{1,000}$

$X = 1.57 \text{ kg} = 1.6 \text{ kg}$

6) $1 \text{ lb} = 16 \text{ oz}$

$\dfrac{1 \text{ lb}}{16 \text{ oz}} \diagdown \dfrac{X \text{ lb}}{10 \text{ oz}}$

$16X = 10$

$\dfrac{16X}{16} = \dfrac{10}{16}$

$X = 0.625 \text{ lb}$

$6 \text{ lb } 10 \text{ oz} = 6.625 \text{ lb}$

$\dfrac{1 \text{ kg}}{2.2 \text{ lb}} \diagdown \dfrac{X \text{ kg}}{6.625 \text{ lb}}$

$2.2X = 6.625$

$\dfrac{2.2X}{2.2} = \dfrac{6.625}{2.2}$

$X = 3.01 \text{ kg} = 3 \text{ kg}$

17) $\dfrac{1 \text{ kg}}{2.2 \text{ lb}} \diagdown \dfrac{X \text{ kg}}{64 \text{ lb}}$

$2.2X = 64$

$\dfrac{2.2X}{2.2} = \dfrac{64}{2.2}$

$X = 29.09 \text{ kg} = 29.1 \text{ kg}$

Minimum daily dosage:

$10 \text{ mg/kg/day} \times 29.1 \text{ kg} = 291 \text{ mg/day}$, or:

$\dfrac{1 \text{ kg}}{10 \text{ mg}} \diagdown \dfrac{29.1 \text{ kg}}{X \text{ mg}}$

$X = 291 \text{ mg (per day)}$

Minimum single dose (based on b.i.d.):

$291 \text{ mg per 2 doses} = 145.5 \text{ mg/dose}$

Maximum daily dosage:

$15 \text{ mg/kg/day} \times 29.1 \text{ kg} = 436.5 \text{ mg/day}$, or:

$\dfrac{1 \text{ kg}}{15 \text{ mg}} \diagdown \dfrac{29.1 \text{ kg}}{X \text{ mg}}$

$X = 436.5 \text{ mg (per day)}$

Maximum single dose (based on b.i.d.):

$436.5 \text{ mg} \div 2 \text{ doses} = 218.25 \text{ mg/dose} =$

218.3 mg/dose

Dosage ordered is safe. Child will receive 300 mg in a 24-hour period in divided doses of 150 mg b.i.d. This falls within the recommended dosage range of 145.5–218.3 mg/dose and does not exceed the maximum recommended single-dosage allowance of 250 mg/dose.

18) $\dfrac{250 \text{ mg}}{5 \text{ mL}} \diagdown \dfrac{150 \text{ mg}}{X \text{ mL}}$

$250X = 750$

$\dfrac{250X}{250} = \dfrac{750}{250}$

$X = 3 \text{ mL}$

19) $\dfrac{1 \text{ kg}}{1,000 \text{ g}} \diagdown \dfrac{X \text{ kg}}{2,500 \text{ g}}$

$1,000X = 2,500$

$\dfrac{1,000X}{1,000} = \dfrac{2,500}{1,000}$

$X = 2.5 \text{ kg}$

Recommended daily dosage:

$50,000 \text{ units/kg/day} \times 2.5 \text{ kg} = 125,000 \text{ units/day}$, or:

$\dfrac{1 \text{ kg}}{50,000 \text{ units}} \diagdown \dfrac{2.5 \text{ kg}}{X \text{ units}}$

$X = 50,000 \times 2.5$

$X = 125,000 \text{ units (per day)}$

Recommended daily and single dosage:

$125,000 \text{ units/dose}$

Ordered dose is safe.

20) Select 250,000 units/mL concentration because the amount to give will be an exact measurement in the 1 mL syringe; this will require you to add 18 mL of diluent.

Solution volume:

$\dfrac{1 \text{ mL}}{250,000 \text{ units}} \diagdown \dfrac{X \text{ mL}}{5,000,000 \text{ units}}$

$250,000X = 5,000,000$

$\dfrac{250,000X}{250,000} = \dfrac{5,000,000}{250,000}$

$X = 20 \text{ mL}$

23)

$$\frac{250{,}000 \text{ units}}{1 \text{ mL}} \times \frac{125{,}000 \text{ units}}{X \text{ mL}}$$

$$250{,}000X = 125{,}000$$

$$\frac{250{,}000X}{250{,}000} = \frac{125{,}000}{250{,}000}$$

$$X = 0.5 \text{ mL}$$

23)

$$\frac{1 \text{ kg}}{2.2 \text{ lb}} \times \frac{X \text{ kg}}{30.5 \text{ lb}}$$

$$2.2X = 30.5$$

$$\frac{2.2X}{2.2} = \frac{30.5}{2.2}$$

$$X = 13.86 \text{ kg} = 13.9 \text{ kg}$$

Recommended daily dosage:

40 mg/kg/day × 13.9 kg = 556 mg/day, or:

$$\frac{1 \text{ kg}}{40 \text{ mg}} \times \frac{13.9 \text{ kg}}{X \text{ mg}}$$

$$X = 556 \text{ mg (per day)}$$

Recommended single dosage:

556 mg ÷ 3 doses = 185.336 mg = 185.3 mg

The ordered dosage of 187 mg p.o. is reasonably

safe for this child.

24)   Order: 187 mg

Supply: 187 mg per 5 mL

Think: It is obvious that you want to give 5 mL.

$$\frac{187 \text{ mg}}{5 \text{ mL}} \times \frac{187 \text{ mg}}{X \text{ mL}}$$

$$187X = 935$$

$$\frac{187X}{187} = \frac{935}{187}$$

$$X = 5 \text{ mL}$$

If we use the exact recommended single dosage of

185.3 mg/dose, the calculation would be:

$$\frac{187 \text{ mg}}{5 \text{ mL}} \times \frac{185.3 \text{ mg}}{X \text{ mL}}$$

$$187X = 926.5$$

$$\frac{187X}{187} = \frac{926.5}{187}$$

X = 4.95 mL; which we would round up to 5 mL to

measure in the pediatric oral syringe; therefore, as

stated above, the ordered dosage is reasonably safe.

25)

$$\frac{1 \text{ kg}}{2.2 \text{ lb}} \times \frac{X \text{ kg}}{22 \text{ lb}}$$

$$2.2X = 22$$

$$\frac{2.2X}{2.2} = \frac{22}{2.2}$$

$$X = 10 \text{ kg}$$

0.01 mg/kg/dose × 10 kg = 0.1 mg/dose, or:

$$\frac{1 \text{ kg}}{10 \text{ mg}} \times \frac{0.01 \text{ kg}}{X \text{ mg}}$$

$$X = 0.1 \text{ mg/dose}$$

$$\frac{1 \text{ mg}}{1{,}000 \text{ mcg}} \times \frac{0.1 \text{ mg}}{X \text{ mcg}}$$

$$X = 100 \text{ mcg}$$

Ordered dose is safe.

29)

$$\frac{1 \text{ kg}}{2.2 \text{ lb}} \times \frac{X \text{ kg}}{20 \text{ lb}}$$

$$2.2X = 20$$

$$\frac{2.2X}{2.2} = \frac{20}{2.2}$$

$$X = 9.09 \text{ kg} = 9.1 \text{ kg}$$

Recommended minimum daily dosage:

50 mg/kg/day × 9.1 kg = 455 mg/day, or:

$$\frac{1 \text{ kg}}{50 \text{ mg}} \times \frac{9.1 \text{ kg}}{X \text{ mg}}$$

$$X = 455 \text{ mg (per day)}$$

Recommended minimum single dosage:

455 mg ÷ 2 doses = 227.5 mg/dose

Recommended maximum daily dosage:

75 mg/kg/day × 9.1 kg = 682.5 mg/day, or:

$$\frac{1 \text{ kg}}{75 \text{ mg}} \times \frac{9.1 \text{ kg}}{X \text{ mg}}$$

$$X = 682.5 \text{ mg/day}$$

Maximum single dosage:

682.5 mg ÷ 2 doses = 341.25 mg = 341.3 mg/dose

The dosage ordered (1 g q.12 h) is not safe. The

recommended range for a child of this weight is

227.5–341.3 mg/dose. Physician should be called for

clarification.

41)

$$\frac{1 \text{ kg}}{2.2 \text{ lb}} \times \frac{X \text{ kg}}{51 \text{ lb}}$$

$$2.2X = 51$$

$$\frac{2.2X}{2.2} = \frac{51}{2.2}$$

$$X = 23.18 \text{ kg} = 23.2 \text{ kg}$$

Recommended daily dosage:

15 mg/kg/day × 23.2 kg = 348 mg/day, or:

$$\frac{1 \text{ kg}}{15 \text{ mg}} \times \frac{23.2 \text{ kg}}{X \text{ mg}}$$

$$X = 348 \text{ mg (per day)}$$

Recommended single dosage:

348 mg ÷ 2 doses = 174 mg/dose

Ordered dosage of 175 mg is reasonably safe as an

oral medication and should be given.

43)

$$\frac{1 \text{ kg}}{2.2 \text{ lb}} \times \frac{X \text{ kg}}{95 \text{ lb}}$$

$$2.2X = 95$$

$$\frac{2.2X}{2.2} = \frac{95}{2.2}$$

$$X = 43.18 \text{ kg} = 43.2 \text{ kg}$$

$$0.5 \text{ mg/kg/day} \times 43.2 \text{ kg} = 21.6 \text{ mg/day, or:}$$

$$\frac{1 \text{ kg}}{0.5 \text{ mg}} \times \frac{43.2 \text{ kg}}{X \text{ mg}}$$

$$X = 21.6 \text{ mg (per day)}$$

Because the recommended dosage is not less than

21.6 mg/day and the order is for 10 mg q.6h for a

total of 40 mg/day, the order is safe.

$$\frac{40 \text{ mg}}{1 \text{ mL}} \times \frac{10 \text{ mg}}{X \text{ mL}}$$

$$40X = 10$$

$$\frac{40X}{40} = \frac{10}{40}$$

$$X = 0.25 \text{ mL}$$

Section 3—Self-Evaluation from pages 349–360

1) C; 2 **2)** F; 1 **3)** J; 1 **4)** B; 2 **5)** H; 12 **6)** I; 2 **7)** E; 2 **8)** K; $\frac{1}{2}$ **9)** M; 1.25 **10)** L; 7.5 **11)** E; 4 **12)** C; 3.5

13) G; 0.2 **14)** A; 0.8 **15)** D; 1.5 **16)** F; 0.75 **17)** B; 0.6 **18)** H; 0.75

19)

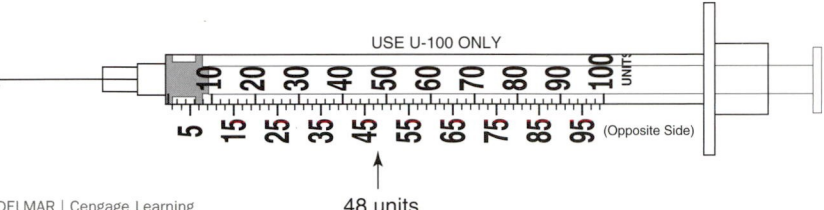

DELMAR | Cengage Learning

48 units

20)

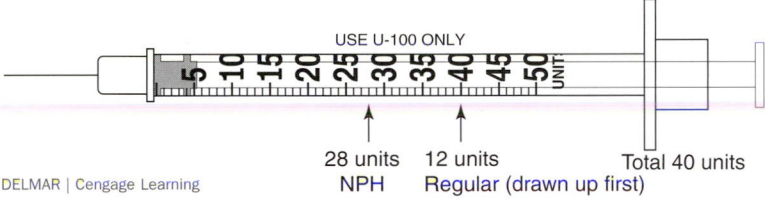

DELMAR | Cengage Learning

28 units   12 units   Total 40 units
NPH   Regular (drawn up first)

21)   4.8; 5; 100; 5

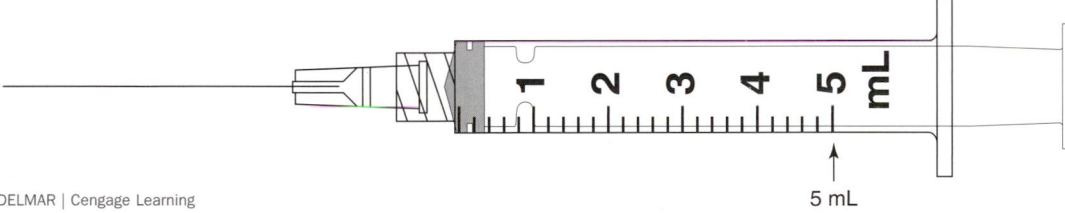

DELMAR | Cengage Learning

5 mL

22)   10; 10; 500 per 10; 8; 1

DELMAR | Cengage Learning

2/6/xx, 0800, reconstituted as 500 mg per 10 mL. Expires 2/10/xx, 0800. Keep refrigerated. G.D.P.

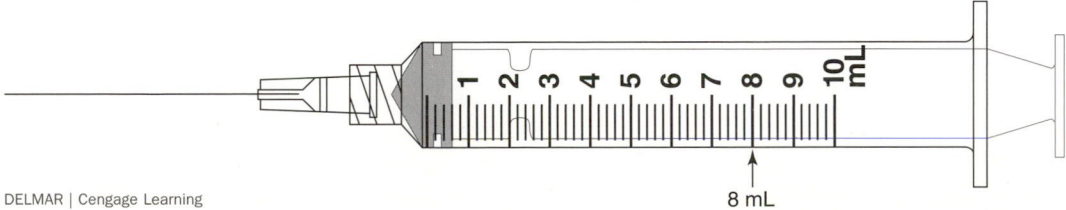

DELMAR | Cengage Learning

8 mL

23)   2.4; 2.5; 100; 1.5

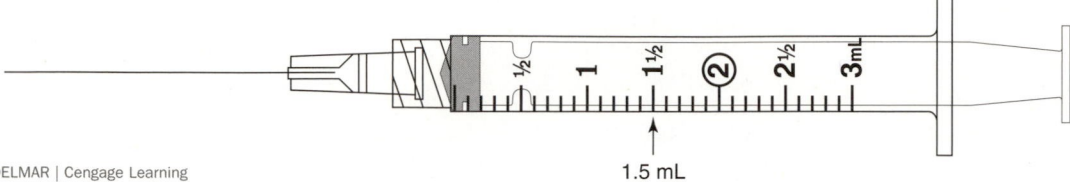

2/6/xx, 0800, reconstituted as
100 mg/mL. Expires 2/9/xx, 0800. Keep
refrigerated. G.D.P.

DELMAR | Cengage Learning

DELMAR | Cengage Learning

1.5 mL

24)   2.5; 3; 330; 2.3

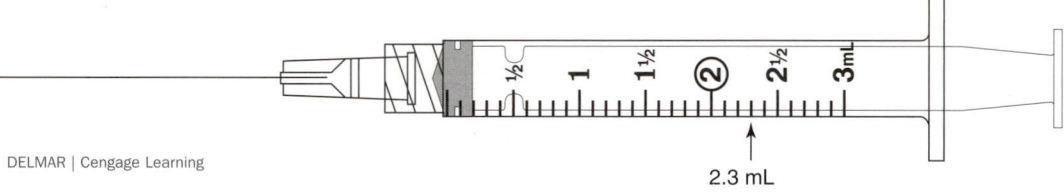

2/6/xx, 0800, reconstituted as
330 mg/mL. Expires 2/7/xx, 0800.
Store at room temperature. G.D.P.

DELMAR | Cengage Learning

DELMAR | Cengage Learning

2.3 mL

25)   8; 8; 62.5; 4; 2

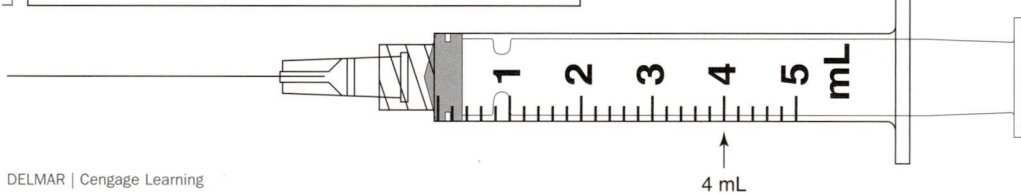

2/6/xx, 0800, reconstituted as
62.5 mg/mL. Expires 2/8/xx, 0800. Keep
at controlled room temperature 20–25°C
(66-77°F). G.D.P.

DELMAR | Cengage Learning

DELMAR | Cengage Learning

4 mL

26)   29; 50; 100 per 5; 20; 5

2/6/xx, 0800, reconstituted as
100 mg per 5 mL. Expires 2/20/xx, 0800.
Keep refrigerated. G.D.P.

DELMAR | Cengage Learning

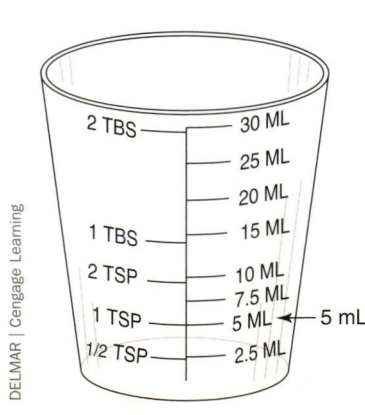

5 mL

DELMAR | Cengage Learning

27)   10

28)   No; the medication supplied will be used up before it expires. It is good for 14 days under refrigeration. The medication is to be given every 12 hours; therefore 10 doses will be administered in 5 days.

29) 120; 240 **30)** 180; 60 **31)** 120 **32)** 1 **33)** 3 **34)** 540 **35)** $\frac{1}{4}$, gr i = 60 mg **36)** 52.3, 1 kg = 2.2 lb **37)** 625,000, 1 mg = 1,000 mcg **38)** 300, 1 g = 1,000 mg **39)** 7 **40)** 1.5 **41)** 10 **42)** 2 **43)** 3 **44)** 3.8

45)   0.75

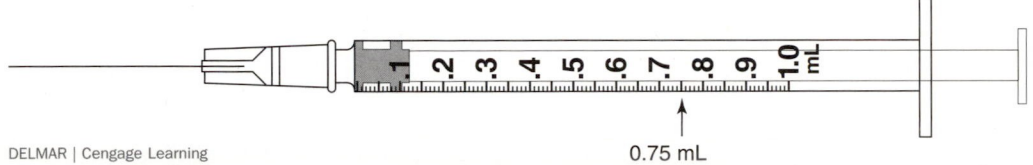

DELMAR | Cengage Learning

0.75 mL

46)   113; 150; 25; 3

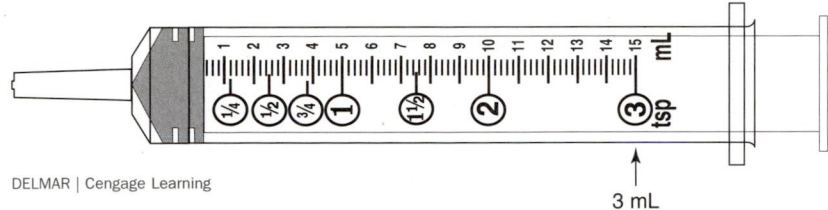

DELMAR | Cengage Learning

3 mL

47)   Order of 100 mg t.i.d. is too high and the maximum recommended dosage is 100 mg/day for this child. The order is not safe. Physician should be called for clarification.

48)   Order is too high and the maximum recommended dosage for this child is 292 mg/day. This order would deliver 748 mg/day. Recommended dosage is also 3 times daily and this order is for 4 times/day. This order is not safe. Physician should be called for clarification.

49)   **(a)** Order is too high and is not safe. Recommended dosage is 109.5 mg/day or 36.5 mg/dose. Physician should be called for clarification.

   (b) 500

50)   **Prevention:** This type of calculation error occurred because the nurse set up the ratio and proportion incorrectly. In this instance the nurse mixed up the values for desired dosage and the dosage on hand.

$$\frac{125 \text{ mg}}{5 \text{ mL}} \times \frac{50 \text{ mg}}{X \text{ mL}}$$

$$125X = 250$$

$$\frac{125X}{125} = \frac{250}{125}$$

$$X = 2 \text{ mL}$$

In addition, **think first.** Then use ratio-proportion to calculate the dosage.

Solutions—Section 3—Self-Evaluation

5) $$\frac{20 \text{ mEq}}{15 \text{ mL}} \times \frac{16 \text{ mEq}}{X \text{ mL}}$$

$$20X = 240$$

$$\frac{20X}{20} = \frac{240}{20}$$

$$X = 12 \text{ mL}$$

$$\frac{25 \text{ mcg}}{1 \text{ tab}} \times \frac{50 \text{ mcg}}{X \text{ tab}}$$

$$25X = 50$$

$$\frac{25X}{25} = \frac{50}{25}$$

$$X = 2 \text{ tabs}$$

7) $$\frac{1 \text{ mg}}{1,000 \text{ mcg}} \times \frac{0.05 \text{ mg}}{X \text{ mcg}}$$

$$X = 1,000 \times 0.05$$

$$X = 50 \text{ mcg}$$

Label N (Synthroid 100 mcg) not selected because it is best to give whole tablets when possible rather than trying to split a tablet in half.

8) Order: gr $\frac{1}{4}$

$$\frac{\text{gr } 1}{60 \text{ mg}} \bowtie \frac{\text{gr } \frac{1}{4}}{\text{X mg}}$$

$$X = 15 \text{ mg}$$

Supply: 30 mg/tab

$$\frac{30 \text{ mg}}{1 \text{ tab}} \bowtie \frac{15 \text{ mg}}{\text{X tab}}$$

$$30X = 15$$

$$\frac{30X}{30} = \frac{15}{30}$$

$$X = \frac{1}{2} \text{ tab}$$

9) Order: 12.5 mg

Supply: 10 mg/mL

$$\frac{10 \text{ mg}}{1 \text{ mL}} \bowtie \frac{12.5 \text{ mg}}{\text{X mL}}$$

$$10X = 12.5$$

$$\frac{10X}{10} = \frac{12.5}{10}$$

$$X = 1.25 \text{ mL}$$

Answer should be left at 1.25 mL and not rounded as the dropper supplied with the medication will measure 1.25 mL. Notice the picture of the dropper on the label.

13) Order: 200 mcg

Supply: 1 mg/mL = 1,000 mcg/mL

$$\frac{1,000 \text{ mcg}}{1 \text{ mL}} \bowtie \frac{200 \text{ mcg}}{\text{X mL}}$$

$$1,000X = 200$$

$$\frac{1,000X}{1,000} = \frac{200}{1,000}$$

$$X = 0.2 \text{ mL}$$

17) Order: gr $\frac{1}{10}$

$$\frac{\text{gr } 1}{60 \text{ mg}} \bowtie \frac{\text{gr } \frac{1}{10}}{\text{X mg}}$$

$$X = 6 \text{ mg}$$

Supply: 10 mg/mL

$$\frac{10 \text{ mg}}{1 \text{ mL}} \bowtie \frac{6 \text{ mg}}{\text{X mL}}$$

$$10X = 6$$

$$\frac{10X}{10} = \frac{6}{10}$$

$$X = 0.6 \text{ mL}$$

22) Order: 400 mg

Supply: 500 mg per 10 mL

$$\frac{500 \text{ mg}}{10 \text{ mL}} \bowtie \frac{400 \text{ mg}}{\text{X mL}}$$

$$500X = 4,000$$

$$\frac{500X}{500} = \frac{4,000}{500}$$

$$X = 8 \text{ mL}$$

$$\frac{400 \text{ mg}}{1 \text{ dose}} \bowtie \frac{500 \text{ mg}}{\text{X dose}}$$

$$400X = 500$$

$$\frac{400X}{400} = \frac{500}{400}$$

$$X = 1.25 \text{ doses (1 full available)}$$

25) $$\frac{62.5 \text{ mg}}{1 \text{ mL}} \bowtie \frac{250 \text{ mg}}{\text{X mL}}$$

$$62.5X = 250$$

$$\frac{62.5X}{62.5} = \frac{250}{62.5}$$

$$X = 4 \text{ mL}$$

500 mg vial:

$$\frac{250 \text{ mg}}{1 \text{ dose}} \bowtie \frac{500 \text{ mg}}{\text{X dose}}$$

$$250X = 500$$

$$\frac{250X}{250} = \frac{500}{250}$$

$$X = 2 \text{ doses (available)}$$

29) $$\frac{1}{3} \bowtie \frac{\text{X mL}}{360 \text{ mL}}$$

$$3X = 360$$

$$\frac{3X}{3} = \frac{360}{3}$$

$$X = 120 \text{ mL (hydrogen peroxide)}$$

360 mL (total) − 120 mL (solute) = 240 mL (solvent)

31) $$\frac{1 \text{ fl oz}}{30 \text{ mL}} \bowtie \frac{8 \text{ fl oz}}{\text{X mL}}$$

$$X = 240 \text{ mL}$$

$$\frac{2}{3} \bowtie \frac{240 \text{ mL}}{\text{X mL}}$$

$$2X = 720$$

$$\frac{2X}{2} = \frac{720}{2}$$

$$X = 360 \text{ mL (total quantity)}$$

360 mL (total) − 240 mL (Ensure) = 120 mL (water)

33) 9 infants require 4 fl oz each; 4 fl oz × 9 = 36 fl oz total

$$\frac{1}{2} \bowtie \frac{\text{X fl oz}}{36 \text{ fl oz}}$$

$$2X = 36$$

$$\frac{2X}{2} = \frac{36}{2}$$

$$X = 18 \text{ fl oz (Isomil)}$$

$$\frac{8 \text{ fl oz}}{1 \text{ can}} \diagup\hspace{-0.9em}\diagdown \frac{18 \text{ fl oz}}{X \text{ can}}$$

$$8X = 18$$

$$\frac{8X}{8} = \frac{18}{8}$$

$$X = 2\frac{1}{4} \text{ cans (you would need to open 3 cans)}$$

34) 36 fl oz total solution − 18 fl oz solute (Isomil) =

18 fl oz solvent (water)

$$\frac{30 \text{ mL}}{1 \text{ fl oz}} \diagup\hspace{-0.9em}\diagdown \frac{X \text{ mL}}{18 \text{ fl oz}}$$

$$X = 540 \text{ mL (water)}$$

35) Equivalent: gr i = 60 mg

$$\text{mg} \rightarrow \text{gr; Smaller} \uparrow \text{Larger} \rightarrow (\div)$$

$$15 \text{ mg} \div 60 \text{ mg/gr} = \text{gr } \frac{1}{4}$$

39) Order: 175 mg

Supply: 25 mg/mL

Formula Method

$$\frac{\overset{7}{\cancel{175} \text{ mg}}}{\underset{1}{\cancel{25} \text{ mg}}} \times 1 \text{ mL} = 7 \text{ mL}$$

Dimensional Analysis

$$X \text{ mL} = \frac{1 \text{ mL}}{25 \text{ mg}} \times 175 \text{ mg} = 7 \text{ mL}$$

41) Order: 500 mg

Supply: 500 mg per 10 mL

It is obvious that you want to give 10 mL.

Formula Method

$$\frac{500 \text{ mg}}{500 \text{ mg}} \times 10 \text{ mL} = 10 \text{ mL}$$

Dimensional Analysis

$$X \text{ mL} = \frac{10 \text{ mL}}{500 \text{ mg}} \times 500 \text{ mg} = 10 \text{ mL}$$

42) Order: gr $\frac{1}{100}$

Supply: 0.3 mg/tab

Formula Method

Convert: gr i = 60 mg

$$\text{gr} \rightarrow \text{mg; Larger} \downarrow \text{Smaller} \rightarrow (\times)$$

$$\text{gr } \frac{1}{100} \times 60 \text{ mg/gr} = 0.6 \text{ mg}$$

$$\frac{\overset{2}{0.6 \text{ mg}}}{\underset{1}{0.3 \text{ mg}}} \times 1 \text{ tab} = 2 \text{ tab}$$

Dimensional Analysis

$$X \text{ tab} = \frac{1 \text{ tab}}{0.3 \text{ mg}} \times \frac{60 \text{ mg}}{\text{gr } 1} \times \frac{\text{gr } 1/100}{1} = \frac{60/100}{0.3} = \frac{0.6}{0.3}$$

$$= 2 \text{ tab}$$

45) $$\frac{1 \text{ kg}}{2.2 \text{ lb}} \diagup\hspace{-0.9em}\diagdown \frac{X \text{ kg}}{67 \text{ lb}}$$

$$2.2X = 67$$

$$\frac{2.2X}{2.2} = \frac{67}{2.2}$$

$$X = 30.45 \text{ kg} = 30.5 \text{ kg}$$

Minimum recommended dosage:

100 mcg/kg/dose × 30.5 kg = 3,050 mcg/dose, or:

$$\frac{1 \text{ kg}}{100 \text{ mcg}} \diagup\hspace{-0.9em}\diagdown \frac{30.5 \text{ kg}}{X \text{ mcg}}$$

$$X = 100 \times 30.5$$

$$X = 3,050 \text{ mcg/dose}$$

Maximum recommended dosage:

200 mcg/kg/dose × 30.5 kg = 6,100 mcg/dose, or:

$$\frac{1 \text{ kg}}{200 \text{ mcg}} \diagup\hspace{-0.9em}\diagdown \frac{30.5 \text{ kg}}{X \text{ mcg}}$$

$$X = 6,100 \text{ mcg/dose}$$

Order: gr $\frac{1}{10}$

$$\frac{\text{gr } 1}{60 \text{ mg}} \diagup\hspace{-0.9em}\diagdown \frac{\text{gr } \frac{1}{10}}{X \text{ mg}}$$

$$X = 6 \text{ mg}$$

$$\frac{1 \text{ mg}}{1,000 \text{ mcg}} \diagup\hspace{-0.9em}\diagdown \frac{6 \text{ mg}}{X \text{ mcg}}$$

$$X = 6,000 \text{ mcg}$$

This dosage is safe.

$$\frac{8 \text{ mg}}{1 \text{ mL}} \diagup\hspace{-0.9em}\diagdown \frac{6 \text{ mg}}{X \text{ mL}}$$

$$8X = 6$$

$$\frac{8X}{8} = \frac{6}{8}$$

$$X = 0.75 \text{ mL}$$

46) $$\frac{1 \text{ kg}}{2.2 \text{ lb}} \diagup\hspace{-0.9em}\diagdown \frac{X \text{ kg}}{15 \text{ lb}}$$

$$2.2X = 15$$

$$\frac{2.2X}{2.2} = \frac{15}{2.2}$$

$$X = 6.81 \text{ kg} = 6.8 \text{ kg}$$

Minimum daily dosage:

20 mg/kg/day × 6.8 kg = 136 mg/day, or:

$$\frac{1 \text{ kg}}{20 \text{ mg}} \diagup\hspace{-0.9em}\diagdown \frac{6.8 \text{ kg}}{X \text{ mg}}$$

$$X = 136 \text{ mg (per day)}$$

Minimum single dosage: 136 mg ÷ 3 doses =

45.33 mg/dose = 45.3 mg/dose

Maximum daily dosage:

40 mg/kg/day × 6.8 kg = 272 mg/day, or:

$$\frac{1 \text{ kg}}{40 \text{ mg}} \diagup\hspace{-0.9em}\diagdown \frac{6.8 \text{ kg}}{X \text{ mg}}$$

$$X = 272 \text{ mg (per day)}$$

Maximum single dosage: 272 mg ÷ 3 doses =

90.66 mg/dose = 90.7 mg/dose

Dosage ordered is safe.

Supply: 125 mg per 5 mL

$$\frac{125 \text{ mg}}{5 \text{ mL}} \diagup\hspace{-0.9em}\diagdown \frac{75 \text{ mg}}{X \text{ mL}}$$

$$125X = 375$$

$$\frac{125X}{125} = \frac{375}{125}$$

$$X = 3 \text{ mL}$$

47) Recommended dosage:

5 mg/kg/day × 20 kg = 100 mg/day, or:

$$\frac{1 \text{ kg}}{5 \text{ mg}} \diagup\hspace{-0.9em}\diagdown \frac{20 \text{ kg}}{X \text{ mg}}$$

$$X = 100 \text{ mg (per day)}$$

100 mg ÷ 3 doses = 33.33 mg/dose = 33.3 mg/dose

Order of 100 mg t.i.d. is not safe. It is higher than the recommended dosage of 33.3 mg/dose.

48)
$$\frac{1 \text{ kg}}{2.2 \text{ lb}} \diagup\hspace{-0.9em}\diagdown \frac{X \text{ kg}}{16 \text{ lb}}$$

$$2.2X = 16$$

$$\frac{2.2X}{2.2} = \frac{16}{2.2}$$

$$X = 7.27 \text{ kg} = 7.3 \text{ kg}$$

Recommended dosage:

40 mg/kg/day × 7.3 kg = 292 mg/day, or:

$$\frac{1 \text{ kg}}{40 \text{ mg}} \diagup\hspace{-0.9em}\diagdown \frac{7.3 \text{ kg}}{X \text{ mg}}$$

$$X = 292 \text{ mg/day}$$

Ordered dosage is not safe. The child would receive 187 mg/dose × 4 doses/day or a total of 748 mg per day, which is over the recommended dosage of 292 mg/day.

49a)
$$\frac{1 \text{ kg}}{2.2 \text{ lb}} \diagup\hspace{-0.9em}\diagdown \frac{X \text{ kg}}{16 \text{ lb}}$$

$$2.2X = 16$$

$$\frac{2.2X}{2.2} = \frac{16}{2.2}$$

$$X = 7.27 \text{ kg} = 7.3 \text{ kg}$$

Recommended dosage:

15 mg/kg/day × 7.3 kg = 109.5 mg/day, or:

$$\frac{1 \text{ kg}}{15 \text{ mg}} \diagup\hspace{-0.9em}\diagdown \frac{7.3 \text{ kg}}{X \text{ mg}}$$

$$X = 109.5 \text{ mg/day}$$

109.5 mg ÷ 3 doses = 36.5 mg/dose

Dosage ordered as 60 mg q.8h, which is over the recommended dosage of 36.5 mg/dose. Although the total daily dosage is within limits, the q.8h dosage is too high and is not safe.

49b)
$$\frac{1 \text{ kg}}{2.2 \text{ lb}} \diagup\hspace{-0.9em}\diagdown \frac{X \text{ kg}}{275 \text{ lb}}$$

$$2.2X = 275$$

$$\frac{2.2X}{2.2} = \frac{275}{2.2}$$

$$X = 125 \text{ kg}$$

15 mg/kg/day × 125 kg = 1,875 mg/day, or:

$$\frac{1 \text{ kg}}{15 \text{ mg}} \diagup\hspace{-0.9em}\diagdown \frac{125 \text{ kg}}{X \text{ mg}}$$

$$X = 1,875 \text{ mg (per day)}$$

Because 1,875 mg/day or 1.9 g/day exceeds the recommended maximum dosage of 1.5 g/day, you would expect the order for this adult to be the maximum recommended dosage of 1.5 g/day or 1,500 mg/day. This could be divided into 3 doses of 0.5 mg q.8h or 500 mg q.8h.

Review Set 32 from pages 367–369

1)   C; sodium chloride 0.9%, 0.9 g per 100 mL; 308 mOsm/L; isotonic

2)   E; dextrose 5%, 5 g per 100 mL; 252 mOsm/L; isotonic

3)   G; dextrose 5%, 5 g per 100 mL; sodium chloride 0.9%, 0.9 g per 100 mL; 560 mOsm/L; hypertonic

4)   D; dextrose 5%, 5 g per 100 mL, sodium chloride 0.45%, 0.45 g per 100 mL; 406 mOsm/L; hypertonic

5)   A; dextrose 5%, 5 g per 100 mL, sodium chloride 0.225%, 0.225 g per 100 mL; 329 mOsm/L; isotonic

6)   H; dextrose 5%, 5 g per 100 mL; sodium lactate 0.31 g per 100 mL, NaCl 0.6 g per 100 mL; KCl 0.03 g per 100 mL; CaCl 0.02 g per 100 mL; 525 mOsm/L; hypertonic

7)   B; dextrose 5%, 5 g per 100 mL; sodium chloride 0.45%; 0.45 g per 100 mL; potassium chloride 20 mEq per liter (0.149 g per 100 mL); 447 mOsm/L; hypertonic

8)   F; sodium chloride 0.45%, 0.45 g per 100 mL; 154 mOsm/L; hypotonic

Review Set 33 from page 371

1) 50; 9 **2)** 25; 2.25 **3)** 25 **4)** 6.75 **5)** 25; 1.125 **6)** 150; 27 **7)** 50; 1.125 **8)** 36; 2.7 **9)** 100; 4.5 **10)** 3.375

Solutions—Review Set 33

1) D_5 NS = 5 g dextrose per 100 mL and 0.9 g NaCl per 100 mL

Dextrose:

$$\frac{5 \text{ g}}{100 \text{ mL}} \diagtimes \frac{X \text{ g}}{1{,}000 \text{ mL}}$$

$$100X = 5{,}000$$

$$\frac{100X}{100} = \frac{5{,}000}{100}$$

$$X = 50 \text{ g (dextrose)}$$

NaCl:

$$\frac{0.9 \text{ g}}{100 \text{ mL}} \diagtimes \frac{X \text{ g}}{1{,}000 \text{ mL}}$$

$$100X = 900$$

$$\frac{100X}{100} = \frac{900}{100}$$

$$X = 9 \text{ g (NaCl)}$$

7) $D_{10} \frac{1}{4}$ NS = 10 g dextrose per 100 mL and 0.225 g NaCl per 100 mL

Dextrose:

$$\frac{10 \text{ g}}{100 \text{ mL}} \diagtimes \frac{X \text{ g}}{500 \text{ mL}}$$

$$100X = 5{,}000$$

$$\frac{100X}{100} = \frac{5{,}000}{100}$$

$$X = 50 \text{ g (dextrose)}$$

NaCl:

$$\frac{0.225 \text{ g}}{100 \text{ mL}} \diagtimes \frac{X \text{ g}}{500 \text{ mL}}$$

$$100X = 112.5$$

$$\frac{100X}{100} = \frac{112.5}{100}$$

$$X = 1.125 \text{ g (NaCl)}$$

Review Set 34 from page 381

1) 100 **2)** 120 **3)** 83 **4)** 200 **5)** 120 **6)** 125 **7)** 125 **8)** 200 **9)** 75 **10)** 125 **11)** 63 **12)** 24 **13)** 150 **14)** 125 **15)** 42

Solutions—Review Set 34

1) 1 L = 1,000 mL

$$\frac{\text{Total mL}}{\text{Total h}} = \frac{1{,}000 \text{ mL}}{10 \text{ h}} = 100 \text{ mL/h}$$

3) $\dfrac{\text{Total mL}}{\text{Total h}} = \dfrac{2{,}000 \text{ mL}}{24 \text{ h}} = 83.3 \text{ mL/h} = 83 \text{ mL/h}$

4) $\dfrac{100 \text{ mL}}{30 \text{ min}} \diagtimes \dfrac{X \text{ mL/h}}{60 \text{ min/h}}$

$$30X = 6{,}000$$

$$\frac{30X}{30} = \frac{6{,}000}{30}$$

$$X = 200 \text{ mL/h}$$

5) $\dfrac{30 \text{ mL}}{15 \text{ min}} \diagtimes \dfrac{X \text{ mL/h}}{60 \text{ min/h}}$

$$15X = 1{,}800$$

$$\frac{15X}{15} = \frac{1{,}800}{15}$$

$$X = 120 \text{ mL/h}$$

6) $\dfrac{1 \text{ L}}{1{,}000 \text{ mL}} \diagtimes \dfrac{2.5 \text{ L}}{X \text{ mL}}$

$$X = 2{,}500 \text{ mL}$$

$$\frac{\text{Total mL}}{\text{Total h}} = \frac{2{,}500 \text{ mL}}{20 \text{ h}} = 125 \text{ mL/h}$$

Review Set 35 from pages 383–384

1) 15 **2)** 10 **3)** 60 **4)** 60 **5)** 10

Review Set 36 from pages 386–387

1) $\frac{V}{T} \times C = R$ **2)** 21 **3)** 50 **4)** 33 **5)** 25 **6)** 83 **7)** 42 **8)** 50 **9)** 50 **10)** 80 **11)** 20 **12)** 30 **13)** 17 **14)** 55 **15)** 40

Solutions—Review Set 36

1) $\dfrac{V}{T} \times C = R$ or $\dfrac{\text{Volume}}{\text{Time in min}} \times \text{Drop Factor} = \text{Rate}$

Volume in mL divided by *time* in minutes, multiplied by the *drop factor calibration* in drops per milliliter, equals the flow *rate* in drops per minute.

2) $\dfrac{V}{T} \times C = \dfrac{\overset{}{125 \text{ mL}}}{\underset{6}{60 \text{ min}}} \times \overset{1}{10} \text{ gtt/mL} = \dfrac{125 \text{ gtt}}{6 \text{ min}} = 20.8 \text{ gtt/min}$

$= 21 \text{ gtt/min}$

3) $\dfrac{V}{T} \times C = \dfrac{\overset{1}{\cancel{50}\text{ mL}}}{\underset{1}{\cancel{60}\text{ min}}} \times \cancel{60}\text{ gtt/}\cancel{\text{mL}} = 50\text{ gtt/min}$

Recall that when drop factor is 60 mL/h, then mL/h = gtt/min.

4) $\dfrac{V}{T} \times C = \dfrac{\overset{1}{\cancel{100}\text{ mL}}}{\underset{3}{\cancel{60}\text{ min}}} \times \cancel{20}\text{ gtt/}\cancel{\text{mL}} = \dfrac{100\text{ gtt}}{3\text{ min}} = 33.3\text{ gtt/min}$

$= 33\text{ gtt/min}$

6) Two 500 mL units of blood = 1,000 mL total volume

mL/h $= \dfrac{1,000\text{ mL}}{4\text{ h}} = 250\text{ mL/h}$

$\dfrac{V}{T} \times C = \dfrac{\overset{1}{\cancel{250}\text{ mL}}}{\underset{3}{\cancel{60}\text{ min}}} \times \cancel{20}\text{ gtt/}\cancel{\text{mL}} = \dfrac{250\text{ gtt}}{3\text{ min}} = 83.3\text{ gtt/min}$

$= 83\text{ gtt/min}$

7) $\dfrac{\text{Total mL}}{\text{total h}} = \dfrac{1,000\text{ mL}}{6\text{ h}} = 166.6\text{ mL/h} = 167\text{ mL/h}$

$\dfrac{V}{T} \times C = \dfrac{\overset{4}{\cancel{167}\text{ mL}}}{\underset{}{\cancel{60}\text{ min}}} \times \overset{1}{\cancel{15}}\text{ gtt/}\cancel{\text{mL}} = \dfrac{167\text{ gtt}}{4\text{ min}} = 41.7\text{ gtt/min}$

$= 42\text{ gtt/min}$

9) $\dfrac{150\text{ mL}}{\underset{3}{\cancel{45}\text{ min}}} \times \overset{1}{\cancel{15}}\text{ gtt/}\cancel{\text{mL}} = \dfrac{\overset{50}{\cancel{150}}\text{ gtt}}{\underset{1}{\cancel{3}}\text{ min}} = 50\text{ gtt/min}$

Review Set 37 from pages 389–390

1) 60 **2)** 1 **3)** 3 **4)** 4 **5)** 6 **6)** $\dfrac{\text{mL/h}}{\text{drop factor constant}}$ = gtt/min **7)** 50 **8)** 42 **9)** 28 **10)** 60 **11)** 8 **12)** 31 **13)** 28 **14)** 25 **15)** 11

Solutions—Review Set 37

4) $\dfrac{60}{15} = 4$

7) $\dfrac{\text{mL/h}}{\text{drop factor constant}}$ = gtt/min: $\dfrac{200\text{ mL/h}}{4} = 50\text{ gtt/min}$

8) $\dfrac{\text{mL/h}}{\text{drop factor constant}}$ = gtt/min: $\dfrac{125\text{ mL/h}}{3} = 41.6\text{ gtt/min}$ $= 42\text{ gtt/min}$

9) $\dfrac{\text{mL/h}}{\text{drop factor constant}}$ = gtt/min: $\dfrac{165\text{ mL/h}}{6} = 27.5\text{ gtt/min}$ $= 28\text{ gtt/min}$

10) $\dfrac{\text{mL/h}}{\text{drop factor constant}}$ = gtt/min: $\dfrac{60\text{ mL/h}}{1} = 60\text{ gtt/min}$

(Set the flow rate at the same number of gtt/min as the number of mL/h when the drop factor is 60 gtt/mL because the drop factor constant is 1.)

14) 0.5 L = 500 mL; $\dfrac{500\text{ mL}}{20\text{ h}} = 25\text{ mL/h}$; because the drop factor is 60 gtt/mL, then mL/h = gtt/min; so the rate is 25 gtt/min

15) $\dfrac{650\text{ mL}}{10\text{ h}} = 65\text{ mL/h}$

$\dfrac{\text{mL/h}}{\text{drop factor constant}}$ = gtt/min: $\dfrac{65\text{ mL/h}}{6} = 10.8\text{ gtt/min}$ $= 11\text{ gtt/min}$

Review Set 38 from pages 390–391

1) 125; 31 **2)** 100 **3)** 100; 33 **4)** 50 **5)** 125; 31 **6)** 125; 125 **7)** 35 **8)** 17 **9)** 25 **10)** 125 **11)** 83 **12)** 125 **13)** 200 **14)** 150 **15)** 200 **16)** 13.5 **17)** 20; 1.8 **18)** 22.5 **19)** 32.5; 2.925 **20)** 50; 2.25

Solutions—Review Set 38

1) $\dfrac{\text{Total mL}}{\text{Total h}} = \dfrac{3,000\text{ mL}}{24\text{ h}} = 125\text{ mL/h}$

$\dfrac{V}{T} \times C = \dfrac{\overset{1}{\cancel{125}\text{ mL}}}{\underset{4}{\cancel{60}\text{ min}}} \times \cancel{15}\text{ gtt/}\cancel{\text{mL}} = \dfrac{125\text{ gtt}}{4\text{ min}} = 31.2\text{ gtt/min}$

$= 31\text{ gtt/min}$

7) $\dfrac{\text{mL/h}}{\text{drop factor constant}}$ = gtt/min: $\dfrac{105\text{ mL/h}}{3} = 35\text{ gtt/min}$

8) $\dfrac{\text{mL/h}}{\text{drop factor constant}}$ = gtt/min: $\dfrac{100\text{ mL/h}}{6} = 16.6\text{ gtt/min}$ $= 17\text{ gtt/min}$

10) $\dfrac{\text{Total mL}}{\text{Total h}} = \dfrac{1,000\text{ mL}}{8\text{ h}} = 125\text{ mL/h}$

13) $\dfrac{100 \text{ mL}}{30 \text{ min}} \diagdown \dfrac{X \text{ mL/h}}{60 \text{ min/h}}$

$30X = 6{,}000$

$\dfrac{30X}{30} = \dfrac{6{,}000}{30}$

$X = 200 \text{ mL/h}$

15) $\dfrac{150 \text{ mL}}{45 \text{ min}} \diagdown \dfrac{X \text{ mL/h}}{60 \text{ min/h}}$

$45X = 9{,}000$

$\dfrac{45X}{45} = \dfrac{9{,}000}{45}$

$X = 200 \text{ mL/h}$

16) $\frac{1}{2}$ NS $= 0.45\%$ NaCl $= 0.45$ g NaCl per 100 mL

$\dfrac{0.45 \text{ g}}{100 \text{ mL}} \diagdown \dfrac{X \text{ g}}{3{,}000 \text{ mL}}$

$100X = 1{,}350$

$\dfrac{100X}{100} = \dfrac{1{,}350}{100}$

$X = 13.5 \text{ g (NaCl)}$

17) $D_{10} = 10\%$ dextrose $= 10$ g dextrose per 100 mL

Dextrose:

$\dfrac{10 \text{ g}}{100 \text{ mL}} \diagdown \dfrac{X \text{ g}}{200 \text{ mL}}$

$100X = 2{,}000$

$\dfrac{100X}{100} = \dfrac{2{,}000}{100}$

$X = 20 \text{ g (dextrose)}$

NS $= 0.9\%$ NaCl $= 0.9$ g NaCl per 100 mL

NaCl:

$\dfrac{0.9 \text{ g}}{100 \text{ mL}} \diagdown \dfrac{X \text{ g}}{200 \text{ mL}}$

$100X = 180$

$\dfrac{100X}{100} = \dfrac{180}{100}$

$X = 1.8 \text{ g (NaCl)}$

Review Set 39 from pages 394–397

1) 42; 6; 142; 47; 12%; reset to 47 gtt/min (12% increase is acceptable).

2) 42; 2; 180; 45; 7%; reset to 45 gtt/min (7% increase is acceptable).

3) 42; 4; 200; 67; 60%; recalculated rate 67 gtt/min (60% increase is unacceptable). Consult physician.

4) 28; 4; 188; 31; 11%; reset to 31 gtt/min (11% increase is acceptable).

5) 21; 4; 188; 31; 48%; (48% increase is unacceptable). Consult physician.

6) 31; 1,350; 10; 135; 34; 10%; reset to 34 gtt/min (10% increase is acceptable).

7) 50; 3; 233; 78; 56%; (56% increase is unacceptable). Consult physician.

8) 33; 3; 83; 28; –15%; (–15% slower is acceptable). IV is ahead of schedule. Slow rate to 28 gtt/min, and observe patient's condition.

9) 13; 10; 60; 15; 15%; reset to 15 gtt/min (15% increase is acceptable).

10) 100; 5; 100; 100; 0%; IV is on time, so no adjustment is needed.

Solutions—Review Set 39

1) $\dfrac{V}{T} \times C = \dfrac{125 \text{ mL}}{\overset{3}{\cancel{60}} \text{ min}} \times \overset{1}{\cancel{20}} \text{ gtt/mL} = \dfrac{125 \text{ gtt}}{3 \text{ min}} = 41.6 \text{ gtt/min} = 42 \text{ gtt/min (ordered rate)}$

$12 \text{ h} - 6 \text{ h} = 6 \text{ h}$

$\dfrac{\text{Remaining volume}}{\text{Remaining hours}} = \text{Recalculated mL/h}; \dfrac{850 \text{ mL}}{6 \text{ h}} = 141.6 \text{ mL/h} = 142 \text{ mL/h}$

$\dfrac{V}{T} \times C = \dfrac{142 \text{ mL}}{\overset{3}{\cancel{60}} \text{ min}} \times \overset{1}{\cancel{20}} \text{ gtt/mL} = \dfrac{142 \text{ gtt}}{3 \text{ min}} = 47.3 \text{ gtt/min} = 47 \text{ gtt/min (adjusted rate)}$

$\dfrac{\text{Adjusted gtt/min} - \text{Ordered gtt/min}}{\text{Ordered gtt/min}} = \% \text{ of variation}; \dfrac{47 - 42}{42} = \dfrac{5}{42} = 0.119 = 0.12 = 12\%$ (within the acceptable % of variation); reset rate to 47 gtt/min

3) $\dfrac{V}{T} \times C = \dfrac{\overset{}{125 \text{ mL}}}{\underset{3}{60 \text{ min}}} \times \overset{1}{20} \text{ gtt/mL} = \dfrac{125 \text{ gtt}}{3 \text{ min}} = 41.6 \text{ gtt/min} = 42 \text{ gtt/min (ordered rate)}$

8 h − 4 h = 4 h

$\dfrac{800 \text{ mL}}{4 \text{ h}} = 200 \text{ mL/h}; \dfrac{V}{T} \times C = \dfrac{\overset{}{200 \text{ mL}}}{\underset{3}{60 \text{ min}}} \times \overset{1}{20} \text{ gtt/mL} = \dfrac{200 \text{ gtt}}{3 \text{ min}} = 66.6 \text{ gtt/min} = 67 \text{ gtt/min (adjusted rate)}$

$\dfrac{\text{Adjusted gtt/min} - \text{Ordered gtt/min}}{\text{Ordered gtt/min}} = \% \text{ of variation}; \dfrac{67 - 42}{42} = \dfrac{25}{42} = 0.595 = 0.6 = 60\% \text{ faster};$

unacceptable % of variation—call physician for a revised order

6) $\dfrac{V}{T} \times C = \dfrac{\overset{}{125 \text{ mL}}}{\underset{4}{60 \text{ min}}} \times \overset{1}{15} \text{ gtt/mL} = \dfrac{125 \text{ gtt}}{4 \text{ min}} = 31.2 \text{ gtt/min} = 31 \text{ gtt/min (ordered rate)}$

2,000 mL − 650 mL = 1,350 mL remaining; 16 h − 6 h = 10 h

$\dfrac{1,350 \text{ mL}}{10 \text{ h}} = 135 \text{ mL/h}; \dfrac{V}{T} \times C = \dfrac{\overset{}{135 \text{ mL}}}{\underset{4}{60 \text{ min}}} \times \overset{1}{15} \text{ gtt/mL} = \dfrac{135 \text{ gtt}}{4 \text{ min}} = 33.7 \text{ gtt/min} = 34 \text{ gtt/min}$

$\dfrac{\text{Adjusted gtt/min} - \text{Ordered gtt/min}}{\text{Ordered gtt/min}} = \% \text{ of variation}; \dfrac{34 - 31}{31} = \dfrac{3}{31} = 0.096 = 0.10 = 10\%$

(within acceptable % of variation); reset rate to 34 gtt/min

8) $\dfrac{V}{T} \times C = \dfrac{\overset{}{100 \text{ mL}}}{\underset{3}{60 \text{ min}}} \times \overset{1}{20} \text{ gtt/mL} = \dfrac{100 \text{ gtt}}{3 \text{ min}} = 33.3 \text{ gtt/min} = 33 \text{ gtt/min (ordered rate)}$

5 h − 2 h = 3 h

$\dfrac{250 \text{ mL}}{3 \text{ h}} = 83.3 \text{ mL/h} = 83 \text{ mL/h}; \dfrac{V}{T} \times C = \dfrac{\overset{}{83 \text{ mL}}}{\underset{3}{60 \text{ min}}} \times \overset{1}{20} \text{ gtt/mL} = \dfrac{83 \text{ gtt}}{3 \text{ min}} = 27.6 \text{ gtt/min} = 28 \text{ gtt/min (adjusted rate)}$

$\dfrac{\text{Adjusted gtt/min} - \text{Ordered gtt/min}}{\text{Ordered gtt/min}} = \% \text{ of variation}; \dfrac{28 - 33}{33} = \dfrac{-5}{33} = -0.151 = -0.15 = -15\%$

(Remember the [−] sign indicates the IV is ahead of schedule and rate must be decreased.) Within the acceptable

% of variation. Slow IV to 28 gtt/min, and closely monitor patient.

Review Set 40 from pages 402–403

1) 133 2) 133 3) 50 4) 200 5) 100 6) 25 7) 50 8) 200 9) 150 10) 167 11) 133 12) 25 13) 120 14) 56 15) 200
16) 12; 3; 1 17) 3; 3; 0.25 18) 0.6; 2; 24; 0.06 19) 2; 18; 10; 2.5 20) 1.5; 0.75; 0.19

Solutions—Review Set 40

1) $\dfrac{V}{T} \times C = \dfrac{\overset{}{100 \text{ mL}}}{\underset{3}{45 \text{ min}}} \times \overset{4}{60} \text{ gtt/mL} = \dfrac{400 \text{ gtt}}{3 \text{ min}} = 133.3 \text{ gtt/min}$

= 133 gtt/min

2)
$\dfrac{100 \text{ mL}}{45 \text{ min}} \diagdown \dfrac{X \text{ mL/h}}{60 \text{ min/h}}$

45X = 6,000

$\dfrac{45X}{45} = \dfrac{6,000}{45}$

X = 133.3 mL/h

X = 133 mL/h

3) $\dfrac{V}{T} \times C = \dfrac{\overset{}{50 \text{ mL}}}{\underset{1}{15 \text{ min}}} \times \overset{1}{15} \text{ gtt/mL} = 50 \text{ gtt/min}$

4)
$\dfrac{50 \text{ mL}}{15 \text{ min}} \diagdown \dfrac{X \text{ mL/h}}{60 \text{ min/h}}$

15X = 3,000

$\dfrac{15X}{15} = \dfrac{3,000}{15}$

X = 200 mL/h

11) $\dfrac{V}{T} \times C = \dfrac{\overset{}{100 \text{ mL}}}{\underset{3}{15 \text{ min}}} \times \overset{4}{20} \text{ gtt/mL} = \dfrac{400 \text{ gtt}}{3 \text{ min}} = 133.3 \text{ gtt/min}$

= 133 gtt/min

16) $\dfrac{10 \text{ mg}}{1 \text{ mL}} \diagup\!\!\!\!\diagdown \dfrac{120 \text{ mg}}{X \text{ mL}}$

$10X = 120$

$\dfrac{10X}{10} = \dfrac{120}{10}$

$X = 12 \text{ mL}$

$\dfrac{40 \text{ mg}}{1 \text{ min}} \diagup\!\!\!\!\diagdown \dfrac{120 \text{ mg}}{X \text{ min}}$

$40X = 120$

$\dfrac{40X}{40} = \dfrac{120}{40}$

$X = 3 \text{ min}$

Administer 12 mL over at least 3 min.

1 min = 60 sec

3 min × 60 sec/min = 180 sec

$\dfrac{12 \text{ mL}}{180 \text{ sec}} \diagup\!\!\!\!\diagdown \dfrac{X \text{ mL}}{15 \text{ sec}}$

$180X = 180$

$\dfrac{180X}{180} = \dfrac{180}{180}$

$X = 1 \text{ mL (per 15 sec)}$

17) $\dfrac{250 \text{ mg}}{5 \text{ mL}} \diagup\!\!\!\!\diagdown \dfrac{150 \text{ mg}}{X \text{ mL}}$

$250X = 750$

$\dfrac{250X}{250} = \dfrac{750}{250}$

$X = 3 \text{ mL}$

$\dfrac{50 \text{ mg}}{1 \text{ min}} \diagup\!\!\!\!\diagdown \dfrac{150 \text{ mg}}{X \text{ min}}$

$50X = 150$

$\dfrac{50X}{50} = \dfrac{150}{50}$

$X = 3 \text{ min}$

Administer 3 mL over 3 min.

1 min = 60 sec

3 min × 60 sec/min = 180 sec

$\dfrac{3 \text{ mL}}{180 \text{ sec}} \diagup\!\!\!\!\diagdown \dfrac{X \text{ mL}}{15 \text{ sec}}$

$180X = 45$

$\dfrac{180X}{180} = \dfrac{45}{180}$

$X = 0.25 \text{ mL (per 15 sec)}$

18) $\dfrac{10 \text{ mg}}{1 \text{ mL}} \diagup\!\!\!\!\diagdown \dfrac{6 \text{ mg}}{X \text{ mL}}$

$10X = 6$

$\dfrac{10X}{10} = \dfrac{6}{10}$

$X = 0.6 \text{ mL}$

$\dfrac{2.5 \text{ mg}}{1 \text{ min}} \diagup\!\!\!\!\diagdown \dfrac{6 \text{ mg}}{X \text{ min}}$

$2.5X = 6$

$\dfrac{2.5X}{2.5} = \dfrac{6}{2.5}$

$X = 2.4 \text{ min}$

1 min = 60 sec

2 min × 60 sec/min = 120 sec; 0.4 min × 60 sec/min = 24 sec

120 sec + 24 sec = 144 sec

$\dfrac{0.6 \text{ mL}}{144 \text{ sec}} \diagup\!\!\!\!\diagdown \dfrac{X \text{ mL}}{15 \text{ sec}}$

$144X = 9$

$\dfrac{144X}{144} = \dfrac{9}{144}$

$X = 0.062 \text{ mL}$

$X = 0.06 \text{ mL (per 15 sec)}$

Review Set 41 from pages 406–407

1) 5 h and 33 min **2)** 6 h and 40 min **3)** 8 **4)** 6; 20 **5)** 4; 20 **6)** Approximately 11; 0300 the next morning

7) 16; 0730 the next morning **8)** 3,000 **9)** 1,152 **10)** 3,024 **11)** 260 **12)** 300 **13)** 600 **14)** 480, 320 **15)** 240, 540

Solutions—Review Set 41

1) $\dfrac{V}{T} \times C = R$; notice T is the missing quantity

$\dfrac{500 \text{ mL}}{T \text{ min}} \times 20 \text{ gtt/mL} = 30 \text{ gtt/min}$

$\dfrac{10,000}{T} \diagup\!\!\!\!\diagdown \dfrac{30}{1}$

$30T = 10,000$

$\dfrac{30T}{30} = \dfrac{10,000}{30}$

$T = 333.3 \text{ min}$

$T = 333 \text{ min}$

333 min ÷ 60 min/h = 5.55 or 5 h and 33 min

2) $\dfrac{V}{T} \times C = R$; notice T is the missing quantity

$\dfrac{1,000 \text{ mL}}{T \text{ min}} \times 10 \text{ gtt/mL} = 25 \text{ gtt/min}$

$\dfrac{10,000}{T} \diagup\!\!\!\!\diagdown \dfrac{25}{1}$

$25T = 10,000$

$\dfrac{25T}{25} = \dfrac{10,000}{25}$

$T = 400 \text{ min}$

400 min ÷ 60 min/h = $6\dfrac{2}{3}$ h or 6 h and 40 min

4) Time: $\frac{\text{Total vol}}{\text{mL/h}} = \text{Total h}$

$\frac{120 \text{ mL}}{20 \text{ mL/h}} = 6 \text{ h}$

$\frac{V}{T} \times C = \frac{20 \text{ mL}}{60 \text{ min}} \times 60 \text{ gtt/mL} = 20 \text{ gtt/min}$

6) $\frac{V}{T} \times C = R$; notice T is the missing quantity

$\frac{1,200 \text{ mL}}{\text{T min}} \times 15 \text{ gtt/mL} = 27 \text{ gtt/min}$

$\frac{18,000}{T} \quad\times\quad \frac{27}{1}$

$27T = 18,000$

$\frac{27T}{27} = \frac{18,000}{27}$

$T = 666.6 \text{ min}$

$T = 667 \text{ min}; 667 \text{ min} \div 60 \text{ min/h} =$
   $11.11 \text{ h or } 11 \text{ h and } 7 \text{ min or } 11 \text{ h (rounded)}$

$2400 \text{ h} - 1600 \text{ h} = 8 \text{ h (until midnight)}$

$11 \text{ h} - 8 \text{ h} = 3 \text{ h (into next day)}$

Completion time: 0300 (the next morning)

7) Time: $\frac{\text{Total vol}}{\text{mL/h}} = \text{Total h}$

$\frac{2,000 \text{ mL}}{125 \text{ mL/h}} = 16 \text{ h}$

$2400 - 1530 = 8\text{h } 30 \text{ min (until midnight)}$

$16\text{h} - 8\text{h } 30 \text{ min} = 7\text{h } 30 \text{ min (into the next day)}$

Completion time: 0730 (the next morning)

8) Total hours $\times$ mL/h $=$ Total volume

$24 \text{ h} \times 125 \text{ mL/h} = 3,000 \text{ mL}$

9) $24 \text{ h} \times 60 \text{ min/h} = 1,440 \text{ min}$

$\frac{V}{T} \times C = R$; notice V is the missing quantity

$\frac{V \text{ mL}}{1,440 \text{ min}} \times 15 \text{ gtt/mL} = 12 \text{ gtt/min}$

$\frac{15V}{1,440} \quad\times\quad \frac{12}{1}$

$15V = 17,280$

$\frac{15V}{15} = \frac{17,280}{15}$

$V = 1,152 \text{ mL}$

11) $65 \text{ mL/h} \times 4 \text{ h} = 260 \text{ mL}$

14) $8 \text{ h} \times 60 \text{ min/h} = 480 \text{ min}$

$\frac{V}{T} \times C = R$; notice V is the missing quantity

$\frac{V \text{ mL}}{480 \text{ min}} \times 60 \text{ gtt/mL} = 40 \text{ gtt/min}$

$\frac{60V}{480} \quad\times\quad \frac{40}{1}$

$60V = 19,200$

$\frac{60V}{60} = \frac{19,200}{60}$

$V = 320 \text{ mL}$

15) $4 \text{ h} \times 60 \text{ min/h} = 240 \text{ min}$

$\frac{V}{T} \times C = R$; notice V is the missing quantity

$\frac{V \text{ mL}}{240 \text{ min}} \times 20 \text{ gtt/mL} = 45 \text{ gtt/min}$

$\frac{20V}{240} \quad\times\quad \frac{45}{1}$

$20V = 10,800$

$\frac{20V}{20} = \frac{10,800}{20}$

$V = 540 \text{ mL}$

Practice Problems—Chapter 15 from pages 410–413

1) 17 **2)** 42 **3)** 42 **4)** 8 **5)** 125 **6)** Assess patient. If stable, recalculate and reset to 114 mL/h; observe patient closely.

7) 31 **8)** 42 **9)** Assess patient. If stable, recalculate and reset to 50 gtt/min; observe patient closely. **10)** 3,000

11) Abbott Laboratories **12)** 15 gtt/mL **13)** 4

14) $\text{mL/h} = \frac{500 \text{ mL}}{4 \text{ h}} = 125 \text{ mL/h}$

$\frac{\text{mL/h}}{\text{drop factor constant}} = \text{gtt/min}: \frac{125 \text{ mL/h}}{4} = 31.2 \text{ gtt/min} = 31 \text{ gtt/min}$

15) $\frac{V}{T} \times C = \frac{125 \text{ mL}}{60 \text{ min}} \times 15 \text{ gtt/mL} = \frac{125 \text{ gtt}}{4 \text{ min}} = 31.2 \text{ gtt/min} = 31 \text{ gtt/min}$

16) 1930 (or 7:30 PM) **17)** 250 **18)** Recalculate 210 mL to infuse over remaining 2 hours. Reset IV to 26 gtt/min and observe patient closely. **19)** 125 **20)** 100 **21)** Dextrose 2.5% (2.5 g per 100 mL) and NaCl 0.45% (0.45 g per 100 mL)

22) 25; 4.5 **23)** A central line is a special catheter inserted to access a large vein in the chest. **24)** A primary line is the IV tubing used to set up a primary IV infusion. **25)** The purpose of a saline/heparin lock is to administer IV medications when the patient does not require continuous IV fluids. **26)** 10; 5; 0.5; 0.13 **27)** The purpose of the PCA pump is to allow the patient to safely self-administer IV pain medication without having to call the nurse for a p.r.n. medication.

28) Advantages of the syringe pump are that a small amount of medication can be delivered directly from the syringe, and a specified time can be programmed in the pump. **29)** Phlebitis and infiltration **30)** q $\frac{1}{2}$ − 1 h, according to hospital policy **31)** This IV tubing has two spikes—one for blood, the other for saline—that join at a common drip chamber or Y connection. **32)** 14 **33)** 21 **34)** 28 **35)** 83 **36)** 17 **37)** 25 **38)** 33 **39)** 100 **40)** 33 **41)** 50 **42)** 67 **43)** 200 **44)** 8 **45)** 11 **46)** 15 **47)** 45 **48)** 150. The IV will finish in 1 hour. Leave a new IV bag in case you are delayed so the relief nurse can spike the new bag and continue the infusion. **49)** 1250 (or 12:50 PM)

50) **Prevention:** This error could have been prevented had the nurse carefully inspected the IV tubing package to determine the drop factor. Every IV tubing set has the drop factor printed on the package, so it is not necessary to memorize or guess the drop factor. The IV calculation should have looked like this:

$$\frac{V}{T} \times C = \frac{125 \text{ mL}}{\overset{}{\underset{3}{60 \text{ min}}}} \times \overset{1}{\cancel{20}} \text{ gtt/mL} = \frac{125 \text{ gtt}}{3 \text{ min}} = 41.6 \text{ gtt/min} = 42 \text{ gtt/min}$$

With the infusion set of 20 gtt/mL, a flow rate of 42 gtt/min would infuse 125 mL/h. At the 125 gtt/min rate the nurse calculated, the patient received three times the IV fluid ordered hourly. Thus, the patient actually received 375 mL/h of IV fluids.

Solutions—Practice Problems—Chapter 15

1) 100 mL/h = 100 mL per 60 min

$$\frac{V}{T} \times C = \frac{100 \text{ mL}}{\underset{6}{60 \text{ min}}} \times \overset{1}{\cancel{10}} \text{ gtt/mL} = \frac{100 \text{ gtt}}{6 \text{ min}} = 16.6 \text{ gtt/min}$$
$$= 17 \text{ gtt/min}$$

2) $\frac{\text{Total mL}}{\text{Total h}} = \frac{1,000 \text{ mL}}{24 \text{ h}} = 41.6 \text{ mL/h} = 42 \text{ mL/h}$

drop factor is 60 gtt/mL: 42 mL/h = 42 gtt/min

5) $\frac{\text{Total mL}}{\text{Total h}} = \frac{1,000 \text{ mL}}{8 \text{ h}} = 125 \text{ mL/h}$

6) $\frac{\text{Total mL}}{\text{Total h}} = \frac{800 \text{ mL}}{7 \text{ h}} = 114.2 \text{ mL/h} = 114 \text{ mL/h}$

$\frac{\text{Adjusted mL/h} - \text{Ordered mL/h}}{\text{Ordered mL/h}} = \%$ variation:

$\frac{114 - 125}{125} = \frac{-11}{125} = -0.088 = -9\%$ (decrease);

within safe limits of 25% variance.

Reset infusion rate to 114 mL/h.

7) 1,000 mL + 2,000 mL = 3,000 mL;

$\frac{\text{Total mL}}{\text{Total h}} = \frac{3,000 \text{ mL}}{24 \text{ h}} = 125 \text{ mL/h}$

$$\frac{V}{T} \times C = \frac{125 \text{ mL}}{\underset{4}{60 \text{ min}}} \times \overset{1}{\cancel{15}} \text{ gtt/mL} = \frac{125 \text{ gtt}}{4 \text{ min}} = 31.2 \text{ gtt/min}$$
$$= 31 \text{ gtt/min}$$

8) $\frac{V}{T} \times C = \frac{125 \text{ mL}}{\underset{3}{60 \text{ min}}} \times \overset{1}{\cancel{20}} \text{ gtt/mL} = \frac{125 \text{ gtt}}{3 \text{ min}}$
$= 41.6 \text{ gtt/min} = 42 \text{ gtt/min}$

9) $\frac{\text{Total mL}}{\text{Total h}} = \frac{1,000 \text{ mL}}{6 \text{ h}} = 166.6 \text{ mL/h} = 167 \text{ mL/h}$

$$\frac{V}{T} \times C = \frac{167 \text{ mL}}{\underset{4}{60 \text{ min}}} \times \overset{1}{\cancel{15}} \text{ gtt/mL} = \frac{167 \text{ gtt}}{4 \text{ min}} = 41.7 \text{ gtt/min}$$
$$= 42 \text{ gtt/min}$$

6 h − 2 h = 4 h remaining; $\frac{\text{Total mL}}{\text{Total h}} = \frac{\overset{200}{\cancel{800} \text{ mL}}}{\underset{1}{4 \text{ h}}}$
$= 200 \text{ mL/h}$

$$\frac{V}{T} \times C = \frac{200 \text{ mL}}{\underset{4}{60 \text{ min}}} \times \overset{1}{\cancel{15}} \text{ gtt/mL} = \frac{\overset{50}{\cancel{200} \text{ gtt}}}{\underset{1}{4 \text{ min}}}$$
$$= 50 \text{ gtt/min}$$

$\frac{\text{Adjusted gtt/min} - \text{Ordered gtt/min}}{\text{Ordered gtt/min}} = \%$ variation:

$\frac{50 - 42}{42} = \frac{8}{42} = 0.19 = 19\%$ increase;

within safe limits of 25% variance

Reset infusion rate to 50 gtt/min.

10) q.4h = 6 times per 24 h; 6 × 500 mL = 3,000 mL

13) $\frac{60}{15} = 4$

16) 1530 + 4 h = 1530 + 0400 = 1930; 1930 − 1200
= 7:30 PM

17) $\frac{\text{Total mL}}{\text{Total h}} = \frac{500 \text{ mL}}{4 \text{ h}} = 125 \text{ mL/h}$

125 mL/h × 2 h = 250 mL

18)

$$\frac{\text{Total mL}}{\text{Total h}} = \frac{210\ \text{mL}}{2\ \text{h}} = 105\ \text{mL/h}$$

$$\frac{V}{T} \times C = \frac{105\ \cancel{\text{mL}}}{\underset{4}{\cancel{60}\ \text{min}}} \times \overset{1}{\cancel{15}}\ \text{gtt/}\cancel{\text{mL}} = \frac{105\ \text{gtt}}{4\ \text{min}} = 26.2\ \text{gtt/min}$$

$$= 26\ \text{gtt/min}$$

$$\frac{\text{Adjusted gtt/min} - \text{Ordered gtt/min}}{\text{Ordered gtt/min}} = \%\ \text{variation:}$$

$$\frac{26 - 31}{31} = \frac{-5}{31} = -0.161 = -0.16 = -16\%\ \text{decrease;}$$

within safe limits

Reset infusion rate to 26 gtt/min.

19)

$$\frac{\text{Total mL}}{\text{Total h}} = \frac{500\ \text{mL}}{4\ \text{h}} = 125\ \text{mL/h}$$

20)

$$\frac{50\ \text{mL}}{30\ \text{min}} \ \diagdown\!\!\!\diagup\ \frac{X\ \text{mL/h}}{60\ \text{min/h}}$$

$$30X = 3,000$$

$$\frac{30X}{30} = \frac{3,000}{30}$$

$$X = 100\ \text{mL/h}$$

22) Dextrose 5% = 5 g per 100 mL   NaCl 0.9% = 0.9 g per 100 mL

Dextrose:

$$\frac{5\ \text{g}}{100\ \text{mL}} \ \diagdown\!\!\!\diagup\ \frac{X\ \text{g}}{500\ \text{mL}}$$

$$100X = 2,500$$

$$\frac{100X}{100} = \frac{2,500}{100}$$

$$X = 25\ \text{g}$$

NaCl:

$$\frac{0.9\ \text{g}}{100\ \text{mL}} \ \diagdown\!\!\!\diagup\ \frac{X\ \text{g}}{500\ \text{mL}}$$

$$100X = 450$$

$$\frac{100X}{100} = \frac{450}{100}$$

$$X = 4.5\ \text{g}$$

26)

$$\frac{5\ \text{mg}}{1\ \text{min}} \ \diagdown\!\!\!\diagup\ \frac{50\ \text{mg}}{X\ \text{min}}$$

$$5X = 50$$

$$\frac{5X}{5} = \frac{50}{5}$$

$$X = 10\ \text{min}$$

$$\frac{10\ \text{mg}}{1\ \text{mL}} \ \diagdown\!\!\!\diagup\ \frac{50\ \text{mg}}{X\ \text{mL}}$$

$$10X = 50$$

$$\frac{10X}{10} = \frac{50}{10}$$

$$X = 5\ \text{mL}$$

Give 50 mg per 10 min or 5 mL per 10 min;

0.5 mL/min

1 min = 60 sec

10 $\cancel{\text{min}}$ × 60 sec/$\cancel{\text{min}}$ = 600 sec

$$\frac{5\ \text{mL}}{600\ \text{sec}} \ \diagdown\!\!\!\diagup\ \frac{X\ \text{mL}}{15\ \text{sec}}$$

$$600X = 75$$

$$\frac{600X}{600} = \frac{75}{600}$$

$$X = 0.125\ \text{mL (per 15 sec)}$$

$$X = 0.13\ \text{mL (per 15 sec)}$$

32)

$$\frac{\text{Total mL}}{\text{Total h}} = \frac{1,000\ \text{mL}}{12\ \text{h}} = 83.3\ \text{mL/h} = 83\ \text{mL/h};\ \frac{V}{T} \times C =$$

$$\frac{83\ \cancel{\text{mL}}}{\underset{6}{\cancel{60}\ \text{min}}} \times \overset{1}{\cancel{10}}\ \text{gtt/}\cancel{\text{mL}} = \frac{83\ \text{gtt}}{6\ \text{min}} = 13.8\ \text{gtt/min} = 14\ \text{gtt/min}$$

33)

$$\frac{V}{T} \times C = \frac{83\ \cancel{\text{mL}}}{\underset{4}{\cancel{60}\ \text{min}}} \times \overset{1}{\cancel{15}}\ \text{gtt/}\cancel{\text{mL}} = \frac{83\ \text{gtt}}{4\ \text{min}} = 20.7\ \text{gtt/min}$$

$$= 21\ \text{gtt/min}$$

34)

$$\frac{V}{T} \times C = \frac{83\ \cancel{\text{mL}}}{\underset{3}{\cancel{60}\ \text{min}}} \times \overset{1}{\cancel{20}}\ \text{gtt/}\cancel{\text{mL}} = \frac{83\ \text{gtt}}{3\ \text{min}} = 27.6\ \text{gtt/min}$$

$$= 28\ \text{gtt/min}$$

35)

$$\frac{V}{T} \times C = \frac{83\ \cancel{\text{mL}}}{\underset{1}{\cancel{60}\ \text{min}}} \times \cancel{60}\ \text{gtt/}\cancel{\text{mL}} = 83\ \text{gtt/min}$$

Remember, if the drop factor is 60 gtt/mL, then

mL/h = gtt/min; so 83 mL/h = 83 gtt/min

48) $\frac{V}{T} \times C = R$; V is the unknown quantity

$$\frac{V\ \text{mL}}{60\ \text{min}} \times 10\ \text{gtt/mL} = 25\ \text{gtt/min}$$

$$\frac{10V}{60} \ \diagdown\!\!\!\diagup\ \frac{25}{1}$$

$$10V = 1,500$$

$$\frac{10V}{10} = \frac{1,500}{10}$$

$$V = 150\ \text{mL}$$

49)

$$\frac{400\ \cancel{\text{mL}}}{75\ \cancel{\text{mL}}\text{/h}} = 5\tfrac{1}{3}\ \text{h or 5 h and 20 min}$$

0730 + 0520 = 1250 (or 12:50 PM)

Review Set 42 from page 419

1) 0.68 **2)** 2.35 **3)** 0.69 **4)** 1.4 **5)** 2.03 **6)** 1 **7)** 1.67 **8)** 0.4 **9)** 1.69 **10)** 0.52 **11)** 1.11 **12)** 0.78 **13)** 0.15 **14)** 0.78
15) 0.39 **16)** 0.64 **17)** 0.25 **18)** 1.08 **19)** 0.5 **20)** 0.88

Solutions—Review Set 42

1) Household: BSA $(m^2) = \sqrt{\dfrac{\text{ht (in)} \times \text{wt (lb)}}{3,131}} = \sqrt{\dfrac{36 \times 40}{3,131}} = \sqrt{\dfrac{1,440}{3,131}} = \sqrt{0.459\ldots} = 0.678\ m^2 = 0.68\ m^2$

2) Metric: BSA $(m^2) = \sqrt{\dfrac{\text{ht (cm)} \times \text{wt (kg)}}{3,600}} = \sqrt{\dfrac{190 \times 105}{3,600}} = \sqrt{\dfrac{19,950}{3,600}} = \sqrt{5.541\ldots} = 2.354\ m^2 = 2.35\ m^2$

Review Set 43 from pages 421–423

1) 1,640,000 **2)** 5.9; 11.8 **3)** 735 **4)** 15.84; 63.36 **5)** 250 **6)** 0.49; 122.5; Yes; 2.5 **7)** 0.89; 2.9; Yes; 1.2 **8)** 66; 22; Yes
9) 198; Yes; 990 **10)** 612; 612; 1,224; 2,448 **11)** 8.1; 24.7 **12)** 67–167.5; 33.5–83.8; Yes **13)** 8–14.4; Yes **14)** 0.82;
2,050; Yes; 2.7; 102.7; 51 **15)** 1.62; 4,050; Yes; 5.4; 105.4; 53

Solutions—Review Set 43

1) 2,000,000 units/m^2 × 0.82 m^2 = 1,640,000 units

2) 10 mg/m^2/day × 0.59 m^2 = 5.9 mg/day (minimum
safe dosage)

20 mg/m^2/day × 0.59 m^2 = 11.8 mg/day
(maximum safe dosage)

3) 500 mg/m^2 × 1.47 m^2 = 735 mg

4) 6 mg/m^2/day × 2.64 m^2 = 15.84 mg/day

15.84 mg/day × 4 days = 63.36 mg

6) Household: BSA $(m^2) = \sqrt{\dfrac{\text{ht (in)} \times \text{wt (lb)}}{3,131}} =$
$\sqrt{\dfrac{30 \times 25}{3,131}} = \sqrt{\dfrac{750}{3,131}} = \sqrt{0.239\ldots} = 0.489\ m^2 =$
0.49 m^2

250 mg/m^2 × 0.49 m^2 = 122.5 mg; dosage is safe

$\dfrac{50\ mg}{1\ mL} \diagdown \dfrac{122.5\ mg}{X\ mL}$

50X = 122.5

$\dfrac{50X}{50} = \dfrac{122.5}{50}$

X = 2.45 mL = 2.5 mL

8) 150 mg/m^2/day × 0.44 m^2 = 66 mg/day

$\dfrac{66\ mg}{3\ doses}$ = 22 mg/dose; dosage is safe

9) 900 mg/m^2/day × 0.22 m^2 = 198 mg/day; dosage
is safe

198 mg/day × 5 days = 990 mg

10) 600 mg/m^2 × 1.02 m^2 = 612 mg, initially

300 mg/m^2 × 1.02 m^2 = 306 mg; (for 2 doses):

306 mg × 2 doses = 612 mg

q.12 h is 2 doses/day and 2 doses/day × 2 days =
4 doses

306 mg × 4 doses = 1,224 mg

612 mg + 612 mg + 1,224 mg = 2,448 mg (total)

11) 10 mg/m^2 × 0.81 m^2 = 8.1 mg (bolus)

30.5 mg/m^2/day × 0.81 m^2 = 24.7 mg/day

14) Metric: BSA $(m^2) = \sqrt{\dfrac{\text{ht (cm)} \times \text{wt (kg)}}{3,600}} = \sqrt{\dfrac{100 \times 24}{3,600}} =$
$\sqrt{\dfrac{2,400}{3,600}} = \sqrt{0.666\ldots} = 0.816\ m^2 = 0.82\ m^2$

2,500 units/m^2 × 0.82 m^2 = 2,050 units; dosage
is safe

$\dfrac{750\ units}{1\ mL} \diagdown \dfrac{2,050\ units}{X\ mL}$

750X = 2,050

$\dfrac{750X}{750} = \dfrac{2,050}{750}$

X = 2.73 = 2.7 mL

2.7 mL (Oncaspar) + 100 mL (D_5W)
= 102.7 mL (total volume)

$\dfrac{102.7\ mL}{2\ h}$ = 51.3 mL/h = 51 mL/h

15) Metric: BSA $(m^2) = \sqrt{\dfrac{\text{ht (cm)} \times \text{wt (kg)}}{3,600}} =$
$\sqrt{\dfrac{58.2 \times 162}{3,600}} = \sqrt{\dfrac{9,428.4}{3,600}} = \sqrt{2.619} = 1.618\ m^2$
= 1.62 m^2

2,500 units/m^2 × 1.62 m^2 = 4,050 units; dosage
is safe

$\dfrac{750\ units}{1\ mL} \diagdown \dfrac{4,050\ units}{X\ mL}$

750X = 4,050

$\dfrac{750X}{750} = \dfrac{4,050}{750}$

X = 5.4 mL

5.4 mL (Oncaspar) + 100 mL (D_5W) = 105.4 mL
(total volume)

$\dfrac{105.4\ mL}{2\ h}$ = 52.7 mL/h = 53 mL/h

Review Set 44 from pages 426–427

1) 87; 2; 48 **2)** 75; 3; 57 **3)** 120; 3; 22 **4)** 80; 6; 44 **5)** 60; 1; 31; 180 **6)** 2; 23 **7)** 2; 8 **8)** 12; 45 **9)** 7.2; 36.8

10) 7.5; 88.5

Solutions—Review Set 44

1) Total volume: 50 mL + 15 mL = 65 mL

$$\frac{V}{T} \times C = \frac{65\ \overset{4}{\cancel{mL}}}{\underset{3}{\cancel{45}}\ min} \times \overset{}{\cancel{60}}\ gtt/mL =$$

$$\frac{260\ gtt}{3\ min} = 86.6\ gtt/min = 87\ gtt/min$$

$$\frac{60\ mg}{2\ mL} \diagdown \frac{60\ mg}{X\ mL}$$

$$60X = 120$$

$$\frac{60X}{60} = \frac{120}{60}$$

$$X = 2\ mL\ (medication)$$

Volume IV fluid to add to chamber:

50 mL − 2 mL = 48 mL

4) Total volume: 50 mL + 30 mL = 80 mL

80 mL per 60 min = 80 mL/h

$$\frac{1\ g}{10\ mL} \diagdown \frac{0.6\ g}{X\ mL}$$

$$X = 6\ mL\ (medication)$$

Volume IV fluid to add to chamber:

50 mL − 6 mL = 44 mL

6) $$\frac{50\ mL}{60\ min} \diagdown \frac{X\ mL}{30\ min}$$

$$60X = 1,500$$

$$\frac{60X}{60} = \frac{1,500}{60}$$

$$X = 25\ mL\ (total\ volume)$$

$$\frac{125\ mg}{1\ mL} \diagdown \frac{250\ mg}{X\ mL}$$

$$125X = 250$$

$$\frac{125X}{125} = \frac{250}{125}$$

$$X = 2\ mL\ (medication)$$

Volume IV fluid to add to chamber:

25 mL − 2 mL = 23 mL

8) $$\frac{85\ mL}{60\ min} \diagdown \frac{X\ mL}{40\ min}$$

$$60X = 3,400$$

$$\frac{60X}{60} = \frac{3,400}{60}$$

$$X = 56.6\ mL = 57\ mL\ (total\ volume)$$

$$\frac{50\ mg}{1\ mL} \diagdown \frac{600\ mg}{X\ mL}$$

$$50X = 600$$

$$\frac{50X}{50} = \frac{600}{50}$$

$$X = 12\ mL\ (medication)$$

Volume IV fluid to add to chamber:

57 mL − 12 mL = 45 mL

9) $$\frac{66\ mL}{60\ min} \diagdown \frac{X\ mL}{40\ min}$$

$$60X = 2,640$$

$$\frac{60X}{60} = \frac{2,640}{60}$$

$$X = 44\ mL\ (total\ volume)$$

$$\frac{1,000\ mg}{10\ mL} \diagdown \frac{720\ mg}{X\ mL}$$

$$1,000X = 7,200$$

$$\frac{1,000X}{1,000} = \frac{7,200}{1,000}$$

$$X = 7.2\ mL\ (medication)$$

Volume IV fluid to add to chamber:

44 mL – 7.2 mL = 36.8 mL

Hint: Add the medication to the volume control chamber, and fill with IV fluid to the 44 mL mark. The chamber measures whole (not fractional) mL.

10) 48 mL/h × 2 h = 96 mL (total volume)

$$\frac{100\ mg}{10\ mL} \diagdown \frac{75\ mg}{X\ mL}$$

$$100X = 750$$

$$\frac{100X}{100} = \frac{750}{100}$$

$$X = 7.5\ mL$$

Volume IV fluid to add to chamber:

96 mL − 7.5 mL = 88.5 mL

Review Set 45 from pages 430–431

1) 4 **2)** 25 **3)** 1,600; 67 **4)** 1,150; 48 **5)** 1,800; 75 **6)** 350; 15 **7)** 3.5 or 4; 11.6 or 12 **8)** 2.6 or 3; 65 **9)** 2.3 or 2; 35

10) This order should be questioned because normal saline is an isotonic solution and appears to be a continuous infusion for this child. This solution does not contribute enough electrolytes for the child and water intoxication may result. Hint: The equipment measures whole mL; therefore, round to the next whole mL.

Solutions—Review Set 45

1)

$$\frac{100 \text{ mg}}{1 \text{ mL}} \times \frac{400 \text{ mg}}{\text{X mL}}$$

$$100\text{X} = 400$$

$$\frac{100\text{X}}{100} = \frac{400}{100}$$

$$\text{X} = 4 \text{ mL}$$

3)

100 mL/kg/day $\times$ 10 kg $=$ 1,000 mL/day for first 10 kg

50 mL/kg/day $\times$ 10 kg $=$ 500 mL/day for next 10 kg

20 mL/kg/day $\times$ 5 kg $=$ 100 mL/day for remaining 5 kg

Total $=$ 1,600 mL/day or per 24 h

$$\frac{1,600 \text{ mL}}{24 \text{ h}} = 66.6 \text{ mL/h} = 67 \text{ mL/h}$$

4)

100 mL/kg/day $\times$ 10 kg $=$ 1,000 mL/day for first 10 kg

50 mL/kg/day $\times$ 3 kg $=$ 150 mL/day for next 10 kg

Total $=$ 1,150 mL/day or per 24 h

$$\frac{1,150 \text{ mL}}{24 \text{ h}} = 47.9 \text{ mL/h} = 48 \text{ mL/h}$$

5)

$$\frac{1 \text{ kg}}{2.2 \text{ lb}} \times \frac{\text{X kg}}{77 \text{ lb}}$$

$$2.2\text{X} = 77$$

$$\frac{2.2\text{X}}{2.2} = \frac{77}{2.2}$$

$$\text{X} = 35 \text{ kg}$$

100 mL/kg/day $\times$ 10 kg $=$ 1,000 mL/day for first 10 kg

50 mL/kg/day $\times$ 10 kg $=$ 500 mL/day for next 10 kg

20 mL/kg/day $\times$ 15 kg $=$ 300 mL/day for remaining 15 kg

Total $=$ 1,800 mL/day or per 24 h

$$\frac{1,800 \text{ mL}}{24 \text{ h}} = 75 \text{ mL/h}$$

7)

$$\frac{100 \text{ mg}}{1 \text{ mL}} \times \frac{350 \text{ mg}}{\text{X mL}}$$

$$100\text{X} = 350$$

$$\frac{100\text{X}}{100} = \frac{350}{100}$$

$$\text{X} = 3.5 \text{ or } 4 \text{ mL (min. dilution volume)}$$

$$\frac{30 \text{ mg}}{1 \text{ mL}} \times \frac{350 \text{ mg}}{\text{X mL}}$$

$$30\text{X} = 350$$

$$\frac{30\text{X}}{30} = \frac{350}{30}$$

$$\text{X} = 11.6 \text{ or } 12 \text{ mL (max. dilution volume)}$$

Practice Problems—Chapter 16 from pages 432–438

1) 1.17; 1.8–2.3; Yes; 2; 0.5 **2)** 0.52; 42; 0.84 **3)** 0.43; 108 **4)** 2.2 **5)** 0.7 **6)** 350 **7)** 1 of each (one 100 mg capsule and one 250 mg capsule) **8)** 0.8; 2,000 **9)** 2.7 **10)** No **11)** 1.3; 26 **12)** 13 **13)** 1.69 **14)** 1.11 **15)** 0.32 **16)** 1.92 **17)** 1.63 **18)** 0.69 **19)** 1.67 **20)** 0.52 **21)** 560,000 **22)** 1,085; 1.09 **23)** 1.9–3.8 **24)** 8 **25)** 40 **26)** 45; 90; 4.2; 25.8 **27)** 58.8

28) 60; 60; 1.9; 43.1 **29)** 22.8 **30)** 10; 33 **31)** 200 **32)** 6.2; 37.8 **33)** 130.2 **34)** 1,000; 42 **35)** 1,520; 63 **36)** 1,810; 75

37) 1,250; 52 **38)** 240; 10 **39)** 1,500–1,875; 250–312.5; Yes; 2.8 **40)** 35; 2.8; 32.2 **41)** 12.3; 1,230; 308; Yes; 6.2

42) 23; 6.2; 16.8 **43)** 330–495; 110–165; Yes; 3.3 **44)** 25; 3.3; 21.7 **45)** 1,800–2,700; 300–450; No; exceeds maximum

dose; do not give dosage ordered. **46)** Consult physician before further action. **47)** 25; 2,500,000–6,250,000;

416,667–1,041,667 **48)** Yes; 2.6 **49)** 20; 2.6; 17.4

50)   **Prevention:** The nurse made several assumptions in trying to calculate and prepare this chemotherapy quickly. The nurse assumed that the weight notation was the same on the two units without verification. The recording of the weights as 20/.45 was confusing. Notice the period before the 45, which later the physician stated was the calculated BSA, 0.45 m^2. Because no unit of measure was identified, it was unclear what those numbers really meant. Never assume; always ask for clarification when notation is unclear. Also, a child who weighs 20 lb and a child who weighs 45 lb are quite different in size, yet the nurse failed to notice such a size difference. This nurse, though, is probably not used to discriminating small children's weight differences but should have realized that weight in lb is approximately two times weight in kg. Additionally, the actual volume drawn up was probably small in comparison to most adult dose volumes that this nurse prepares. The amount of 1.6 mL likely seemed reasonable to the nurse. Finally, this is an instance in which the person giving the medication, the physician, prevented a medication error by stopping and thinking what is a reasonable amount for this child and questioning the actual calculation of the dose. Remember, the person who administers the medication is the last point at which a potential error can be avoided.

Solutions—Practice Problems—Chapter 16

1)   Household: BSA $(m^2) = \sqrt{\dfrac{ht\,(in) \times wt\,(lb)}{3,131}} = \sqrt{\dfrac{50 \times 85}{3,131}}$

$= \sqrt{\dfrac{4,250}{3,131}} = \sqrt{1.357...} = 1.165\ m^2 = 1.17\ m^2$

Recommended dosage range:

$1.5\ mg/m^2 \times 1.17\ m^2 = 1.8\ mg$

$2\ mg/m^2 \times 1.17\ m^2 = 2.3\ mg$

Ordered dosage is safe.

$\dfrac{1\ mg}{1\ mL} \diagdown \dfrac{2\ mg}{X\ mL}$

$X = 2\ mL$

Give 2 mL/min

$\dfrac{2\ mL}{60\ sec} \diagdown \dfrac{X\ mL}{15\ sec}$

$60X = 30$

$\dfrac{60X}{60} = \dfrac{30}{60}$

$X = 0.5\ mL\ (per\ 15\ sec)$

2)   BSA = 0.52 m^2

$80\ mg/m^2/day \times 0.52\ m^2 = 41.6\ mg/day = 42\ mg/day$

$\dfrac{50\ mg}{1\ mL} \diagdown \dfrac{42\ mg}{X\ mL}$

$50X = 42$

$\dfrac{50X}{50} = \dfrac{42}{50}$

$X = 0.84\ mL$

3)   BSA = 0.43 m^2

$250\ mcg/m^2/day \times 0.43\ m^2 = 107.5\ mcg/day$

$= 108\ mcg/day$

4) $\dfrac{500\ mcg}{10\ mL} \diagdown \dfrac{108\ mcg}{X\ mL}$

$500X = 1,080$

$\dfrac{500X}{500} = \dfrac{1,080}{500}$

$X = 2.16\ mL = 2.2\ mL$

6) $0.5\ g/m^2 \times 0.7\ m^2 = 0.35\ g$

$0.35\ g = 0.350. = 350\ mg$

8)   BSA = 0.8 m^2

$2,500\ units/m^2 \times 0.8\ m^2 = 2,000\ units$

9) $\dfrac{750\ units}{1\ mL} \diagdown \dfrac{2,000\ units}{X\ mL}$

$750X = 2,000$

$\dfrac{750X}{750} = \dfrac{2,000}{750}$

$X = 2.66\ mL = 2.7\ mL$

10)   Dose amount exceeds child maximum IM volume per injection site; give in 2 injections.

11)   Metric: BSA $(m^2) = \sqrt{\dfrac{ht\,(cm) \times wt\,(kg)}{3,600}} =$

$\sqrt{\dfrac{140 \times 43.5}{3,600}} = \sqrt{\dfrac{6,090}{3,600}} = \sqrt{1.691...} = 1.30\ m^2$

$= 1.3\ m^2$

$20\ mg/m^2 \times 1.3\ m^2 = 26\ mg$

12)
$$\frac{2\ mg}{1\ mL} \diagdown\!\!\!\diagup \frac{26\ mg}{X\ mL}$$

$$2X = 26$$

$$\frac{2X}{2} = \frac{26}{2}$$

$$X = 13\ mL$$

13) 1 ft = 12 in

$$\frac{1\ ft}{12\ in} \diagdown\!\!\!\diagup \frac{5\ ft}{X\ in}$$

$$X = 60\ in$$

Convert 5 ft 6 in to total in:

60 in + 6 in = 66 in

Household: BSA (m^2) = $\sqrt{\dfrac{ht\ (in) \times wt\ (lb)}{3,131}}$ =

$\sqrt{\dfrac{66 \times 136}{3,131}} = \sqrt{\dfrac{8,976}{3,131}} = \sqrt{2.866...} = 1.693\ m^2 =$

1.69 m^2

15) Metric: BSA (m^2) = $\sqrt{\dfrac{ht\ (cm) \times wt\ (kg)}{3,600}} = \sqrt{\dfrac{60 \times 6}{3,600}}$

$= \sqrt{\dfrac{360}{3,600}} = \sqrt{0.1} = 0.316\ m^2 = 0.32\ m^2$

19) 1 in = 2.5 cm

$$\frac{1\ in}{2.5\ cm} \diagdown\!\!\!\diagup \frac{64\ in}{X\ cm}$$

$$X = 160\ cm$$

Metric: BSA (m^2) = $\sqrt{\dfrac{ht\ (cm) \times wt\ (kg)}{3,600}}$ =

$\sqrt{\dfrac{160 \times 63}{3,600}} = \sqrt{\dfrac{10,080}{3,600}}$

$= \sqrt{2.8} = 1.673\ m^2 = 1.67\ m^2$

22) 500 mg/m^2 × 2.17 m^2 = 1,085 mg

1,085 mg = 1.085. = 1.085 g = 1.09 g

24) 6 mg/m^2 × 1.34 m^2 = 8.04 mg = 8 mg

25) 8 mg/day × 5 days = 40 mg

26) Total volume = 30 mL + 15 mL = 45 mL

Flow rate:

$$\frac{45\ mL}{30\ min} \diagdown\!\!\!\diagup \frac{X\ mL}{60\ min}$$

$$30X = 2,700$$

$$\frac{30X}{30} = \frac{2,700}{30}$$

$$X = 90\ mL$$

$$\frac{500\ mg}{5\ mL} \diagdown\!\!\!\diagup \frac{420\ mg}{X\ mL}$$

$$500X = 2,100$$

$$\frac{500X}{500} = \frac{2,100}{500}$$

$$X = 4.2\ mL\ (medication)$$

30 mL (total solution) − 4.2 mL (med)

= 25.8 mL (D$_5$NS)

Note: Add 4.2 mL med. to chamber and fill with

D$_5$NS to 30 mL.

27) 4.2 mL/dose × 2 doses/day = 8.4 mL/day

8.4 mL/day × 7 days = 58.8 mL (total)

28) Total volume: 45 mL + 15 mL = 60 mL

Flow rate: $\dfrac{60\ mL}{60\ min}$ = 60 mL/h

$$\frac{75\ mg}{0.5\ mL} \diagdown\!\!\!\diagup \frac{285\ mg}{X\ mL}$$

$$75X = 142.5$$

$$\frac{75X}{75} = \frac{142.5}{75}$$

$$X = 1.9\ mL\ (medication)$$

Volume of IV fluid: 45 mL − 1.9 mL = 43.1 mL

29) 1.9 mL/dose × 3 doses/day = 5.7 mL/day

5.7 mL/day × 4 days = 22.8 mL (total)

30)
$$\frac{50\ mg}{1\ mL} \diagdown\!\!\!\diagup \frac{500\ mg}{X\ mL}$$

$$50X = 500$$

$$\frac{50X}{50} = \frac{500}{50}$$

$$X = 10\ mL\ (medication)$$

$$\frac{65\ mL}{60\ min} \diagdown\!\!\!\diagup \frac{X\ mL}{40\ min}$$

$$60X = 2,600$$

$$\frac{60X}{60} = \frac{2,600}{60}$$

$$X = 43.3\ mL = 43\ mL$$

43 mL (total solution) − 10 mL (med) =

33 mL (D$_5$ 0.33% NaCl)

31) 10 mL/dose × 4 doses/day = 40 mL/day

40 mL/day × 5 days = 200 mL

35)

100 mL/kg/day × 10 kg	=	1,000 mL/day for first 10 kg
50 mL/kg/day × 10 kg	=	500 mL/day for next 10 kg
20 mL/kg/day × 1 kg	=	20 mL/day for remaining 1 kg
Total	=	1,520 mL/day or per 24 h

$$\frac{1,520\ mL}{24\ h} = 63.3\ mL/h = 63\ mL/h$$

36)
$$\frac{1\ kg}{2.2\ lb} \diagdown\!\!\!\diagup \frac{X\ kg}{78\ lb}$$

$$2.2X = 78$$

$$\frac{2.2X}{2.2} = \frac{78}{2.2}$$

$$X = 35.45\ kg = 35.5\ kg$$

100 mL/kg/day × 10 kg	=	1,000 mL/day for first 10 kg
50 mL/kg/day × 10 kg	=	500 mL/day for next 10 kg
20 mL/kg/day × 15.5 kg	=	310 mL/day for remaining 15.5 kg
Total	=	1,810 mL/day or per 24 h

$$\frac{1,810\ mL}{24\ h} = 75.4\ mL/h = 75\ mL/h$$

38) 2,400 g = 2.400. = 2.4 kg

100 mL/kg/day × 2.4 kg = 240 mL/day

$\dfrac{240 \text{ mL}}{24 \text{ h}}$ = 10 mL/h

39) Safe daily dosage range:

100 mg/kg × 15 kg = 1,500 mg

125 mg/kg × 15 kg = 1,875 mg

Safe single dosage range:

$\dfrac{1,500}{6 \text{ doses}}$ = 250 mg/dose

$\dfrac{1,875}{6 \text{ doses}}$ = 312.5 mg/dose

Yes, the dosage is safe.

1 g = 1,000 mg

$\dfrac{1,000 \text{ mg}}{10 \text{ mL}} \bowtie \dfrac{275 \text{ mg}}{X \text{ mL}}$

1,000X = 10 × 275

$\dfrac{1,000X}{1,000} = \dfrac{2,750}{1,000}$

X = 2.75 mL = 2.8 mL (med)

40) IV fluid volume:

$\dfrac{53 \text{ mL}}{60 \text{ min}} \bowtie \dfrac{X \text{ mL}}{40 \text{ min}}$

60X = 2,120

$\dfrac{60X}{60} = \dfrac{2,120}{60}$

X = 35.3 mL = 35 mL

35 mL (total) − 2.8 mL (med) =

32.2 mL (D$_5$ 0.45% NaCl)

45) Safe daily dosage range:

200 mg/kg × 9 kg = 1,800 mg

300 mg/kg × 9 kg = 2,700 mg

Safe single dosage range:

$\dfrac{1,800 \text{ mg}}{6 \text{ doses}}$ = 300 mg/dose

$\dfrac{2,700 \text{ mg}}{6 \text{ doses}}$ = 450 mg/dose

Dosage is *not* safe; exceeds maximum safe dosage.

Do not give dosage ordered; consult with physician.

47) $\dfrac{1 \text{ kg}}{2.2 \text{ lb}} \bowtie \dfrac{X \text{ kg}}{55 \text{ lb}}$

2.2X = 55

$\dfrac{2.2X}{2.2} = \dfrac{55}{2.2}$

X = 25 kg

Safe daily dosage:

100,000 units/kg × 25 kg = 2,500,000 units

250,000 units/kg × 25 kg = 6,250,000 units

Safe single dosage:

$\dfrac{2,500,000 \text{ units}}{6 \text{ doses}}$ = 416,666.6 units/dose

= 416,667 units/dose

$\dfrac{6,250,000 \text{ units}}{6 \text{ doses}}$ = 1,041,666.6 units/dose

= 1,041,667 units/dose

48) Yes, dosage is safe.

$\dfrac{200,000 \text{ units}}{1 \text{ mL}} \bowtie \dfrac{525,000 \text{ units}}{X \text{ mL}}$

200,000X = 525,000

$\dfrac{200,000X}{200,000} = \dfrac{525,000}{200,000}$

X = 2.62 mL = 2.6 mL

49) $\dfrac{60 \text{ mL}}{60 \text{ min}} \bowtie \dfrac{X \text{ mL}}{20 \text{ min}}$

60X = 1,200

$\dfrac{60X}{60} = \dfrac{1,200}{60}$

X = 20 mL

20 mL (total) − 2.6 mL (med) = 17.4 mL (D$_5$NS)

Review Set 46 from pages 445–446

1) 40 **2)** 14 **3)** 10 **4)** 19 **5)** 48; Consult physician; per policy, you may be directed to stop this infusion if physician does not respond immediately. **6)** 16 **7)** 75; 6,000; 6; 1,350; 14 **8)** 6,000; 6; 300; 3; 17 **9)** 3,000; 3; 150; 1.5; 19

10) Continue the rate at 19 mL/h. **11)** 10 **12)** 50 **13)** 4 **14)** 20 **15)** 8

Solutions—Review Set 46

1)

$$\frac{25{,}000 \text{ units}}{1{,}000 \text{ mL}} \times \frac{1{,}000 \text{ units/h}}{X \text{ mL/h}}$$

$$25{,}000X = 1{,}000{,}000$$

$$\frac{25{,}000X}{25{,}000} = \frac{1{,}000{,}000}{25{,}000}$$

$$X = 40 \text{ mL/h}$$

4)

$$\frac{40{,}000 \text{ units}}{500 \text{ mL}} \times \frac{1{,}500 \text{ units/h}}{X \text{ mL/h}}$$

$$40{,}000X = 750{,}000$$

$$\frac{40{,}000X}{40{,}000} = \frac{750{,}000}{40{,}000}$$

$$X = 18.7 \text{ mL/h} = 19 \text{ mL/h}$$

5)

$$\frac{25{,}000 \text{ units}}{1{,}000 \text{ mL}} \times \frac{1{,}200 \text{ units/h}}{X \text{ mL/h}}$$

$$25{,}000X = 1{,}200{,}000$$

$$\frac{25{,}000X}{25{,}000} = \frac{1{,}200{,}000}{25{,}000}$$

$$X = 48 \text{ mL/h}$$

The IV is infusing too rapidly. The physician should be called immediately for further action.

6)

$$\frac{25{,}000 \text{ units}}{500 \text{ mL}} \times \frac{800 \text{ units/h}}{X \text{ mL/h}}$$

$$25{,}000X = 400{,}000$$

$$\frac{25{,}000X}{25{,}000} = \frac{400{,}000}{25{,}000}$$

$$X = 16 \text{ mL/h}$$

7)

$$\frac{1 \text{ kg}}{2.2 \text{ lb}} \times \frac{X \text{ kg}}{165 \text{ lb}}$$

$$2.2X = 165$$

$$\frac{2.2X}{2.2} = \frac{165}{2.2}$$

$$X = 75 \text{ kg}$$

Initial heparin bolus: 80 units/kg × 75 kg = 6,000 units

$$\frac{1{,}000 \text{ units}}{1 \text{ mL}} \times \frac{6{,}000 \text{ units}}{X \text{ mL}}$$

$$1{,}000X = 6{,}000$$

$$\frac{1{,}000X}{1{,}000} = \frac{6{,}000}{1{,}000}$$

$$X = 6 \text{ mL}$$

Initial Heparin infusion rate: 18 units/kg/h × 75 kg = 1,350 units/h

$$\frac{25{,}000 \text{ units}}{250 \text{ mL}} \times \frac{1{,}350 \text{ units/h}}{X \text{ mL/h}}$$

$$25{,}000X = 337{,}500$$

$$\frac{25{,}000X}{25{,}000} = \frac{337{,}500}{25{,}000}$$

$$X = 13.5 \text{ mL/h}$$

$$= 14 \text{ mL/h (on infusion pump)}$$

8) Rebolus: 80 units/kg × 75 kg = 6,000 units

$$\frac{1{,}000 \text{ units}}{1 \text{ mL}} \times \frac{6{,}000 \text{ units}}{X \text{ mL}}$$

$$1{,}000X = 6{,}000$$

$$\frac{1{,}000X}{1{,}000} = \frac{6{,}000}{1{,}000}$$

$$X = 6 \text{ mL}$$

Reset infusion rate: 4 units/kg/h × 75 kg = 300 units/h (increase)

$$\frac{25{,}000 \text{ units}}{250 \text{ mL}} \times \frac{300 \text{ units/h}}{X \text{ mL/h}}$$

$$25{,}000X = 75{,}000$$

$$\frac{25{,}000X}{25{,}000} = \frac{75{,}000}{25{,}000}$$

$$X = 3 \text{ mL/h}$$

14 mL/h + 3 mL/h = 17 mL/h

Reset infusion rate to 17 mL/h

9) Rebolus: 40 units/kg × 75 kg = 3,000 units

$$\frac{1{,}000 \text{ units}}{1 \text{ mL}} \times \frac{3{,}000 \text{ units}}{X \text{ mL}}$$

$$1{,}000X = 3{,}000$$

$$\frac{1{,}000X}{1{,}000} = \frac{3{,}000}{1{,}000}$$

$$X = 3 \text{ mL}$$

Reset infusion rate: 2 units/kg/h × 75 kg = 150 units/h (increase)

$$\frac{25{,}000 \text{ units}}{250 \text{ mL}} \times \frac{150 \text{ units/h}}{X \text{ mL/h}}$$

$$25{,}000X = 37{,}500$$

$$\frac{25{,}000X}{25{,}000} = \frac{37{,}500}{25{,}000}$$

$$X = 1.5 \text{ mL/h}$$

17 mL/h + 1.5 mL/h = 18.5 mL/h = 19 mL/h (on infusion pump)

Reset infusion rate to 19 mL/h

11) $\dfrac{500 \text{ units}}{500 \text{ mL}} \diagdown \dfrac{10 \text{ units/h}}{\text{X mL/h}}$

$500\text{X} = 5{,}000$

$\dfrac{500\text{X}}{500} = \dfrac{5{,}000}{500}$

$\text{X} = 10 \text{ mL/h}$

$\dfrac{125\text{X}}{125} = \dfrac{500}{125}$

$\text{X} = 4 \text{ mL/h}$

14) $\dfrac{125 \text{ mg}}{250 \text{ mL}} \diagdown \dfrac{10 \text{ mg/h}}{\text{X mL/h}}$

$125\text{X} = 2{,}500$

$\dfrac{125\text{X}}{125} = \dfrac{2{,}500}{125}$

$\text{X} = 20 \text{ mL/h}$

13) $\dfrac{125 \text{ mg}}{100 \text{ mL}} \diagdown \dfrac{5 \text{ mg/h}}{\text{X mL/h}}$

$125\text{X} = 500$

Review Set 47 from pages 455–456

1) 2; 120 **2)** 1; 60 **3)** 1.5; 90 **4)** 90; 360; 0.4; 24 **5)** 1,050; 0.66; 40 **6)** 142–568 **7)** 0.14–0.57 **8)** Yes **9)** 4 **10)** Yes
11) 100; 25 **12)** 1 **13)** 0.025 **14)** 25 **15)** Yes

Solutions—Review Set 47

1) $\dfrac{2{,}000 \text{ mg}}{1{,}000 \text{ mL}} \diagdown \dfrac{4 \text{ mg/min}}{\text{X mL/min}}$

$2{,}000\text{X} = 4{,}000$

$\dfrac{2{,}000\text{X}}{2{,}000} = \dfrac{4{,}000}{2{,}000}$

$\text{X} = 2 \text{ mL/min}$

$\dfrac{2 \text{ mL}}{1 \text{ min}} \diagdown \dfrac{\text{X mL/h}}{60 \text{ min/h}}$

$\text{X} = 120 \text{ mL/h}$

2) $\dfrac{500 \text{ mg}}{250 \text{ mL}} \diagdown \dfrac{2 \text{ mg/min}}{\text{X mL/min}}$

$500\text{X} = 500$

$\dfrac{500\text{X}}{500} = \dfrac{500}{500}$

$\text{X} = 1 \text{ mL/min}$

$\dfrac{1 \text{ mL}}{1 \text{ min}} \diagdown \dfrac{\text{X mL/h}}{60 \text{ min/h}}$

$\text{X} = 60 \text{ mL/h}$

3) $\dfrac{2{,}000 \text{ mcg}}{500 \text{ mL}} \diagdown \dfrac{6 \text{ mcg/min}}{\text{X mL/min}}$

$2{,}000\text{X} = 3{,}000$

$\dfrac{2{,}000\text{X}}{2{,}000} = \dfrac{3{,}000}{2{,}000}$

$\text{X} = 1.5 \text{ mL/min}$

$\dfrac{1.5 \text{ mL}}{1 \text{ min}} \diagdown \dfrac{\text{X mL/h}}{60 \text{ min/h}}$

$\text{X} = 90 \text{ mL/h}$

4) $\dfrac{1 \text{ kg}}{2.2 \text{ lb}} \diagdown \dfrac{\text{X kg}}{198 \text{ lb}}$

$2.2\text{X} = 198$

$\dfrac{2.2\text{X}}{2.2} = \dfrac{198}{2.2}$

$\text{X} = 90 \text{ kg}$

$4 \text{ mcg/kg/min} \times 90 \text{ kg} = 360 \text{ mcg/min}$

$\dfrac{1{,}000 \text{ mcg}}{1 \text{ mg}} \diagdown \dfrac{360 \text{ mcg/min}}{\text{X mg/min}}$

$1{,}000\text{X} = 360$

$\dfrac{1{,}000\text{X}}{1{,}000} = \dfrac{360}{1{,}000}$

$\text{X} = 0.36 \text{ mg/min}$

$\dfrac{450 \text{ mg}}{500 \text{ mL}} \diagdown \dfrac{0.36 \text{ mg/min}}{\text{X mL/min}}$

$450\text{X} = 180$

$\dfrac{450\text{X}}{450} = \dfrac{180}{450}$

$\text{X} = 0.4 \text{ mL/min}$

$\dfrac{0.4 \text{ mL}}{1 \text{ min}} \diagdown \dfrac{\text{X mL/h}}{60 \text{ min/h}}$

$\text{X} = 24 \text{ mL/h}$

5) $15 \text{ mcg/kg/min} \times 70 \text{ kg} = 1{,}050 \text{ mcg/min}$

$\dfrac{1 \text{ mg}}{1{,}000 \text{ mcg}} \diagdown \dfrac{\text{X mg/min}}{1{,}050 \text{ mcg/min}}$

$1{,}000\text{X} = 1{,}050$

$\dfrac{1{,}000\text{X}}{1{,}000} = \dfrac{1{,}050}{1{,}000}$

$\text{X} = 1.05 \text{ mg/min}$

$\dfrac{800 \text{ mg}}{500 \text{ mL}} \diagdown \dfrac{1.05 \text{ mg/min}}{\text{X mL/min}}$

$800\text{X} = 525$

$\dfrac{800\text{X}}{800} = \dfrac{525}{800}$

$\text{X} = 0.656 \text{ mL/min} = 0.66 \text{ mL/min}$

$\dfrac{0.66 \text{ mL}}{1 \text{ min}} \diagdown \dfrac{\text{X mL/h}}{60 \text{ min/h}}$

$\text{X} = 39.6 = 40 \text{ mL/h}$

6) $\dfrac{1 \text{ kg}}{2.2 \text{ lb}} \diagdown \dfrac{\text{X kg}}{125 \text{ lb}}$

$2.2\text{X} = 125$

$$\frac{2.2X}{2.2} = \frac{125}{2.2}$$

X = 56.8 kg

Minimum: 2.5 mcg/kg/min × 56.8 kg = 142 mcg/min

Maximum: 10 mcg/kg/min × 56.8 kg = 568 mcg/min

7) Minimum:

$$\frac{1 \text{ mg}}{1,000 \text{ mcg}} \bowtie \frac{X \text{ mg/min}}{142 \text{ mcg/min}}$$

1,000X = 142

$$\frac{1,000X}{1,000} = \frac{142}{1,000}$$

X = 0.142 mg/min = 0.14 mg/min

Maximum:

$$\frac{1 \text{ mg}}{1,000 \text{ mcg}} \bowtie \frac{X \text{ mg/min}}{568 \text{ mcg/min}}$$

1,000X = 568

$$\frac{1,000X}{1,000} = \frac{568}{1,000}$$

X = 0.568 mg/min = 0.57 mg/min

8)

$$\frac{500 \text{ mg}}{500 \text{ mL}} \bowtie \frac{X \text{ mg/h}}{15 \text{ mL/h}}$$

500X = 7,500

$$\frac{500X}{500} = \frac{7,500}{500}$$

X = 15 mg/h

$$\frac{15 \text{ mg}}{60 \text{ min}} \bowtie \frac{X \text{ mg}}{1 \text{ min}}$$

60X = 15

$$\frac{60X}{60} = \frac{15}{60}$$

X = 0.25 mg (per min) or 0.25 mg/min

Yes, the order is within the safe range of 0.14–0.57 mg/min.

9)

$$\frac{2,000 \text{ mg}}{500 \text{ mL}} \bowtie \frac{X \text{ mg/h}}{60 \text{ mL/h}}$$

500X = 120,000

$$\frac{500X}{500} = \frac{120,000}{500}$$

X = 240 mg/h

$$\frac{240 \text{ mg/h}}{60 \text{ min/h}} \bowtie \frac{X \text{ mg}}{1 \text{ min}}$$

60X = 240

$$\frac{60X}{60} = \frac{240}{60}$$

X = 4 mg (per min) or 4 mg/min

10) Yes, 4 mg/min is within the normal range of 2–6 mg/min.

11) Bolus:

$$\frac{2 \text{ g}}{30 \text{ min}} \bowtie \frac{X \text{ g}}{60 \text{ min}}$$

30X = 120

X = 4 g (per 60 min or 4 g/h)

$$\frac{20 \text{ g}}{500 \text{ mL}} \bowtie \frac{4 \text{ g/h}}{X \text{ mL/h}}$$

20X = 2,000

$$\frac{20X}{20} = \frac{2,000}{20}$$

X = 100 mL/h

Continuous:

$$\frac{20 \text{ g}}{500 \text{ mL}} \bowtie \frac{1 \text{ g/h}}{X \text{ mL/h}}$$

20X = 500

$$\frac{20X}{20} = \frac{500}{20}$$

X = 25 mL/h

12)

$$\frac{1 \text{ unit}}{1,000 \text{ milliunits}} \bowtie \frac{X \text{ units}}{1 \text{ milliunit}}$$

1,000X = 1

$$\frac{1,000X}{1,000} = \frac{1}{1,000}$$

X = 0.001 units

$$\frac{15 \text{ units}}{250 \text{ mL}} \bowtie \frac{0.001 \text{ units/min}}{X \text{ mL/min}}$$

15X = 0.25

$$\frac{15X}{15} = \frac{0.25}{15}$$

X = 0.0166 mL/min = 0.017 mL/min

$$\frac{0.017 \text{ mL}}{1 \text{ min}} \bowtie \frac{X \text{ mL/h}}{60 \text{ min/h}}$$

X = 1.02 mL/h = 1 mL/h

13)

$$\frac{10 \text{ mg}}{1,000 \text{ mL}} \bowtie \frac{X \text{ mg/h}}{150 \text{ mL/h}}$$

1,000X = 1,500

$$\frac{1,000X}{1,000} = \frac{1,500}{1,000}$$

X = 1.5 mg/h

$$\frac{1.5 \text{ mg/h}}{60 \text{ min/h}} \bowtie \frac{X \text{ mg}}{1 \text{ min}}$$

60X = 1.5

$$\frac{60X}{60} = \frac{1.5}{60}$$

X = 0.025 mg (per min) or 0.025 mg/min

14)

$$\frac{1 \text{ mg}}{1,000 \text{ mcg}} \diagdown \diagup \frac{0.025 \text{ mg/min}}{X \text{ mcg/min}}$$

$$X = 25 \text{ mcg/min}$$

Review Set 48 from pages 458–460

1) 33; 19 **2)** 40; 42 **3)** 25; 32 **4)** 50; 90 **5)** 50; 40 **6)** 100; 100 **7)** 200; 76 **8)** 200; 122 **9)** 17; 21 **10)** 120; 112

Solutions—Review Set 48

1) Step 1.

IV PB rate: $\frac{V}{T} \times C = \frac{\overset{}{100 \text{ mL}}}{\underset{3}{30 \text{ min}}} \times \overset{1}{10} \text{ gtt/mL} =$

$\frac{100}{3} \text{ gtt/min} = 33.3 \text{ gtt/min} = 33 \text{ gtt/min}$

Step 2. Total IV PB time: q.4h $\times$ 30 min = 6 $\times$ 30 min = 180 min; 180 min $\div$ 60 min/h = 3 h

Step 3. Total IV PB volume: 6 $\times$ 100 mL = 600 mL

Step 4. Total Regular IV volume: 3,000 mL − 600 mL = 2,400 mL

Step 5. Total Regular IV time: 24 h − 3 h = 21 h

Step 6. Regular IV rate:

$\frac{2,400 \text{ mL}}{21 \text{ h}} = 114.2 \text{ mL/h} = 114 \text{ mL/h}$

$\frac{\text{mL/h}}{\text{drop factor constant}} = \text{gtt/min}; \frac{114 \text{ mL/h}}{6} = 19 \text{ gtt/min}$

2) Step 1. IV PB rate: When drop factor is 60 gtt/mL, then mL/h = gtt/min. Rate is 40 gtt/min.

Step 2. Total IV PB time: q.i.d. $\times$ 1 h = 4 $\times$ 1 h = 4 h

Step 3. Total IV PB volume: 4 $\times$ 40 mL = 160 mL

Step 4. Total Regular IV volume: 1,000 mL − 160 mL = 840 mL

Step 5. Total Regular IV time: 24 h − 4 h = 20 h

Step 6. Total Regular IV rate: mL/h = $\frac{840 \text{ mL}}{20 \text{ h}}$ = 42 mL/h. When drop factor is 60 gtt/mL, then mL/h = gtt/min. Rate is 42 gtt/min.

3) Step 1.

IV PB rate: $\frac{V}{T} \times C = \frac{\overset{}{50 \text{ mL}}}{\underset{2}{30 \text{ min}}} \times \overset{1}{15} \text{ gtt/mL} = \frac{50}{2} \text{ gtt/min} = 25 \text{ gtt/min}$

Step 2. Total IV PB time: q.6h $\times$ 30 min = 4 $\times$ 30 min = 120 min; 120 min $\div$ 60 min/h = 2 h

Step 3. Total IV PB volume: 4 $\times$ 50 mL = 200 mL

Step 4. Total Regular IV volume: 3,000 mL − 200 mL = 2,800 mL

Step 5. Total Regular IV time: 24 h − 2 h = 22 h

Step 6. Total Regular IV rate:

$\frac{2,800}{22 \text{ h}} = 127.2 \text{ mL/h} = 127 \text{ mL/h}$

$\frac{\text{mL/h}}{\text{drop factor constant}} = \text{gtt/min}; \frac{127 \text{ mL/h}}{4} = 31.7 \text{ gtt/min} = 32 \text{ gtt/min}$

4) Step 1. IV PB rate: 50 mL/h or 50 gtt/min (because drop factor is 60 gtt/mL)

Step 2. Total IV PB time: q.6h $\times$ 1 h = 4 $\times$ 1 h = 4 h

Step 3. Total IV PB volume: 4 $\times$ 50 mL = 200 mL

Step 4. Total Regular IV volume: 2,000 mL − 200 mL = 1,800 mL

Step 5. Total Regular IV time: 24 h − 4 h = 20 h

Step 6. Regular IV rate: $\frac{1,800 \text{ mL}}{20 \text{ h}}$ = 90 mL/h or 90 gtt/min (because drop factor is 60 gtt/mL)

5) Step 1. IV PB rate: 50 mL/h or 50 gtt/min (because drop factor is 60 gtt/mL)

Step 2. IV PB time: q.8h $\times$ 1 h = 3 $\times$ 1 h = 3 h

Step 3. IV PB volume: 3 $\times$ 50 mL = 150 mL

Step 4. Total Regular IV volume: 1,000 mL $-$ 150 mL = 850 mL

Step 5. Total Regular IV time: 24 h $-$ 3 h = 21 h

Step 6. Regular IV rate: $\frac{850 \text{ mL}}{21 \text{ h}}$ = 40.4 mL/h = 40 mL/h or 40 gtt/min (because drop factor is 60 gtt/mL)

6) Step 1. IV PB rate:

$$\frac{50 \text{ mL}}{30 \text{ min}} \quad\diagdown\diagup\quad \frac{X \text{ mL}}{60 \text{ min}}$$

$$30X = 3,000$$

$$\frac{30X}{30} = \frac{3,000}{30}$$

$$X = 100 \text{ mL}; \; 100 \text{ mL per 60 min} = 100 \text{ mL/h}$$

Step 2. IV PB time: q.6h $\times$ 30 min = 4 $\times$ 30 min = 120 min; 120 min $\div$ 60 min/h = 2 h

Step 3. IV PB volume: 4 $\times$ 50 mL = 200 mL

Step 4. Total Regular IV volume: 2,400 mL $-$ 200 mL = 2,200 mL

Step 5. Total Regular IV time: 24 h $-$ 2 h = 22 h

Step 6. Regular IV rate: $\frac{2,200 \text{ mL}}{22 \text{ h}}$ = 100 mL/h

7) Step 1. IV PB rate:

$$\frac{100 \text{ mL}}{30 \text{ min}} \quad\diagdown\diagup\quad \frac{X \text{ mL}}{60 \text{ min}}$$

$$30X = 6,000$$

$$\frac{30X}{30} = \frac{6,000}{30}$$

$$X = 200 \text{ mL}; \; 200 \text{ mL per 60 min} = 200 \text{ mL/h}$$

Step 2. IV PB time: q.8h $\times$ 30 min = 3 $\times$ 30 min = 90 min; 90 min $\div$ 60 min/h = $1\frac{1}{2}$ h

Step 3. IV PB volume: 3 $\times$ 100 mL = 300 mL

Step 4. Total Regular IV volume: 2,000 mL $-$ 300 mL = 1,700 mL

Step 5. Total Regular IV time: 24 h $-$ $1\frac{1}{2}$ h = $22\frac{1}{2}$ h

Step 6. Regular IV rate: $\frac{1,700 \text{ mL}}{22.5 \text{ h}}$ = 75.5 mL/h = 76 mL/h

8) Step 1. IV PB rate

$$\frac{50 \text{ mL}}{15 \text{ min}} \quad\diagdown\diagup\quad \frac{X \text{ mL}}{60 \text{ min}}$$

$$15X = 3,000$$

$$\frac{15X}{15} = \frac{3,000}{15}$$

$$X = 200 \text{ mL}; \; 200 \text{ mL per 60 min} = 200 \text{ mL/h}$$

Step 2. IV PB time: q.6h $\times$ 15 min = 4 $\times$ 15 min = 60 min = 1 h

Step 3. IV PB volume: 4 $\times$ 50 mL = 200 mL

Step 4. Total Regular IV volume: 3,000 mL $-$ 200 mL = 2,800 mL

Step 5. Total Regular IV time: 24 h $-$ 1 h = 23 h

Step 6. Regular IV rate: $\frac{2,800}{23 \text{ h}}$ = 121.7 mL/h = 122 mL/h

Practice Problems—Chapter 17 from pages 461–466

1) 60 2) 5 3) 20 4) 50 5) 1 6) 12 7) 50 8) 63 9) 35 10) 6; 15 11) 60 12) 45 13) 60 14) 24 15) Yes 16) 17; 22

17) 100; 127 18) 102 19) 8 mEq 20) 2 21) 15 22) 50 23) 25 24) 7.4 25) 12; 18 26) 150; 50 27) 2 28) 35 29) 8

30) 63 31) 80 32) 0.4 33) 4 34) 4 35) 100 36) 0.2; 200 37) 30 38) 200; 50 39) 5 40) 550 41) 2,450 42) 19

43) 129 44) 13; 39 45) 100; 80 46) 8,000; 1,000; 8 47) 18; 1,800; 100; 18 48) 6; 40; 4,000; 4; increase; 2; 200;

2; 20 49) Decrease rate by 2 units/kg/h; 18

STANDARD WEIGHT-BASED HEPARIN PROTOCOL WORKSHEET

Round Patient's Total Body Weight to Nearest 10 kg: _100_ kg
DO NOT Change the Weight Based on Daily Measurements

FOUND ON THE ORDER FORM
Initial Bolus (80 units/kg) _8,000_ units __8__ mL
Initial Infusion Rate (18 units/kg/h) _1,800_ units/h __18__ mL/h

Make adjustments to the heparin drip rate as directed by the order form.
ALL DOSES ARE ROUNDED TO THE NEAREST 100 UNITS

| Date | Time | APTT | Bolus | Rate Change | | New Rate | RN 1 | RN 2 |
				Units/h	mL/h			
5/10/XX	1730	37 sec	4,000 units (4 mL)	+200 units/h	+2 mL/h	20 mL/h	G.P.	M.S.
5/10/XX	2330	77 sec		−200 units/h	−2 mL/h	18 mL/h	G.P.	M.S.

Signatures	Initials
G. Pickar, R.N.	G.P.
M. Smith, R.N.	M.S.

50)   **Prevention:** The nurse who prepares any IV solution with an additive should *carefully* compare the order and medication three times: before beginning to prepare the dose, after the dosage is prepared, and just before it is administered to the patient. Further, the nurse should verify the safety of the dosage using the three-step method (convert, think, and calculate). It was clear that the nurse realized the error when a colleague questioned what was being prepared and the nurse verified the actual order. Also, taking the time to do the calculation on paper helps the nurse to "see" the answer and avoid a potentially life-threatening error. The precriber should also write out units and milliunits (U and mU are not permitted abbreviations). The nurse should contact the prescriber to clarify an order when unacceptable notation is used.

Solutions—Practice Problems—Chapter 17

1) Volume control sets are microdrip infusion sets calibrated for 60 gtt/mL.

2) 1 g is ordered and it is prepared as a supply dosage of 1 g per 5 mL. Add 5 mL.

3) $\dfrac{50 \text{ mL}}{60 \text{ min}} \diagdown \dfrac{X \text{ mL}}{30 \text{ min}}$

$$60X = 1,500$$

$$\frac{60X}{60} = \frac{1,500}{60}$$

$$X = 25 \text{ mL total volume}$$

25 mL total − 5 mL med = 20 mL D_5W

4) $\dfrac{\text{mL/h}}{\text{drop factor constant}} = \dfrac{50 \text{ mL/h}}{1} = 50 \text{ gtt/min};$

when drop factor is 60 gtt/mL, then mL/h = gtt/min

5) once (at 1200 hours)

6) $\dfrac{25,000 \text{ units}}{250 \text{ mL}} \diagdown \dfrac{1,200 \text{ units/h}}{X \text{ mL/h}}$

$$25,000X = 300,000$$

$$\frac{25,000X}{25,000} = \frac{300,000}{25,000}$$

$$X = 12 \text{ mL/h}$$

7) $\dfrac{100 \text{ mg}}{1,000 \text{ mL}} \diagdown \dfrac{5 \text{ mg/h}}{X \text{ mL/h}}$

$$100X = 5,000$$

$$\frac{100X}{100} = \frac{5,000}{100}$$

$$X = 50 \text{ mL/h}$$

8) $\dfrac{4,000 \text{ mg}}{500 \text{ mL}} \diagdown \dfrac{500 \text{ mg/h}}{X \text{ mL/h}}$

$$4,000X = 250,000$$

$$\frac{4,000X}{4,000} = \frac{250,000}{4,000}$$

$$X = 62.5 \text{ mL/h} = 63 \text{ mL/h}$$

9) $\dfrac{20,000 \text{ units}}{500 \text{ mL}} \diagdown \dfrac{1,400 \text{ units/h}}{X \text{ mL/h}}$

$$20,000X = 700,000$$

$$\frac{20,000X}{20,000} = \frac{700,000}{20,000}$$

$$X = 35 \text{ mL/h}$$

10) $\dfrac{1 \text{ L}}{1,000 \text{ mL}} \diagdown \dfrac{1.5 \text{ L}}{X \text{ mL}}$

$$X = 1,500 \text{ mL}$$

$$\frac{1,500 \text{ mL}}{4 \text{ mL/min}} = 375 \text{ min}$$

$375 \text{ min} \div 60 \text{ min/h} = 6.25 \text{ h} = 6\frac{1}{4} \text{ h} = 6 \text{ h } 15 \text{ min}$

11) $\dfrac{2,000 \text{ mg}}{500 \text{ mL}} \diagdown \dfrac{4 \text{ mg/min}}{X \text{ mL/min}}$

$$2,000X = 2,000$$

$$\frac{2,000X}{2,000} = \frac{2,000}{2,000}$$

$$X = 1 \text{ mL/min}$$

which is the same as 60 mL per 60 min or 60 mL/h

12) $\dfrac{1,000 \text{ mg}}{250 \text{ mL}} \diagdown \dfrac{3 \text{ mg/min}}{X \text{ mL/min}}$

$$1,000X = 750$$

$$\frac{1,000X}{1,000} = \frac{750}{1,000}$$

$$X = 0.75 \text{ mL/min}$$

$\dfrac{0.75 \text{ mL}}{1 \text{ min}} \diagdown \dfrac{X \text{ mL/h}}{60 \text{ min/h}}$

$$X = 45 \text{ mL/h}$$

13) $\dfrac{1,000 \text{ mg}}{500 \text{ mL}} \diagdown \dfrac{2 \text{ mg/min}}{X \text{ mL/min}}$

$$1,000X = 1,000$$

$$\frac{1,000X}{1,000} = \frac{1,000}{1,000}$$

$$X = 1 \text{ mL/min}$$

which is the same as 60 mL per 60 min or 60 mL/h

14) 5 mcg/kg/min × 80 kg = 400 mcg/min

$\dfrac{1 \text{ mg}}{1,000 \text{ mcg}} \diagdown \dfrac{X \text{ mg/min}}{400 \text{ mcg/min}}$

$$1,000X = 400$$

$$\frac{1,000X}{1,000} = \frac{400}{1,000}$$

$$X = 0.4 \text{ mg/min}$$

$\dfrac{250 \text{ mg}}{250 \text{ mL}} \diagdown \dfrac{0.4 \text{ mg/min}}{X \text{ mL/min}}$

$$250X = 100$$

$$\frac{250X}{250} = \frac{100}{250}$$

$$X = 0.4 \text{ mL/min}$$

$\dfrac{0.4 \text{ mL}}{1 \text{ min}} \diagdown \dfrac{X \text{ mL/h}}{60 \text{ min/h}}$

$$X = 24 \text{ mL/h}$$

15) $\dfrac{2,000 \text{ mg}}{1,000 \text{ mL}} \diagdown \dfrac{X \text{ mg/h}}{75 \text{ mL/h}}$

$$1,000X = 150,000$$

$$\frac{1,000X}{1,000} = \frac{150,000}{1,000}$$

$$X = 150 \text{ mg/h}$$

$\dfrac{150 \text{ mg/h}}{60 \text{ min/h}} \diagdown \dfrac{X \text{ mg}}{1 \text{ min}}$

$$60X = 150$$

$$\frac{60X}{60} = \frac{150}{60}$$

$$X = 2.5 \text{ mg (per min)} = 2.5 \text{ mg/min}$$

within normal range of 1–4 mg/min

16) IV PB flow rate: $\dfrac{\text{mL/h}}{\text{drop factor constant}} = \dfrac{100 \text{ mL/h}}{6} =$

16.6 gtt/min = 17 gtt/min

Total IV PB time: q.6h $\times$ 1 h = 4 $\times$ 1 h = 4 h

Total IV PB volume: 4 $\times$ 100 mL = 400 mL

Total Regular IV volume: 3,000 mL $-$ 400 mL = 2,600 mL

Total Regular IV time: 24 h $-$ 4 h = 20 h

Regular IV rate: mL/h = $\dfrac{2,600 \text{ mL}}{20\text{h}} = 130$ mL/h;

$\dfrac{\text{mL/h}}{\text{drop factor constant}} = \dfrac{130 \text{ mL/h}}{6} = 21.6$ gtt/min = 22 gtt/min

17) IV PB rate:

$$\dfrac{50 \text{ mL}}{30 \text{ min}} \times\!\!\!\times \dfrac{X \text{ mL}}{60 \text{ min}}$$

$$30X = 3,000$$

$$\dfrac{30X}{30} = \dfrac{3,000}{30}$$

$$X = 100 \text{ mL}; 100 \text{ mL per 60 min}$$
$$= 100 \text{ mL/h}$$

Total IV PB time: q.i.d. $\times$ 30 min = 4 $\times$ 30 min = 120 min; 120 min $\div$ 60 min/h = 2 h

Total IV PB volume: 4 $\times$ 50 mL = 200 mL

Total Regular IV volume: 3,000 mL $-$ 200 mL = 2,800 mL

Total Regular IV time: 24 h $-$ 2 h = 22 h

Regular IV rate: $\dfrac{2,800 \text{ mL}}{22 \text{ h}} = 127.2$ mL/h = 127 mL/h

18) $\dfrac{1 \text{ kg}}{2.2 \text{ lb}} \times\!\!\!\times \dfrac{X \text{ kg}}{125 \text{ lb}}$

$$2.2X = 125$$

$$\dfrac{2.2X}{2.2} = \dfrac{125}{2.2}$$

$$X = 56.8 \text{ kg}$$

3 mcg/kg/min $\times$ 56.8 kg = 170.4 mcg/min

$$\dfrac{1 \text{ mg}}{1,000 \text{ mcg}} \times\!\!\!\times \dfrac{X \text{ mg/min}}{170.4 \text{ mcg/min}}$$

$$1,000X = 170.4$$

$$\dfrac{1,000X}{1,000} = \dfrac{170.4}{1,000}$$

$$X = 0.17 \text{ mg/min}$$

$$\dfrac{50 \text{ mg}}{500 \text{ mL}} \times\!\!\!\times \dfrac{0.17 \text{ mg/min}}{X \text{ mL/min}}$$

$$50X = 85$$

$$\dfrac{50X}{50} = \dfrac{85}{50}$$

$$X = 1.7 \text{ mL/min}$$

$$\dfrac{1.7 \text{ mL}}{1 \text{ min}} \times\!\!\!\times \dfrac{X \text{ mL/h}}{60 \text{ min/h}}$$

$$X = 102 \text{ mL/h}$$

19) 1,000 mL $-$ 800 mL = 200 mL infused

$$\dfrac{40 \text{ mEq}}{1,000 \text{ mL}} \times\!\!\!\times \dfrac{X \text{ mEq}}{200 \text{ mL}}$$

$$1,000X = 8,000$$

$$\dfrac{1,000X}{1,000} = \dfrac{8,000}{1,000}$$

$$X = 8 \text{ mEq}$$

20) $\dfrac{125 \text{ mL}}{60 \text{ min}} = 2$ mL/min

21) $\dfrac{1,500 \text{ mL}}{100 \text{ mL/h}} = 15$ h

22) $\dfrac{40 \text{ mEq}}{1,000 \text{ mL}} \times\!\!\!\times \dfrac{2 \text{ mEq/h}}{X \text{ mL/h}}$

$$40X = 2,000$$

$$\dfrac{40X}{40} = \dfrac{2,000}{40}$$

$$X = 50 \text{ mL/h}$$

23) $\dfrac{50,000 \text{ units}}{1,000 \text{ mL}} \times\!\!\!\times \dfrac{1,250 \text{ units/h}}{X \text{ mL/h}}$

$$50,000X = 1,250,000$$

$$\dfrac{50,000X}{50,000} = \dfrac{1,250,000}{50,000}$$

$$X = 25 \text{ mL/h}$$

24) $\dfrac{5 \text{ mg}}{1 \text{ mL}} \times\!\!\!\times \dfrac{37 \text{ mg}}{X \text{ mL}}$

$$5X = 37$$

$$\dfrac{5X}{5} = \dfrac{37}{5}$$

$$X = 7.4 \text{ mL}$$

25) $\dfrac{1 \text{ unit}}{1,000 \text{ milliunits}} \times\!\!\!\times \dfrac{10 \text{ units}}{X \text{ milliunits}}$

$$X = 10,000 \text{ milliunits}$$

$$\dfrac{10,000 \text{ milliunits}}{500 \text{ mL}} \times\!\!\!\times \dfrac{4 \text{ milliunits/min}}{X \text{ mL/min}}$$

$$10,000X = 2,000$$

$$\dfrac{10,000X}{10,000} = \dfrac{2,000}{10,000}$$

$$X = 0.2 \text{ mL/min (for first 20 minutes)}$$

$$\dfrac{0.2 \text{ mL}}{1 \text{ min}} \times\!\!\!\times \dfrac{X \text{ mL/h}}{60 \text{ min/h}}$$

$$X = 12 \text{ mL/h}$$

$$\frac{10{,}000 \text{ milliunits}}{500 \text{ mL}} \times \frac{6 \text{ milliunits/min}}{X \text{ mL/min}}$$

$$10{,}000X = 3{,}000$$

$$\frac{10{,}000X}{10{,}000} = \frac{3{,}000}{10{,}000}$$

$$X = 0.3 \text{ mL/min (for next 20 minutes)}$$

$$\frac{0.3 \text{ mL}}{1 \text{ min}} \times \frac{X \text{ mL/h}}{60 \text{ min/h}}$$

$$X = 18 \text{ mL/h}$$

26) Bolus:

$$\frac{3 \text{ g}}{30 \text{ min}} \times \frac{X \text{ g/h}}{60 \text{ min/h}}$$

$$\frac{30X}{30} = \frac{180}{30}$$

$$X = 6 \text{ g/h}$$

$$\frac{20 \text{ g}}{500 \text{ mL}} \times \frac{6 \text{ g/h}}{X \text{ mL/h}}$$

$$20X = 3{,}000$$

$$\frac{20X}{20} = \frac{3{,}000}{20}$$

$$X = 150 \text{ mL/h}$$

Continuous infusion:

$$\frac{20 \text{ g}}{500 \text{ mL}} \times \frac{2 \text{ g/h}}{X \text{ mL/h}}$$

$$20X = 1{,}000$$

$$\frac{20X}{20} = \frac{1{,}000}{20}$$

$$X = 50 \text{ mL/h}$$

29) $\dfrac{\overset{8}{\cancel{4{,}000}} \text{ mg}}{\underset{1}{\cancel{500}} \text{ mL}} = 8 \text{ mg/mL}$

30) $\dfrac{4{,}000 \text{ mg}}{500 \text{ mL}} \times \dfrac{500 \text{ mg/h}}{X \text{ mL/h}}$

$$4{,}000X = 250{,}000$$

$$\frac{4{,}000X}{4{,}000} = \frac{250{,}000}{4{,}000}$$

$$X = 62.5 \text{ mL/h} = 63 \text{ mL/h}$$

31) $\dfrac{1 \text{ unit}}{1{,}000 \text{ milliunits}} \times \dfrac{80 \text{ units}}{X \text{ milliunits}}$

$$X = 80{,}000 \text{ milliunits}$$

$$\frac{80{,}000 \text{ milliunits}}{1{,}000 \text{ mL}} \times \frac{X \text{ milliunits}}{1 \text{ mL}}$$

$$1{,}000X = 80{,}000$$

$$\frac{1{,}000X}{1{,}000} = \frac{80{,}000}{1{,}000}$$

$$X = 80 \text{ milliunits (per mL) or 80 milliunits/mL}$$

33) $\dfrac{1 \text{ mg}}{1{,}000 \text{ mcg}} \times \dfrac{4 \text{ mg}}{X \text{ mcg}}$

$$X = 4{,}000 \text{ mcg}$$

$$\frac{4{,}000 \text{ mcg}}{1{,}000 \text{ mL}} \times \frac{X \text{ mcg}}{1 \text{ mL}}$$

$$1{,}000X = 4{,}000$$

$$\frac{1{,}000X}{1{,}000} = \frac{4{,}000}{1{,}000}$$

$$X = 4 \text{ mcg (per mL) or 4 mcg/mL}$$

36) $\dfrac{20 \text{ mg}}{100 \text{ mL}} \times \dfrac{X \text{ mg}}{1 \text{ mL}}$

$$100X = 20$$

$$\frac{100X}{100} = \frac{20}{100}$$

$$X = 0.2 \text{ mg (per mL) or 0.2 mg/mL}$$

$$\frac{1 \text{ mg}}{1{,}000 \text{ mcg}} \times \frac{0.2 \text{ mg}}{X \text{ mcg}}$$

$$X = 200 \text{ mcg (per mL) or 200 mcg/mL}$$

37) $1 \text{ mcg/kg/min} \times 100 \text{ kg} = 100 \text{ mcg/min}$

$$\frac{20{,}000 \text{ mcg}}{100 \text{ mL}} \times \frac{100 \text{ mcg/min}}{X \text{ mL/min}}$$

$$20{,}000X = 10{,}000$$

$$\frac{20{,}000X}{20{,}000} = \frac{10{,}000}{20{,}000}$$

$$X = 0.5 \text{ mL/min}$$

$$\frac{0.5 \text{ mL}}{1 \text{ min}} \times \frac{X \text{ mL/h}}{60 \text{ min/h}}$$

$$X = 30 \text{ mL/h}$$

38) IV PB rates:

$$\frac{100 \text{ mL}}{30 \text{ min}} \times \frac{X \text{ mL}}{60 \text{ min}}$$

$$30X = 6{,}000$$

$$\frac{30X}{30} = \frac{6{,}000}{30}$$

$$X = 200 \text{ mL (per 60 min)}$$

200 mL per 60 min = 200 mL/h (ampicillin)

gentamicin: 50 mL/h

39) ampicillin: q.6h $\times$ 30 min = 4 $\times$ 30 min = 120 min

120 min $\div$ 60 min/h = 2 h

gentamicin: q.8h $\times$ 1 h = 3 $\times$ 1 h = 3 h

Total IV PB time: 2 h + 3 h = 5 h

40) ampicillin: 4 doses $\times$ 100 mL/dose = 400 mL

gentamicin: 3 doses $\times$ 50 mL/dose = 150 mL

Total IV PB volume: 400 mL + 150 mL = 550 mL

41) 3,000 mL − 550 mL = 2,450 mL

42) 24 h − 5 h = 19 h

43) $\dfrac{2{,}450 \text{ mL}}{19 \text{ h}} = 128.9 \text{ mL/h} = 129 \text{ mL/h}$

44) $\dfrac{1 \text{ kg}}{2.2 \text{ lb}} \times \dfrac{X \text{ kg}}{190 \text{ lb}}$

$$2.2X = 190$$

$$\frac{2.2X}{2.2} = \frac{190}{2.2}$$

$$X = 86.36 \text{ kg} = 86.4 \text{ kg}$$

$$4 \text{ mcg/kg/min} \times 86.4 \text{ kg} = 345.6 \text{ mcg/min}$$

$$\frac{345.6 \text{ mcg}}{1 \text{ min}} \diagdown \frac{X \text{ mcg/h}}{60 \text{ min/h}}$$

$$X = 20,736 \text{ mcg/h}$$

$$\frac{1 \text{ mg}}{1,000 \text{ mcg}} \diagdown \frac{X \text{ mg}}{20,736 \text{ mcg}}$$

$$1,000X = 20,736$$

$$\frac{1,000X}{1,000} = \frac{20,736}{1,000}$$

$$X = 20.7 \text{ mg/h} = 21 \text{ mg/h}$$

$$\frac{800 \text{ mg}}{500 \text{ mL}} \diagdown \frac{21 \text{ mg/h}}{X \text{ mL/h}}$$

$$800X = 10,500$$

$$\frac{800X}{800} = \frac{10,500}{800}$$

$$X = 13.1 \text{ mL/h} = 13 \text{ mL/h (initial rate)}$$

$$12 \text{ mcg/kg/min} \times 86.4 \text{ kg} = 1,036.8 \text{ mcg/min}$$

$$\frac{1,036.8 \text{ mcg}}{1 \text{ min}} \diagdown \frac{X \text{ mcg/h}}{60 \text{ min/h}}$$

$$X = 62,208 \text{ mcg/h}$$

$$\frac{1 \text{ mg}}{1,000 \text{ mcg}} \diagdown \frac{X \text{ mg}}{62,208 \text{ mcg}}$$

$$1,000X = 62,208$$

$$\frac{1,000X}{1,000} = \frac{62,208}{1,000}$$

$$X = 62 \text{ mg/h}$$

$$\frac{800 \text{ mg}}{500 \text{ mL}} \diagdown \frac{62 \text{ mg/h}}{X \text{ mL/h}}$$

$$800X = 31,000$$

$$\frac{800X}{800} = \frac{31,000}{800}$$

$$X = 38.7 \text{ mL/h} = 39 \text{ mL/h (after titration)}$$

45)
$$\frac{1 \text{ kg}}{2.2 \text{ lb}} \diagdown \frac{X \text{ kg}}{225 \text{ lb}}$$

$$2.2X = 225$$

$$\frac{2.2X}{2.2} = \frac{225}{2.2}$$

$$X = 102.27 \text{ kg} = 100 \text{ kg (rounded)}$$

80 units/kg bolus dosage

46) 80 units/kg $\times$ 100 kg = 8,000 units

1,000 units/mL

$$\frac{1,000 \text{ units}}{1 \text{ mL}} \diagdown \frac{8,000 \text{ units}}{X \text{ mL}}$$

$$1,000X = 8,000$$

$$\frac{1,000X}{1,000} = \frac{8,000}{1,000}$$

$$X = 8 \text{ mL}$$

47) 18 units/kg/h $\times$ 100 kg = 1,800 units/h

$$\frac{25,000 \text{ units}}{250 \text{ mL}} \diagdown \frac{X \text{ units}}{1 \text{ mL}}$$

$$250X = 25,000$$

$$\frac{250X}{250} = \frac{25,000}{250}$$

$$X = 100 \text{ units (per mL)}$$

$$\frac{100 \text{ units}}{1 \text{ mL}} \diagdown \frac{1,800 \text{ units/h}}{X \text{ mL/h}}$$

$$100X = 1,800$$

$$\frac{100X}{100} = \frac{1,800}{100}$$

$$X = 18 \text{ mL/h}$$

48) q.6h

40 units/kg $\times$ 100 kg = 4,000 units

$$\frac{1,000 \text{ units}}{1 \text{ mL}} \diagdown \frac{4,000 \text{ units}}{X \text{ mL}}$$

$$1,000X = 4,000$$

$$\frac{1,000X}{1,000} = \frac{4,000}{1,000}$$

$$X = 4 \text{ mL}$$

Increase rate: 2 units/kg/h $\times$ 100 kg = 200 units/h

Increase rate:

$$\frac{100 \text{ units}}{1 \text{ mL}} \diagdown \frac{200 \text{ units/h}}{X \text{ mL/h}}$$

$$100X = 200$$

$$\frac{100X}{100} = \frac{200}{100}$$

$$X = 2 \text{ mL/h}$$

18 mL/h + 2 mL/h = 20 mL/h (new infusion rate)

49) Decrease rate by 2 units/kg/h

2 units/kg/h $\times$ 100 kg = 200 units/h (decrease)

$$\frac{100 \text{ units}}{1 \text{ mL}} \diagdown \frac{200 \text{ units/h}}{X \text{ mL/h}}$$

$$100X = 200$$

$$\frac{100X}{100} = \frac{200}{100}$$

$$X = 2 \text{ mL/h (decrease)}$$

20 mL/h − 2 mL/h = 18 mL/h (new infusion rate)

Section 4—Self-Evaluation from pages 467–471

1) 0.9% NaCl **2)** 0.9 g NaCl per 100 mL **3)** 0.45 g NaCl per 100 mL **4)** 50 **5)** 4.5 **6)** 2.25 **7)** 75 **8)** 6.75 **9)** mL/h **10)** 21 **11)** 83 **12)** 1940 **13)** 1,536 **14)** Give a total of 3,000 mL IV solution per day to include normal saline (0.9% NaCl) with 20 milliequivalents of potassium chloride added per liter (1,000 mL) *and* an IV piggyback solution of 250 mg cefazolin added to 100 mL of normal saline (0.9% NaCl) over 30 min administered every 8 hours. To administer the order each day, give 900 mL NS with KCl over $7\frac{1}{2}$ hours $\times$ 3 administrations and 100 mL NS with cefazolin over $\frac{1}{2}$ hour $\times$ 3 administrations **15)** 120 **16)** 200 **17)** Reset rate to 118 gtt/min, if policy and patient's condition permit. **18)** 1,410 **19)** 59 **20)** 120 **21)** 5 **22)** 0.48 **23)** 1.3 **24)** 1.04 **25)** 0.5 **26)** 18.5–37.5 **27)** Yes **28)** 18.5 **29)** 37 mL **30)** 120 **31)** 18.5 **32)** 0.8 **33)** 1.6 **34)** Yes **35)** 1.6 **36)** 18; 2 **37)** 7.5 **38)** 43 **39)** 200 **40)** 43 **41)** 200 **42)** 50 **43)** 12 **44)** 15 **45)** 0.13 **46)** 8 **47)** 80 **48)** 20 **49)** 61 **50)** 38

Solutions—Section 4—Self-Evaluation

4) D_5 0.45% NaCl = 5% dextrose =

5 g dextrose per 100 mL

$$\frac{5\text{ g}}{100\text{ mL}} \diagup\!\!\!\!\diagdown \frac{X\text{ g}}{1000\text{ mL}}$$

$$100X = 5,000$$

$$\frac{100X}{100} = \frac{5,000}{100}$$

$$X = 50\text{ g}$$

5) D_5 0.45% NaCl = 0.45% NaCl =

0.45 g NaCl per 100 mL

$$\frac{0.45\text{ g}}{100\text{ mL}} \diagup\!\!\!\!\diagdown \frac{X\text{ g}}{1,000\text{ mL}}$$

$$100X = 450$$

$$\frac{100X}{100} = \frac{450}{100}$$

$$X = 4.5\text{ g}$$

10) $\frac{2,000\text{ mL}}{24\text{ h}} = 83.3\text{ mL/h} = 83\text{ mL/h}$

$$\frac{\text{mL/h}}{\text{drop factor constant}} = \text{gtt/min}$$

$$\frac{83\text{ mL/h}}{4} = 20.8 = 21\text{ gtt/min}$$

12) $\frac{V}{T} \times C = R$: $\frac{400\text{ mL}}{T\text{ min}} \times 15\text{ gtt/mL} = 24\text{ gtt/min}$

$$\frac{400}{T} \times 15 = 24$$

$$\frac{6,000}{T} \diagup\!\!\!\!\diagdown \frac{24}{1}$$

$$24T = 6,000$$

$$\frac{24T}{24} = \frac{6,000}{24}$$

$$T = 250\text{ min}$$

$$250\text{ min} \div 60\text{ min/h} = 4\frac{1}{6}\text{ h} = 4\text{ h }10\text{ min}$$

$$\begin{array}{r} 1530\text{ hours} \\ +\ 410\text{ hours} \\ \hline 1940\text{ hours} \end{array}$$

13) $\frac{V}{T} \times C = R$: $\frac{V\text{ mL}}{60\text{ min}} \times 10\text{ gtt/mL} = 32\text{ gtt/min}$

$$\frac{10V}{60} \diagup\!\!\!\!\diagdown \frac{32}{1}$$

$$10V = 1,920$$

$$\frac{10V}{10} = \frac{1,920}{10}$$

$$V = 192\text{ mL/h};\ 192\text{ mL/h} \times 8\text{ h} = 1,536\text{ mL}$$
$$\text{(administered during your 8 h shift)}$$

15) IVPB total volume: 100 mL $\times$ 3 = 300 mL

IVPB total time: 30 min $\times$ 3 = 90 min = $1\frac{1}{2}$ h

Regular IV total volume: 3,000 mL − 300 mL =

2,700 mL

Regular IV total time: 24h − $1\frac{1}{2}$ h =

$22\frac{1}{2}$ h (22.5 h)

$$\frac{2,700\text{ mL}}{22.5\text{ h}} = 120\text{ mL/h}$$

16) $\frac{100\text{ mL}}{30\text{ min}} \diagup\!\!\!\!\diagdown \frac{X\text{ mL/h}}{60\text{ min/h}}$

$$30X = 6,000$$

$$\frac{30X}{30} = \frac{6,000}{30}$$

$$X = 200\text{ mL/h}$$

17) $\frac{1,200\text{ mL}}{100\text{ mL/h}} = 12$ h (total time ordered to infuse

1,200 mL)

2200 hours (10:00 PM; current time) and 1530

(3:30 PM; start time); 6 h 30 min (elapsed time)

$6\frac{1}{2}$ h $\times$ 100 mL/h = 650 mL (expected to be infused)

After $6\frac{1}{2}$ h, 650 mL should have been infused, with

550 mL remaining. IV is behind schedule.

1,200 mL − 650 mL = 550 mL (should be remaining)

$$\frac{\text{Remaining volume}}{\text{Remaining time}} = \frac{650\text{ mL}}{5.5\text{ h}} = 118\text{ mL/h (adjusted rate)}$$

$$\frac{\text{Adjusted gtt/min − Ordered gtt/min}}{\text{Ordered gtt/min}} = \%\text{ of variation};$$

$$\frac{118 - 100}{100} = \frac{18}{100} = 0.18 = 18\%\text{ (variance is safe)}$$

If policy and patient's condition permit, reset rate to

118 mL/h.

18) $\dfrac{1 \text{ kg}}{2.2 \text{ lb}} \diagdown\diagup \dfrac{X \text{ kg}}{40 \text{ lb}}$

$2.2X = 40$

$\dfrac{2.2X}{2.2} = \dfrac{40}{2.2}$

$X = 18.18 \text{ kg} = 18.2 \text{ kg}$

First 10 kg: 100 mL/kg/day $\times$ 10 kg = $\quad$ 1,000 mL/day

Remaining 8.2 kg: 50 mL/kg/day $\times$ 8.2 kg = $\underline{410 \text{ mL/day}}$

$\qquad\qquad\qquad\qquad\qquad\qquad\qquad$ 1,410 mL/day

19) $\dfrac{1,410 \text{ mL}}{24 \text{ h}} = 58.7 \text{ mL/h} = 59 \text{ mL/h}$

20) 1,185 g = 1.185. = 1.185 kg = 1.2 kg

First 10 kg: 100 mL/kg/day $\times$ 1.2 kg = 120 mL/day

21) $\dfrac{120 \text{ mL}}{24 \text{ h}} = 5 \text{ mL/h}$

22) Household:

BSA (m^2) = $\sqrt{\dfrac{\text{ht (in)} \times \text{wt (lb)}}{3,131}} = \sqrt{\dfrac{30 \times 24}{3,131}} = \sqrt{\dfrac{720}{3,131}}$

$= \sqrt{0.229...} = 0.479 \text{ m}^2 = 0.48 \text{ m}^2$

23) Metric:

BSA (m^2) = $\sqrt{\dfrac{\text{ht (cm)} \times \text{wt (kg)}}{3,600}} = \sqrt{\dfrac{155 \times 39}{3,600}} =$

$\sqrt{\dfrac{6,045}{3,600}} = \sqrt{1.679...} = 1.295 \text{ m}^2 = 1.3 \text{ m}^2$

26) Minimum safe dosage: 37 mg/m^2 $\times$ 0.5 m^2 = 18.5 mg

Maximum safe dosage: 75 mg/m^2 $\times$ 0.5 m^2 = 37.5 mg

28) 1 mL/mg $\times$ 18.5 mg = 18.5 mL

29) 2 mL/mg $\times$ 18.5 mg = 37 mL

30) $\dfrac{18.5 \text{ mg}}{37 \text{ mL}} \diagdown\diagup \dfrac{1 \text{ mg/min}}{X \text{ mL/min}}$

$18.5X = 37$

$\dfrac{18.5X}{18.5} = \dfrac{37}{18.5}$

$X = 2 \text{ mL/min}$

$\dfrac{2 \text{ mL}}{1 \text{ min}} \diagdown\diagup \dfrac{X \text{ mL/h}}{60 \text{ min/h}}$

$X = 120 \text{ mL/h}$

31) Think: At 1 mg/min, 18.5 mg will infuse in 18.5 min.

$\dfrac{1 \text{ mg}}{1 \text{ min}} \diagdown\diagup \dfrac{18.5 \text{ mg}}{X \text{ min}}$

$X = 18.5 \text{ min}$

33) 2 mg/m^2 $\times$ 0.8 m^2 = 1.6 mg

36) $\dfrac{125 \text{ mg}}{1 \text{ mL}} \diagdown\diagup \dfrac{250 \text{ mg}}{X \text{ mL}}$

$125X = 250$

$\dfrac{125X}{125} = \dfrac{250}{125}$

$X = 2 \text{ mL (Ancef)}$

$\dfrac{40 \text{ mL}}{60 \text{ min}} \diagdown\diagup \dfrac{X \text{ mL}}{30 \text{ min}}$

$60X = 1,200$

$\dfrac{60X}{60} = \dfrac{1,200}{60}$

$X = 20 \text{ mL}$

20 mL (total IV solution) $-$ 2 mL (Ancef) = 18 mL (NS)

37) $\dfrac{100 \text{ mg}}{1 \text{ mL}} \diagdown\diagup \dfrac{750 \text{ mg}}{X \text{ mL}}$

$100X = 750$

$\dfrac{100X}{100} = \dfrac{750}{100}$

$X = 7.5 \text{ mL}$

7.5 mL IV solution to be used with the 750 mg of Timentin for minimal dilution.

38) Total IV PB volume: 100 mL $\times$ 6 = 600 mL

Regular IV volume: 1,500 mL $-$ 600 mL = 900 mL

Total IV PB time of q.4h $\times$ 30 min: 6 $\times$ 30 min = 180 min; 180 min $\div$ 60 min/h = 3 h

Total Regular IV time: 24 h $-$ 3 h = 21 h

Regular IV rate: mL/h = $\dfrac{900 \text{ mL}}{21 \text{ h}}$ = 42.8 mL/h = 43 mL/h or 43 gtt/min (because drop factor is 60 gtt/mL)

$\dfrac{\text{mL/h}}{\text{drop factor constant}}$ = gtt/min; $\dfrac{42.8 \text{ mL/h}}{1}$ = 42.8 gtt/min = 43 gtt/min

39) $\dfrac{100 \text{ mL}}{30 \text{ min}} \diagdown\diagup \dfrac{X \text{ mL}}{60 \text{ min}}$

$30X = 6,000$

$\dfrac{30X}{30} = \dfrac{6,000}{30}$

$X = 200 \text{ mL/h or 200 gtt/min (because}$ drop factor is 60 gtt/mL)

40) See #38, Regular IV rate calculated at 43 mL/h.

41) See #39, IV PB rate calculated at 200 mL/h.

42) $\dfrac{40\ mEq}{1{,}000\ mL} \bowtie \dfrac{2\ mEq/h}{X\ mL/h}$

$40X = 2{,}000$

$\dfrac{40X}{40} = \dfrac{2{,}000}{40}$

$X = 50\ mL/h$

43) $1\ L = 1{,}000\ mL$

$1\ mg = 1{,}000\ mcg$

$\dfrac{1\ mg}{1{,}000\ mcg} \bowtie \dfrac{25\ mg}{X\ mcg}$

$X = 25{,}000\ mcg$

25 mg per L = 25,000 mcg per 1,000 mL

$\dfrac{25{,}000\ mcg}{1{,}000\ mL} \bowtie \dfrac{X\ mcg}{1\ mL}$

$1{,}000X = 25{,}000$

$\dfrac{1{,}000X}{1{,}000} = \dfrac{25{,}000}{1{,}000}$

$X = 25\ mcg/mL$

$\dfrac{25\ mcg}{1\ mL} \bowtie \dfrac{5\ mcg/min}{X\ mL/min}$

$25X = 5$

$\dfrac{25X}{25} = \dfrac{5}{25}$

$X = 0.2\ mL/min$

$\dfrac{0.2\ mL}{1\ min} \bowtie \dfrac{X\ mL/h}{60\ min/h}$

$X = 12\ mL/h$

44) $1\ L = 1{,}000\ mL$

$1\ unit = 1{,}000\ milliunits$

$\dfrac{1\ unit}{1{,}000\ milliunits} \bowtie \dfrac{15\ units}{X\ milliunits}$

$X = 15{,}000\ milliunits$

$\dfrac{15{,}000\ milliunits}{1{,}000\ mL} \bowtie \dfrac{X\ milliunits}{1\ mL}$

$1{,}000X = 15{,}000$

$\dfrac{1{,}000X}{1{,}000} = \dfrac{15{,}000}{1{,}000}$

$X = 15\ milliunits/mL$

45) $\dfrac{15\ milliunits}{1\ mL} \bowtie \dfrac{2\ milliunits/min}{X\ mL/min}$

$15X = 2$

$\dfrac{15X}{15} = \dfrac{2}{15}$

$X = 0.13\ mL/min$

46) $\dfrac{0.13\ mL}{1\ min} \bowtie \dfrac{X\ mL/h}{60\ min/h}$

$X = 7.8\ mL/h = 8\ mL/h$

47) $\dfrac{15\ milliunits}{1\ mL} \bowtie \dfrac{20\ milliunits/min}{X\ mL/min}$

$15X = 20$

$\dfrac{15X}{15} = \dfrac{20}{15}$

$X = 1.33\ mL/min$

$\dfrac{1.33\ mL}{1\ min} \bowtie \dfrac{X\ mL/h}{60\ min/h}$

$X = 80\ mL/h$

48) $\dfrac{1\ kg}{2.2\ lb} \bowtie \dfrac{X\ kg}{150\ lb}$

$2.2X = 150$

$\dfrac{2.2X}{2.2} = \dfrac{150}{2.2}$

$X = 68.18\ kg = 68.2\ kg$

4 mcg/kg/min × 68.2 kg = 272.8 mcg/min = 273 mcg/min

$\dfrac{273\ mcg}{1\ min} \bowtie \dfrac{X\ mcg/h}{60\ min/h}$

$X = 16{,}380\ mcg/h$

$\dfrac{1\ L}{1{,}000\ mL} \bowtie \dfrac{0.5\ L}{X\ mL}$

$X = 500\ mL$

$\dfrac{400\ mg}{500\ mL} \bowtie \dfrac{X\ mg}{1\ mL}$

$500X = 400$

$\dfrac{500X}{500} = \dfrac{400}{500}$

$X = 0.8\ mg\ (per\ mL)$

$\dfrac{1\ mg}{1{,}000\ mcg} \bowtie \dfrac{0.8\ mg}{X\ mcg}$

$X = 800\ mcg\ (per\ mL)$

$\dfrac{800\ mcg}{1\ mL} \bowtie \dfrac{16{,}380\ mcg/h}{X\ mL/h}$

$800X = 16{,}380$

$\dfrac{800X}{800} = \dfrac{16{,}380}{800}$

$X = 20.4\ mL/h = 20\ mL/h$

49) 12 mcg/kg/min × 68.2 kg = 818.4 mcg/min = 818 mcg/min

$\dfrac{818\ mcg}{1\ min} \bowtie \dfrac{X\ mcg/h}{60\ min/h}$

$X = 49{,}080\ mcg/h$

$\dfrac{800\ mcg}{1\ mL} \bowtie \dfrac{49{,}080\ mcg/h}{X\ mL/h}$

$800X = 49{,}080$

$\dfrac{800X}{800} = \dfrac{49{,}080}{800}$

$X = 61.4\ mL/h = 61\ mL/h$

50) $\dfrac{10{,}000\ units}{500\ mL} \bowtie \dfrac{750\ units/h}{X\ mL/h}$

$10{,}000X = 375{,}000$

$\dfrac{10{,}000X}{10{,}000} = \dfrac{375{,}000}{10{,}000}$

$X = 37.5\ mL/h = 38\ mL/h$

Essential Skills Evaluation from pages 473–486

1) 0.5

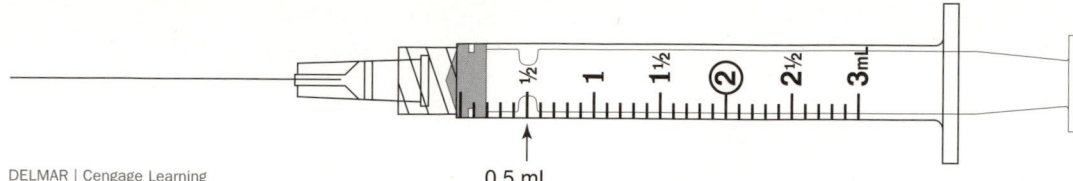

0.5 mL

2) 0.88

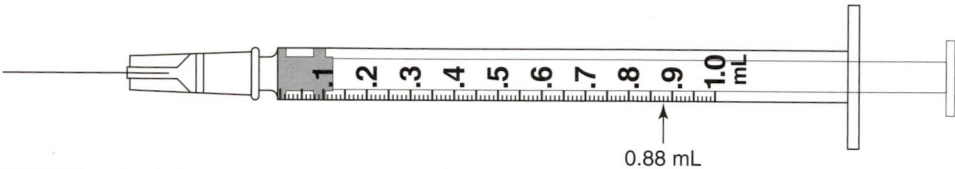

0.88 mL

3) 1, 1, 0.25

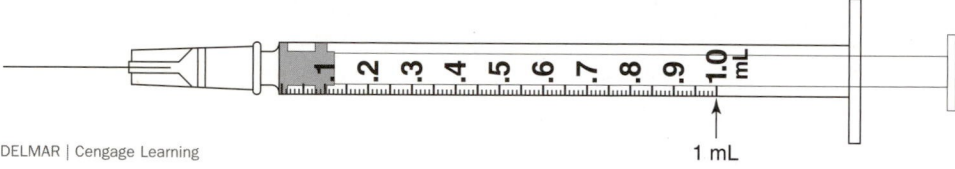

1 mL

4) 1

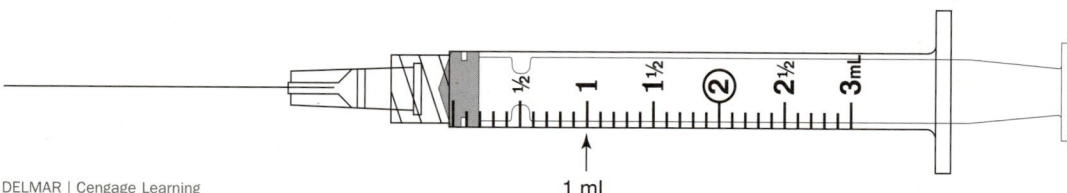

1 mL

5) $1\frac{1}{2}$

6) 0.5

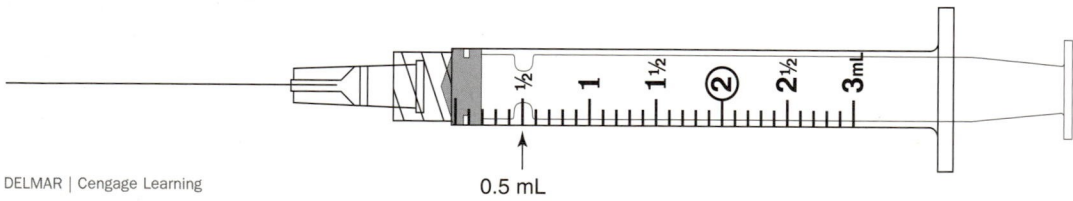

0.5 mL

7) 0.4 mL

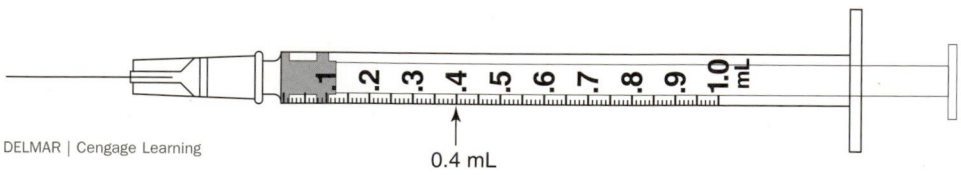

0.4 mL

8) 1.4

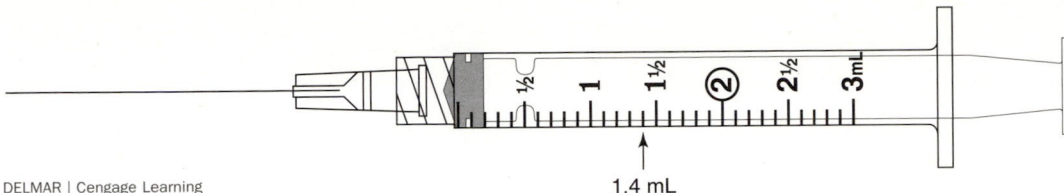

1.4 mL

9) 68

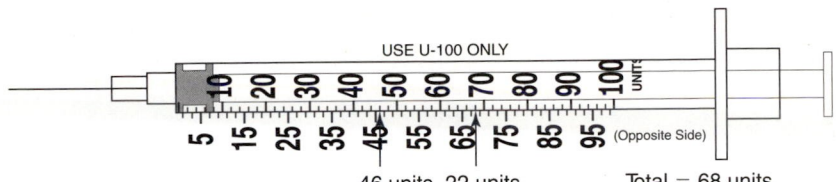

USE U-100 ONLY

(Opposite Side)

46 units 22 units   Total = 68 units

NPH   Regular (drawn up first)

10) 2 **11)** $\frac{1}{2}$ **12)** $1\frac{1}{2}$

13) 0.8

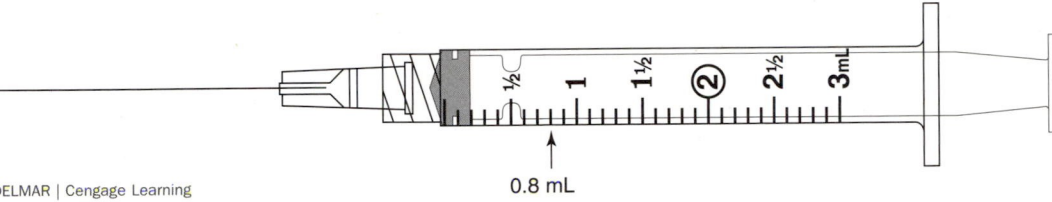

0.8 mL

14) 1.5

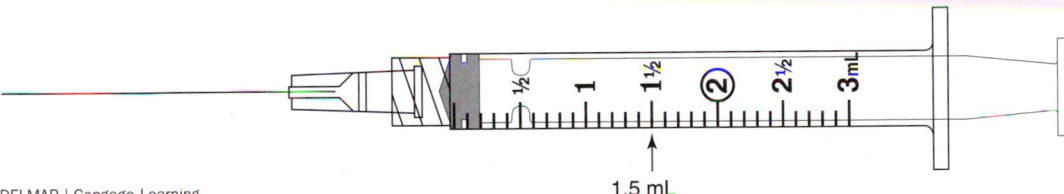

1.5 mL

15) 2.5

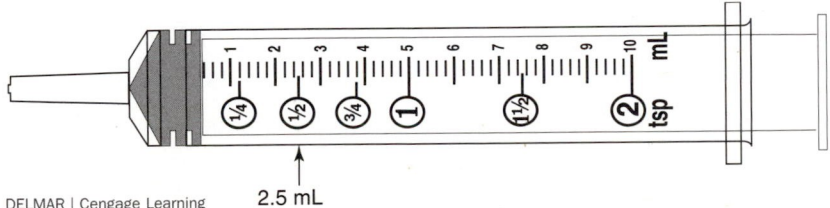

2.5 mL

16) 4

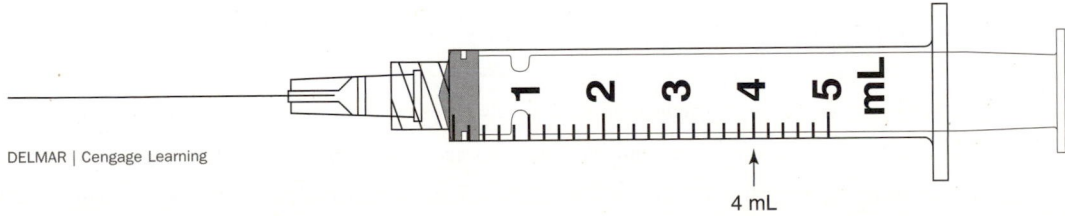

4 mL

17)   1.4; 75

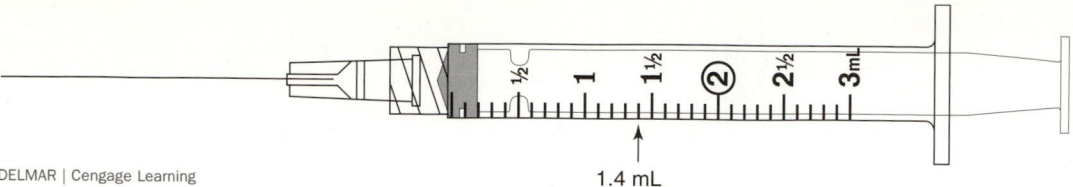

1.4 mL

18)   Yes. Her temperature is 102.2°F. Tylenol is indicated for fever greater than 101°F every 4 hours. It has been 5 hours and 5 minutes since her last dose.

19) 2 **20)** $\frac{1}{2}$ (one half)

21)   Benadryl; 0.7

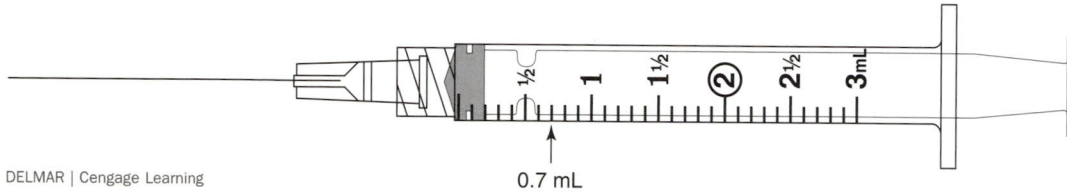

0.7 mL

22)   Narcan; 1

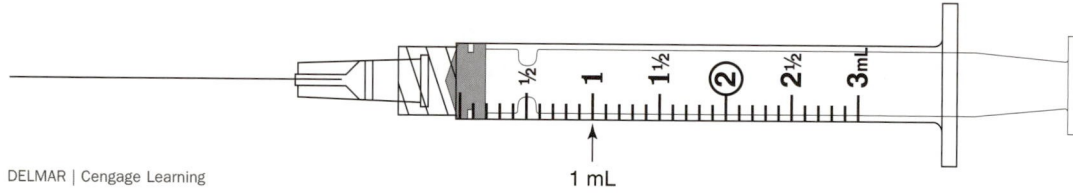

1 mL

23) 18.8; 138 **24)** 138 **25)** 8; 2 **26)** 1; 0745, 1145, 1745, 2200

27)   18; subcutaneous

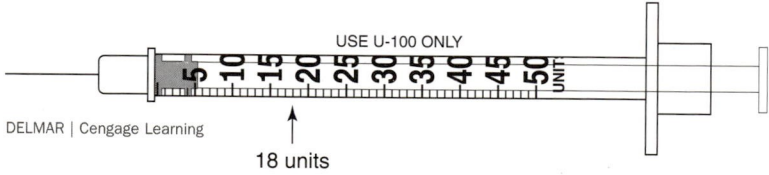

18 units

28) 113 **29)** Yes. The usual dosage is 20–40 mg/kg/day divided into 3 doses q.8h, which is equivalent to 66.7–133.3 mg per dose for a 22 lb (10 kg) child. **30)** 4 **31)** 4 mL line; every 8 hours **32)** 250–500; Yes; 1.7; 25 **33)** 1,000 **34)** Yes **35)** 3; dosage is safe **36)** 25 **37)** 280; 420 **38)** 13 **39)** 30; No **40)** Do not administer; consult with physician before giving drug. **41)** 1 **42)** 5; 5 **43)** 50 **44)** 0030; 12:30 AM **45)** 200 **46)** 10 **47)** 1,000; 10; 100 **48)** 5

49)

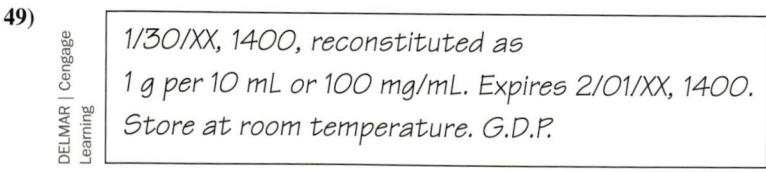

1/30/XX, 1400, reconstituted as 1 g per 10 mL or 100 mg/mL. Expires 2/01/XX, 1400. Store at room temperature. G.D.P.

50)   **Prevention:** The importance of checking a medication label at least three times to verify supply dosage cannot be overemphasized. It is also important NEVER to assume that the supply dosage is the same as a supply dosage used to calculate previously. Always read the label carefully. Writing the calculation down will also help improve accuracy.

Solutions—Essential Skills Evaluation

1) $\dfrac{25 \text{ mg}}{1 \text{ mL}} \bowtie \dfrac{12.5 \text{ mg}}{X \text{ mL}}$

$$25X = 12.5$$

$$\dfrac{25X}{25} = \dfrac{12.5}{25}$$

$$X = 0.5 \text{ mL}$$

2) $\dfrac{40 \text{ mg}}{1 \text{ mL}} \bowtie \dfrac{35 \text{ mg}}{X \text{ mL}}$

$$40X = 35$$

$$\dfrac{40X}{40} = \dfrac{35}{40}$$

$$X = 0.875 \text{ mL} = 0.88 \text{ mL}$$

3) $\dfrac{250 \text{ mg}}{5 \text{ mL}} \bowtie \dfrac{50 \text{ mg}}{X \text{ mL}}$

$$250X = 250$$

$$\dfrac{250X}{250} = \dfrac{250}{250}$$

$$X = 1 \text{ mL}$$

$\dfrac{1 \text{ mL}}{60 \text{ sec}} \bowtie \dfrac{X \text{ mL}}{15 \text{ sec}}$

$$60X = 15$$

$$\dfrac{60X}{60} = \dfrac{15}{60}$$

$$X = 0.25 \text{ mL (per 15 sec)}$$

Note: 1 mL syringe is a better choice because measurement of 0.25 mL increments is clearly visible.

4) 0.2 mg = 0.200. = 200 mcg; *Or*

$\dfrac{1 \text{ mg}}{1,000 \text{ mcg}} \bowtie \dfrac{0.2 \text{ mg}}{X \text{ mcg}}$

$$1X = 200 \text{ mcg}$$

$$X = 200 \text{ mcg}$$

It is now obvious that you want to give 1 mL.

5) $\dfrac{5 \text{ mg}}{1 \text{ tab}} \bowtie \dfrac{7.5 \text{ mg}}{X \text{ tab}}$

$$5X = 7.5$$

$$\dfrac{5X}{5} = \dfrac{7.5}{5}$$

$$X = 1\tfrac{1}{2} \text{ tab}$$

6) $\dfrac{0.25 \text{ mg}}{1 \text{ mL}} \bowtie \dfrac{0.125 \text{ mg}}{X \text{ mL}}$

$$0.25X = 0.125$$

$$\dfrac{0.25X}{0.25} = \dfrac{0.125}{0.25}$$

$$X = 0.5 \text{ mL}$$

7) $\dfrac{\text{gr } 1}{60 \text{ mg}} \bowtie \dfrac{\text{gr } \tfrac{1}{15}}{X \text{ mg}}$

$$X = \dfrac{60}{1} \times \dfrac{1}{15}$$

$$X = \dfrac{60}{15}$$

$$X = 4 \text{ mg}$$

$\dfrac{10 \text{ mg}}{1 \text{ mL}} \bowtie \dfrac{4 \text{ mg}}{X \text{ mL}}$

$$10X = 4$$

$$\dfrac{10X}{10} = \dfrac{4}{10}$$

$$X = 0.4 \text{ mL}$$

8) $\dfrac{500 \text{ mg}}{2 \text{ mL}} \bowtie \dfrac{350 \text{ mg}}{X \text{ mL}}$

$$500X = 700$$

$$\dfrac{500X}{500} = \dfrac{700}{500}$$

$$X = 1.4 \text{ mL}$$

9) 46 units + 22 units = 68 units (total)

10) $\dfrac{0.15 \text{ mg}}{1 \text{ tab}} \bowtie \dfrac{0.3 \text{ mg}}{X \text{ tab}}$

$$0.15X = 0.3$$

$$\dfrac{0.15X}{0.15} = \dfrac{0.3}{0.15}$$

$$X = 2 \text{ tabs}$$

11) $\dfrac{80 \text{ mg}}{1 \text{ tab}} \bowtie \dfrac{40 \text{ mg}}{X \text{ tab}}$

$$80X = 40$$

$$\dfrac{80X}{80} = \dfrac{40}{80}$$

$$X = \tfrac{1}{2} \text{ tab}$$

12) $\dfrac{250 \text{ mg}}{1 \text{ tab}} \bowtie \dfrac{375 \text{ mg}}{X \text{ tab}}$

$$250X = 375$$

$$\dfrac{250X}{250} = \dfrac{375}{250}$$

$$X = 1\tfrac{1}{2} \text{ tab}$$

13) $\dfrac{50 \text{ mg}}{1 \text{ mL}} \bowtie \dfrac{40 \text{ mg}}{X \text{ mL}}$

$$50X = 40$$

$$\dfrac{50X}{50} = \dfrac{40}{50}$$

$$X = 0.8 \text{ mL}$$

14) $\dfrac{2 \text{ mg}}{1 \text{ mL}} \bowtie \dfrac{3 \text{ mg}}{X \text{ mL}}$

$$2X = 3$$

$$\dfrac{2X}{2} = \dfrac{3}{2}$$

$$X = 1.5 \text{ mL}$$

You will need 2 vials of the drug, because each vial contains 1 mL.

15) $\dfrac{200 \text{ mg}}{5 \text{ mL}} \diagdown \dfrac{100 \text{ mg}}{X \text{ mL}}$

$200X = 500$

$\dfrac{200X}{200} = \dfrac{500}{200}$

$X = 2.5 \text{ mL}$

16) $\dfrac{\text{gr } 1}{60 \text{ mg}} \diagdown \dfrac{\text{gr } \frac{1}{150}}{X \text{ mg}}$

$X = 60 \times \dfrac{1}{150} = \dfrac{60}{150}$

$X = 0.4 \text{ mg}$

$\dfrac{0.1 \text{ mg}}{1 \text{ mL}} \diagdown \dfrac{0.4 \text{ mg}}{X \text{ mL}}$

$0.1X = 0.4$

$\dfrac{0.1X}{0.1} = \dfrac{0.4}{0.1}$

$X = 4 \text{ mL}$

17) $\dfrac{50 \text{ mg}}{2 \text{ mL}} \diagdown \dfrac{35 \text{ mg}}{X \text{ mL}}$

$50X = 70$

$\dfrac{50X}{50} = \dfrac{70}{50}$

$X = 1.4 \text{ mL}$

$\dfrac{V}{T} \times C = \dfrac{\overset{5}{\cancel{100}} \text{ mL}}{\underset{1}{\cancel{20}} \text{ min}} \times 15 \text{ gtt/mL} = 75 \text{ gtt/min}$

18) $°F = 1.8°C + 32 = (1.8 \times 39) + 32 = 70.2 + 32$

$= 102.2°F$

102.2°F is greater than 101°F; difference between 2400 and 2110 hours is 2 h 50 min;

0215 = 2 h 15 min after 2400;

2 h 50 min + 2 h 15 min = 4 h 65 min or 5 h 5 min

19) $\dfrac{325 \text{ mg}}{1 \text{ tab}} \diagdown \dfrac{650 \text{ mg}}{X \text{ tab}}$

$325X = 650$

$\dfrac{325X}{325} = \dfrac{650}{325}$

$X = 2 \text{ tab}$

20) $\dfrac{\overset{1}{\cancel{30}} \text{ mg}}{\underset{2}{\cancel{60}} \text{ mg}} = \dfrac{1}{2} \text{ (one half)}$

21) $\dfrac{50 \text{ mg}}{1 \text{ mL}} \diagdown \dfrac{35 \text{ mg}}{X \text{ mL}}$

$50X = 35$

$\dfrac{50X}{50} = \dfrac{35}{50}$

$X = 0.7 \text{ mL}$

23) $\dfrac{80 \text{ mg}}{15 \text{ mL}} \diagdown \dfrac{100 \text{ mg}}{X \text{ mL}}$

$80X = 1,500$

$\dfrac{80X}{80} = \dfrac{1,500}{80}$

$X = 18.75 \text{ mL} = 18.8 \text{ mL}$

$50 \text{ mL} + 18.8 \text{ mL} = 68.8 \text{ mL}$

$\dfrac{V}{T} \times C = \dfrac{68.8 \text{ mL}}{\underset{1}{\cancel{30}} \text{ min}} \times \overset{2}{\cancel{60}} \text{ gtt/mL}$

$= 137.6 \text{ gtt/min} = 138 \text{ gtt/min}$

24) 138 gtt/min = 138 mL/h because gtt/min = mL/h when the drop factor is 60 gtt/mL

25) $\dfrac{500 \text{ mg}}{8 \text{ mL}} \diagdown \dfrac{125 \text{ mg}}{X \text{ mL}}$

$500X = 1,000$

$\dfrac{500X}{500} = \dfrac{1,000}{500}$

$X = 2 \text{ mL}$

29) $\dfrac{1 \text{ kg}}{2.2 \text{ lb}} \diagdown \dfrac{X \text{ kg}}{22 \text{ lb}}$

$2.2X = 22$

$\dfrac{2.2X}{2.2} = \dfrac{22}{2.2}$

$X = 10 \text{ kg}$

Yes, it is safe.

Minimum dosage: $20 \text{ mg/kg/day} \times 10 \text{ kg} = 200 \text{ mg/day}$

$\dfrac{200 \text{ mg}}{3 \text{ doses}} \diagdown \dfrac{X \text{ mg}}{1 \text{ dose}}$

$3X = 200$

$\dfrac{3X}{3} = \dfrac{200}{3}$

$X = 66.66 \text{ mg (per dose) or } 66.7 \text{ mg/dose}$

Maximum dosage: $40 \text{ mg/kg/day} \times 10 \text{ kg} = 400 \text{ mg/day}$

$\dfrac{400 \text{ mg}}{3 \text{ doses}} \diagdown \dfrac{X \text{ mg}}{1 \text{ dose}}$

$3X = 400$

$\dfrac{3X}{3} = \dfrac{400}{3}$

$X = 133.33 \text{ mg (per dose) or } 133.3 \text{ mg/dose}$

30) $\dfrac{125 \text{ mg}}{5 \text{ mL}} \diagdown \dfrac{100 \text{ mg}}{X \text{ mL}}$

$125X = 500$

$\dfrac{125X}{125} = \dfrac{500}{125}$

$X = 4 \text{ mL}$

32) $\dfrac{1 \text{ kg}}{2.2 \text{ lb}} \diagdown \dfrac{X \text{ kg}}{110 \text{ lb}}$

$2.2X = 110$

$\dfrac{2.2X}{2.2} = \dfrac{110}{2.2}$

$X = 50 \text{ kg}$

Minimum dosage: $20 \text{ mg/kg/day} \times 50 \text{ kg} = 1,000 \text{ mg/day}$

$$\frac{1{,}000 \text{ mg}}{4 \text{ doses}} \diagdown \frac{X \text{ mg}}{1 \text{ dose}}$$

$$4X = 1{,}000$$

$$\frac{4X}{4} = \frac{1{,}000}{4}$$

$$X = 250 \text{ mg (per dose) or } 250 \text{ mg/dose}$$

Maximum dosage: $40 \text{ mg/kg/day} \times 50 \text{ kg} =$ 2,000 mg/day

$$\frac{2{,}000 \text{ mg}}{4 \text{ doses}} \diagdown \frac{X \text{ mg}}{1 \text{ dose}}$$

$$4X = 2{,}000$$

$$\frac{4X}{4} = \frac{2{,}000}{4}$$

$$X = 500 \text{ mg (per dose) or } 500 \text{ mg/dose}$$

$$\frac{300 \text{ mg}}{2 \text{ mL}} \diagdown \frac{250 \text{ mg}}{X \text{ mL}}$$

Yes, dosage is safe.

$$300X = 500$$

$$\frac{300X}{300} = \frac{500}{300}$$

$$X = 1.7 \text{ mL}$$

$$\frac{V}{T} \times C = \frac{50 \text{ mL}}{\overset{}{\underset{2}{20 \text{ min}}}} \times \overset{1}{\cancel{10}} \text{ gtt/mL} = \frac{50 \text{ gtt}}{2 \text{ min}} = 25 \text{ gtt/min}$$

33)

	IV fluid =	200 mL
gelatin:	$4 \text{ fl oz} \times 30 \text{ mL/fl oz} =$	120 mL
water:	$3 \text{ fl oz} \times 2 \times 30 \text{ mL/fl oz} =$	180 mL
apple juice:	$16 \text{ fl oz} = \text{pt i} =$	500 mL
	Total =	1,000 mL

(16 fl oz could also be converted as 16 fl oz $\times$ 30 mL/oz = 480 mL for 980 mL total volume. Remember: These are approximate equivalents.)

34)

$$\frac{1 \text{ kg}}{2.2 \text{ lb}} \diagdown \frac{X \text{ kg}}{40 \text{ lb}}$$

$$2.2X = 40$$

$$\frac{2.2X}{2.2} = \frac{40}{2.2}$$

$$X = 18.18 \text{ kg} = 18.2 \text{ kg}$$

$40 \text{ mg/kg/day} \times 18.2 \text{ kg} = 728 \text{ mg/day}$

$$\frac{728 \text{ mg}}{3 \text{ doses}} \diagdown \frac{X \text{ mg}}{1 \text{ dose}}$$

$$3X = 728$$

$$\frac{3X}{3} = \frac{728}{3}$$

$X = 242.6 \text{ mg} = 243 \text{ mg (per dose) or}$
243 mg/dose; close approximation to ordered dosage of 240 mg/dose; dosage is safe

35)

$$\frac{400 \text{ mg}}{5 \text{ mL}} \diagdown \frac{240 \text{ mg}}{X \text{ mL}}$$

$$400X = 1{,}200$$

$$\frac{400X}{400} = \frac{1{,}200}{400}$$

$$X = 3 \text{ mL}$$

36)

$$\text{mL/h} = \frac{\overset{150}{\cancel{600} \text{ mL}}}{\underset{1}{\cancel{4} \text{ h}}} = 150 \text{ mL/h}$$

$$\frac{V}{T} \times C = \frac{150 \text{ mL}}{\underset{6}{\cancel{60} \text{ min}}} \times \overset{1}{\cancel{10}} \text{ gtt/mL} = \frac{150 \text{ gtt}}{6 \text{ min}} = 25 \text{ gtt/min}$$

37)

$$\frac{1 \text{ lb}}{16 \text{ oz}} \diagdown \frac{X \text{ lb}}{8 \text{ oz}}$$

$$16X = 8$$

$$\frac{16X}{16} = \frac{8}{16}$$

$$X = \frac{1}{2} = 0.5 \text{ lb}$$

61 lb 8 ounces = 61.5 lb

$$\frac{1 \text{ kg}}{2.2 \text{ lb}} \diagdown \frac{X \text{ kg}}{61.5 \text{ lb}}$$

$$2.2X = 61.5$$

$$\frac{2.2X}{2.2} = \frac{61.5}{2.2}$$

$$X = 27.95 \text{ kg} = 28 \text{ kg}$$

Minimum dosage: $10 \text{ mg/kg} \times 28 \text{ kg} = 280 \text{ mg}$
Maximum dosage: $15 \text{ mg/kg} \times 28 \text{ kg} = 420 \text{ mg}$

38)

$$\frac{80 \text{ mg}}{2.5 \text{ mL}} \diagdown \frac{420 \text{ mg}}{X \text{ mL}}$$

$$80X = 1{,}050$$

$$\frac{80X}{80} = \frac{1{,}050}{80}$$

$$X = 13.1 \text{ mL} = 13 \text{ mL}$$

39)

$$\frac{1 \text{ kg}}{2.2 \text{ lb}} \diagdown \frac{X \text{ kg}}{52 \text{ lb}}$$

$$2.2X = 52$$

$$\frac{2.2X}{2.2} = \frac{52}{2.2}$$

$$X = 23.63 \text{ kg} = 23.6 \text{ kg}$$

$5 \text{ mg/kg/day} \times 23.6 \text{ kg} = 118 \text{ mg/day}$

$$\frac{118 \text{ mg}}{4 \text{ doses}} \diagdown \frac{X \text{ mg}}{1 \text{ dose}}$$

$$4X = 118$$

$$\frac{4X}{4} = \frac{118}{4}$$

$X = 30 \text{ mg (per dose)}$; dosage is too low to
be therapeutic and is not safe

41)

$$\frac{50 \text{ mg}}{50 \text{ mL}} \diagdown \frac{1 \text{ mg}}{X \text{ mL}}$$

$$50X = 50$$

$$\frac{50X}{50} = \frac{50}{50}$$

$$X = 1 \text{ mL}$$

42) $1 \text{ mg/dose} \times 5 \text{ doses} = 5 \text{ mg}$
$1 \text{ mL/dose} \times 5 \text{ doses} = 5 \text{ mL}$

43) $\dfrac{50 \text{ mg}}{1 \text{ mg/dose}} = 50 \text{ doses}$

44) $\dfrac{50 \text{ doses}}{5 \text{ doses/h}} = 10 \text{ h}$

$\begin{array}{l} 1430 \text{ h} \\ +1000 \text{ h} \\ \hline 2430 \text{ h (0030 hours)} \end{array}$ $\begin{array}{l} 2430 \\ -1200 \\ \hline 12{:}30 \text{ AM} \end{array}$

45) $\dfrac{100 \text{ mL}}{30 \text{ min}} \bowtie \dfrac{X \text{ mL/h}}{60 \text{ min/h}}$

$30X = 6{,}000$

$\dfrac{30X}{30} = \dfrac{6{,}000}{30}$

$X = 200 \text{ mL/h}$

48) $0.5 \text{ g} = 0.500. = 500 \text{ mg}$

$\dfrac{100 \text{ mg}}{1 \text{ mL}} \bowtie \dfrac{500 \text{ mg}}{X \text{ mL}}$

$100X = 500$

$\dfrac{100X}{100} = \dfrac{500}{100}$

$X = 5 \text{ mL}$

Comprehensive Skills Evaluation from pages 487–500

1) 2 **2)** Sublingual. The medication is to be administered under the tongue.

3) 2; 2; 0.5

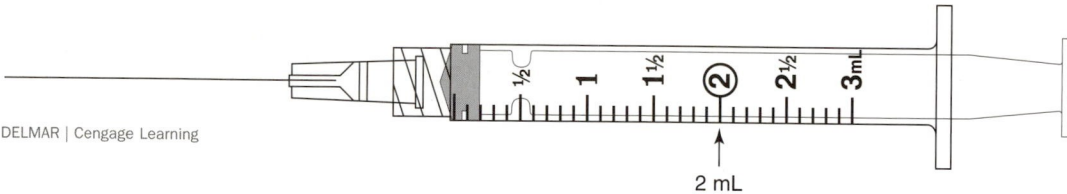

2 mL

4) 1

5) 1; 1; 0.25

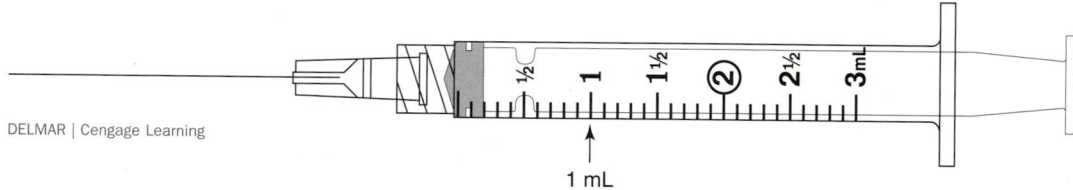

1 mL

6) $\frac{1}{2}$ **7)** 80 **8)** 0.8 **9)** 19.2 **10)** 1,920 **11)** 0500; 9/4/XX **12)** 2 **13)** 80 **14)** nitroglycerin, furosemide, digoxin, and KCl
15) 5

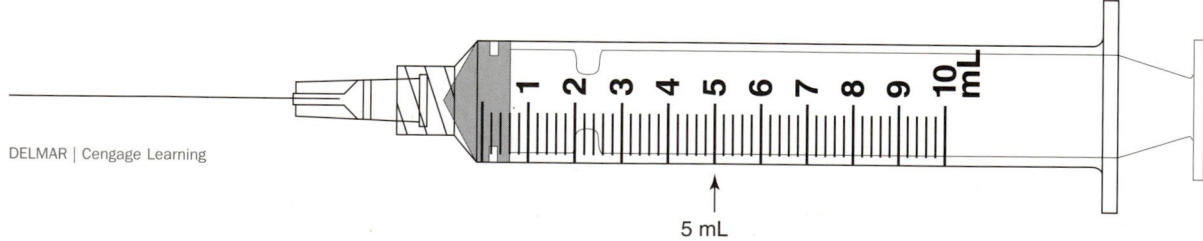

5 mL

16)　30

17)　Dosage ordered is safe; 5

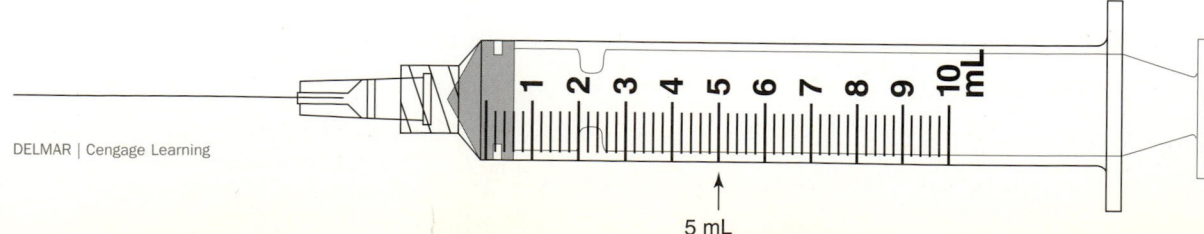

5 mL

18) 19 **19)** 30,000; 30 **20)** 60 **21)** Yes, the recommended dosage for this child is 225 mg/day in 3 divided doses or 75 mg/dose. This is the same as the order; 2; 23; 40 **22)** 12 **23)** Yes, safe dosage for this child is 300 mg/dose, which is the same as the order; 6; 44; 1,200 **24)** 1,700; 71; No. The ordered rate of 50 mL per hour is less than the recommended hourly maintenance IV rate. **25)** 3.2

26)

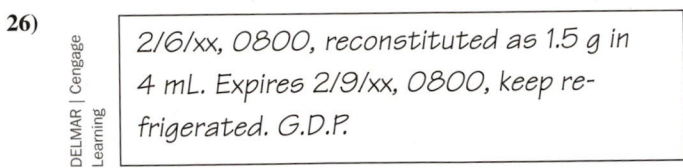

2/6/xx, 0800, reconstituted as 1.5 g in 4 mL. Expires 2/9/xx, 0800, keep refrigerated. G.D.P.

27) 1.3

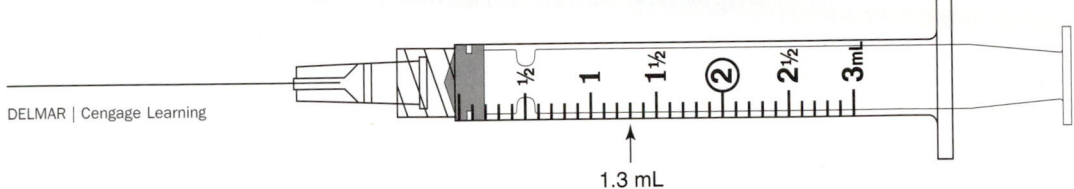

1.3 mL

28) 102

29) 2; 60

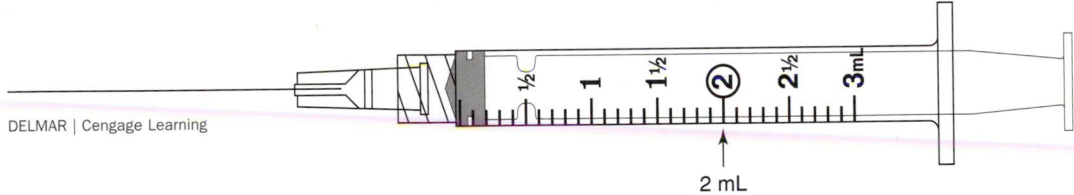

2 mL

30) 56.8; 4,544; 4.5; 1,022; 10 **31)** Decrease rate by 2 units/kg/h; 114; 1; 9

32) 8; 0.08; Insulin should be administered with an insulin syringe. This question and answer are provided to evaluate your understanding of the insulin syringe and insulin concentration. 8 units of U100 insulin equals a volume of 0.08 mL.

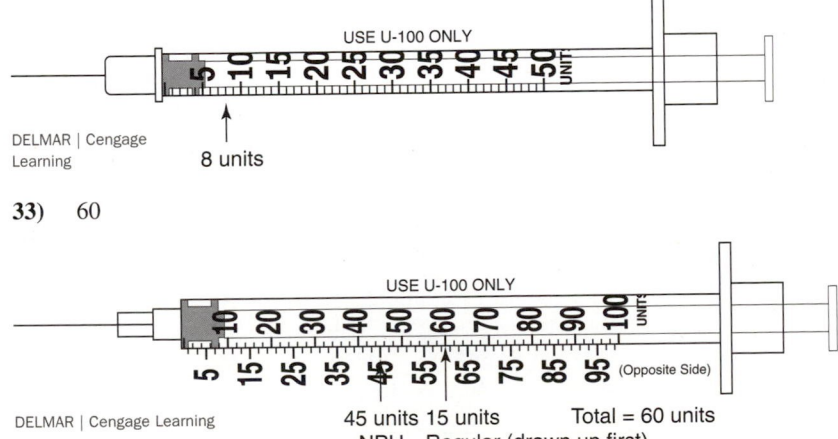

8 units

33) 60

USE U-100 ONLY

45 units 15 units Total = 60 units
NPH Regular (drawn up first)

34) 20 **35)** 720; 960 **36)** 730; 30 **37)** 1.43 **38)** 14.3–28.6; Yes **39)** 0.5; 56; 5.6; 1.4 **40)** 50; 4.5 **41)** 6; 44

42) Yes; the recommended amount of IV fluid to safely dilute this med is 15–60 mL. The order calls for 50 mL total, or 44 mL of IV fluid. **43)** 1,600,000; Yes, the minimum daily dosage is 1,500,000 units/day and the maximum is 2,500,000 units/day. The ordered dosage falls within this range; 1.8; 500,000; 0.8

Reconstitution label

DELMAR | Cengage Learning

> 1/14/xx; 0800, reconstituted as 500,000 units/mL. Expires 1/21/xx; 0800. Keep refrigerated. G.D.P.

44) 101 **45)** 2145 **46)** 0.5; 0.13 **47)** 15 **48)** 230

49) **Prevention:** Either the route or the frequency of this order is missing or is unclear. If the student actually gave this medication in the eye, it would cause a severe reaction. The medication particles could scratch the eyes or cause a worse reaction, such as blindness.

To prevent this from occurring, the student/nurse should always ensure that each medication order is complete. Every order should include the name of the drug, the dose, the route, and the time (with the patient, prescriber, and licensure identified). When any of these are missing, the order should be clarified. Further, the "od" abbreviation is obsolete and discouraged by The Joint Commission. The student nurse should also look medications up and know the safe use for each medication ordered. Had this student looked Lanoxin up in a drug guide, the student would have discovered that the medication is never given in the eye.

50) **Prevention:** The student nurse took the correct action with this order. The nurses who had given the medication previously should have looked up the medication if they were unfamiliar with it to safely identify whether it was ordered by an appropriate route, correct dosage, and correct time. There was also an error made by the pharmacist who supplied the medication to the nursing unit. It is extremely important to be familiar with the medications being given. If there's a question or any doubt, the medication should be looked up in a drug guide and/or the prescriber should be questioned. Also, close reading of the label and matching it to the order is also extremely important. Remember the Six Rights of medication administration.

Solutions—Comprehensive Skills Evaluation

1)
$$\frac{6.5 \text{ mg}}{1 \text{ cap}} \times \frac{13 \text{ mg}}{X \text{ cap}}$$
$$6.5X = 13$$
$$\frac{6.5X}{6.5} = \frac{13}{6.5}$$
$$X = 2 \text{ cap}$$

3)
$$\frac{10 \text{ mg}}{1 \text{ mL}} \times \frac{20 \text{ mg}}{X \text{ mL}}$$
$$10X = 20$$
$$\frac{10X}{10} = \frac{20}{10}$$
$$X = 2 \text{ mL}$$

$$\frac{40 \text{ mg}}{2 \text{ min}} \times \frac{20 \text{ mg}}{X \text{ min}}$$
$$40X = 40$$
$$\frac{40X}{40} = \frac{40}{40}$$
$$X = 1 \text{ min} \quad \text{Give 2 mL over 1 min}$$

$$\frac{2 \text{ mL}}{60 \text{ sec}} \times \frac{X \text{ mL}}{15 \text{ sec}}$$
$$60X = 30$$
$$\frac{60X}{60} = \frac{30}{60}$$
$$X = 0.5 \text{ mL} \quad \text{Give 0.5 mL over 15 sec}$$

4)
$$\frac{20 \text{ mg}}{1 \text{ tab}} \times \frac{20 \text{ mg}}{X \text{ tab}}$$
$$20X = 20$$
$$\frac{20X}{20} = \frac{20}{20}$$
$$X = 1 \text{ tab}$$

5) 0.25 mg is ordered and the supply dosage is 0.25 mg/mL. It is obvious that you want to give 1 mL.

1 mL added to 4 mL NS = 5 mL total

$$\frac{\overset{1}{\cancel{5}} \text{ mL}}{\underset{1}{\cancel{5}} \text{ min}} = 1 \text{ mL/min}$$

$$\frac{1 \text{ mL}}{60 \text{ sec}} \times \frac{X \text{ mL}}{15 \text{ sec}}$$
$$60X = 15$$
$$\frac{60X}{60} = \frac{15}{60}$$
$$X = 0.25 \text{ mL (per 15 sec)}$$

6)

$$\frac{0.25 \text{ mg}}{1 \text{ tab}} \times \frac{0.125 \text{ mg}}{X \text{ tab}}$$

$$0.25X = 0.125$$

$$\frac{0.25}{0.25} = \frac{0.125}{0.25}$$

$$X = \frac{1}{2} \text{ tab}$$

Daily; means you will need $\frac{1}{2}$ tab per 24 h.

7)

$$\frac{\text{mL/h}}{\text{drop factor constant}} = \text{gtt/min}$$

$$\frac{80 \text{ mL/h}}{1} = 80 \text{ gtt/min or}$$

$$80 \text{ mL/h} = 80 \text{ gtt/min (because drop factor is}$$

$$60 \text{ gtt/mL)}$$

8) The total fluid volume is:

$$1,000 \text{ mL (D}_5 \tfrac{1}{2} \text{ NS)} + 5 \text{ mL (KCl)} = 1,005 \text{ mL}$$

$$\frac{10 \text{ mEq}}{1,005 \text{ mL}} \times \frac{X \text{ mEq/h}}{80 \text{ mL/h}}$$

$$1,005X = 800$$

$$\frac{1,005X}{1,005} = \frac{800}{1,005}$$

$$X = 0.79 \text{ mEq/h} = 0.8 \text{ mEq/h}$$

9) $0.8 \text{ mEq/h} \times 24 \text{ h} = 19.2 \text{ mEq}$

10) $80 \text{ mL/h} \times 24 \text{ h} = 1,920 \text{ mL}$

11) $\frac{1,000 \text{ mL}}{80 \text{ mL/h}} = 12.5 \text{ h} = 12 \text{ h } 30 \text{ min}$

1630 hours + 12 h 30 min later = 0500 hours the

next day (9/4/xx)

12) $1 \text{ g} = 1,000 \text{ mg}$

$$\frac{500 \text{ mg}}{1 \text{ tab}} \times \frac{1,000 \text{ mg}}{X \text{ tab}}$$

$$500X = 1,000$$

$$\frac{500X}{500} = \frac{1,000}{500}$$

$$X = 2 \text{ tabs}$$

13) Order is for 80 mL/h—this is the setting for the

infusion pump.

15)

$$\frac{10 \text{ mg}}{1 \text{ mL}} \times \frac{50 \text{ mg}}{X \text{ mL}}$$

$$10X = 50$$

$$\frac{10X}{10} = \frac{50}{10}$$

$$X = 5 \text{ mL}$$

16)

$$\frac{2,000 \text{ mg}}{500 \text{ mL}} \times \frac{2 \text{ mg/min}}{X \text{ mL/min}}$$

$$2,000X = 1,000$$

$$\frac{2,000X}{2,000} = \frac{1,000}{2,000}$$

$$X = 0.5 \text{ mL/min}$$

16)

$$\frac{0.5 \text{ mL}}{1 \text{ min}} \times \frac{X \text{ mL/h}}{60 \text{ min/h}}$$

$$X = 30 \text{ mL/h}$$

17)

$$\frac{1 \text{ kg}}{2.2 \text{ lb}} \times \frac{X \text{ kg}}{110 \text{ lb}}$$

$$2.2X = 110$$

$$\frac{2.2X}{2.2} = \frac{110}{2.2}$$

$$X = 50 \text{ kg}$$

Minimum: 5 mcg/kg/min × 50 kg = 250 mcg/min

Maximum: 10 mcg/kg/min × 50 kg = 500 mcg/min

Ordered dosage is safe.

$$\frac{80 \text{ mg}}{1 \text{ mL}} \times \frac{400 \text{ mg}}{X \text{ mL}}$$

$$80X = 400$$

$$\frac{80X}{80} = \frac{400}{80}$$

$$X = 5 \text{ mL}$$

18)

$$\frac{1 \text{ mg}}{1,000 \text{ mcg}} \times \frac{X \text{ mg/min}}{500 \text{ mcg/min}}$$

$$1,000X = 500$$

$$\frac{1,000X}{1,000} = \frac{500}{1,000}$$

$$X = 0.5 \text{ mg/min}$$

$$\frac{400 \text{ mg}}{250 \text{ mL}} \times \frac{0.5 \text{ mg/min}}{X \text{ mL/min}}$$

$$400X = 125$$

$$\frac{400X}{400} = \frac{125}{400}$$

$$X = 0.312 \text{ mL/min} = 0.31 \text{ mL/min}$$

$$\frac{0.31 \text{ mL}}{1 \text{ min}} \times \frac{X \text{ mL/h}}{60 \text{ min/h}}$$

$$X = 18.6 \text{ mL/h} = 19 \text{ mL/h}$$

19)

$$\frac{500 \text{ mcg}}{1 \text{ min}} \times \frac{X \text{ mcg/h}}{60 \text{ min/h}}$$

$$X = 30,000 \text{ mcg/h}$$

$$\frac{1 \text{ mg}}{1,000 \text{ mcg}} \times \frac{X \text{ mg/h}}{30,000 \text{ mcg/h}}$$

$$1,000X = 30,000$$

$$\frac{1,000X}{1,000} = \frac{30,000}{1,000}$$

$$X = 30 \text{ mg/h}$$

20)

$$\frac{2,000 \text{ mg}}{500 \text{ mL}} \times \frac{4 \text{ mg/min}}{X \text{ mL/min}}$$

$$2,000X = 2,000$$

$$\frac{2,000X}{2,000} = \frac{2,000}{2,000}$$

$$X = 1 \text{ mL/min}$$

$$\frac{1 \text{ mL}}{1 \text{ min}} \times \frac{X \text{ mL/h}}{60 \text{ min/h}}$$

$$X = 60 \text{ mL/h}$$

21)
$$\frac{1\text{ kg}}{2.2\text{ lb}} \diagup\diagdown \frac{X\text{ kg}}{33\text{ lb}}$$

$$2.2X = 33$$

$$\frac{2.2X}{2.2} = \frac{33}{2.2}$$

$$X = 15\text{ kg}$$

15 mg/kg/day $\times$ 15 kg = 225 mg/day

Maximum:

$$\frac{225\text{ mg}}{3\text{ doses}} \diagup\diagdown \frac{X\text{ mg}}{1\text{ dose}}$$

$$3X = 225$$

$$\frac{3X}{3} = \frac{225}{3}$$

$$X = 75\text{ mg (per dose)}$$

The order is safe. It is obvious you want to give 2 mL.

25 mL (total IV solution) − 2 mL (Kantrex) = 23 mL

$(D_5 \frac{1}{2} NS)$

25 mL (total solution) + 15 mL (flush) = 40 mL

(total in 1 h)

40 mL over 1 h is 40 mL/h.

22)
$$\frac{125\text{ mg}}{100\text{ mL}} \diagup\diagdown \frac{15\text{ mg/h}}{X\text{ mL/h}}$$

$$125X = 1,500$$

$$\frac{125X}{125} = \frac{1,500}{125}$$

$$X = 12\text{ mL/h}$$

23)
$$\frac{1\text{ kg}}{2.2\text{ lbs}} \diagup\diagdown \frac{X\text{ kg}}{66\text{ lbs}}$$

$$2.2X = 66$$

$$\frac{2.2X}{2.2} = \frac{66}{2.2}$$

$$X = 30\text{ kg}$$

40 mg/kg/day $\times$ 30 kg = 1,200 mg/day

$$\frac{1,200\text{ mg}}{4\text{ doses}} \diagup\diagdown \frac{X\text{ mg}}{1\text{ dose}}$$

$$4X = 1,200$$

$$\frac{4X}{4} = \frac{1,200}{4}$$

$$X = 300\text{ mg (per dose)}$$

$$\frac{500\text{ mg}}{10\text{ mL}} \diagup\diagdown \frac{300\text{ mg}}{X\text{ mL}}$$

$$500X = 3,000$$

$$\frac{500X}{500} = \frac{3,000}{500}$$

$$X = 6\text{ mL}$$

50 mL (total IV volume) − 6 mL (Vancomycin) =

44 mL $(D_5 \frac{1}{2} NS)$; 50 mL/h $\times$ 24 h = 1,200 mL

24) weight = 30 kg

100 mL/kg/day $\times$ 10 kg = 1,000 mL/day for first 10 kg

50 mL/kg/day $\times$ 10 kg = 500 mL/day for next 10 kg

20 mL/kg/day $\times$ 10 kg = 200 mL/day for remaining 10 kg

Total: 1,000 mL/day + 500 mL/day + 200 mL/day =

1,700 mL/day or per 24 hours

1,700 mL/day ÷ 24 h/day = 70.8 mL/h = 71 mL/h

The ordered rate is less than the recommended daily

rate of maintenance fluids. The nurse should

consider possible clinical reasons for the difference

and consult the physician as needed for clarification.

25) The vial size is 1.5 g. Choose the diluent that

corresponds to the vial chosen. Adding 3.2 mL will

yield a total of 4.0 mL containing 1.5 g.

27)
$$\frac{1,500\text{ mg}}{4\text{ mL}} \diagup\diagdown \frac{500\text{ mg}}{X\text{ mL}}$$

$$1,500X = 2,000$$

$$\frac{1,500X}{1,500} = \frac{2,000}{1,500}$$

$$X = 1.33\text{ mL} = 1.3\text{ mL}$$

28) 50 mL (total IV PB) + 1 mL (med) = 51 mL (total

to infuse in 30 min)

$$\frac{51\text{ mL}}{30\text{ min}} \diagup\diagdown \frac{X\text{ mL/h}}{60\text{ min/h}}$$

$$30X = 3,060$$

$$\frac{30X}{30} \diagup\diagdown \frac{3,060}{30}$$

$$X = 102\text{ mL/h}$$

29)
$$\frac{5,000\text{ units}}{1\text{ mL}} \diagup\diagdown \frac{10,000\text{ units}}{X\text{ mL}}$$

$$5,000X = 10,000$$

$$\frac{5,000X}{5,000} = \frac{10,000}{5,000}$$

$$X = 2\text{ mL}$$

$$\frac{10,000\text{ units}}{500\text{ mL}} \diagup\diagdown \frac{1,200\text{ units/h}}{X\text{ mL/h}}$$

$$10,000X = 600,000$$

$$\frac{10,000X}{10,000} = \frac{600,000}{10,000}$$

$$X = 60\text{ mL/h}$$

30)
$$\frac{1\text{ kg}}{2.2\text{ lb}} \diagup\diagdown \frac{X\text{ kg}}{125\text{ lb}}$$

$$2.2X = 125$$

$$\frac{2.2X}{2.2} = \frac{125}{2.2}$$

$$X = 56.81\text{ kg} = 56.8\text{ kg}$$

80 units/kg $\times$ 56.8 kg = 4,544 units

$$\frac{1,000 \text{ units}}{1 \text{ mL}} \diagdown \frac{4,544 \text{ units/h}}{X \text{ mL}}$$

$$1,000X = 4,544$$

$$\frac{1,000X}{1,000} = \frac{4,544}{1,000}$$

$$X = 4.544 \text{ mL} = 4.5 \text{ mL}$$

18 units/kg × 56.8 kg = 1,022.4 units = 1,022 units

$$\frac{25,000 \text{ units}}{250 \text{ mL}} \diagdown \frac{1,022 \text{ units/h}}{X \text{ mL/h}}$$

$$25,000X = 255,500$$

$$\frac{25,000X}{25,000} = \frac{255,500}{25,000}$$

$$X = 10.2 \text{ mL/h} = 10 \text{ mL/h}$$

31) Decrease rate by 2 units/kg/h

2 units/kg/h × 56.8 kg = 113.6 units/h = 114 units/h

$$\frac{25,000 \text{ units}}{250 \text{ mL}} \diagdown \frac{114 \text{ units/h}}{X \text{ mL/h}}$$

$$25,000X = 28,500$$

$$\frac{25,000X}{25,000} = \frac{28,500}{25,000}$$

$$X = 1.14 \text{ mL/h} = 1 \text{ mL/h}$$

10 mL/h − 1 mL/h = 9 mL/h

32)

$$\frac{100 \text{ units}}{1 \text{ mL}} \diagdown \frac{8 \text{ units}}{X \text{ mL}}$$

$$100X = 8$$

$$\frac{100X}{100} = \frac{8}{100}$$

$$X = 0.08 \text{ mL}$$

Insulin should be administered with an insulin syringe. This question and solution are provided to evaluate your understanding of the insulin syringe and insulin concentration. 8 units of U-100 insulin equals a volume of 0.08 mL.

33) 15 units + 45 units = 60 units

34) U 100 insulin: 100 units/mL

$$\frac{100 \text{ units}}{1 \text{ mL}} \diagdown \frac{300 \text{ units}}{X \text{ mL}}$$

$$100X = 300$$

$$\frac{100X}{100} = \frac{300}{100}$$

$$X = 3 \text{ mL}$$

Total IV volume: 150 mL (NS) + 3 mL (insulin) = 153 mL

$$\frac{300 \text{ units}}{153 \text{ mL}} \diagdown \frac{X \text{ units/h}}{10 \text{ mL/h}}$$

$$153X = 3,000$$

$$\frac{153X}{153} = \frac{3,000}{153}$$

$$X = 19.6 \text{ units/h} = 20 \text{ units/h}$$

35)

$$\frac{1 \text{ fl oz}}{30 \text{ mL}} \diagdown \frac{8 \text{ fl oz}}{X \text{ mL}}$$

$$X = 240 \text{ mL}$$

$$\frac{1}{4} \diagdown \frac{240}{X \text{ mL}}$$

$X = 960 \text{ mL}$ (total volume of reconstituted $\frac{1}{4}$ strength Isomil)

960 mL total solution − 240 mL (solute or Isomil) = 720 mL (solvent or water)

36)

$$\frac{1 \text{ kg}}{2.2 \text{ lb}} \diagdown \frac{X \text{ kg}}{16 \text{ lb}}$$

$$2.2X = 16$$

$$\frac{2.2X}{2.2} = \frac{16}{2.2}$$

$$X = 7.27 \text{ kg} = 7.3 \text{ kg}$$

100 mL/kg/day × 7.3 kg = 730 mL/day

730 mL/day ÷ 24 h/day = 30 mL/h

37)

$$\frac{1 \text{ ft}}{12 \text{ in}} \diagdown \frac{5 \text{ ft}}{X \text{ in}}$$

$$X = 60 \text{ in}$$

60 in + 2 in = 62 in

Household:

$$\text{BSA (m}^2\text{)} = \sqrt{\frac{\text{ht (in)} \times \text{wt (lb)}}{3,131}} = \sqrt{\frac{62 \times 103}{3,131}} = \sqrt{2.039...} = 1.428 \text{ m}^2 = 1.43 \text{ m}^2$$

38) 10 mg/m² × 1.43 m² = 14.3 mg

20 mg/m² × 1.43 m² = 28.6 mg

Yes, the order is safe.

39) Concentration: 40 mg per 80 mL

$$\frac{40 \text{ mg}}{80 \text{ mL}} \diagdown \frac{X \text{ mg}}{1 \text{ mL}}$$

$$80X = 40$$

$$\frac{80X}{80} = \frac{40}{80}$$

$X = 0.5 \text{ mg}$ (per mL or 0.5 mg/mL)

$$\frac{0.5 \text{ mg}}{1 \text{ mL}} \diagdown \frac{28 \text{ mg}}{X \text{ mL}}$$

$$0.5X = 28$$

$$\frac{0.5X}{0.5} = \frac{28}{0.5}$$

$$X = 56 \text{ mL}$$

$$\frac{56 \text{ mL}}{10 \text{ min}} \diagdown \frac{X \text{ mL}}{1 \text{ min}}$$

$$10X = 56$$

$$\frac{10X}{10} = \frac{56}{10}$$

$X = 5.6 \text{ mL}$ (per min or 5.6 mL/min or 5.6 mL per 60 sec)

$$\frac{5.6 \text{ mL}}{60 \text{ sec}} \times \frac{X \text{ mL}}{15 \text{ sec}}$$

$$60X = 84$$

$$\frac{60X}{60} = \frac{84}{60}$$

$$X = 1.4 \text{ mL (per 15 sec)}$$

40) Dextrose: NaCl:

$$\frac{5 \text{ g}}{100 \text{ mL}} \times \frac{X \text{ g}}{1,000 \text{ mL}} \qquad \frac{0.45 \text{ g}}{100 \text{ mL}} \times \frac{X \text{ g}}{1,000 \text{ mL}}$$

$$100X = 5,000 \qquad\qquad 100X = 450$$

$$\frac{100X}{100} = \frac{5,000}{100} \qquad\qquad \frac{100X}{100} = \frac{450}{100}$$

$$X = 50 \text{ g} \qquad\qquad\qquad X = 4.5 \text{ g}$$

41)

$$\frac{100 \text{ mg}}{1 \text{ mL}} \times \frac{600 \text{ mg}}{X \text{ mL}}$$

$$100X = 600$$

$$\frac{100X}{100} = \frac{600}{100}$$

$$X = 6 \text{ mL}$$

50 mL (total fluid) − 6 mL (med) = 44 mL (IV fluid). Note: Add the med to the chamber and then add IV fluid up to the 50 mL mark.

42) Maximal dilution:

$$\frac{10 \text{ mg}}{1 \text{ mL}} \times \frac{600 \text{ mg}}{X \text{ mL}}$$

$$10X = 600$$

$$\frac{10X}{10} = \frac{600}{10}$$

$$X = 60 \text{ mL (per 600 mg)}$$

Minimal dilution:

$$\frac{40 \text{ mg}}{1 \text{ mL}} \times \frac{600 \text{ mg}}{X \text{ mL}}$$

$$40X = 600$$

$$\frac{40X}{40} = \frac{600}{40}$$

$$X = 15 \text{ mL (per 600 mg)}$$

43) 400,000 units/dose × 4 doses/day = 1,600,000 units/day

Minimum: 150,000 units/kg/day × 10 kg = 1,500,000 units/day

Maximum: 250,000 units/kg/day × 10 kg = 2,500,000 units/day

Reconstitute with 1.8 mL for a concentration of 500,000 units/mL. This concentration is selected because it will be further diluted.

$$\frac{500,000 \text{ units}}{1 \text{ mL}} \times \frac{400,000 \text{ units}}{X \text{ mL}}$$

$$500,000X = 400,000$$

$$\frac{500,000X}{500,000} = \frac{400,000}{500,000}$$

$$X = 0.8 \text{ mL (penicillin)}$$

44) 100 mL (NS) + 0.8 mL (penicillin) = 100.8 or 101 mL to be infused in 60 min or 1 h. Set IV pump at 101 mL/h.

45) The primary IV will infuse for 8 hours. The IV PB will infuse for 30 minutes. Therefore, the primary IV will be interrupted by the IV PB and then will resume. The IV will be completely infused in 8 hours and 30 min.

(1315 + 8 h 30 min = 1315 + 0830 = 2145)

46)

$$\frac{25 \text{ mg}}{1 \text{ mL}} \times \frac{12.5 \text{ mg}}{X \text{ mL}}$$

$$25X = 12.5$$

$$\frac{25X}{25} = \frac{12.5}{25}$$

$$X = 0.5 \text{ mL}$$

Give 0.5 mL/min or

$$\frac{0.5 \text{ mL}}{60 \text{ sec}} \times \frac{X \text{ mL}}{15 \text{ sec}}$$

$$60X = 7.5$$

$$\frac{60X}{60} = \frac{7.5}{60}$$

$$X = 0.125 \text{ mL} = 0.13 \text{ mL (per 15 sec)}$$

47)

$$\frac{100 \text{ mg}}{1 \text{ mL}} \times \frac{1,500 \text{ mg}}{X \text{ mL}}$$

$$100X = 1,500$$

$$\frac{100X}{100} = \frac{1,500}{100}$$

$$X = 15 \text{ mL}$$

48) 100 mL (IV PB) + 15 mL (med) = 115 mL (total to infuse in 30 min)

$$\frac{115 \text{ mL}}{30 \text{ min}} \times \frac{X \text{ mL/h}}{60 \text{ min/h}}$$

$$30X = 6,900$$

$$\frac{30X}{30} = \frac{6,900}{30}$$

$$X = 230 \text{ mL/h}$$

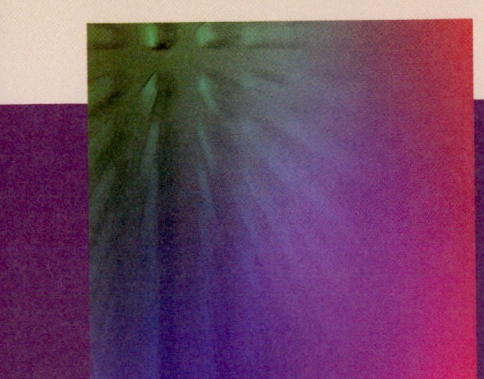

Index

Drug Label Index

8.7 *Acknowledgment.* By opening this package and/or by accessing the Licensed Content on this Web site, THE END USER ACKNOWLEDGES THAT IT HAS READ THIS AGREEMENT, UNDERSTANDS IT, AND AGREES TO BE BOUND BY ITS TERMS AND CONDITIONS. IF YOU DO NOT ACCEPT THESE TERMS AND CONDITIONS, YOU MUST NOT ACCESS THE LICENSED CONTENT AND RETURN THE LICENSED PRODUCT TO CENGAGE LEARNING (WITHIN 30 CALENDAR DAYS OF THE END USER'S PURCHASE) WITH PROOF OF PAYMENT ACCEPTABLE TO CENGAGE LEARNING, FOR A CREDIT OR A REFUND. Should the End User have any questions/comments regarding this Agreement, please contact Cengage Learning at Delmar.help@cengage.com.

Set Up Instructions for Windows:

1. Insert disc into CD-ROM drive. The CD installation program should start automatically. If it does not, go to step 2.
2. From My Computer, double-click the icon for the CD drive.
3. Double click the PickarDosage.exe file to start the program.

Set Up Instructions for Mac:

1. Insert disc into CD-ROM drive. A CD-ROM image will appear on the desktop.
2. Click the CD-ROM image on the desktop. The Finder program will display the contents of the CD.
3. Double click the *PickarDosage.app* file to start the program.

MINIMUM SYSTEM REQUIREMENTS

Windows

- Operating System: Windows XP (SP2, SP3); Windows Vista (SP1)
- Processor: Pentium 4, 1.4 MHz or higher
- Memory: 512 MB *(FMI strongly recommends 1 GB memory when using Windows Vista)*

Macintosh

- Mac OS X 10.4 (Tiger) or 10.5 (Leopard)